BSAVA Manual of Canine and Feline Haematology and Transfusion Medicine

Editors:

Michael J. Day
˙S(Hons) PhD FASM DipECVP MRCPath FRCVS
Department of Pathology and Microbiology
School of Veterinary Science, University of Bristol
Langford House, Langford, Bristol BS40 5DU

Andrew Mackin
BSc BVMS MVS DVSc FACVSc DSAM DipACVIM MRCVS
College of Veterinary Medicine
Mississippi State University
Mississippi State, MS 39762-9825, USA

Janet D. Littlewood
MA PhD BVSc(Hons) DVR CertSAD MRCVS
Department of Clinical Studies
Animal Health Trust, Lanwades Park
Newmarket, Suffolk CB8 7DW

Published by:

British Small Animal Veterinary Association
Woodrow House, 1 Telford Way,
Waterwells Business Park, Quedgeley,
Gloucester GL2 4AB

A Company Limited by Guarantee in England.
Registered Company No. 2837793.
Registered as a Charity.

A catalogue record for this book is available from the British Library.

ISBN 0 905214 39 0

The publishers and contributors cannot take responsibility for information
provided on dosages and methods of application of drugs mentioned in this
publication. Details of this kind must be verified by individual users from the
appropriate literature.

Typeset by: Fusion Design, Fordingbridge, Hampshire, UK

Printed by: Lookers, Upton, Poole, Dorset, UK

Other titles in the BSAVA Manuals series:

Coming soon:

For further information on BSAVA publications, visit our website at: www.bsava.com

Contents

Contributors

Anthony CG Abrams-Ogg DVM DVSc DipACVIM
Department of Clinical Studies, Ontario Veterinary College, University of Guelph, Guelph, Ontario,
Canada N1G 2W1

Dorothee Bienzle DVM MSc PhD DipACVP
Department of Pathobiology, Ontario Veterinary College, University of Guelph, Guelph, Ontario, N1G 2W1,
Canada

Michael J. Day BSc BVMS(Hons) PhD FASM DipECVP MRCPath FRCVS
Department of Pathology and Microbiology, School of Veterinary Science, University of Bristol,
Langford House, Langford, Bristol BS40 5DU

Jane Dobson MA BVetMed DVetMed DipECVIM-CA MRCVS
Department of Clinical Veterinary Medicine, University of Cambridge, Madingley Road, Cambridge CB3 0ES

John K. Dunn MA MVetSc BVM&S DipECVIM DSAM MRCVS
AXIOM Veterinary Laboratories Ltd, George Street, Teignmouth, Devon TQ14 8AH

Darren J. Foster BSc BVMS PhD FACVSc
Veterinary Specialist Centre, Corner Delhi and Plassey Roads, PO Box 307, North Ryde, NSW 1670, Australia

Krystyna Grodecki DVM DVSc MRCVS
Département de Pathologie Clinique, Faculté de Médecine Vétérinaire, Université de Montréal,
3200 rue Sicotte, C.P. 5000, Saint-Hyacinthe, Québec, J2S 7C5, Canada

Tim Gruffydd-Jones BVetMed PhD DipECVIM MRCVS
Department of Clinical Veterinary Science, University of Bristol, Langford House, Langford, Bristol BS40 5DU

Andreas Hans Hasler Dr.vet.med. DipACVIM DipECVIM
Tierärztliches Uberweisungs Zentrum, Hauptstrasse 21, CH-4456 Tenniken, Switzerland

Steven A. Holloway BVSc PhD MVS MACVSc DipACVIM
Small Animal Medicine Department, University of Melbourne Veterinary Clinical Centre, Princes Highway,
Werribee, Vic 3030, Australia

David C. Lewis BVSc DipVetClinStud PhD DipACVIM
Antech Diagnostics, 12616 SE Stark, Portland, OR 97233, USA

Janet D. Littlewood MA PhD BVSc(Hons) DVR CertSAD MRCVS
Department of Clinical Studies, Animal Health Trust, Lanwades Park, Newmarket, Suffolk CB8 7DW

Remo Lobetti BVSc MMedVet DipECVIM
Department of Companion Animal Medicine, Faculty of Veterinary Science, University of Pretoria,
Private Bag X04, Onderstepoort, 0110, South Africa

Andrew Mackin BSc BVMS MVS DVSc FACVSc DSAM DipACVIM MRCVS
College of Veterinary Medicine, Box 9825, Spring Street, Mississippi State University, Mississippi State,
MS 39762-9825, USA

Mary F. McConnell BVSc DipClinPath PhD
VETPATH Laboratory Services, PO Box 18, Belmont, WA 6984, Australia

Jennifer N. Mills BVSc DipVetClinPath MSc PhD
Division of Veterinary Clinical Sciences, Murdoch University, South Street, Murdoch, WA 6150, Australia

Joanna Morris BSc BVSc PhD FRCVS
Department of Clinical Veterinary Medicine, University of Cambridge, Madingley Road, Cambridge CB3 0ES

Kostas Papasouliotis DVM PhD MRCVS
Department of Clinical Veterinary Science, University of Bristol, Langford House, Langford, Bristol BS40 5DU

Andrew Sparkes BVetMed PhD DipECVIM MRCVS
Department of Clinical Veterinary Science, University of Bristol, Langford House, Langford, Bristol BS40 5DU

Tracy Stokol BVSc PhD DipACVP
Department of Population Medicine and Diagnostic Science, College of Veterinary Medicine,
Cornell University, Ithaca, NY 14853-6401, USA

Michael Stone DVM DipACVIM
Tufts University School of Veterinary Medicine, Department of Small Animal Medicine, 200 Westboro Road,
North Grafton, MA 01536, USA

Andrew G.T. Torrance MA VetMB PhD DipACVIM DipACVP MRCVS
AXIOM Veterinary Laboratories Ltd, George Street, Teignmouth, Devon TQ14 8AH

Elizabeth Villiers BVSc CertSAM CertVR MRCVS
Department of Clinical Veterinary Medicine, University of Cambridge, Madingley Road, Cambridge CB3 0ES

Foreword

The demands of modern small animal practice, and the greater understanding by clients of what can be achieved for their pets requires more in depth knowledge by the veterinary surgeon working in primary health care and in referral practice.

Taking a blood sample for haematological analysis is one of the most common diagnostic procedures in practice, either for analysis within the practice or outside the practice in specialist laboratories. Correct interpretation of the results is essential.

The *BSAVA Manual of Canine and Feline Haematology and Transfusion Medicine* combines both clinical pathology and the diagnosis and management of a range of haematological diseases. It also includes those diseases that may become more commonly diagnosed in the UK with the introduction of the PETS Travel Scheme.

The final section of the manual gives detailed practical guidance on blood transfusion techniques in the dog and cat including collection, storage, blood typing, cross matching and administration.

The Editors and the BSAVA Publishing Manager are to be congratulated on this excellent manual. They have drawn together the specialist knowledge of authors from around the world for this comprehensive guide. The chapters are fully illustrated with tables, diagrams and colour photographs and those on technique will be of particular use to many of us in practice.

We have waited some time for this manual but I am sure you will agree with me that our patience has been amply rewarded with this very welcome new addition to the BSAVA manual series.

Lynn Turner MA VetMB MRCVS
BSAVA President 2000–2001

Preface

The *BSAVA Manual of Canine and Feline Haematology and Transfusion Medicine* is a unique publication that bridges the disciplines of clinical pathology, internal medicine and critical care in a single volume.

Haematological analysis is probably the single most commonly performed laboratory diagnostic test in small animal practice, so much so that many practices have now established in-house analysis facilities. Moreover, in recent years more sophisticated haematology analytical techniques have also become available through specialist laboratories. This book reviews the basics of sample collection, test performance and interpretation for routine haematology, together with assessment of haemostatic function and bone marrow analysis. In addition, newer developments such as the application of flow cytometry to the phenotyping of leukaemias, and molecular genetics to the diagnosis of haemostatic disorders are discussed.

However, this volume is more than just a clinical pathology manual. The diagnosis and management of a selected range of major haematological diseases are discussed by specialists in internal medicine and oncology. These chapters cover the major infectious, immune-mediated and neoplastic diseases of the haemopoietic system. Of particular relevance to UK practitioners is the realization that 'new' haematological diseases such as babesiosis, ehrlichiosis and leishmaniasis will be increasingly recognized in their country following the lifting of quarantine. Indeed, in the first months of the Pet Travel Scheme, two cases of canine babesiosis have been documented in the *Veterinary Record*, and this manual specifically includes a chapter on this disease. The growing specialty of feline medicine is reflected by the inclusion of a number of chapters dedicated to conditions specific to the cat.

The final section of the manual is devoted to the field of transfusion medicine. These chapters provide a detailed and very practical guide to performing blood transfusion in the dog and cat - including donor blood collection and storage, blood typing and cross-matching, administration of the transfusion and management of transfusion reactions.

This manual is the sum of a series of excellent contributions from internationally recognized specialists from Europe, the United States, Canada, Australia and South Africa. Each chapter is designed as a self-contained review, and there is inevitably some limited overlap in content. However, as this is often presented from a different perspective it can only add to the value of the manual. The text is supported throughout by tables, diagrams and colour photographs. The photographic guides to performing bone marrow collection, catheter insertion and blood transfusion will be of particular value in the practice setting.

The *BSAVA Manual of Canine and Feline Haematology and Transfusion Medicine* has been a long time in gestation, and the Editors are grateful for the patience of all contributors who readily updated their chapters in the few months preceding publication. This has meant that the final product is very much a state-of-the-art volume that will serve readers for many years to come. The rapid final production stages of the manual are due in no small part to the dedication and efforts of Marion Jowett (BSAVA Publishing Manager), Liz Payne (copy editor), Jill Greenway (proof reader) and Graeme Kowalewicz (design and layout) who have worked beyond the call of duty in the last months.

Michael Day
Andrew Mackin
Janet Littlewood
August 2000

PART ONE

Haematology

CHAPTER ONE

Overview of Haematological Diagnostic Techniques

Andrew Torrance

INTRODUCTION

Haematological diagnostic techniques are an essential part of the data base for diagnostic investigation. The haematological profile includes haemoglobin, haematocrit or packed cell volume (PCV), red cell indices, total cell counts, differential counts and comments by a veterinary haematologist on the morphology of the erythrocyte, leucocyte and platelet populations. Microscopic examination of a blood film alone may reveal the diagnosis in some cases. More often, interpretation of the haematological profile in conjunction with biochemistry, urinalysis, history and physical findings directs the clinician in the selection of subsequent, ultimately diagnostic, imaging and sampling techniques. Dogs and cats exhibit a wider range of haematological pathology than other species, making diagnostic haematology particularly important in small animal medicine.

BLOOD SAMPLING AND THE USE OF ANTICOAGULANTS

To be of diagnostic value, a sample of blood must truly reflect the impact of disease processes on the blood cells and platelets. The composition of blood is constantly changing and there is a rapid response to physiological phenomena such as splenic contraction or demargination of neutrophils. These processes are readily induced by stressing the patient at the time of sampling and will produce physiological alterations that may confuse interpretation of the haematological profile. Stress-induced neutrophilia may be mistaken for an inflammatory leucogram in cats and increased PCV by splenic contraction may be mistaken for dehydration in dogs. Sedatives and analgesics have profound haematological effects, which mask disease processes.

   Physical damage to blood constituents during collection is the most common and frustrating cause of poor blood samples. The fragility of erythrocytes and the aggregability of platelets are quite unpredictable and vary between individuals and pathological processes. These problems can be minimized by using consistent, excellent technique. The slow flow and application of variable vacuum that occurs during collection of blood from a peripheral vein tests the resilience of blood cells and encourages platelet aggregation. Extraction with consistent vacuum from a large central vein is less damaging and therefore preferable. Jugular venepuncture is easy in dogs (Figures 1.1 and 1.2) and cats (Figures 1.3 and 1.4), is often less stressful than the use of peripheral veins and undoubtedly yields the most reliable results.

Requirements
Needles: 18–21 gauge 2 cm needles Syringe: 5–20 ml or evacuated tubes 2–5 ml
Positioning and preparation
Most dogs will sit for this procedure. Large dogs should be placed with their back to a wall. The holder usually stands astride the dog with his or her legs behind the dog's shoulders. The sampler squats in front of the dog. Small dogs will usually sit near the edge of the table. Clip the hair over the jugular groove and prepare the skin for venepuncture. The dog's head is tipped back, exposing the jugular groove, and the sampler occludes one jugular vein just cranial to the thoracic inlet
Procedure
In most cases the vein is located by palpation rather than by sight. The vein is raised and lowered, and the jugular groove is palpated to locate the vein. The needle is inserted with the tip pointing cranially, and blood is withdrawn by gentle suction

Figure 1.1: Jugular venepuncture in dogs.

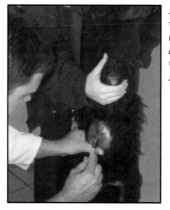

Figure 1.2: Jugular venepuncture in the dog. (Courtesy of Jacob Hayes and Karen Gerber. © AXIOM Veterinary Laboratories.)

Requirements
Needles: 21 or 20 gauge 1-2 cm needles
Syringe: 5-10 ml or evacuated tubes 2-3 ml
Positioning and preparation
Bring the cat to the edge of a table. Hold the front legs down over the edge of the table. Tip the neck back and the nose up. The front legs and neck up to the point of the mandible should then make a vertical plane. Clip the hair over one jugular groove and prepare for venepuncture
Procedure
The blood sampler takes a position in front of the cat and occludes one jugular vein by compressing the jugular groove. The needle is then inserted with the tip pointing cranially, and gentle suction is applied as soon as the tip of the needle enters the lumen of the vein

Figure 1.3: Jugular venepuncture in cats.

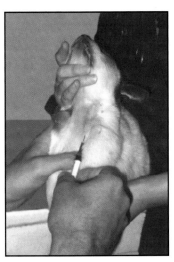

Figure 1.4: Jugular venepuncture in the cat. (Courtesy of Jacob Hayes and Karen Gerber. © AXIOM Veterinary Laboratories.)

Evacuated tubes or syringes are equally efficient in skilled hands but should not be used together. Samples are ruined when blood is extracted with a syringe and needle and the needle pushed through the cap of an evacuated tube. Blood cells are then forced through the lumen of the needle twice under pressure, and damage results. When blood has been collected into a syringe, the needle should be removed and the blood gently pushed out into an open tube containing the appropriate anticoagulant. The tube should then be capped and rolled gently to ensure adequate mixing.

The anticoagulant of choice for the haematological profile is ethylenediamine tetra-acetic acid (EDTA) because it preserves cell morphology. Tubes containing sodium citrate are used for any tests involving clotting times and clotting factors. Both sodium citrate and EDTA prevent coagulation by complexing calcium, but sodium citrate is favoured for tests of coagulation because calcium binding is more readily reversed by addition of calcium. Heparinized blood is of little use for haematology because leucocyte staining is

poor and Wright's-stained films develop a blue background, which impairs evaluation of morphology. Basic erythrocyte counts and indices, however, can be assessed in heparinized samples.

BASIC QUANTIFICATION TECHNIQUES

The measurement of PCV and cell counts can be performed manually by using microhaematocrit tubes and a haemocytometer.

Microhaematocrit
The microhaematocrit method for calculating PCV is the simplest way to assess red cell mass manually. It is widely used in practices, intensive care units and haematology laboratories. The PCV is determined by centrifuging anticoagulated blood in a small capillary tube to separate cells from plasma. The PCV is calculated by dividing the length of the packed erythrocytes by the total length of the packed erythrocytes, buffy coat and plasma. Various simple devices are available to perform this measurement (Figure 1.5).

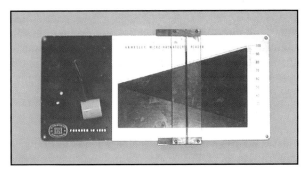

Figure 1.5: Sliding device for measuring the haematocrit in a microhaematocrit tube. (© AXIOM Veterinary Laboratories.)

The minimal errors that occur with measurement of microhaematocrit are usually associated with centrifugation. Microhaematocrit centrifuges operate at high speeds (11,500-15,000 rpm), which ensure adequate packing of erythrocytes. Multipurpose centrifuges may not rotate fast enough to pack the cells, and increased duration of centrifugation will not compensate for this. Adequate cell packing is achieved with 5 minutes of centrifugation at the appropriate speed. At a PCV above 50%, packing is not as complete after 5 minutes, leading to overestimation of red cell mass. In such cases an additional period of 5 minutes centrifugation at appropriate speed may be necessary. Overfilling the microhaematocrit tube by more than 75% of its length will also reduce the rate of packing and increase the centrifugation time. When the PCV is below 25%, the packing of erythrocytes will be tighter and may exaggerate the decrease in PCV, making the animal appear more anaemic than it really is. Small variations in PCV may also occur with different anticoagulants.

Manual cell counts

Manual cell counts are done with an improved Neubauer-ruled haemocytometer, calibrated coverglass, disposable capillary pipette and plastic reservoir chamber containing a premeasured volume of diluent.

The haemocytometer is a transparent glass chamber that holds a cell suspension beneath the microscope for counting. The chamber is 0.1 mm deep and has a well defined space of known volume. The volume is subdivided by a grid of 9 x 1 square mm engraved on the base of the chamber. The central 1 mm square of the grid is further subdivided into 25 squares of suitable size for counting red cells at an appropriate dilution.

Blood is diluted to achieve appropriate density of cells for counting with the diluent container. For erythrocyte counting the dilution is 1:200, for leucocytes 1:20 and for platelets 1:100. The total counts are then calculated by using a correction factor that takes into account the counting volume and the dilution factors.

The count is performed in duplicate on different sides of the haemocytometer grid. The erythrocyte and leucocyte counts from the two sites should only vary by 20% and 10%, respectively, if performed correctly. If the two cell counts are consistent, the average of the two is multiplied by the conversion factor to obtain the count per litre.

Manual counts with a haemocytometer have a significant error compared with automated counts (± 20% on leucocyte counts). This is particularly important in monitoring changes in leucocyte number over time, for example a change of 20% can simply be an intercount variation rather than a true alteration.

AUTOMATED QUANTIFICATION TECHNIQUES

Measurement of erythrocyte counts, haemoglobin, haematocrit, mean cell volume (MCV), mean cell haemoglobin (MCH), mean cell haemoglobin concentration (MCHC) and leucocyte counts are now fully automated in most laboratories and in many practices. Differential leucocyte counts are usually assessed visually because of the diversity of leucocyte patterns in dogs and cats. Examination of a blood film for the differential leucocyte count also provides an opportunity for the haematologist to comment on erythrocyte morphology and the presence of any abnormal cells. The diagnostic value of the haematological profile is seriously compromised when cell counts are interpreted without such morphological examination, or vice versa. Interpretive comments programmed into automated analysers are frequently irrelevant and can be extremely misleading.

Factors affecting the quality of automatic counts include analyser type, sample damage, sample ageing, platelet aggregation and abnormalities in platelet size. The presence of microclots in damaged and poorly anticoagulated samples renders automated counts useless, and will also block the counting channels in some analysers. Damaged erythrocytes often swell during storage and transport, and this may increase the MCV measured by automatic counters, which in turn will artefactually increase the calculated haematocrit.

Samples that contain large numbers of metarubricytes and rubricytes (nucleated red blood cells or nRBCs) will tend to cause artefactually elevated leucocyte counts because the counter will mistake nRBCs for leucocytes. In such cases, manual examination of the film will be required to produce corrected leucocyte counts. This correction is done if more than 5 nRBCs are noted while counting 100 leucocytes in a differential count. The leucocyte count is corrected as follows:

$$\text{Corrected leucocyte count} = \frac{100}{100 + \text{nRBCs}} \times \text{nucleated cell count (automated)}$$

Poor sample collection and sample ageing may result in platelet aggregation, and the platelet clumps may be counted as red or white cells, or missed altogether, leading to an erroneous platelet count. For this reason, it is always recommended that platelet counts are checked by manual estimation, and abnormal counts from automatic cell counters should always be regarded with suspicion. Variations in platelet size may also lead to erroneous platelet counts. This was conspicuously shown in a study of breed-associated thrombocytopenia in Cavalier King Charles Spaniels in which manual platelet counts and automated counts were discordant. Affected dogs had a combination of large platelets (macrothrombocytes) and mild thrombocytopenia. The automated counts exaggerated the thrombocytopenia by counting macrothrombocytes as erythrocytes thus artefactually decreasing the platelet count (Ecksell *et al.*, 1994).

Haemoglobin

Three methods for measuring haemoglobin are currently used by different haematology analysers. The cyanmethaemoglobin method has been used as the international standard for many years, but the reagent contains potassium cyanide, which can cause problems with disposal and handling.

The oxyhaemoglobin method tends to underestimate total haemoglobin because it only measures the oxyhaemoglobin fraction. This can cause problems with external quality control because the oxyhaemoglobin in samples converts to methaemoglobin with time. This is also a problem in samples from patients with significant methaemoglobinaemia.

Recently, the use of a less toxic reagent, sodium lauryl sulphate (SLS), has replaced the cyanmethaemoglobin method. The erythrocytes are lysed, haemoglobin is converted to SLS–haemoglobin by a four-step reaction and then quantified colorimetrically.

Blood cell counts

Three major principles are currently used for cell counting by different haematology analysers: electronic cell counting by the Coulter principle, electronic-optical counting using laser detection systems and quantitative buffy coat analysis (QBC).

The Coulter principle

A stream of red blood cells (RBCs) diluted in electrolyte solution is focused on an aperture across which there is an electric current. As each individual cell passes through the aperture, the electrical resistance increases, generating a pulse. The pulse height is proportional to the cell volume (MCV), and the pulse frequency is proportional to cell numbers. Cumulative pulse height detection enables computation of the haematocrit. MCH and MCHC are then computed as follows:

$$\text{MCH (pg)} = \text{haemoglobin} \times \frac{10}{\text{RBC count}}$$

$$\text{MCHC (g/dl)} = \text{haemoglobin} \times \frac{100}{\text{haematocrit}}$$

In this system the haematocrit is a calculated variable and therefore should not be referred to as the PCV. The PCV measured by the microhaematocrit method and the calculated haematocrit often differ slightly. If the variation is greater than 3–5%, a technical problem should be suspected. The Coulter counter identifies cells to be counted from electronic thresholds, which depend on cell size. This causes errors when counting erythrocytes of different sizes from different species. Most analysers that are calibrated for human use are adequate for canine use because the MCVs of these two species are similar. Cats have much smaller erythrocytes and more platelet clumping, which leads to significant errors on Coulter counters calibrated for human use.

The same principle is applied to Coulter leucocyte counts. Minor adjustments must be made to electronic thresholds in conversion of human counters for feline and canine use. Macrothrombocytes and nRBCs may be erroneously counted as leucocytes. Differential leucocyte counts can be performed by some of these analysers by a process of elimination. Samples of blood are treated with reagents that lyse specific leucocyte types. Alkaline diluent, for example, will lyse and enucleate neutrophils, monocytes and lymphocytes while leaving eosinophils intact due to the stability of eosinophil granules in alkaline conditions. The count is then performed on the eosinophil-rich sample.

Laser cell counters

Laser cell counters use an electronic-optical laser detection system to measure the size and internal complexity of each cell on the basis of light scatter.

Compared with Coulter techniques, this method provides greatly expanded information about each cell type. The great advantage of laser counters is that the size and haemoglobin concentration of each erythrocyte is measured and then presented in a scattergram, which shows the distribution of MCV and haemoglobin throughout the erythrocyte population rather than just providing a mean value. The shape of the scattergram yields important diagnostic information about erythrocyte morphology, and exposes hidden subpopulations of cells that would otherwise disappear into the mean value.

Laser counters are also able to perform differential white cell counts and scattergram distributions on the basis of cell size and cytoplasmic characteristics, such as peroxidase content of granules. This can cause problems when assessing leucocytes from different species due to variable peroxidase content. The elimination process with lysing reagents, described previously for Coulter techniques, is used in conjunction with laser counting techniques in some analysers.

Quantitative buffy coat analysis

The QBC analysis system is based on the principle that erythrocytes, leucocytes and platelets will layer according to density upon centrifugation. The various layers are expanded by a plastic float and are identified by their acridine orange staining patterns as observed under blue–violet light. The widths of the various layers or bands are measured and used to predict the total leucocyte count, the absolute non-granulocyte and granulocyte counts, the platelet count and the PCV. The accuracy is excellent for PCV, total leucocyte count and granulocyte count, good for non-granulocyte count and fair for platelets (Tvedten and Weiss, 1999). The precision (based on coefficient of variation) is better than that for manual counts but worse than that for electronic counters. Indistinct separation of the granulocyte and erythrocyte layers occurs in some cases, especially with leucocytosis, and in these circumstances leucocytes cannot be counted. The QBC system cannot detect left shifts, morphological leucocyte abnormalities or red blood cell morphology. Manual examination of a blood film in addition to the QBC screen is, therefore, essential.

BLOOD FILMS

Whenever blood cannot be analysed within 2–3 hours it should be refrigerated at 4°C because erythrocyte swelling after 6–24 hours of storage at room temperature increases the PCV and MCV and lowers the MCHC. These variables are unchanged for at least 24 hours in refrigerated blood. Samples sent to a laboratory by post can be expected to have artefacts due to RBC swelling. The magnitude of these artefacts is unpredictable and in many samples changes are minimal. Exposure to high or very low temperatures and damage during collection are highly detrimental to stored and transported blood samples. Samples must never be frozen because the thawing process completely destroys the cells.

Production of high quality blood smears (Figure 1.6) is a skill that can only be acquired with constant practice and is a matter of pride for most haematologists. Evenly spread blood films are an absolute necessity for generating reliable differential cell counts. Veterinary surgeons are encouraged to submit a blood film (fixed by air drying) to accompany the EDTA sample. Although these films tend to have variable thickness and are rarely used for differential cell counts, they can be extremely useful for distinguishing between changes in cell morphology due to sample ageing and genuine diagnostic findings.

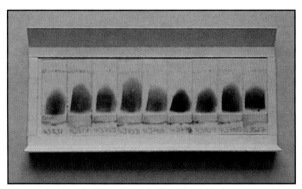

Figure 1.6: *A tray of well made blood smears stained with Wright's stain. (© AXIOM Veterinary Laboratories.)*

Staining

Blood films are stained with Romanowsky stains such as Leishman's stain or Wright's/Giemsa. Staining must be consistent because the learned skills involved in morphological interpretation depend on examination of very large numbers of films stained in exactly the same way. Staining can be done manually, but in laboratories with high turnover this becomes impractical and automatic stainers are used. Automatic staining is consistent as long as blood smears are well made and homogeneous.

The Romanowsky stains are compound dyes consisting of a mixture of methylene blue and eosin, with several contaminating dyes that can alter staining characteristics. Methylene blue stains the acidic cell components such as nuclei and cytoplasmic RNA. Eosin is red and stains more basic components such as haemoglobin. The dyes are dissolved in methyl alcohol, which also acts as a fixative. Contamination of methyl alcohol with water will spoil the fixation and lead to loss of cell detail. The stain solutions must therefore be kept absolutely free of water vapour in storage. This is a frequent cause of poor quality smears in laboratories where stains are made up in damp glassware and not stoppered.

Diff-Quik is a simple haematological stain to use in practice. It is not strictly a Romanowsky stain but works on a similar principle, by using blue and orange dyes to give appropriate staining characteristics. The two dyes are in separate jars, and the intensity of blue and orange staining can be altered manually with the number of dips of the slide in each stain.

One further stain that is frequently used in haematology is 1% new methylene blue in citrate saline. This is a vital stain, which precipitates and dyes the residual RNA in immature red cells identifying them as reticulocytes. Blood anticoagulated with EDTA is mixed with new methylene blue and allowed to stand for 15–20 minutes. The blood is then remixed and smeared for examination. RNA within reticulocytes stains blue-black, whereas mature erythrocytes stain pale green.

Examination

Blood films are routinely scanned without a cover slip with a 20X dry objective and then examined in detail with a 50X oil immersion objective. Details of intracellular morphology, such as red cell parasites and toxic granulation in the cytoplasm of neutrophils, may require a 100X oil immersion objective.

Routine differential leucocyte counts are based on 100 cells counted in a specific area of the film. The area of the film selected is critical because different sized cells spread at different rates and the largest tend to be found in the tail of the smear. The cells are counted in the body of the film where the smear is one cell thick and where the individual cells are sufficiently separated to make individual cell morphology and abnormal aggregation absolutely clear. The rest of the smear, including the tail, is then scanned for atypical or neoplastic cells and platelet clumps. The percentage differential leucocyte counts are multiplied by the total nucleated cell count to obtain the total differential counts.

Morphological comments on erythrocytes and leucocytes are recorded as an annotation to the haematological profile. Usually only abnormal morphological features are noted.

BLOOD CELL MORPHOLOGY AND INTERPRETATION

Erythrocyte morphology

The size, colour, shape and stage of development of erythrocytes can all be assessed microscopically and have great interpretive and diagnostic significance.

Macrocytes

Macrocytes are large erythrocytes. They are often hypochromic (deficient in haemoglobin) (Figure 1.7) immature erythrocytes produced in a regenerative response to blood loss or haemolysis. Breed-related macrocytosis is a normal finding in some poodles. Macrocytes can be associated with feline leukaemia virus (FeLV) subgroup A infection in kittens and with myeloproliferative disorders of both dogs and cats. Abnormal numbers of macrocytes can be seen in damaged or aged samples as an artefact of erythrocyte swelling.

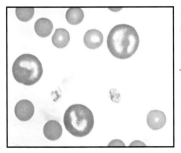

Figure 1.7: Three polychromatic macrocytes in a regenerative response from a dog with immune-mediated haemolytic anaemia (Wright's stain; original magnification ×1000). (© AXIOM Veterinary Laboratories.)

Microcytes

Microcytes are small erythrocytes. They may be normochromic or hypochromic. Microcytes with a normal haemoglobin content occur in anaemia of chronic inflammation. Hypochromic microcytes (Figure 1.8) are important markers of altered iron metabolism and are present in dogs with iron deficiency and also in dogs with portosystemic shunts. The most common cause of iron deficiency in dogs is chronic occult blood loss from the gastrointestinal tract. The abnormality of iron metabolism in portosystemic shunts is currently under investigation. Akitas have unusually small erythrocytes and also have a particularly high potassium content compared with other dog breeds.

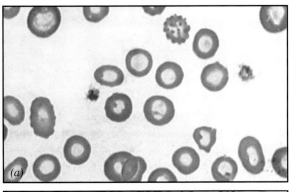

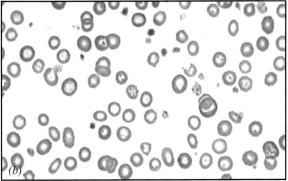

Figure 1.8: Microcytic hypochromic cells from a case of iron deficiency in a dog (Wright's stain; (a) original magnification ×1000, (b) original magnification ×500). (© AXIOM Veterinary Laboratories.)

Anisocytosis

Anisocytosis is a term applied when the erythrocytes in a film are of variable, rather than consistent, volume. This is frequently seen in both regenerative and non-regenerative anaemias.

Spherocytes

Spherocytes are small, densely staining spherical erythrocytes denoted by lack of central pallor (Figure 1.9). These cells adopt a spherical shape after reduction in the cell membrane area (and hence surface to volume ratio) due to partial phagocytosis by mononuclear phagocytes. The presence of spherocytes in a smear implies that the erythrocytes have surface-bound antibody or complement, which is recognized by cell surface receptors on phagocytes. Spherocytes are less deformable than normal erythrocytes and consequently are osmotically fragile. The presence of spherocytes is a sensitive indicator of immune-mediated haemolytic anaemia in dogs. Feline RBCs have a lower MCV and less appreciable central pallor than canine RBCs. Consequently spherocytes are rarely recognized in cats.

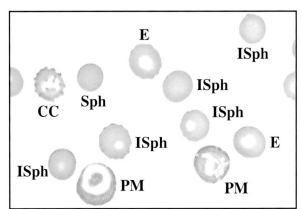

Figure 1.9: One spherocyte (Sph) and five erythrocytes showing various stages of incomplete spherocyte formation (ISph) (reducing area of central pallor) accompanied by two normal erythrocytes (E), one crenated cell (CC) and two polychromatic macrocytes (PM) (Wright's stain; original magnification ×1000). (© AXIOM Veterinary Laboratories.)

Codocytes (target cells)

Codocytes are bell-shaped erythrocytes which, when viewed in two dimensions, have a dense centre surrounded by a clear area and a peripheral haemoglobin rim (Figure 1.10). This bizarre shape is adopted because of increases in the cholesterol:phopholipid ratio within the cell membrane. Codocytes are seen in iron deficiency anaemia, liver disease with cholestasis and after splenectomy in dogs. Reticulocytes have increased surface to volume ratio and can also appear as target cells in two dimensions, but this is not indicative of any underlying process other than the presence of red blood cell regeneration.

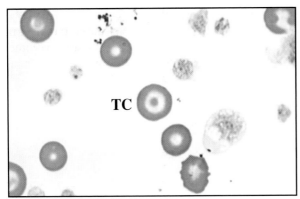

Figure 1.10: A target cell (codocyte) (TC) (Wright's stain; original magnification ×1000). (Courtesy of AXIOM Veterinary Laboratories.)

Acanthocytes

Acanthocytes are irregularly spiculated erythrocytes with a few unevenly distributed surface projections of variable diameter and length (Figure 1.11). Similar to codocytes, acanthocytes may occur as a result of alterations in the cholesterol:phospholipid ratio of the cell membrane but can also be seen in association with RBC fragmentation. Acanthocytes are seen in dogs with diseases of capillary beds such as splenic haemangioma/haemangiosarcoma, diffuse liver disease or portosystemic shunts. They have also been observed in association with high cholesterol diets.

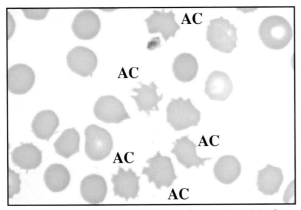

Figure 1.11: Acanthocytes (AC) (Wright's stain; original magnification ×1000). (© AXIOM Veterinary Laboratories.)

Echinocytes (Burr cells)

Echinocytes are regularly spiculated erythrocytes, which usually arise as an artefact due to crenation. Echinocytes that are not due to crenation are seen in some dogs with lymphoma, chronic renal disease, glomerulonephritis or chronic doxorubicin toxicosis.

Schistocytes

Schistocytes are irregular erythrocyte fragments resulting from mechanical trauma to circulating erythrocytes (Figure 1.12). They are markers of disseminated intravascular coagulation (DIC) and other microvascular angiopathies and are seen in patients with immune-mediated anaemia, thrombosis, splenic haemangiosarcoma, hypersplenism, glomerulonephritis, congestive heart failure, valvular heart disease, doxorubicin toxicosis and myelofibrosis.

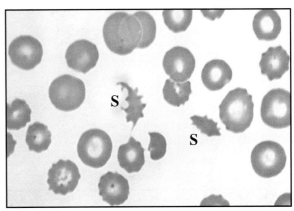

Figure 1.12: Schistocytes (S) (Wright's stain; original magnification ×1000). (© AXIOM Veterinary Laboratories.)

Eccentrocytes

Eccentrocytes are erythrocytes in which oxidative damage causes fusion of opposing cell membranes on one edge of the erythrocyte (Figure 1.13). This has the effect of squeezing haemoglobin into a smaller volume. When viewed in two dimensions the fused membranes appear as a clear zone whereas the compressed haemoglobin appears eccentric and darker than normal. Eccentrocytes are a sensitive indicator of oxidative damage in dogs, and eccentrocytic anaemias are often associated with onion poisoning in this species. Cats are more sensitive than dogs to oxidative erythrocyte damage, which is manifested by the formation of numerous Heinz bodies rather than eccentrocytes.

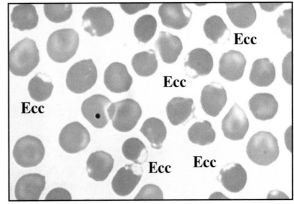

Figure 1.13: Eccentrocytes (Ecc) (Wright's stain; original magnification ×1000). (© AXIOM Veterinary Laboratories.)

Erythrocyte inclusions

Erythrocyte inclusions of importance include parasites, Howell–Jolly Bodies, Heinz bodies and basophilic stippling.

Haemobartonella felis: *Haemobartonella felis* organisms are highly pleomorphic and stain with variable intensity, appearing as chains, discs or rods on the surface of erythrocytes (Figure 1.14).

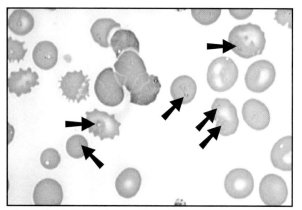

Figure 1.14: Haemobartonella *organisms (arrowed) in the erythrocytes of a ferret with fatal haemolytic anaemia (Wright's stain; original magnification ×1000). (© AXIOM Veterinary Laboratories.)*

Babesia: *Babesia* is an intracellular parasite of canine erythrocytes, which causes major morbidity in tropical and subtropical areas of the world (see Chapter 5). It is transmitted by various species of tick, particularly *Rhipicephalus sanguineous*. It is not endemic in the United Kingdom but is likely to be of increasing importance in imported dogs.

Howell–Jolly bodies: Howell–Jolly bodies are deeply staining spherical structures within the erythrocyte. They are remnants of the incompletely extruded metrarubricyte nucleus and usually reflect reticuloendothelial dysfunction.

Heinz bodies: Heinz bodies are small highly refractile bodies that stain poorly with Wrights stain and well with supravital stains. They are eccentrically located beneath the erythrocyte cell membrane or protrude through it. Heinz bodies are formed by irreversible precipitation of oxidatively denatured haemoglobin. They are markers of oxidative damage, for example in paracetamol toxicosis in cats.

Basophilic stippling: Basophilic stippling of erythrocytes and metarubricytes occurs in lead poisoning and is characterized by the presence of punctate or reticulated basophilic granules (clumped ribosomes) within the erythrocyte. Basophilic stippling may also be a feature of marked regenerative responses in cats.

Nucleated red blood cells

The nRBCs seen most frequently in the peripheral circulation are metarubricytes. They have a condensed pyknotic nucleus and abundant polychromatic (bluish staining) or orthochromic (the colour of mature erythrocytes) cytoplasm. Rubricytes, which have a round viable nucleus and are larger than the metarubricytes, are sometimes seen.

The presence of nRBCs in circulation is always important (see Figure 1.15). Metarubricytes appear during bone marrow regenerative responses to haemolysis or blood loss. They may also be liberated after extramedullary haematopoiesis in the reticuloendothelial system. They are typically present in dogs with splenic haemangiosarcoma and also occur in splenectomized individuals. The presence of earlier erythrocyte precursors (rubricytes/prorubricytes) in circulation usually implies quite severe bone marrow or reticuloendothelial disease but can occasionally be seen in association with very marked regenerative responses.

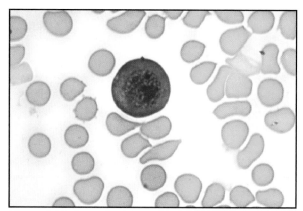

Figure 1.15: An erythroblastoid cell (primitive nucleated red blood cell) in the peripheral blood of a cat with myelodysplasia due to FeLV infection (Wright's stain; original magnification ×1000). (© AXIOM Veterinary Laboratories.)

Reticulocytes

The normal morphological response to blood loss is a regenerative pattern with reticulocytes and metarubricytes. In a normal Wright's/Giemsa-stained blood smear reticulocytes appear as large polychromatic cells. When stained with new methylene blue, the reticulocytes show an internal reticulated pattern of nuclear material and condensed organelles. The new methylene blue-stained smear is used for the reticulocyte count, which is an objective index of the degree of regeneration.

In cats, reticulocytes show punctate (dots) or aggregate (clusters and lines) patterns of condensed organelles. This is a unique feature of the maturation of reticulocytes in the cat. In feline regenerative responses, aggregate reticulocytes are released first. After a short maturation time of around 12 hours, the aggregate form becomes a punctate reticulocyte, which has a maturation time of 10–12 days. Aggregate reticulocytes therefore reflect active regeneration whereas punctate reticulocytes reflect recent cumulative regeneration.

Leucocyte morphology

Important morphological features of leucocytes include immaturity, abnormal cytoplasmic granulation and infectious inclusions.

Neutrophils

Mature neutrophils have a long thin segmented/lobulated nucleus, uneven but well defined nuclear margins and abundant, lightly basophilic or eosinophilic, slightly granulated cytoplasm. Immature neutrophils are termed bands and are recognizable because the nucleus is elongated but parallel-sided and not lobulated (Figure 1.16). Metamyelocytes may also be seen; these are larger than mature neutrophils and have a similar cytoplasm but the nucleus is kidney bean-shaped and not lobulated (Figure 1.17). Metamyelocytes can be difficult to distinguish from monocytes, but in general are smaller and more discrete.

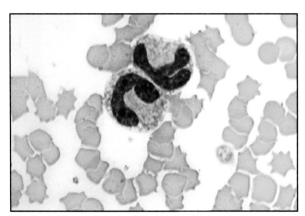

Figure 1.16: *Two neutrophilic bands. These cells are showing evidence of toxic change; note the coarse basophilic 'foaminess' of the cytoplasm (Wright's stain; original magnification ×1000). (© AXIOM Veterinary Laboratories.)*

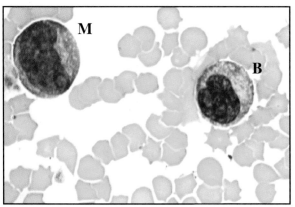

Figure 1.17: *A metamyelocyte (M) and a band (B) with a folded nucleus. These cells are showing evidence of toxic change; note the coarse basophilic 'foaminess' of the cytoplasm (Wright's stain; original magnification ×1000). (© AXIOM Veterinary Laboratories.)*

The presence of immature neutrophils (band neutrophils and metamyelocytes) in the peripheral circulation is termed a 'left shift' and is either a response to increased neutrophil consumption by inflammatory and infectious processes or an abnormal increase in neutrophil production. When mature neutrophils greatly outnumber the immature forms and the mature neutrophil count is increased, the left shift is termed 'regenerative' and indicates that the immune system is coping with the inflammatory or infectious process. If the immature forms outnumber the mature forms, the left shift is termed 'degenerative,' and is a poor prognostic sign. The combination of a low mature neutrophil count with a degenerative left shift is a grave prognostic sign. Toxic cytoplasmic changes in mature and immature neutrophils are often present at the same time as a degenerative left shift and frequently indicate an overwhelming septic process. The appearance of metamyelocytes in a left shift suggests a potent inflammatory or regenerative stimulus. If even earlier granulocyte forms appear, myeloproliferative disease and other disorders of bone marrow should be suspected (Figure 1.18).

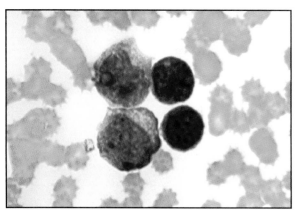

Figure 1.18: *Two myeloblasts (smaller round cells) and two monoblasts from a myelomonocytic leukaemia in a dog (Wright's stain; original magnification ×1000). (© AXIOM Veterinary Laboratories.)*

Regenerative left shifts are nearly always associated with systemic inflammation but under certain conditions this interpretation may be misleading. The observation that anaemias with marked regeneration, such as immune-mediated haemolytic anaemia, are very frequently accompanied by a significant left shift has often been interpreted as a reflection of non-specific stimulation of the granulocyte cell line by mediators of RBC regeneration. There is continuing debate about this, but current research suggests that the left shift is actually associated with neutrophil consumption due to tissue damage and the systemic inflammatory response which either initiates, or is induced by, the haemolytic anaemia (McManus and Craig, 1999).

Occasionally, the regenerative response to an inflammatory stimulus is so excessive that enormously high neutrophil counts with a primitive left shift are generated. This is termed a 'leukaemoid response' and can be impossible to distinguish from myeloid leukaemia on morphological grounds alone.

'Toxic change' is a collective term for morphological features that develop in neutrophils as a result of disturbed cellular maturation in the bone marrow associated with marked inflammatory or septic processes

(Figure 1.19). The spectrum of toxic changes in dog and cat neutrophils approximately correlates with the severity and duration of the stimulus. One of the earliest changes is the presence of Doehle bodies (lamellar aggregates of rough endoplasmic reticulum) in the cytoplasm (Figure 1.20). As 'toxicity' becomes more severe, the cytoplasm becomes more basophilic and develops a foamy appearance. Intensely stained primary granules may also be apparent. Finally, the nucleus swells and the nuclear envelope appears ragged. Doehle bodies are less useful for indicating early toxicity in cats than in dogs because they can be present in up to 30% of normal cat neutrophils.

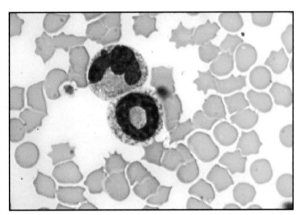

Figure 1.19: Two toxic bands. Note the cell with the 'doughnut' nucleus; this is a feature of abnormal nuclear maturation and is part of the spectrum of toxicity. Both cells show coarse basophilic foaminess of the cytoplasm (Wright's stain; original magnification ×1000). (© AXIOM Veterinary Laboratories.)

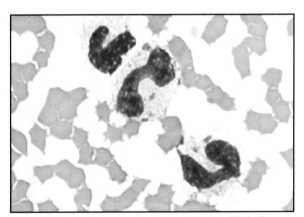

Figure 1.20: Three toxic bands containing Doehle bodies (Wright's stain; original magnification ×1000). (© AXIOM Veterinary Laboratories.)

Hereditary abnormalities of neutrophils occur occasionally in dogs and cats. Pelger–Huet anomaly has been reported in both species. This is a failure of the normal nuclear maturation of neutrophils. The mature cells have a parallel-sided nucleus and mimic bands. Chediak–Higashi syndrome has been reported in Persian cats and is characterized by poorly functioning neutrophils with giant intracytoplasmic granules. Vacuolation of neutrophils may be seen in storage disorders such as α-mannosidosis.

Eosinophils

Eosinophils have very recognizable morphology with bright pinkish-red uniformly stained cytoplasmic granules and a polymorphic nucleus, which is smoother and less segmented than that of a neutrophil (Figure 1.21). Feline eosinophils usually have rod-shaped granules. Canine eosinophils often have an orange hue and may have vacuolated granules. Greyhound eosinophils are highly vacuolated. Occasional canine eosinophils have very large red cell-sized granules. Toxic eosinophils sometimes have purplish-black granules.

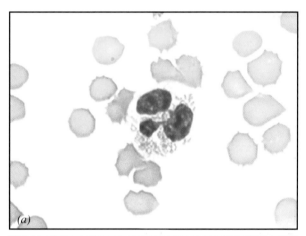

(a)

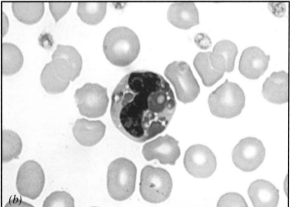

(b)

Figure 1.21: (a) A feline eosinophil; (b) a canine eosinophil (Wright's stain; original magnification ×1000). (© AXIOM Veterinary Laboratories.)

Basophils

Dog and cat basophils have rather unusual morphology and can easily be missed by inexperienced haematologists. The canine mature basophil is usually larger than a neutrophil and has a lobulated or strap-like nucleus. The cytoplasm is basophilic with occasional large dark purple granules (Figure 1.22). Immature basophils tend to have more marked granulation. Canine basophils can be mistaken for highly toxic neutrophils, leading to errors in interpretation. Feline basophils have similar nuclear features but the cytoplasm contains large numbers of pale grey granules that can be mistaken for eosinophil granules (Figure 1.23).

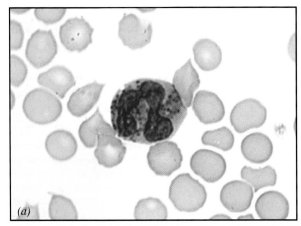

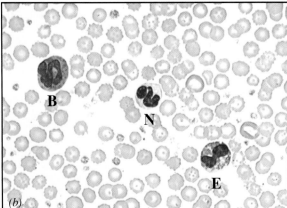

Figure 1.22: *(a) A canine basophil (Wright's stain; original magnification x1000). (b) A canine basophil (B), neutrophil (N) and eosinophil (E) in the same high power field. Note the relative sizes of the cells (Wright's stain; original magnification ×500). (© AXIOM Veterinary Laboratories.)*

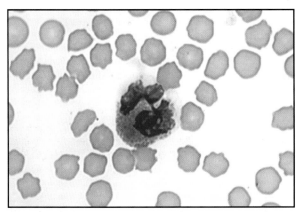

Figure 1.23: *A feline basophil (Wright's stain; original magnification ×1000). (© AXIOM Veterinary Laboratories.)*

Monocytes

Monocytes are large cells with variable amoeboid morphology, which can be differentiated from other large blood cells such as metamyelocytes by their blue ground-glass cytoplasm and reticulated or ribbon-like nuclear chromatin (Figure 1.24). Transformation of monocytes to active vacuolated macrophages in circulation can be seen in severe chronic inflammatory processes such as bacterial endocarditis.

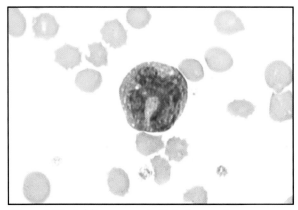

Figure 1.24: *A feline monocyte. Note the ropy/lacy chromatin pattern (Wright's stain; original magnification ×1000). (© AXIOM Veterinary Laboratories.)*

Lymphocytes

Circulating lymphocytes have very variable size and morphology. They can be small, medium or large, with nuclei varying from round to cleaved and convoluted (Figure 1.25). The most consistent features of lymphocytes are the coarsely clumped chromatin pattern and the presence of small quantities of basophilic cytoplasm.

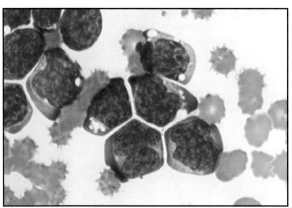

Figure 1.25: *Cleaved lymphocytes in a dog with lymphocytic leukaemia (Wright's stain; original magnification ×1000). (© AXIOM Veterinary Laboratories.)*

The typical small lymphocyte has a round- or bean-shaped nucleus approximately the diameter of an RBC, with a thin rim of basophilic cytoplasm. Reactive lymphocytes (Figure 1.26) are larger and have an increased volume of more basophilic cytoplasm than quiescent lymphocytes. Large granular lymphocytes (Figure 1.27) in low numbers are also a normal finding. These have increased lightly basophilic cytoplasm containing small azurophilic granules and are thought to represent cytotoxic T cells or natural killer (NK) cells.

Lymphoblasts are large lymphocytes containing one or more prominent nucleoli (Figure 1.28) and their presence in the peripheral circulation is always abnormal and usually due to stage V lymphoma or lymphoid

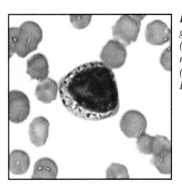

Figure 1.26: *A reactive lymphocyte. This is a medium sized lymphocyte with increased cytoplasmic volume and basophilia. The pale area close to the nucleus is the Golgi zone. (Wright's stain; original magnification ×1000.) (© AXIOM Veterinary Laboratories.)*

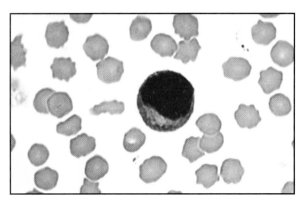

Figure 1.27: *A large granular lymphocyte (Wright's stain; original magnification ×1000). (© AXIOM Veterinary Laboratories.)*

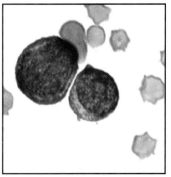

Figure 1.28: *Two lymphoblasts in the circulation of a cat with stage V lymphoma (Wright's stain; original magnification ×1000). (© AXIOM Veterinary Laboratories.)*

leukaemia. Neoplastic lymphocytes can be fragile and are often damaged during blood film preparation. The damaged cells are referred to as 'smear cells' or 'basket cells' and should be viewed with suspicion when observed in large numbers.

Infectious inclusions in leucocytes

Infection by *Leishmania* spp., *Ehrlichia* spp., *Hepatozoon* spp. or canine distemper virus can lead to the presence of recognizable inclusions in leucocytes. *Ehrlichia* spp. form cytoplasmic bodies known as morulae, which occur in monocytes and sometimes neutrophils. *Leishmania* spp. parasitize monocytes and macrophages but are more often seen in bone marrow and lymph node samples than in blood smears. Canine distemper virus forms distinctive purple cytoplasmic inclusions in neutrophils and also in RBCs. *Hepatozoon* spp. occur as large lozenge-shaped non-staining inclusions that fill the cytoplasm of neutrophils.

Platelet morphology

Platelets are anucleate structures, which have a lightly basophilic granular staining pattern and range from 2 to 4 μm in diameter. They have poorly defined cytoplasmic margins and often appear to have small hair-like projections from the surface. Giant platelets, often larger than RBCs, occur in platelet regenerative responses and are a normal finding in some breeds, notably the Cavalier King Charles Spaniel. Platelets (especially feline platelets) tend to form clumps in anticoagulants such as EDTA, which cause artefactually low automated platelet counts. The presence of platelet clumps in the tail of a blood film is an indication that the automated platelet count may be erroneous. Unclumped platelets are normally scattered among the other blood cells in the film. Feline platelets are larger (twice the volume) than most canine platelets.

INTERPRETING THE HAEMATOLOGICAL PROFILE

The haematological profile includes measurements of the variables listed in Figure 1.29. The profile must be interpreted as a whole, noting normal as well as abnormal values. A systematic approach to interpretation is important, aided by consistent presentation of the information. Data in an unusual format can lead to human error.

Variable	Units
Haemoglobin concentration	g/l
Haematocrit (or packed cell volume; PCV)	l/l or %
Erythrocyte count (RBC)	x10^{12}/l
Mean corpuscular volume (MCV)	fl
Mean corpuscular haemoglobin (MCH)	pg
Mean corpuscular haemoglobin concentration (MCHC)	g/l
Platelet count	x10^9/l
Nucleated RBCs	%
Total nucleated cell count (WBC)	x10^9/l
Segmented neutrophils (% and total count)	x10^9/l
Band neutrophils (% and total count)	x10^9/l
Lymphocytes (% and total count)	x10^9/l
Monocytes (% and total count)	x10^9/l
Eosinophils (% and total count)	x10^9/l
Basophils (% and total count)	x10^9/l
Erythrocyte morphology and comment on count	
Leucocyte morphology and comment on count	
Platelet morphology and comment on count	
Description of any abnormal cell	

Figure 1.29: *Components of the haematological profile.*

Erythrocyte variables

First note the haemoglobin concentration as this is the most direct assessment of anaemia. Then check the haematocrit. If the haematocrit is increased, compare with the erythrocyte numbers and MCV. Genuine polycythaemia is unlikely if the erythrocyte numbers are within the reference range. Increased MCV is quite a common cause of an increased haematocrit and is typical of aged samples with erythrocyte swelling. Frequently, increase of the haematocrit is due to haemoconcentration (splenic contraction) or dehydration.

Anaemia is present if the haemoglobin concentration is below the reference range regardless of the erythrocyte numbers and the haematocrit, but in the majority of anaemias all three variables will be low. If anaemia is present, attempt to classify it by studying the MCV, MCHC and the comments on erythrocyte morphology. Many standard texts use the MCV as the primary index for the presence or absence of regeneration. This is surprising, since this varies unpredictably with sample ageing, and many regenerative anaemias do not have MCVs above reference intervals. The presence or absence of polychromasia in the stained smear is a much more reliable index of regeneration. If there is polychromasia, then regeneration is present. The amount of polychromasia and the nRBC count usually reflect the adequacy of regeneration accurately, but in occasional cases a reticulocyte count will be needed to provide an objective index of regeneration.

It is now customary to use the absolute reticulocyte count for the quantitative assessment of regeneration in dogs and cats. In cats the aggregate reticulocyte count is used to indicate current regeneration, whereas the punctate reticulocyte count is more indicative of the recent history of regeneration. Reticulocyte counts above 60 x 10⁹/l in dogs and 50 x 10⁹/l aggregate reticulocytes in cats indicate regeneration. The degree of regeneration is approximately proportional to the absolute count, and the adequacy of regeneration is interpreted in the context of the RBC variables and the clinical features of each case of anaemia. The adequacy of regeneration in any individual case can also be assessed quantitatively by using the reticulocyte production index (RPI), which is a ratio examining the reticulocyte count in relation to the haematocrit (Figure 1.30).

In most regenerative anaemias, MCV is normal or high. One exception to this is the special situation of chronic blood loss in which the patient begins to become iron deficient. Such cases will have mixed erythrocyte morphology featuring increased polychromasia and also a progressively increasing percentage of microcytic cells. The MCV in such cases may be below the reference interval. In non-regenerative anaemias MCV is usually normal or low. Rare cases of non-regenerative anaemia with increased MCV may be associated with myeloproliferative disease, especially FeLV-related disease in cats.

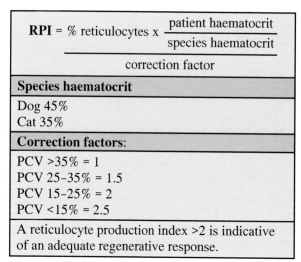

$$\text{RPI} = \%\ \text{reticulocytes} \times \cfrac{\cfrac{\text{patient haematocrit}}{\text{species haematocrit}}}{\text{correction factor}}$$

Species haematocrit
Dog 45%
Cat 35%

Correction factors:
PCV >35% = 1
PCV 25–35% = 1.5
PCV 15–25% = 2
PCV <15% = 2.5

A reticulocyte production index >2 is indicative of an adequate regenerative response.

Figure 1.30: *Calculation and interpretation of the reticulocyte production index (RPI). PCV, packed cell volume.*

The MCHC is a calculated variable expressing the mean haemoglobin concentration per erythrocyte. Hypochromic anaemias will have a low MCHC. The MCH is a calculated variable expressing the mean quantity of haemoglobin per erythrocyte and does not take into account the volume of the erythrocyte. Thus microcytes will automatically have low MCH but may not be hypochromic.

Careful assessment of the morphology of the erythrocytes is of critical importance in the classification of anaemia. Morphological abnormalities such as the formation of spherocytes and acanthocytes are highly sensitive indicators of underlying diseases such as immune-mediated haemolytic anaemia and haemangiosarcoma. The blood film examination also checks the interpretive validity of changes in the RBC indices; for example, if the MCHC and MCV are low then the film should contain microcytic hypochromic erythrocytes.

Erythrocyte morphology should also be noted when anaemia is not present. Polychromasia and nRBCs may indicate ongoing mild blood loss, which is balanced by erythrocyte production and therefore does not decrease the haemoglobin concentration and PCV below the reference range. The presence of nRBCs in the absence of anaemia may also be an indicator of splenic or bone marrow disorders.

Automated platelet count

If the automated platelet count is low, the tail of the blood film should be examined for the presence of platelet clumps, which are a common cause of pseudothrombocytopenia. The presence of large clumps usually indicates a normal platelet count. When platelets are not clumped a count of 8–29 per high power (100X) field indicates adequate platelet numbers in dogs. Macrothrombocytes may also cause erroneously low counts. Genuine thrombocytopenia rarely causes the classic signs of petechiation and ecchymoses unless the count is below 30 x 10⁹/l.

Thrombocytosis occurs relatively frequently in both dogs and cats and may be due to several different processes. Mild thrombocytosis is often non-specific and seems to be associated with inflammatory processes. In dogs it is also a feature of the haematological pattern of iron deficiency, and erythrocyte variables should be checked carefully for evidence of hypochromia and microcytosis. Thrombocytosis is the first change seen in some cases of myeloproliferative disease.

Total leucocyte count

It is important to remember that the leucocyte count is actually a count of nucleated cells, and large numbers of nRBCs can produce an erroneously increased count. If a high percentage of nRBCs is present, the leucocyte count is corrected by the appropriate factor.

Differential leucocyte counts

Differential leucocyte counts should always be interpreted as total counts rather than percentage counts. Percentage counts should be regarded as a means for calculating the total counts, and have little inherent interpretive value. Each differential leucocyte count should first be classified as normal, increased or decreased (e.g. absolute neutrophilia or neutropenia), then the overall leucocyte pattern can be assessed. The major patterns are the inflammatory leucogram, the stress leucogram, the leukaemoid response, various cytopenias and genuine leukaemias. Leucocyte counts and morphology must be assessed together.

Leucocyte patterns

Inflammatory patterns

The classic inflammatory pattern is neutrophilia with a left shift and monocytosis. This pattern is typically seen in sepsis, severe localized infections and tissue necrosis. Neutrophilia with a left shift but no monocytosis often reflects a less well established or more acute inflammatory process. In longstanding inflammatory and/or infectious processes such as granulomatous disease and draining sinus tracts, the inflammatory pattern may evolve into a mature neutrophilia without a left shift but with monocytosis and lymphocytosis. Occasionally the only evidence for chronic inflammation is monocytosis. Regenerative and degenerative left shifts and leukaemoid responses discussed are above. The presence or absence of the morphological signs of neutrophil 'toxicity' is critical in patients with inflammatory leucograms because toxicity is quite a reliable marker for the presence of underlying bacterial infection. Toxicity is also a significant prognostic factor.

Absolute eosinophilia is an inflammatory pattern with several different associations. Eosinophilia can be seen as an adjunct to neutrophilia, left shift and monocytosis in non-specific inflammatory processes, particularly in cats. Other causes of eosinophilia include hypersensitivity, parasitism, eosinophilic diseases and systemic mastocytosis. Eosinophilic diseases of importance in dogs include eosinophilic bronchitis and enteritis. The cat shares these diseases, with the addition of the eosinophilic granuloma complex. German Shepherd Dogs often have eosinophil counts above the reference range for other breeds. The cause of this phenomenon is not known, but the increased eosinophil counts rarely seem to have any clinical importance.

Stress patterns

Stress leucograms are associated with the influence of stress hormones such as catecholamines and glucocorticoids. During acute stress, cats may develop lymphocytosis and/or neutrophilia, due to catecholamine release. Lymphopenia may subsequently develop as a result of corticosteroid release during chronic stress. Dogs are less prone to catecholamine-induced haematological responses than cats but are more sensitive to glucocorticoids. The canine stress leucogram has several patterns. Perhaps the most common pattern is absolute eosinopenia, followed by lymphopenia and then a combination of both. Less frequently, dogs can develop quite massive mature neutrophilia in response to glucocorticoids, and this response may mimic a chronic inflammatory pattern. It is quite common for dogs to have combined inflammatory and stress leucograms (e.g. neutrophilia with a left shift, monocytosis, lymphopenia and eosinopenia).

Cytopenias

The stress leucogram, described above, is the most common cause of lymphopenia and eosinopenia. Neutropenia is a highly significant haematological finding. The short intravascular life span of neutrophils (7–14 hours) makes them early markers of bone marrow dysfunction. The combination of non-regenerative anaemia, thrombocytopenia and granulocytopenia is termed pancytopenia and is invariably associated with severe bone marrow disease. Cytopenias involving any two cell lines should also be regarded as suspicious of bone marrow disease.

Neutropenia is a feature of acute viral infections (e.g. parvovirus or distemper). Non-specific reversible neutropenia occurs quite commonly in dogs with gastroenteritis and is probably associated with margination of neutrophils in the gastrointestinal tract in response to the presence of local enterotoxins. Neutropenia can also be seen in patients with severe degenerative left shifts due to overwhelming infectious or inflammatory processes. In such cases neutrophils often exhibit toxic morphology.

Leukaemia

Acute leukaemia can usually be differentiated from an inflammatory response by the presence of blast cells in peripheral circulation, although occasionally leukaemoid responses may also have blast cells.

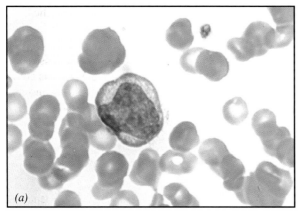

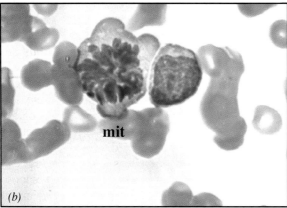

Figure 1.31: (a) A monoblast and (b) two monoblasts, one of which is undergoing mitosis (mit), in the circulation of a dog with monocytic leukaemia (Wright's stain; original magnification ×1000). (© AXIOM Veterinary Laboratories.)

Genuine leukaemia may also present a rather monotonous leucocyte morphology, often with inappropriate numbers of cells at each stage of maturation (Figure 1.31). Chronic granulocytic leukaemia can be indistinguishable from a leukaemoid response on the basis of haematological features alone.

REFERENCES AND FURTHER READING

Eksell P, Haggstrom J, Kvart C and Karlsson A (1994) Thrombocytopenia in the Cavalier King Charles Spaniel. *Journal of Small Animal Practice* **35**, 153-155

Giger U *et al.* (2000) Haematology and Immunology Section In: *Textbook of Veterinary Internal Medicine, 5th edn*, ed. SJ Ettinger and EC Feldman, pp. 1784-1857. WB Saunders, Philadelphia

Jain NC (1993) Examination of the blood and bone marrow. In: *Essentials of Veterinary Haematology, 1st edn*, ed. NC Jain, pp. 1-19. Lea and Febiger, Philadelphia

Latimer KS (1995) Leukocytes in health and disease. In: *Textbook of Veterinary Internal Medicine, 4th edn*, ed. SJ Ettinger and EC Feldman, pp. 1892-1929. WB Saunders, Philadelphia

McManus P and Craig L (1999) Correlation between leukocytosis and necropsy findings in canine immune mediated haemolytic anemia (IMHA) patients. *Veterinary Pathology* **36**, 484

Tvedten H (1994) The complete blood count and bone marrow examination: general comments and selected techniques. In: *Small Animal Clinical Diagnosis by Laboratory Methods, 2nd edn*, ed. MD Willard, H Tvedten and G Turnwald, pp. 11-31. WB Saunders, Philadelphia

Tvedten H and Weiss D (1999) *Small Animal Clinical Diagnosis by Laboratory Methods, 3rd edn*, ed. MD Willard, H Tvedten and G Turnwald, p. 20. WB Saunders, Philadelphia

Weiser MG (1995) Erythrocyte responses and disorders. In: *Textbook of Veterinary Internal Medicine, 4th edn*, ed. SJ Ettinger and EC Feldman, pp. 1864-1891. WB Saunders, Philadelphia

Collection and Interpretation of Bone Marrow Samples

Dorothee Bienzle

INTRODUCTION

Bone marrow is a complex and highly specialized tissue that gives rise to cells with such discrete functions as distribution of essential oxygen, defence against microbial agents, confinement of haemorrhage, and initiation of wound healing. It is a unique tissue whereby undifferentiated precursor cells perpetually generate myriads of new cells. These cells mature in an orderly sequence through an intricate environment of cells and growth factors to become mature functional erythrocytes, leucocytes, and platelets. Terminally differentiated cells are released into the circulation where they execute their varied functions until their predestined short life span has been reached and they are removed by the haemophagocytic component of the spleen. The bone marrow is in a dynamic equilibrium with the requirements of the animal and continually and rapidly adjusts to variable demands. Impairment of any element of the bone marrow has distinct and severe clinical manifestations, and lack of a functional marrow is incompatible with life.

INDICATIONS FOR BONE MARROW EXAMINATION

In contemporary veterinary medicine a haemogram or complete blood count (CBC) is part of the routine evaluation of small animal patients. Any abnormalities that are detected may be appropriate responses to a disease in another tissue, such as an eosinophilia noted in some allergic responses or a responsive anaemia secondary to blood loss. Where deviations from reference values cannot be accounted for, further investigation is required. In general, when haematological abnormalities in an animal cannot be correlated with an apparent disease process, the bone marrow should be evaluated. Figure 2.1 outlines specific indications for examination of the bone marrow.

The decision to examine bone marrow is usually based on findings on the CBC or on potential involvement of the marrow in a systemic disease process. Contraindications for the procedure are few and can be addressed with special precautions: particular attention should be paid to sterile procedure in neutropenic

Persistent and unexplained changes in one cell line
Decreased cell number (anaemia, neutropenia, thrombocytopenia)
Increased cell number (polycythaemia, neutrophilia, lymphocytosis, thrombocytosis)
Any change affecting more than one cell line, e.g. anaemia and thrombocytopenia, anaemia and neutropenia
Abnormal cells in circulation:
Rubricytosis in the absence of a responsive anaemia
Left shift (increased immature neutrophils) without neutrophilia or toxic changes
Immature cells of any cell lineage
Mast cells, macrophages, neoplastic, or unidentifiable cells
Fever of unknown origin
Suspected systemic ehrlichiosis, leishmaniasis or mycotic infection
Staging of mast cell tumours, lymphomas or carcinomas
Hyperproteinaemia or monoclonal gammopathies that may be associated with multiple myeloma, feline plasmacytoma, ehrlichiosis, leishmaniasis, pyoderma, lymphoma, systemic fungal disease or feline infectious peritonitis
Unexplained hypercalcaemia

***Figure 2.1:** Indications for examination of bone marrow.*

or immunosuppressed patients, and soft tissue trauma should be minimized in animals with coagulation deficiencies. Sedation, analgesia or anaesthesia should be tailored to the temperament of the patient or completely omitted in debilitated animals. Although profound thrombocytopenia may seem to be a contraindication for bone marrow biopsy, clinically significant bleeding in such cases is rare. Once an indication for examination of the bone marrow has been established, essentially the procedure can be performed in all patients.

COLLECTING A BONE MARROW SAMPLE

Types of sample

Two types of bone marrow sample can be collected: a cellular aspirate of the non-adherent bone marrow elements (these can be smeared similarly to a blood smear) or a solid core of tissue consisting of bony trabeculae, fat and haematopoietic tissue. The latter biopsy requires fixation and processing like other tissue samples containing bone (Weiss, 1987). For complete evaluation both samples are required, although sometimes a diagnosis may be established from a cellular aspirate alone. Exceptions are cytopenias in the blood, which frequently reflect lack of the corresponding precursor cells in the bone marrow. In these cases an aspirate may contain insufficient cells to yield a diagnosis, and a bone marrow core biopsy is necessary. Similarly, focal lesions or cancer metastases are best evaluated by core samples, which should incorporate areas that are shown as lytic on radiography in addition to apparently unaffected bone marrow. Furthermore, bone marrow disorders such as myelofibrosis or osteosclerosis frequently preclude successful aspiration, and the diagnosis depends on examination of a tissue core. On the other hand, investigation of blood samples with abnormal or excessive numbers of cells or the search for an infectious organism can often be performed satisfactorily by cytological examination alone. Finally, inability to aspirate bone marrow may indicate improper needle placement or a structural abnormality, and necessitates acquisition of a core sample.

Biopsy needles

Figure 2.2 shows the types of needles commonly used for collecting biopsy specimens. The large combination needles may be used for aspirates as well as biopsies. The smaller needles are less expensive, but can be used only for bone marrow aspirates. As solid cortical bone is penetrated for collecting a bone marrow sample, it is important to use appropriate and sharp needles. A 13 gauge 9 cm (3.5 inch) combined aspiration and biopsy needle or a 15 gauge 4.8 cm (1 $^7/_8$ inch) aspiration needle is adequate for most small animal patients, and the disposable types can be sterilized and reused.

Biopsy techniques

Active bone marrow is distributed equally throughout the body, and many sites are suitable for collecting samples (Gulati *et al.*, 1988). In elderly animals the marrow cavity of long bones is more likely to consist of fatty tissue, hence sampling flat bones such as the pelvis or sternum may provide a better yield. Aspirates from the costochondral junction may be useful for evaluation of organisms infecting marrow macrophages (e.g. *Leishmania* spp.); however, core samples cannot

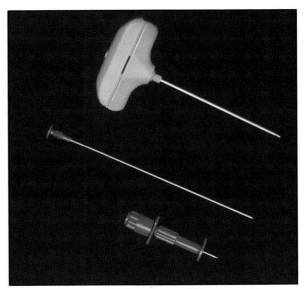

Figure 2.2: Disposable Illinois sternal/iliac bone marrow aspiration needle (bottom) with stylet (middle), and disposable bone marrow biopsy/aspiration needle (top).

be obtained from this site. For the purposes of this chapter, landmarks for aspirates from the pelvis, proximal humerus and femur will be described. Operator familiarity with one particular site is likely to be just as important as the actual origin of the sample.

The biopsy site is clipped and surgically prepared. If the patient is awake, a small area of skin and the periosteum at the chosen site are infiltrated with local anaesthetic containing adrenaline (epinephrine), with a 25 gauge needle. A small skin incision is made with the tip of a hypodermic needle or with a scalpel blade, and the bone marrow needle is inserted through the skin. The needle, with stylet firmly in place, is positioned against bone and then gradually advanced into the marrow cavity using a 'drilling' (forth and back) motion and steady pressure. For needle placement into the femur the animal should be placed in lateral recumbency, the greater trochanter palpated and the needle inserted medial to the trochanter and parallel to the shaft of the femur. Humeral samples are collected by palpating the greater tubercle and inserting the needle lateral to medial on the flat surface of the craniolateral aspect, distal to the greater tubercle. Aspiration from the iliac crest is accomplished by making the animal stand squarely or placing it in sternal recumbency (Figure 2.3), palpating the crest and introducing the needle parallel to the long axis of the wing of the ilium. The wing of the ilium itself can be aspirated in a similar fashion, keeping the needle angled slightly ventral. The ilium can be aspirated anywhere it is clearly palpable, but because the bone is flat the needle should be oriented nearly parallel to the bone surface. Needles and stylets that are seated properly in bone should feel as if they are 'cemented in place' and should be difficult to move.

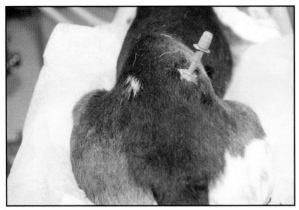

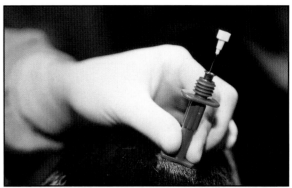

Figure 2.4: Needle cap removed, stylet withdrawn and syringe attached.

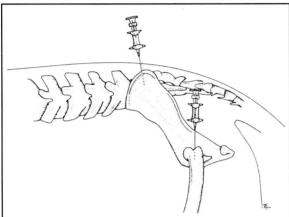

Figure 2.3: Aspiration needle firmly placed in the wing of the ilium of a dog in sternal recumbency and diagram showing placement of needle in detail. Diagram reproduced from Allen (1991) Small Animal Medicine *with the permission of Lippincott Williams & Wilkins.*

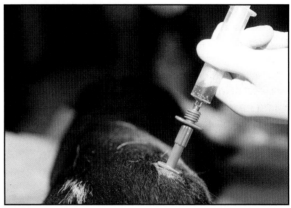

Figure 2.5: Several forceful aspirations with syringe yield thick sanguineous fluid.

Smear preparation from marrow aspirates

As bone marrow samples clot more quickly than peripheral blood, equipment for preparing smears should be ready before a sample is collected: six to eight glass slides on absorbent paper, sterile gloves (and a sterile field) and a jar with fixative.

Once the aspiration needle is firmly seated in the marrow cavity, the stylet is removed (Figure 2.4) and a 12 ml syringe is firmly attached to the needle hub. Bone marrow (which normally resembles thick blood) should appear in the hub of the syringe after several rapid and forceful aspirations (Figure 2.5). When about 0.5 ml of bone marrow has been collected, the syringe is detached and the stylet replaced in the aspiration needle which has remained in the bone marrow. One large drop of bone marrow is placed on each of about five glass slides (Figure 2.6). The slides are tilted sideways to 45 degrees to allow excess blood to run off on to the absorbent paper, leaving marrow particles, which are adherent to the glass (Figure 2.7). A clean glass slide is backed into the remaining bone marrow and the marrow is allowed to spread along the edge of the spreader glass slide, which is then swiftly pushed forward to produce a thin smear with a feathered edge (Figure 2.8). Two further smears are prepared by

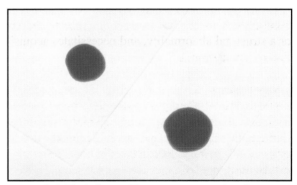

Figure 2.6: Thick drops of bone marrow are placed near frosted edge of glass slides.

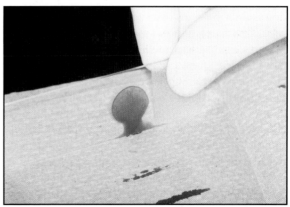

Figure 2.7: Slides are tilted to allow blood to run off on to absorbent tissue paper, leaving marrow particles attached to glass.

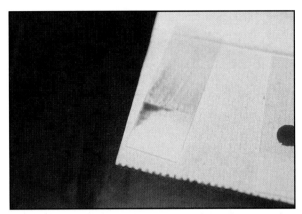

Figure 2.8: Another glass slide is backed into the remainder of the bone marrow drop, and the top glass slide is swiftly pushed forward to produce smears with feathered edges. Smears are air dried quickly.

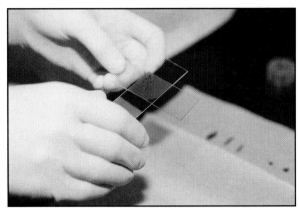

Figure 2.9: Another set of smears is prepared by gently laying a glass slide at right angles across the remainder of the bone marrow drop, pulling the slides apart and rapidly drying them in air.

removing excess blood in the same manner, laying a clean glass slide at right angles on top of the remaining drop of marrow (Figure 2.9) and gently pulling the slides apart. All smears should be quickly air dried. The goal of preparing bone marrow smears is to concentrate the marrow components and to remove much of the contaminating blood. Rapid drying of smears greatly preserves cytological features. Because the sample clots quickly, speed is essential, and preparation of all the smears should take less than one minute. Alternatively, the bone marrow needle and syringe may be rinsed with 10% ethylenediamine tetra-acetic acid (EDTA), or the whole aspirate may be mixed with EDTA in a 3 ml tube before preparing the smears.

A satisfactory aspirate is characterized by the presence of small granules, which are particularly visible after excess blood has been drained off the slide. These are the marrow particles. Fat globules are frequently noted and are a normal component of bone marrow aspirates. Inability to aspirate bone marrow is often due to bone or muscle fragments occluding the needle or the needle being lodged in cortical bone. Retracting the needle a small distance may permit sample collection. Alternatively, the needle should be removed, inspected for blockage and clots and reinserted, with stylet firmly in place, at a different site. Myelofibrosis or certain neoplasms involving the bone marrow may preclude successful aspiration, yielding hypocellular smears despite a hypercellular marrow.

Air-dried smears may be either submitted to a laboratory for staining and evaluation by a pathologist or stained directly. Romanowsky-type stains are most commonly employed, but 'quick' versions will yield adequate staining in many instances. Smears of bone marrow are generally of sufficient cellularity to require prolonged exposure to stain or two staining cycles in an automated stainer.

Obtaining a core biopsy

As marrow architecture is distorted in the immediate vicinity of an aspirate, it is important that either the biopsy needle is completely redirected after aspiration or that another site is sampled. The biopsy needle is inserted into bone in the same manner as for an aspirate. Again, the needle, with stylet in place, is seated firmly in cortical bone. The stylet is removed and the needle is advanced with a gentle 'drilling' motion and steady pressure. The sharp edge of the biopsy needle cuts a cylinder of tissue consisting of thin bony spicules with interspersed marrow. Once the needle has been advanced about 2.5 cm (a little less in cats and small dogs and more in large dogs), the needle is moved swiftly sideways a few times to break off the distal part of the core biopsy and is then retracted. Biopsy needles have tapered tips to retain the core inside the lumen of the needle as it is withdrawn. To retrieve the specimen with minimal distortion, the blunt ended (probe) part of the biopsy needle should be inserted in a retrograde fashion and the core should be carefully pushed from the tapered end backwards to the hub of the needle (Figure 2.10). If an aspirate was not obtained, the core may be gently rolled on a glass slide for a cytological imprint, and then placed in buffered formalin or freshly prepared B-5 fixative. Formalin provides adequate fixation, but B-5 fixative is preferable for optimal histological preparation (Weiss, 1987). An adequate bone marrow core should be at least 1.5 cm long, preferably 2.5 cm (Figure 2.11). If only a small sample is obtained, another core specimen should be collected. All slides and biopsy samples should be labelled and submitted.

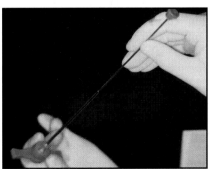

Figure 2.10: Bone marrow core in lumen of biopsy needle is pushed out backwards with the blunt stylet to minimize distortion of the sample.

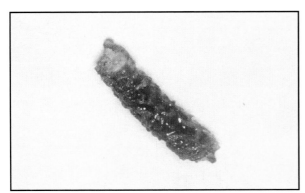

Figure 2.11: *Normal bone marrow core appears red and should measure at least 1.5 cm.*

In conclusion, a complete submission for examination of bone marrow consists of an exact history, three to six prepared smears, a bone marrow core and a concurrent blood sample for a CBC. The history should include details on drugs, physical and laboratory findings and previous or current illness.

INTERPRETATION OF BONE MARROW SAMPLES

Proficient interpretation of bone marrow samples requires a thorough knowledge of haematopoiesis, the stages of cell development, and different disease processes. The skill required for accurate interpretation of bone marrow is difficult to acquire with only occasional practice. Practitioners wanting to examine smears themselves are advised to seek confirmation from experienced haematopathologists until proficient. Detailed description of interpretative principles is beyond the scope of this text; however, basic concepts and deviations from normal findings are reviewed.

To evaluate bone marrow samples accurately, smears must be examined in a systematic and consistent manner. All normal marrow components are assessed sequentially, changes are described, unusual elements are noted and then a composite interpretation and correlation with the hematological and clinical picture are formulated. Figure 2.12 outlines the principles of interpretation.

Low magnification

An adequate marrow smear should have several particles and areas where the cells are sufficiently spread out to enable morphology to be evaluated. Marrow particles from young animals are very cellular, but with age there is progressive replacement of the active marrow with fat: particles containing 25–75% cells are considered normal for adult animals, whereas those containing 80–90% fat are typical for healthy elderly animals (Weiss, 1986). On smears prepared with Wright's stain megakaryocytes are readily identifiable as giant multinucleated cells, which have a dark basophilic cytoplasm if young. With progressive maturity

megakaryocytes have increased cytoplasmic volume, show more eosinophilic staining and have a granular cytoplasm. On average 5–10 megakaryocytes are associated with a particle, although occasionally megakaryocytes are present only at the feathered edge of a smear. Accurate estimates of megakaryocyte numbers are best derived from biopsy specimens, as the variable cellularity of aspirates may preclude objective evaluation. Megakaryocyte hyperplasia is commonly observed with immune-mediated thrombocytopenia (IMT) (Lewis and Meyers, 1996) whereas a lack of megakaryocytes has been reported in cases of IMT where the immune response is thought to be directed against both platelets and their precursors in the marrow (Williams and Maggio-Price, 1984). Iron stains dark brown to black with Wright's stain and should be evident on marrow smears from adult dogs, but not cats. Lack of stainable iron is a consistent finding in the marrow of animals with iron deficiency (Weeks *et al.*, 1987). Increased iron stores have been associated with anaemia of chronic disease. Finally, an area of the smear where the cells are spread apart, usually the 'tail' of a particle, should be selected for closer examination.

High magnification

Normal erythropoiesis and myelopoiesis are characterized by a predominance of the maturing stages of cell development. Granulocyte maturation proceeds

Low magnification
Assess adequacy of specimen
Estimate cellularity of marrow particles
Estimate megakaryocyte numbers and maturity
Assess iron stores
Identify areas for further examination
High magnification
Assess erythroid and myeloid numbers, morphology and synchronicity of maturation
Determine myeloid to erythroid ratio
Identify other cell types: plasma cells, lymphocytes, histiocytes
Identify abnormal cells: mast cells, neoplastic cells
Identify infectious agents: fungal elements, *Ehrlichia* spp.
Assess the presence of myelofibrosis, necrosis and inflammation
Interpretation
Correlate bone marrow with results from the complete blood count, and with other physical and laboratory findings

Figure 2.12: *Evaluation of bone marrow smears.*

from undifferentiated round myeloblasts with nucleoli to promyelocytes containing azurophilic granules to myelocytes with gradually decreasing nuclear size and increasing chromatin condensation. Metamyelocytes have indented nuclei that progress to become band shaped and eventually segmented as in mature neutrophils (Figure 2.13). The three stages of metamyelocytes and band and segmented neutrophils normally comprise 70–80% of all cells in the myeloid series and are the maturing stages of myelopoiesis. Myeloblasts, promyelocytes and myelocytes are able to undergo mitosis and therefore constitute the proliferating component. Development from rubriblast to metarubricyte is distinguished by a progressive decrease in cell size, loss of cytoplasmic basophilia, and increased haemoglobin synthesis, imparting the characteristic pink colour of mature red cells (Figure 2.14). The nucleus gradually condenses and is extruded from metarubricytes before the polychromatophilic erythrocyte stage and exit from the marrow. Where rubricytes and metarubricytes comprise about 90% of all erythroid cells, with the later stages predominating, this indicates synchronicity of maturation. The ratio of myeloid to nucleated erythroid cells (M/E ratio) ranges from 3:1 to 5:1 in healthy dogs and cats.

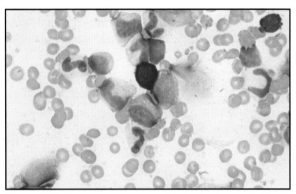

Figure 2.13: Bone marrow smear with developing myeloid cells surrounding a rubriblast. Round nuclei, a prominent nucleolus, and lack of granules characterize myeloblasts. Promyelocytes have azurophilic granules whereas myelocyte granules are poorly visible. Metamyelocytes have indented nuclei that progress to become band shaped and eventually segmented.

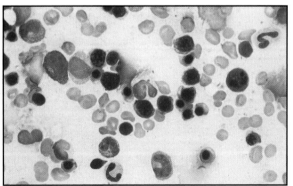

Figure 2.14: Bone marrow smear with erythroid maturation stages. Increasing nuclear condensation and acquisition of an orange cytoplasmic colour concurrent with haemoglobin synthesis indicates progressive maturity in rubricytes.

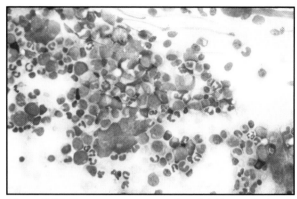

Figure 2.15: Bone marrow smear of myeloid hyperplasia with a predominance of the maturing stages and an increased myeloid to erythroid ratio as seen in chronic suppurative dermatitis. Scattered plasma cells and rubricytes are observed.

An appropriate marrow response to peripheral tissue demand for increased neutrophils or erythrocytes is characterized by an overall increase in the proportion of the particular cell line, concurrent with retained orderly maturation and a predominance of maturing stages (hyperplasia). Therefore, the marrow of a dog with a responsive anaemia has a decreased M/E ratio and an absolute increase in erythroid cells, but a predominance of late stage rubricytes. A chronic inflammatory disease with suppuration, such as pyoderma, increases the M/E ratio by stimulating increased neutrophil production, albeit that most of the granulocytes will be metamyelocytes and band and segmented neutrophils (Figure 2.15). However, early recovery from a nonspecific cytotoxic insult to the bone marrow (canine or feline parvoviral infection, chemotherapy or radiation) consists of increased proportions of immature forms that are easily mistaken for a neoplastic process. Myeloid cells will be most affected, as the longer life span of red cells entails a slower rate of production. In these cases, resampling bone marrow after one week should indicate a progressive return to orderly maturation, with accumulation of late erythroid and myeloid cells.

Pure red cell aplasia is characterized by profound anaemia, near complete lack of erythroid cells in the bone marrow, normal myelopoiesis and thrombopoiesis and a profoundly increased M/E ratio. Aplastic anaemia, however, manifests as a reduction in all cellular elements, and commonly only reticular cells and plasma cells are observed in the bone marrow (Figure 2.16). In myelofibrosis, proliferation of the stromal components in the bone marrow, with excessive production of extracellular matrix, leads to gradual destruction of the normal haematopoietic space. Myelofibrosis may accompany or precede neoplastic diseases of the bone marrow (Blue, 1988) or may occur subsequent to chronically stimulated erythropoiesis in some cases of severe haemolytic anaemia (Reagan, 1993). Aspirating marrow in these instances is difficult or impossible, and the diagnosis is based on histopathological findings.

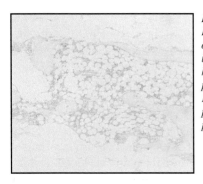

Figure 2.16:
Histological section
of aplastic anaemia
in a cat, with lack of
haematopoietic
precursor cells.
Reticular and
plasma cells are
present.

Neoplasms of haematopoietic cells

Neoplasms of the haematopoietic cells are broadly divided into acute and chronic leukaemias (Jain *et al.*, 1991). Generally, acute leukaemias manifest with profound cytopenias in the peripheral blood, and bone marrow aspirates have a predominance of immature (blast) cells (Figure 2.17) that are difficult to classify by morphological criteria. Remnants of normal haematopoiesis may be present, and the M/E ratio may be normal, but the synchronicity of maturation of the neoplastic cell line will be severely disturbed. Immunophenotypically, most canine acute leukaemias seem to be of granulocytic origin (Figure 2.18), followed by lymphocytic and undifferentiated leukaemias (Vernau and Moore, 1999). In most cases special cytochemical or immunochemical stains or electron microscopy are required to identify the origin of the neoplasm. The prognosis for acute leukaemias in small animals is grave.

In contrast, chronic leukaemias frequently resemble an overaccumulation of morphologically benign and relatively mature cells. Changes on the haemogram consist of a moderate to noticeable increase in cells of the neoplastic lineage, and possibly mild anaemia, neutropenia or thrombocytopenia. A bone marrow aspirate may be difficult to obtain in cases where the core biopsy nevertheless shows profound hypercellularity. Morphologically, maturation of the affected cell line may be synchronous; however, the M/E ratio will be noticeably increased owing to an absolute increase in cells of the neoplastic lineage. Granulocytic and lymphocytic leukaemias (Figure 2.19) with gradual progression have been described in small animals. Most chronic lymphocytic leukaemias in dogs morphologically are large granular lymphocytes (LGL) and express a T-cell receptor (Vernau and Moore, 1999). It has been suggested that a blast cell count of more than 30% in the blood or bone marrow indicates an acute leukaemia, whereas a count of less than 30% in the bone marrow suggests chronic leukaemia, myelodysplastic syndrome or a leukaemoid reaction (Jain *et al.*, 1991). Compared with humans, however, dogs and cats generally present at a later stage of the disease process, and distinction of acute from chronic leukaemia may be difficult. Survival times exceeding four years have been reported in dogs with chronic lymphocytic leukaemia treated with chemotherapy (Leifer and Matus, 1986; Vernau and Moore, 1999).

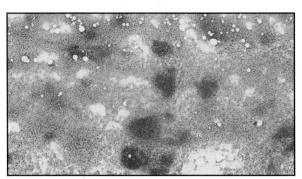

Figure 2.17: Bone marrow smear with profound hypercellularity consisting of immature blast cells. The dog had acute leukaemia and manifested with pancytopenia in the haemogram.

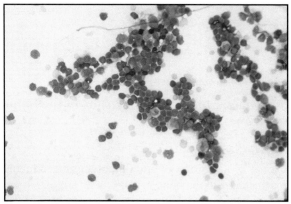

Figure 2.19: Bone marrow smear with predominant small lymphocytes, similar in size to red cells. There is a relative paucity of myeloid and erythroid precursors. The dog had chronic lymphocytic leukaemia and only mild anaemia.

Erythremic myelosis and polycythaemia

Erythremic myelosis is a neoplastic proliferation of rubricytes observed in cats infected with feline leukaemia virus (FeLV) presenting with a rubricytosis consisting of immature and mature rubricytes and with variable leucopenia and thrombocytopenia. Bone marrow smears indicate profoundly disturbed erythroid maturation, granulocytopenia and severely decreased M/E ratios. Chronic tissue hypoxia and ectopic production of erythropoietin result in physiological

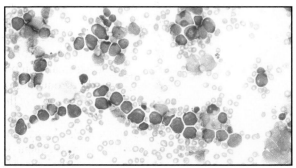

Figure 2.18: Higher magnification of Figure 2.17. Most of the cells are blasts with a small perinuclear clearing (Golgi zone). Two cells are in mitosis and normal haematopoietic elements are severely reduced.

and paraneoplastic polycythaemia, respectively. The peripheral blood picture is characterized by persistently increased red cell counts and concomitant erythroid hyperplasia in the bone marrow. Primary polycythaemia vera is, however, a neoplastic proliferation of either erythrocytes or all mature bone marrow elements, independent of erythropoietin stimulation (Khanna and Bienzle, 1994). In the latter case, the bone marrow is profoundly hypercellular owing to a relatively synchronous increase in all cell lineages (Figure 2.20), which is reflected by an increased haematocrit and granulocytosis and thrombocytosis in the blood. The myelodysplastic syndrome encompasses a variety of abnormal haematopoietic processes: peripheral blood cytopenia with abnormal cell maturation, myelofibrosis and a blast cell count of less than 30% in the bone marrow (Jain *et al.*, 1991). The syndrome occurs predominantly in FeLV-infected cats, and frequently precedes acute leukaemia (Blue, 1988).

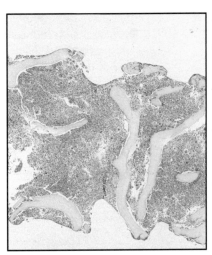

Figure 2.20: Histological section of hypercellular bone marrow from an 11-year-old cat with polycythaemia vera. All haemopoietic elements are present, and the myeloid to erythroid ratio was 3:1.

Non-haematopoietic neoplasms in the bone marrow

Multiple myeloma

Clonal proliferation of immunoglobulin-producing plasma cells in the bone marrow, with a monoclonal gammopathy and lytic bone lesions, characterize most forms of multiple myeloma (Matus *et al.*, 1986). The diagnosis of the neoplasm is based on identifying clusters of monomorphic plasma cells in aspirates or core biopsies from lytic bone lesions, the presence of monoclonal immunoglobulin in serum, or monoclonal light chains in urine. Haematologically normal animals may have 5% to 10% plasma cells in the marrow, and increased proportions of plasma cells have been observed in myelofibrosis, anaemia of renal failure, and aplastic anaemia (Weiss, 1986). In cases of anaemia of renal failure and aplastic anaemia, however, the plasma cells are morphologically mature and dispersed throughout the marrow, and lytic lesions are not observed.

Lymphoma

Lymphoma in the dog has been reported to involve the bone marrow in about 50% of cases, regardless of the histological type (Raskin and Krehbiel, 1988). Therefore, staging of dogs with lymphoma includes assessment of bone marrow involvement and should ideally be based on histological evaluation of core biopsies in order to detect focal involvement and architectural changes. Concurrent evaluation of the primary tumour helps to identify neoplastic lymphocytes as a small number of benign lymphocytes are common in normal haematopoietic tissue. Low-grade diffuse involvement of the marrow in lymphoma is difficult to detect, and the clinician ought to be aware that morphological evaluation of one marrow biopsy is not a sensitive indicator of neoplastic involvement.

Mast cell tumours

Mast cell tumours in the dog may metastasize via the haemolymphatic system to the bone marrow (Rogers, 1996). Buffy coat smears and bone marrow aspirates are commonly examined to detect systemic malignant mastocytosis. Morphologically indistinguishable benign mastocytosis may, however, occur in a variety of non-neoplastic conditions (Bookbinder *et al.*, 1992; Walker *et al*, 1997). Hence, a diagnosis of metastatic mast cell tumour must be based on the detection of clusters of mast cells in bone marrow biopsies or aspirates in the absence of inflammatory diseases such as dermatitis or enteritis, which have been associated with benign mastocytosis (Figures 2.21 and 2.22).

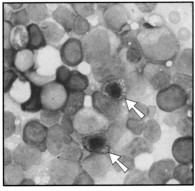

Figure 2.21: Bone marrow smear showing two mast cells (arrowed) among erythroid and myeloid cells. This sample originated from a dog with a cutaneous mast cell tumour.

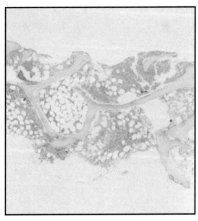

Figure 2.22: Histological section from the case described in Figure 2.21 showing foci with increased cellular density consisting of mast cells. The dog had mast cell tumours in the bone marrow. The extent of the metastatic process was not apparent on aspirates.

Histiocytosis

The bone marrow commonly is involved in proliferative diseases of histiocytic cells. Clusters of large vacuolated, frequently multinucleated, cells with phagocytosed red cells or haemosiderin in the bone marrow and other tissues are characteristic of malignant histiocytosis. This disease must be distinguished from the haemophagocytic syndrome, which is a rare proliferation of morphologically normal histiocytes observed in association with systemic infectious diseases (Walton *et al.*, 1996). Whereas malignant histiocytosis has a rapidly progressive disease course, the haemophagocytic syndrome may spontaneously resolve. Histiocytic hyperplasia is observed in mycotic, protozoal or mycobacterial infections that induce granulomatous inflammation, and in storage diseases resulting in cytoplasmic accumulation of non-degradable metabolic products.

Metastatic carcinomas

Lastly, neoplasms of epithelial origin may metastasize to the bone marrow, although this seems to be an infrequent or a clinically inapparent occurrence in animals. Clusters of adherent non-haematopoietic cells in smears or histological sections of marrow suggest metastatic carcinoma. The prognostic significance of metastatic carcinomas is undetermined for most small animal neoplasms.

Involvement of the bone marrow in metastatic neoplasia affects prognosis and treatment. Most attempts to diagnose metastasis rely solely on morphological identification of neoplastic cells and thus are limited by the size of the sample, the relative presence of the neoplastic cell population and the expertise of the pathologist. Newer diagnostic methods that are currently not routinely available such as immunostaining and assessment of immune receptor clonality or chromosomal abnormalities, will greatly aid in deriving an accurate diagnosis.

SUMMARY

Examination of the bone marrow is an essential tool in the diagnosis of most haematological diseases, and aids in the assessment of many other systemic and neoplastic conditions. Providing adequate specimens is paramount for accurate interpretation, and pathological findings must be interpreted in conjunction with physical and laboratory data, and with the peripheral blood picture. Communication between the clinician and the pathologist is an invaluable component in deriving a diagnosis from a bone marrow sample.

REFERENCES AND FURTHER READING

Blue JT (1988) Myelofibrosis in cats with myelodysplastic syndrome and acute myelogenous leukemia. *Veterinary Pathology* **25**, 154–160

Bookbinder PF, Butt MT and Harvey HJ (1992) Determination of the number of mast cells in lymph node, bone marrow, and buffy coat cytological specimens from dogs. *Journal of the American Veterinary Medical Association* **200**, 1648–1650

Duncan JR, Prasse KW and Mahaffey EA (1994) Hematopoietic neoplasms. In: *Veterinary Laboratory Medicine, 3rd edn*, ed. JR Duncan, KW Prasse and EA Mahaffey, pp 63–73. Iowa State University Press, Ames

Grindem CB (1989) Bone marrow biopsy and evaluation. *Veterinary Clinics of North America* **19**, 669–696

Gulati GL, Ashton JK and Hyun BH (1988) Structure and function of the bone marrow and hematopoiesis. *Hematology/Oncology Clinics of North America* **2**, 495–511

Jacobs RM and Valli VEO (1988) Bone marrow biopsies: principles and perspectives of interpretation. *Seminars in Veterinary Medicine and Surgery* **3**, 176–182

Jain NC, Blue JT, Grindem CB, Harvey JW, Kociba GJ, Krehbiel JD, Latimer KS, Raskin RE, Thrall MA and Zinkl JG (1991) Proposed criteria for classification of acute myeloid leukemia in dogs and cats. *Veterinary Clinical Pathology* **20**, 63–82

Khanna C and Bienzle D (1994) Polycythemia vera in a cat: bone marrow culture in erythropoietin-deficient medium. *Journal of the American Animal Hospital Association* **30**, 45–49

Leifer CE and Matus RE (1986) Chronic lymphocytic leukemia in the dog: 22 cases (1974–1984). *Journal of the American Veterinary Medical Association* **189**, 214–217

Lewis DC and Meyers KM (1996) Canine idiopathic thrombocytopenia purpura. *Journal of Veterinary Internal Medicine* **10**, 207–218

Matus RE, Leiger CE, MacEwen EG and Hurvitz AI (1986) Prognostic factors for multiple myeloma in the dog. *Journal of the American Veterinary Medical Association* **188**, 1288–1292

Raskin RE and Krehbiel JD (1988) Histopathology of canine bone marrow in malignant lymphoproliferative disorders. *Veterinary Pathology* **25**, 83–88

Reagan WJ (1993) A review of myelofibrosis in dogs. *Toxicological Pathology* **21**, 164–169

Rogers KS (1996) Mast cell tumors. *Veterinary Clinics of North America* **26**, 87–102

Vernau W and Moore PF (1999) An immunophenotypic study of canine leukemias and preliminary assessment of clonality by polymerase chain reaction. *Veterinary Immunology and Immunopathology* **69**, 145–164

Walker D, Cowell RL, Clinkenbeard KD, Feder B and Meinkoth JH (1997) Bone marrow mast cell hyperplasia in dogs with aplastic anemia. *Veterinary Clinical Pathology* **26**, 106–111

Walton RM, Modiano J, Wheeler S and Thrall MA (1996) Bone marrow cytological findings in 4 dogs and a cat with hemophagocytic syndrome. *Journal of Veterinary Internal Medicine* **10**, 7–13

Weeks BR, Smith JE and Northrop JK (1987) Relationship of serum ferritin and iron concentration and serum total iron-binding capacity to nonheme iron stores in dogs. *American Journal of Veterinary Research* **50**, 198–200

Weiss DJ (1986) Histopathology of canine non-neoplastic bone marrow. *Veterinary Clinical Pathology* **15**, 7–11

Weiss DJ (1987) A review of the techniques for preparation of histopathologic sections of bone marrow. *Veterinary Clinical Pathology* **16**, 90–94

Williams DA and Maggio-Price L (1984) Canine idiopathic thrombocytopenic purpura: clinical observations and long-term follow-up in 54 cases. *Journal of the American Veterinary Medical Association* **185**, 660–663

Anaemia

Jenny Mills

INTRODUCTION

Anaemia is a common clinical and laboratory test finding, which in itself does not constitute a diagnosis. The ultimate aim for the veterinary practitioner is to determine the pathogenesis of the anaemia in order to deliver the most appropriate therapy for the patient and to instigate steps that may prevent the condition occurring again.

This chapter looks at ways of unravelling the enigma of anaemia in dogs and cats. Steps are described to diagnose the pathogenesis of anaemia in a patient. The astute diagnostician uses various clinical and laboratory clues from the haematological report and the blood film to arrive at a useful pathological diagnosis of the underlying problem. If the initial blood test is not fully revealing, the clinician may need to undertake further tests to achieve a more definitive diagnosis. This chapter describes the process of investigation of anaemia.

RED CELL PRODUCTION

The process of erythropoiesis involves the three basic components of stem cells, cytokines and an appropriate microenvironment. The latter includes factors such as supply of oxygen, nutrients, iron and amino acids (Figure 3.1). In adult mammals, erythropoiesis proceeds within the bone marrow under the influence of specific cytokines, which act directly on surface receptors of the erythroid stem cells: BFU-E (burst-forming unit – erythroid) and CFU-E (colony-forming unit – erythroid). These cytokines include interleukin 3, 'burst-forming activity' and erythropoietin. The effect of erythropoietin is to increase the number of committed erythroid stem cells, to enhance the survival of developing erythroid cells, to promote the release of maturing red cells and to ultimately increase the number of red cells produced by the bone marrow. The effect of erythropoietin on stem cells is modulated and enhanced by other hormones such as androgens, thyroxine, growth hormone, corticosteroids and prostaglandins E_1 and E_2.

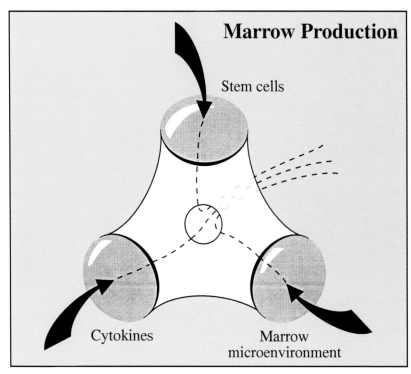

Marrow Production

Stem cells

Cytokines

Marrow microenvironment

Figure 3.1: *Three essential components required for haematopoiesis are stem cells, cytokines and an appropriate marrow microenvironment. The last may consist of an adequate supply of oxygen and nutrients such as iron, amino acids, glycine and vitamins B12, B6 and folate. The nutrients required for red cell production may be considered in two categories; those needed for nucleotide synthesis and those for haemoglobin synthesis. The end product, mature red cells, are then released into the peripheral blood circulation by migration through vascular sinusoids.*

Other factors act to inhibit erythropoiesis by down-regulating the expression of receptors on the surface of the erythroid stem cells. Suppressive factors include interleukin 1 and tumour necrosis factor (TNF), both of which are released from macrophages during inflammation. Oestrogen and prostaglandin $F_{2\alpha}$ also suppress erythropoiesis. In cats, the p15E component of the feline leukaemia virus also acts to inhibit erythropoiesis.

DEFINITION OF ANAEMIA

Anaemia is defined as a situation in which the total erythron mass in peripheral blood is depleted below reference values for animals of the same species that are of similar age. The three basic variables of the erythron that determine whether an animal is anaemic are haemoglobin, packed cell volume (PCV) or haematocrit and red blood cell (RBC) count.

In interpreting any laboratory values, an awareness of factors that influence the results is needed. Of the variables above, RBC count is likely to be the least accurate because of the method of measurement. The concentration of haemoglobin will be falsely high in lipaemic samples. Haemoglobin concentration, PCV and RBC count will be affected by the total plasma volume of the animal. Dehydrated animals will have a contracted plasma volume and therefore may show haemoconcentration and high erythron values. If the resting erythron values were originally low, a dehydrated animal may have a masked anaemia, with the contracted plasma volume masking the measurement of low haemoglobin concentration, PCV or RBC count to the extent that these variables may fall within reference range.

Anaemia may be relative or absolute. In relative anaemia, there is a normal total red cell mass but an expanded plasma volume. Examples of relative anaemia are haemodilution after administration of intravenous fluids and sequestration of red cells due to splenomegaly. In absolute anaemia the total red cell mass is decreased while the plasma volume is normal. The remainder of this chapter deals only with absolute anaemia.

VARIABLES THAT CHARACTERIZE ANAEMIA

Once the presence of anaemia is established from the primary haematological examination, the first step in defining the pathophysiology of the problem involves assessing:

- The regenerative response; reticulocyte count
- Red cell indices; mean corpuscular volume (MCV) and mean corpuscular haemoglobin concentration (MCHC)
- Red cell morphology on a blood smear.

The regenerative response

The physiological limit on the extent of the bone marrow regenerative response to an anaemia is an eightfold or even tenfold increase in red cell production. The greatest regenerative responses are seen with haemolytic anaemia (six- to eightfold increase), and moderate regenerative responses are usually seen with haemorrhagic anaemia (two- to fourfold increase). Exceptions do, however, occur. Anaemias seen within 3 to 4 days after blood loss or haemolysis will show no signs of regeneration in peripheral blood, because of the 4-day production time for red cells. Such conditions are termed preregenerative. An absence of reticulocytes in an ongoing anaemia indicates a defect in production and warrants further investigation. The degree of polychromasia and the reticulocyte count are used to assess the extent of the regenerative response of the erythron, subjectively and objectively, respectively. The reticulocyte count is determined by using a supravital stain and by quantifying those red cells that contain blue-staining RNA in a reticular network. This is usually done manually, but some haematological instruments have the capacity to quantify these cells directly. The percentage reticulocyte count is then compared to, and adjusted for, the degree of anaemia, and conclusions are drawn on the adequacy of the bone marrow response to the anaemia.

The degree of response is represented by the corrected reticulocyte count. The most reliable method of expressing this count is to calculate the absolute reticulocyte count by multiplying the raw reticulocyte percentage by the total RBC count. This calculation expresses the response per unit volume of whole blood and is therefore more appropriate than a percentage value. The normal absolute reticulocyte count for a dog is about $60 \times 10^9/l$. Increases to $360 \times 10^9/l$ will therefore represent a sixfold increase in erythroid production in the bone marrow.

Cats differ from dogs in that they may have punctate reticulocytes, as well as normal aggregate or reticular forms. The punctate forms represent aged reticulocytes, but only the aggregate forms should be counted when assessing the regenerative response.

Red cell indices

Red cell indices define the quality of the red cells produced by describing the average red cell size (MCV) and average red cell haemoglobin content (MCHC). In a very regenerative response, a macrocytic (high MCV) hypochromic (low MCHC) population of red cells is expected. Microcytic (low MCV) hypochromic (low MCHC) populations, however, are likely to occur in conditions of defective haemoglobin synthesis such as iron deficiency.

Macrocytosis may also be seen in myelodysplasia in cats, in association with the administration of antiepileptic drugs, and rarely in some Poodles (toy and miniature breeds) as a dyscrasia resembling vitamin B12 and folate deficiency in humans. The condition in Poodles does not require treatment. Microcytosis may be seen normally in the Japanese Akita and Shiba Inu breeds of dog and in some dogs with portosystemic shunts.

Red cell morphology

Red cell morphology is evaluated by examination of a stained blood smear. Any changes in shape from the classic biconcave disc are identified and semiquantified and may lead to a specific diagnosis or interpretation (Figure 3.2). Compared with red cells from a dog those from a cat are smaller, not as biconcave and show less central pallor on smears.

Feature	Interpretation
Large numbers of spherocytes	Immune-mediated haemolysis
Schistocytes (fragmented cells)	Intravascular red cell injury
Keratocytes (horn shapes)	Intravascular red cell injury
Heinz bodies	Heinz body haemolysis, oxidant injury
Dacryocytes (tear-drop shape)	Iron deficiency, myelofibrosis
Echinocytes (burr cell)	Renal azotaemia, chemotherapy
Acanthocytes (spur cells)	Splenic neoplasia, liver disease, etc

Figure 3.2: Examples of changes in red cell morphology from the classic biconcave disc and their interpretation.

ERYTHRON DISORDERS WITHOUT ANAEMIA

Anaemia occurs when the rate of red cell loss or destruction exceeds the rate of red cell production (Figure 3.3).

Changes in red cell production and/or loss may occur without significant reductions in PCV, haemoglobin concentration or RBC count. Compensated anaemia may be seen in some haemolytic states where the rate of production matches the rate of red cell destruction. In these cases, there are obvious signs of erythroid regeneration in the peripheral blood, with high levels of reticulocytes and possibly some morphological change in the red cells. Examples of this have been reported with immune-mediated haemolysis (Mills, 1997) and in an hereditary defect in the red cells of a dog (Mills and Marsden, 1999).

Defects in bone marrow production and disorders affecting the haemoglobinization process, which lead to ineffective erythropoiesis, may temporarily be asso-

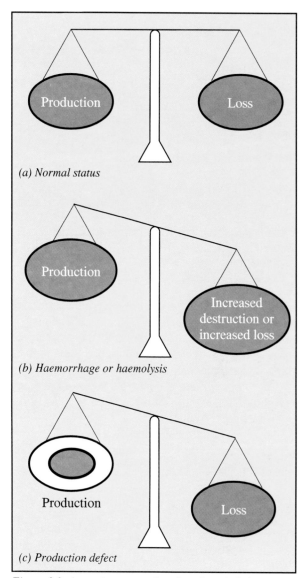

(a) Normal status

(b) Haemorrhage or haemolysis

(c) Production defect

Figure 3.3: Anaemia occurs when there is an imbalance between production and loss of red cells. (a) Normal status. (b) With haemolysis or haemorrhage, the rate of loss or lysis usually exceeds the rate of increase in production for a time, before equilibrium is restored. (c) With production deficits, such as aplastic anaemia, the rate of loss is normal but exceeds the rate of production.

ciated with normal erythron values, before anaemia develops. This condition will be described later. Examples in this category are lead poisoning, folic acid and vitamin B12 deficiencies and iron deficiency.

The spleen plays a role in the red cell life cycle, in that in most domestic animal species it contains narrow vascular sinusoids through which the red cells traverse (Figure 3.4). Senescent red cells lose their deformability and consequently are phagocytosed by macrophages in the spleen. In this way the spleen acts as the 'rubbish sorter' of blood, removing other particles such as Howell–Jolly bodies or nuclei of immature red cells. Consequently, enlargement of the spleen for any reason can trap or sequester more red cells, contributing to an apparent anaemia due mainly to redistribution

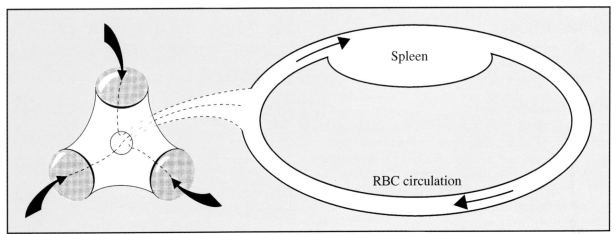

Figure 3.4: *Following production, the red cells circulate in peripheral blood until they are destroyed by macrophages in the spleen, after their nominal lifespan (about 70 days in the cat and 120 days in the dog). Any enlargement of the spleen may cause sequestration of blood or increased destruction of red cells.*

of the cells in this organ. However, the effect of adrenalin release in causing splenic enlargement is minor in the dog and cat compared with that in the horse, where up to 30% of the blood volume may be trapped in an enlarged spleen. However, the spleen of cats does not contain a sinusoidal structure, thereby permitting longer survival of particles such as Heinz bodies within red cells.

If the rate of red cell production exceeds the rate of loss, a state of erythrocytosis (secondary polycythaemia) with high PCV, haemoglobin concentration or RBC count may eventually develop. Increased erythroid production – and consequently reticulocytosis – may occur in response to the high erythropoietin concentrations that follow tissue anoxia. Conditions associated with erythrocytosis include obstructive pulmonary disease, cardiovascular disorders (ventricular septal defects, patent ductus arteriosus), high altitude states or renal hypoxia or renal abnormalities (e.g. embryonal nephroma, renal cysts). Autonomous production of mature red cells, irrespective of erythropoietin concentrations, represents a neoplastic state of haematopoiesis known as polycythaemia vera (primary polycythaemia).

CLASSIFICATION OF ANAEMIA

The classification of anaemia according to basic pathophysiological mechanisms provides a useful approach to the diagnosis of the underlying problem.

Anaemias of bone marrow dysfunction involve reduced red cell production, defects in nucleotide synthesis, defects in haemoglobin synthesis and myelodysplastic syndromes. Anaemias of increased red cell destruction involve haemolysis of normal red cells or haemolysis due to either genetic defects of red cells or acquired defects of red cells. Anaemias of increased red cell loss involve internal or external haemorrhage.

Figure 3.5 shows an outline of causes of anaemia based on diagnostic decisions or observations.

Anaemias of bone marrow dysfunction
The basic requirements for production of red cells are stem cells, cytokines and an appropriate marrow environment, which includes blood supply, oxygen and nutrients. When any of these components are lacking, erythropoiesis will be affected.

Reduced red cell production
Anaemias in this category will be non-regenerative, normocytic (normal MCV) and normochromic (normal MCHC). A concurrent leucopenia and thrombocytopenia should alert the clinician to the possibility of aplastic anaemia or myelophthisis. In these two conditions, multipotential stem cells may be injured, suppressed (aplasia; no growth) or displaced (myelophthisis; marrow wasting). Some of these effects may be mediated by cytokines or regulatory lymphocytes, which may alter the marrow microenvironment. These anaemias can be severe and difficult to treat, but in some instances the administration of cytokines has been found to be helpful in promoting cell development and maturation. Examples of causes of marrow aplasia include the injurious effects of irradiation, toxic plants (bracken fern in cattle), viruses (feline leukaemia virus; FeLV), hormones (oestrogen, particularly in dogs), drugs (e.g. phenylbutazone, chloramphenicol, sulpha drugs), chemicals that accumulate in fat (e.g. DDT, trichlorethylene, cyclic hydrocarbons) and the infectious agent *Ehrlichia canis.*

Myelophthisis represents a space-occupying lesion in bone marrow that inhibits or displaces normal haematopoietic cells. Examples are marrow neoplasms, leukaemias, metastatic neoplasms (carcinomas, melanomas), myelofibrosis and granulomatous inflammatory disease of marrow, such as systemic fungal infections, histoplasmosis and miliary tuberculosis.

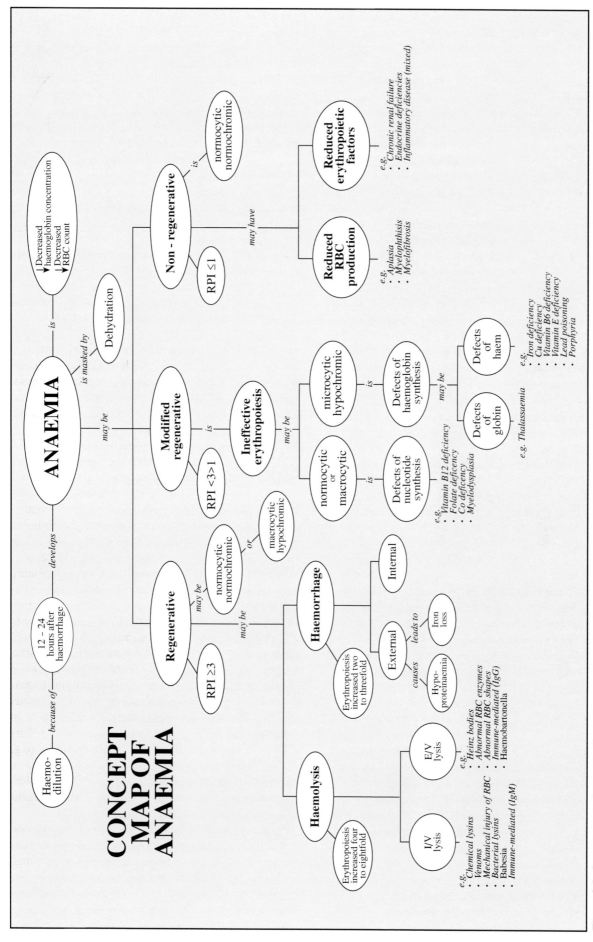

Figure 3.5: *Concept map of anaemia illustrating a pathway for diagnosing anaemia. Linking words are italicized. RBC, red blood cell; RPI, reticulocyte production index; Cu, copper; Co, cobalt; I/V, intravascular; E/V, extravascular.*

The development of myelofibrosis may be idiopathic or occur after prolonged marrow stimulation or as a terminal event in myelproliferative disease. Myelofibrosis is considered to be associated with megakaryocyte-derived growth factors, and marrow mastocytosis may be seen in these patients.

Pure red cell aplasia refers to reductions in committed (unipotential) erythroid stem cells only. Leucocytes and platelets are unaffected. This condition may be caused by FeLV, by direct suppression of BFU-E stem cells or may be immune-mediated in dogs, in which antibody may be specifically directed at epitopes on the immature erythroid cells. In the last case, some spherocytes may be seen in peripheral blood, and the Coombs' test may give a positive result.

Reductions in the concentrations of erythropoietin or cytokines affecting erythropoiesis have a role in the production of non-regenerative anaemias associated with chronic renal failure or endocrine dysfunction (e.g. hypothyroidism, hyperoestrogenism, hypoadrenocorticism or pituitary hypofunction). The dog is particularly prone to suppression of haematopoiesis by oestrogen, from either hyperoestrogenism in sertoli cell tumours or after excessive stilboestrol administration. The suppression is mediated by an inhibitor produced by the thymus in response to oestrogen and which suppresses haematopoiesis at the stem cell level (Brockus, 1998).

The anaemia of chronic renal failure is usually mild to moderate and non-regenerative. It is primarily due to the inabiljy of erythropoietin to be produced from the kidneys. Other factors that contribute to the anaemia of chronic renal failure include:

- Reduced half-life of red cells due to uraemic toxins
- Haemorrhagic loss from gastrointestinal ulcers
- Increased bleeding tendency due to reduced platelet function
- Suppression of erythropoiesis by high concentrations of parathyroid hormone
- Reduced nutrient intake due to inappetance
- Injury of red cells due to glomerular pathology and renal fibrosis.

Echinocytes and some schistocytes or keratocytes can be seen in the anaemia of renal failure.

The anaemia of inflammatory disease – the commonest form of anaemia in domestic animals – is associated with both acute and chronic inflammation. The pathogenesis involves a complex of changes triggered by the cytokines tumour necrosis factor (TNF) and interleukin-1 (IL-1) released from activated macrophages. These proinflammatory cytokines suppress erythropoiesis by downregulating the surface erythropoietin receptors of committed erythroid stem cells. At the same time, other cytokines stimulate granulocyte production to produce leucocytes required to combat the infection. Under the influence of IL-1, storage iron is converted from ferritin to the less available form of haemosiderin; iron is tightly bound to haptoglobin and lactoferrin in leucocytes at the site of infection, becoming unavailable for both red cell production and bacterial use. The concentration of circulating serum iron is consequently reduced but so is its transport protein, transferrin. In addition, red cells from affected patients bind increased surface immunoglobulin and consequently have a shortened life span, being phagocytosed more readily than normal.

Other conditions causing non-regenerative anaemia include dietary protein deficiency or suppression of erythropoiesis by TNF in some parasitic infections. An example of the latter occurs in trypanosomiasis (*Trypanosoma congolense*) where expression of erythropoietin receptors is reduced (Suliman et al., 1999).

Chronic liver disease may also be associated with anaemia for a variety of reasons but usually there is a degree of red cell regeneration, possibly associated with some haemorrhagic loss and red cell injury. In about 60% of dogs with portosystemic shunts, microcytosis may be evident. Disturbances to iron metabolism, copper storage/toxicity and chronic inflammation are likely to contribute to the pathogenesis of the anaemia in chronic liver disorders. Poikilocytosis (abnormal erythrocyte shape) is expected in hepatic disease, with acanthocytosis and ovalocytes (elliptical erythrocytes) seen in many cats with hepatic lipidosis.

Defects in nucleotide synthesis

In conditions of this category, stem cells and cytokines are adequate, but the microenvironment is deficient, lacking a supply of nutrients essential for nucleotide synthesis. Erythropoietin concentrations are increased and cell production proceeds abnormally. Defects in DNA or RNA synthesis cause delays in nuclear synthesis, resulting in asynchrony in cell development. Consequently, nuclear development lags behind cytoplasmic development and the cells produced may be large or megaloblastic. Many cells are recognized as abnormal and are destroyed in the bone marrow. This results in ineffective erythropoiesis. The problem extends to all cells attempting to undergo mitosis.

Examples of this form of anaemia occur with deficiencies of folic acid, vitamin B12, cobalt and intrinsic factor. These conditions are rare in animals but may be induced by administration of folate antagonists such as methotrexate or may occur in patients with malignancies, in which the stores of these nutrients may be exhausted. Administration of sulpha drugs and potentiated sulpha drugs can inhibit folate metabolism and thymidine synthesis. Long-term administration of antiepileptic drugs (mysoline, phenobarbitone and dilantin) can also deplete serum folate concentrations. Macrocytosis may be found in humans with these conditions but has rarely been described in animals.

Defects in haemoglobin synthesis

In a similar way, defects in the production of components essential for haemoglobin manufacture can lead to ineffective erythropoiesis. In this case, cytoplasmic development lags behind nuclear development. These conditions may be considered as defects of either haem or globin synthesis. Examples of defects of globin synthesis are the genetic abnormalities affecting the production of the α or β amino acid chains of haemoglobin, thalassemia and sickle cell anaemia in humans; none of which have been recorded to date in animals. There are many variants of thalassemia in humans, which may result in red cells being more fragile than normal, having a shortened lifespan, being abnormal in shape and showing microcytosis and hypochromasia. Similarly, red cells of patients with sickle cell anaemia have abnormal crescent shapes and a shortened life span.

Iron deficiency anaemia is a classic example of a defect in haem synthesis. In this condition erythropoietin concentrations are high and stem cells are adequate, but the lack of available iron leads to delayed and defective cytoplasmic maturation of red cells. The developing cells may undergo an additional mitosis at the basophilic rubricyte stage while awaiting the haemoglobinization process, consequently becoming smaller (microcytic) and hypochromic. The resulting cells are more fragile than normal, some show tear-drop shapes (dacryocytes) and many are destroyed prematurely.

About 50% of patients with iron deficiency anaemia may have concurrent thrombocytosis, with large numbers of small platelets and consequently a tendency to form microthrombi. Thrombocytosis may occur in patients that have concurrent chronic external blood loss, which has led to the development of the iron-deficient state. Reduced intake of iron may be seen in young animals around the time of weaning, in older animals with defective function of the gastrointestinal tract or in animals with neoplasms of the gastrointestinal tract, affecting absorption of iron and other nutrients.

Deficiencies of copper and vitamin B6 may show similar haematological signs to iron deficiency in humans, with microcytosis and hypochromasia, but rarely cause anaemia in animals. Copper in the enzyme ferroxidase (ceruloplasmin) is essential for the utilization of iron, converting ferrous to ferric iron, in which form it is transported by transferrin to the bone marrow. Within the marrow it is converted back to the ferrous form to be incorporated in red cell production at the haem synthetase step.

Other conditions leading to defects in haem synthesis in small animals are lead poisoning and erythropoietic porphyria. Lead blocks sulphydryl groups within enzymes involved in haem synthesis. Characteristically, large numbers of metarubricytes are found in the peripheral blood of animals with acute lead poisoning,

but there is no concurrent anaemia or polychromasia. Basophilic stippling may be seen in about 30% of affected dogs but is not a specific finding.

Hereditary porphyria has been reported in anaemic Siamese cats as a dominant trait and in some non-anaemic domestic shorthaired cats. Affected animals will have ineffective erythropoiesis in which large quantities of isomer I of protoporphyrin are produced instead of isomer III. Isomer I is unable to combine normally with iron to form haem. There may be some haemolysis of red cells with 'port wine'-coloured urine, photosensitization, and fluorescence of teeth and urine in ultraviolet light due to oxidized porphyrins in these tissues. It is interesting to note that hereditary porphyria in humans is thought to have given rise to the legends of werewolves.

Myelodysplastic syndromes

These conditions are characterized by dysplasia (abnormal development) in one or more haematopoietic cell lines in a hypercellular bone marrow, with concurrent cytopenias in peripheral blood. By definition, there will be fewer than 30% blastic cells in the bone marrow in this condition. Myelodysplasia is often associated with a poorly regenerative refractory anaemia, and the cells produced may be dysfunctional.

In dogs, the conditions may be primary, resulting from a genetic transformation in a multipotential stem cell, or secondary and associated with administration of a drug. The secondary conditions usually resolve on withdrawal of the offending drug. The primary conditions are considered unlikely to respond satisfactorily to haematopoietic cytokines acting as maturation factors, although one exception has been described (Boone *at al.*, 1996). Some cases may transform into overt leukaemia at a later date (McManus and Hess, 1998) but many do not.

These conditions need to be distinguished from ineffective erythropoiesis due to nutrient deficiencies (vitamin B12, folic acid, iron), lead toxicity or drug reaction by bone marrow examination, biochemical assays and clinical history.

Myelodysplasia is rare in dogs and therefore is incompletely categorized. It is clear that the condition does not fit well into the French–American–British classification of myelodysplasia for humans. One of the recently proposed systems of classification for myelodysplasia in dogs (Weiss and Lulich, 1999) is summarized as:

- Dyserythropoiesis
- Sideroblastic dyserythropoiesis
- Dyserythropoiesis with an excess of blasts
- Myelodysplasia
- Sideroblastic myelodysplasia.

It is possible that some of these categories may represent progressive developmental stages of the disorder.

In cats, myelodysplasia is often associated with FeLV infection and may manifest with a macrocytosis. Bone marrow examination is essential to characterize the pathology. A refractory anaemia with an excess of myeloblasts but no marrow granulocyte reserve has been described in young cats with FeLV infection. Secondary infections may occur.

Myelofibrosis and myeloid metaplasia: In this dysplastic condition there is hyperplasia of the myeloid and megakaryocytic series, with asynchrony in the early developmental cells but maturation through to the end-stage cells. The erythroid cells are reduced and many dacryocytes appear in the peripheral blood. Ineffective granulopoiesis occurs leading to leucopenia. In due course, fibrosis of the marrow develops and is closely associated with megakaryocyte hyperplasia. Mast cells are usually plentiful in the marrow in this condition. Core biopsies of marrow may be more revealing than marrow aspirates once myelofibrosis develops.

Anaemias of increased red cell destruction

Haemolysis may be considered the result of an intrinsic or extrinsic defect of the red cell, which causes the cells to be destroyed at a higher rate than normal. Consequently these cells have a short half-life and may show some morphological change. Specific changes in red cell shape may provide clues to the cause of the haemolysis. Examples include immune-mediated haemolytic anaemia (IMHA; spherocytes), signs of intravascular injury (schistocytes, keratocytes), biochemical change (Heinz bodies; poikilocytes) or cellular parasites (e.g. *Haemobartonella*, *Babesia*). The mechanism of destruction of the red cells may be by direct lysis within the blood stream (intravascular haemolysis) or by erythrophagia by macrophages in the spleen, liver, marrow or lymph nodes (extravascular haemolysis), or both.

Clinically, intravascular haemolysis may have a more deleterious effect on the patient than extravascular haemolysis, as, in addition to the effects of low tissue oxygenation, there are also fragments of free red cell membrane in circulation, which may trigger disseminated intravascular coagulation (DIC). The presence of free haemoglobin released from red cells is injurious to tissues and some may appear in urine when concentrations exceed renal thresholds. In addition, the rate of destruction of cells may also exceed the capacity of the liver to process bilirubin, and combined with poor oxygenation, reduced liver function contributes to the appearance of clinical jaundice in many patients with intravascular haemolysis.

Extravascular haemolysis may proceed within macrophages in the spleen, liver or marrow and consequently splenic enlargement due to haemosiderosis may be detected on abdominal palpation. Although affected patients show all the signs of anaemia, there are no signs of haemoglobinaemia, haemoglobinuria or tissue injury usually associated with the other form of haemolysis. In addition, jaundice is rare in extravascular haemolysis.

The anaemia in haemolytic conditions will usually be very regenerative, with large numbers of polychromatic cells. Maximum marrow response may be an eight- to tenfold increase in red cell production, as detected by the absolute reticulocyte count. In the long term, however, continued haemolysis and marrow stimulation, particularly with hereditary haemolytic disorders, can eventually lead to myelofibrosis and in some cases osteosclerosis.

Haemolysis due to genetic defects of red cells

Mechanisms: In these rare conditions, red cells may have an abnormal shape or membrane (elliptocytes, stomatocytes) or a biochemical defect (e.g. deficiency in pyruvate kinase, phosphofructokinase, methaemoglobin reductase, calcium pump ATPase), which acts to shorten their lifespan. Other inherited haemolytic conditions may be associated with copper storage defects, malabsorption of vitamin B12 and hepatic disorders.

Breeds affected: Hereditary stomatocytosis has been described in some dwarf Alaskan Malamutes, and hereditary elliptocytosis has been reported in a cross-bred line of dogs and a Silky Terrier (Mills and Marsden, 1999). Both conditions were associated with either minimal anaemia or compensated anaemia and were discovered incidentally.

Pyruvate kinase deficiency of red cells has been described in Basenjis, Beagles, West Highland White Terriers, a Cairn Terrier and an Abyssinian cat. Affected cells are unable to maintain normal shape, lose potassium and have reduced oxygen affinity. They become sphero-echinocytic and have a lifespan reduced to about 20 days. Pyruvate kinase concentrations in red cells of affected dogs are reduced to about half that of normal dogs.

A non-spherocytic haemolytic anaemia of Beagles is due to a defect in the ATPase calcium pump system. The defect affects older red cells more than young cells. Other non-spherocytic anaemias have been recorded in Miniature Poodles and Beagles. In those cases, chronic haemolysis led to myelofibrosis and osteosclerosis.

A compensated intravascular haemolysis and bilirubinuria have been described in two male English Springer Spaniels with phosphofructokinase (PFK) deficiency of red cells. The affected cells showed increased fragility in alkaline conditions. PFK is a rate-limiting enzyme in glycolysis. A separate polysystemic disorder involving dyserythropoiesis, polymyopathy, megaoesophagus and cardiomegaly has been described in English Spaniels. The exact mechanism causing these defects has not been defined.

Methaemoglobin reductase deficiency has been described in a cat and two dogs (Miniature Poodle and Toy Alaskan Eskimo bitch). The affected animals showed persistent cyanosis of mucous membranes and occasional seizures. Methaemoglobin concentrations were increased to 19–25% of total haemoglobin concentration. In contrast to the condition in humans, these dogs did not respond to oral riboflavin therapy.

Macrocytosis may be seen in some toy and miniature Poodles, with MCVs of 85–95 fl (normal range 60–77 fl). Although marrow examination will reveal abnormal nucleated erythrocytes and incomplete mitosis with some dyserythropoiesis, no therapy is indicated. Similarly, Japanese Akita and Shiba Inu dogs will have smaller red cells than other breeds with MCVs as low as 55–64 fl. Their red cells contain a higher level of intracellular potassium than those of other dogs, thereby causing spurious hyperkalaemia in haemolysed blood samples.

A congenital selective malabsorption of vitamin B12 in Giant Schnauzers has been reported to cause a non-regenerative anaemia with poikilocytosis and neutropenia with hypersegmentation. The condition was inherited as an autosomal recessive trait. Affected dogs showed a dramatic response to injections of vitamin B12. A similar condition in Border Collies was characterized by haematological abnormalities with other metabolic disturbances and ketonuria.

Haemolysis due to acquired defects of red cells

Acquired defects of red cells are the most common cause of haemolysis. The ultimate mechanism of lysis is usually either direct membrane injury or osmotic lysis. Morphological changes to red cells are usually seen in haemolytic anaemia. Causes include:

- Biochemical changes (Heinz bodies, hypophosphataemia)
- Exposure to chemical haemolysins (heavy metals such as lead, zinc, silver; arsenicals; excessive copper and cyclic hydrocarbons)
- Bacterial, animal or plant haemolysins (such as lysins from *Leptospira icterohaemorrhagica*, *Clostridium haemolyticum*; some spider and snake venoms, particularly black snake; and the ricin from castor oil beans, which causes direct lysis)
- Coating of red cells by antibody and or complement (this will shorten their lifespan and lead to IMHA, with the appearance of marked spherocytosis and anisocytosis)
- Mechanical injury of red cells (cell injury that occurs while in circulation may result in intravascular haemolysis: examples are conditions associated with vascular and valvular lesions or some malignancies)

- Parasites: infection with intracellular or extracellular parasites such as *Babesia canis* or *Haemobartonella felis* or *H. canis* will cause haemolytic anaemia, which may be compounded by immune-mediated haemolysis.

Biochemical changes: Prolonged exposure to oxidant drugs or chemicals may lead to exhaustion of reduced glutathione and the rate-limiting enzyme, glutathione 6-phosphate dehydrogenase, within red cells, causing denaturation of haemoglobin. As a result, Heinz bodies form in the older red cells first, making them more rigid than normal, and these cells are either phagocytosed as they pass through the splenic sinuses or lysed directly within the circulation. Heinz bodies are 0.5–1 µm in diameter and their presence may be shown by a supravital stain such as new methylene blue. The methaemoglobin reductase (diaphorase) system is also vulnerable to oxidant injury, resulting in the formation of methaemoglobin. In this state, iron within red cells is oxidized to the ferric form, which cannot transport oxygen. As a result, affected animals may not only have severe anaemia but also hypoxaemia. Ingestion of onions and garlic are common causes of Heinz body formation in dogs. The toxic agent in the onions and garlic is n-propyl disulphide. High doses of vitamins K1 and K3 have also resulted in Heinz body formation.

Cats are more prone to Heinz body formation because their haemoglobin molecules contain eight to ten sulphydryl groups compared with only two or three groups in other species. However, the spleen in cats is non-sinusoidal, allowing longer survival of red cells containing Heinz bodies. Cats with diabetes mellitus, lymphoma and hyperthyroidism have a higher incidence of Heinz bodies than normal cats and this is exacerbated in cats fed a semisolid diet of tinned food containing the preservative, propylene glycol.

Cats are particularly prone to haemolysis associated with severe hypophosphataemia (Adams *et al.*, 1993). For this reason, phosphate supplementation is recommended for cats with serum phosphate concentrations less than 0.48 mmol/l.

Immune-mediated haemolysis: Anaemias in this category are mediated by antibody and/or complement on the surface of red cells. Erythrolysis may occur either within the blood stream or extravascularly. Intravascular lysis is more likely to be associated with IgM antibody or with high concentrations of IgG antibody, and more severe clinical signs. The distinguishing features of immune-mediated haemolysis include a biphasic population of red cells (many small spherocytes and large polychromatic cells), a positive result with a direct Coombs' test and, in some cases, gross agglutination. Spherocytes form as a result of loss by phagocytosis of red cell membrane and attached immune complexes. The injured cell is able to reseal its membrane without loss of internal contents but loses surface area in the process.

In some cases, the antibody is directed against immature developing red cells within bone marrow, rather than against mature erythrocytes. Patients with this phenomenon will have little polychromasia, but some spherocytes should be observed within the peripheral blood. This condition is equivalent to pure red cell aplasia.

Some animals with IMHA may also have antibody specific for platelet epitopes, and in these cases destruction of red cells and platelets (immune-mediated thrombocytopenia) results in both haemolytic and haemorrhagic anaemia.

Anti-red cell antibody may be actively produced by the patient or acquired passively by transfusion or colostral ingestion. The appearance of antibody may be genetically modulated and occur spontaneously or may follow cell injury or adsorption of foreign proteins or haptens on the red cell surface. Examples of the latter are virus particles, drugs (e.g. antibiotics, tranquillizers), chemicals or red cell parasites. In conditions in which a specific causative agent or underlying disease process cannot be identified, the term autoimmune haemolytic anaemia may be applied. Conditions in which a causative agent or underlying disease can be identified are termed immune-mediated haemolytic anaemia.

The immune-mediated haemolytic condition in the dog may be classified into one of five categories on the basis of the type of antibody present. Class I and II are associated with gross agglutination and intravascular haemolysis, respectively, and require aggressive therapy. Class III is the most common, does not spontaneously agglutinate and requires a Coombs' test for verification of the diagnosis. Class IV and V involve cold-reacting antibodies, causing agglutination and lysis, respectively, at 4°C.

Mechanical injury: Mechanical injury of red cells was recognized in humans receiving the early heart valve transplants that consisted of a mechanical ball valve prosthesis. Cells were damaged as they collided at high velocity with the obstacle in their path. Injured cells were recognized on the blood film as fragmented schistocytes and keratocytes. Similar cells may be found in animals with DIC, severe heart worm infection, vasculitis, splenic haemangiosarcoma, patent ductus arteriosus, myelofibrosis, malignancies, the haemolytic-uraemic syndrome and, to some extent, glomerulonephritis. Many of these conditions are associated with microangiopathy.

Haemolysis of normal red cells
Any condition that results in hypersplenism may be associated with increased phagocytosis of red cells by splenic macrophages. The microenvironment within an enlarged spleen will expose cells to high pH and low glucose concentrations, resulting in premature ageing of the cells. Patients with this condition will have a regenerative anaemia with increased metarubricytes, Howell–Jolly bodies, poikilocytes and usually a mild thrombocytopenia.

Anaemias of increased red cell loss
Haemorrhage is a passive loss of whole blood and may involve internal or external blood loss, or both. Both forms can be severe and life threatening depending on the extent of the blood loss. Loss of 30–40% of total blood volume leads to hypovolaemic shock, and death is likely after loss of more than 40% of total blood volume. Total blood volume in dogs is about 84 ml/kg (range 78–88 ml/kg) and in cats 64 ml/kg (range 62–66 ml/kg).

In internal haemorrhage, most red cells are reabsorbed via the lymphatics within a few days and re-enter the circulation in a slightly damaged form. Other cells are phagocytosed and their iron recycled via haemosiderin deposition in the macrophages. External haemorrhage involves loss of both iron and plasma protein from the body, thereby depleting body stores of iron and diminishing the potential for the erythron to regenerate successfully in the long term. The availability of iron is a rate-limiting step in red cell production. Consequently, in managing animals with external haemorrhage, the administration of iron should be considered.

Compared with haemolysis, patients with haemorrhage show noticeable changes in haemodynamics. After a peracute haemorrhagic episode there may be hypotension with a normal PCV. Anaemia and hypoproteinaemia may not develop until 4–24 hours after the haemorrhagic episode, following haemodilution from fluid shifts. Interstitial fluid shifts occur within a few hours, causing mild reductions in erythron values after 4 hours. Significant reductions in plasma protein, PCV and haemoglobin concentration occur after 12–24 hours, when plasma volume has expanded to approximately normal levels.

Haemorrhagic anaemia is classically regenerative, but this response is seen only after 3–4 days. In the interim period, the anaemia may be considered preregenerative. The degree of response depends on the availability of iron. Iron is less readily available in the ferric form in haemorrhagic anaemia than in haemolytic anaemia. This accounts for the lower average increase in red cell production of two- to fourfold normal seen in haemorrhagic anaemias, as assessed by absolute reticulocyte counts. Exceptions to these general guidelines will occur. Peak reticulocyte counts may be seen a week after the haemorrhagic episode.

Plasma protein concentration will be reduced in haemorrhagic patients, particularly those with external haemorrhage. A decrease in plasma protein concentration may occur as early as 4 hours after haemorrhage. A persistently low plasma protein concentration should lead to a suspicion of ongoing external haemorrhage. After a single episode of severe haemorrhage, plasma protein should return to normal levels by 5–7 days.

Platelets in patients with haemorrhage initially decrease in number and then may increase. A thrombocytosis is usually expected in haemorrhagic anaemia of several days' duration. Thrombocytosis is initially caused by movement of platelets from the spleen due to adrenalin response, but general marrow stimulation or stimulation of the erythroid and megakaryocytic cell lines may occur. Leucocyte numbers are not decreased in haemorrhage and in fact are likely to be increased in acute haemorrhage due to adrenalin effects. Mild neutrophilia may occur in the dog concurrently with a marked regenerative erythron response. This may be due to marrow stimulation by haematopoietic cytokines.

Some very regenerative anaemias may be macrocytic and hypochromic in the early stages. With continuing external haemorrhage, the anaemia is classically normocytic and normochromic and protein concentration remains low; and if iron deficiency develops due to continued external haemorrhagic loss, the anaemia may become microcytic and hypochromic.

Causes of haemorrhagic anaemia include:

- Trauma
- Parasitism: internal/external, e.g. fleas, ticks, lice, *Ancylostoma*, *Uncinaria* (dogs)
- Coagulation factor defect: haematomas, haemarthroses and haemorrhage into body cavities (diagnosis may be aided by fine-needle aspiration of the masses, paracentesis and measuring coagulation profiles)
- Platelet defects: petechial and ecchymotic haemorrhages, often flecks of blood in faeces, epistaxis and hyphaema
- Ruptured neoplasm, aneurysm, e.g. haemangiosarcoma.

WHEN TO COLLECT BONE MARROW SAMPLES AND DO FURTHER TESTS

Bone marrow aspirates or core biopsies are advocated in the following situations:

- Cases of pancytopenia
- Non-regenerative or poorly regenerative anaemias
- Neutropenias or thrombocytopenias where the cause is not obvious
- Cases of suspected haematopoietic neoplasia, myelodysplasia or marrow dysfunction as indicated by ineffective cytopoiesis or erythropoiesis
- Cases in which the degree of regenerative response is insufficient for the degree of anaemia.

Marrow biopsy can also be used to assess the amount of storage iron and to evaluate the regenerative erythroid response.

In short, marrow biopsies are recommended if any defect of production of cells is suspected, with either excessive or insufficient numbers of mature cells. Core biopsies are particularly recommended in patients suspected of having myelofibrosis, as aspiration biopsies may be unrewarding.

HAEMATOPOIETIC NEOPLASIA

Neoplasia of the haematopoietic system involves haematopoietic cell lines in bone marrow that have undergone a genetic neoplastic transformation and are proliferating autonomously. The end result is leukaemia. The cells produced may accumulate in bone marrow before appearing in the circulation. There is evidence to suggest that some leukaemic cells have a longer life span in circulation than normal and may have functional defects such as altered adhesive properties, reduced phagocytic and bactericidal capabilities and altered chemotaxis (in the case of neoplastic neutrophils). Neoplastic platelets may have reduced adhesive and functional properties, paradoxically resulting in bleeding.

Clinical signs of haematopoietic neoplasia may include generalized bone pain, lethargy, anorexia, vomiting, diarrhoea, weight loss, fever and bleeding. On clinical examination, affected animals may have pale mucous membranes, splenomegaly and hepatomegaly. These last two changes are likely to be due to metastatic spread to spleen and liver and may provide diagnostic clues to the condition, which otherwise has poorly specific signs. Other metastatic sites occasionally affected are lymph nodes, lungs and meninges. Neurological signs may occur in cases of metastases to the central nervous system or with hyperviscosity syndrome, as seen in some cases of multiple myeloma.

From a haematological perspective, neoplasms of the haematopoietic system may be suspected when either blastic haematopoietic cells appear in circulation or an unexplained pancytopenia or bicytopenia or a marked leucocytosis is present in peripheral blood. The presence of haematopoietic neoplasia will cause variable degrees of myelophthisis, and consequently the peripheral blood will show some degree of cytopenia and mild to moderate poorly regenerative anaemia. Myelophthisis may be due to the physical presence of the neoplasm as well as the effects of marrow suppressive factors associated with the tumour. Thrombocytopenia may also occur due to reduced platelet production and some splenic sequestration, resulting in haemorrhage.

Figures 3.6 and 3.7 show a system of classification of haematopoietic neoplasms. In general terms, haematopoietic neoplasms may be myeloproliferative (covering erythroid, granulocytic, monocytic, megakaryocytic cells) or lymphoproliferative (lymphoid leukaemia). Some visceral lymphomas may metastasize to bone marrow and blood at a late stage of disease (leukaemic lymphoma). Some lymphoid tumours (multiple myeloma, B-cell lymphoma) may be immunosecretory and produce a paraprotein (monoclonal gammopathy). Note that neoplastic plasma cells rarely circulate in multiple myeloma.

Type	Findings in blood and bone marrow
AUL	Acute undifferentiated leukaemia: blast cells non-reactive for myeloid or lymphoid cytochemical markers or antibodies
M1	Myeloblastic leukaemia without maturation: type I myeloblasts are >90% of all nucleated cells in bone marrow
M2	Myeloblastic leukaemia with maturation: myeloblasts are 30% to >90% of all nucleated cells
M3	Promyelocytic leukaemia: abnormal promyelocytes are >30% of nucleated cells in bone marrow
M4	Myelomonocytic leukaemia: myeloblasts and monoblasts are >30% of all nucleated cells in bone marrow
M5	Monocytic leukaemia: monocytic cells are >80% in bone marrow. Two forms exist: M5a >80% monoblasts and M5b <80% monoblasts with a predominance of differentiated monocytic cells
M6	Erythroleukaemia: marrow erythroid cells are >50% of nucleated cells in bone marrow, myeloblasts and monoblasts are <30% in blood but >30% in bone marrow. A variant, M6Er, is defined by a predominance of rubriblasts (>30%) in the erythroid component
M7	Megakaryoblastic leukaemia: megakaryoblasts are >30% of all nucleated cells in bone marrow. Myelofibrosis may be present in marrow core biopsies. Abnormal megakaryoblasts may be found in blood

Figure 3.6: *Classification of acute myeloid leukaemias. Based on the French–American–British (FAB) Scheme and National Cancer Institute Criteria of classification. Jain et al. (1991).*

Type	Findings in blood and bone marrow
MDS:	Blast cells are <30% of all nucleated cells, with <50% erythroid cells. Marrow may be normocellular to hypercellular, with dyshaematopoiesis. Blood shows refractory anaemia, often with increased mean corpuscular volume in cats, and leucopenia. A variant, MDS-Er, is defined by a predominance of erythroid cells in bone marrow
CMLs:	Blast cells are <30% of all nucleated cells, and erythroid cells are 50% in marrow. Absence of dyshaematopoiesis and presence of noticeable leucocytosis in blood. Several variants exist: • Chronic myelogenous leukaemia (CML): neutrophils with a disorderly left shift • Chronic monocytic leukaemia (CMoL): absolute monocytosis • Chronic myelomonocytic leukaemia (CMMoL): absolute monocytosis and neutrophilia, with disorderly left shift (may have dysplastic granulocytes and megakaryocytes and may have <20% blast cells)
Other leukaemias:	Primary thrombocythaemia (also called essential thrombocythaemia). Mature platelets are noticeably increased; marrow dysplasia present. Polycythaemia vera (also called primary polycythaemia). Mature red blood cells are noticeably increased, with increase in white blood cell and platelets numbers. Eosinophilic leukaemia Basophilic leukaemia Mast cell leukemia
Lymphoid leukaemias:	Acute lymphoblastic leukaemia (ALL): predominantly lymphoblasts Chronic lymphocytic leukaemia (CLL): predominantly lymphocytes Granular lymphocytic leukaemia: neoplasm of granular natural killer cells or cytotoxic T cells, which contain metachromatic cytoplasmic granules. These patients usually have an abdominal or thoracic mass containing neoplastic large granular lymphoid cells (LGLs) which may be of splenic origin Multiple myeloma: plasma cell tumour usually located throughout the bone marrow, secreting an immunoglobulin (Ig) or component of Ig, causing a monoclonal gammopathy (the neoplastic plasma cells rarely circulate in this condition)

Figure 3.7: *Classification of myelodysplastic syndrome (MDS) and other leukaemias.*

Identification of the neoplastic cell line involved is based on a variety of cellular attributes such as morphology, surface antigenic markers, biochemical content, histochemical stain reactions, electron microscopic morphology, isoenzymes and chromosomal changes. The last two features are rarely used in veterinary medicine at this time. Morphological identification alone is frequently insufficient for a specific diagnosis, as neoplastic cells may be poorly differentiated.

Haematopoietic neoplasms are classified as either acute or chronic on the basis of the maturity of the cells involved. Acute leukaemias are defined as having more than 30% blastic cells in bone marrow, and the cells show maturation arrest. Acute leukaemia generally has a rapid clinical course of 1–2 months and carries a poor prognosis. Chronic leukaemias have less than 30% blastic cells in bone marrow and involve well differentiated cells with no maturation arrest. Chronic leukaemia generally has a slower clinical course of 1–3 years. For example, the life expectancy of patients with acute lymphoblastic leukaemia is about 65 days compared with 450 days for patients with chronic lymphocytic leukaemia. An animal with chronic leukaemia, particularly chronic myelogenous leukaemia, may develop a 'blastic crisis,' which then may be rapidly fatal.

The stem cell giving rise to the neoplastic clone in acute and chronic leukaemia is different. In humans, chronic myelogenous leukemia has been shown to originate from the pluripotential stem cell, and patients with this condition have similar chromosomal (Philadelphia chromosome) and biochemical (G6PD) changes in the neoplastic cell populations. In contrast, acute myelogenous leukaemia was found to originate from the committed granulocytic stem cell.

One American study has shown the incidence rates for all leukaemias per 100 000 cats or dogs to be 224 and 30, respectively. Cats had 6.1 times more lymphomas, including leukaemias, and 15.7 times more myeloproliferative disorders than dogs. Neutered animals, particularly neutered queens and castrated dogs, had the lowest risk of leukaemia.

Leukaemias can occur in animals of any age, but acute granulocytic leukaemias are more common in young dogs (average age 3–5 years). Acute lymphoblastic leukemia (ALL) is seen in middle-aged dogs (average age 6.2 years) whereas chronic lymphocytic leukemia (CLL) is a disease of relatively older dogs (average age 9.4 years). Many CLLs in dogs are of T cell lineage (Verneau and Moore, 1999).

The lymphoid leukaemias of dogs are more common in males than females; male to female incidence ratios for ALL and CLL are 3:2 and 2:1, respectively. Lymphoproliferative disease is ten times more common than myeloproliferative disease in the dog. In a survey of 30 dogs with ALL, 27% were of the German Shepherd breed.

Ionizing radiation is known to lead to ALL and chronic myelogenous leukemia but not to CLL. There is a suggested association between genetic factors, autoimmune disorders and CLL.

CAUSES OF ANAEMIA IN PERSPECTIVE

The commonest cause of anaemia in all domestic animal species is the anaemia of inflammatory disease. This usually causes only a mild to moderate anaemia and is normocytic, normochromic and non-regenerative. Published surveys have shown that dogs are likely to have non-regenerative and haemorrhagic anaemias in about equal proportions, whereas about 70% of reported anaemias in cats are non-regenerative. It is possible that this may be associated with factors unique to the cat such as the prevalence of viral infections, shorter life span of the red cells and reduced amounts of iron stored in the bone marrow.

REFERENCES

Adams LG, Hardy RM, Weiss DJ and Bartges JW (1993) Hypophosphatemia and hemolytic anemia associated with diabetes mellitus and hepatic lipidosis in cats. *Journal of Veterinary Internal Medicine* **7**, 226–271

Brockus CW (1998) Endogenous estrogen myelotoxicosis associated with functional cystic ovaries in a dog. *Veterinary Clinical Pathology* **27**, 55–56

Boone L, Moriano J and Knauer K (1996) Treatment of dyserythropoiesis with refractory anaemia and excess of blasts in a dog using human recombinant erythropoietin (abstract). *Veterinary Pathology* **33**, 573

Jain NC, Blue JT, Grindem CB, Harvey JW, *et al.* (1991) Proposed criteria for classification of acute myeloid leukaemia in dogs and cats. *Veterinary Clinical Pathology* **20**, 63–82

McManus PM and Hess RS (1998) Myelodysplastic changes in a dog with subsequent acute myeloid leukaemia. *Veterinary Clinical Pathology* **27**, 112–115

Mills JN (1997) Compensated haemolytic anaemia in a dog. *Australian Veterinary Journal* **75**, 24–26

Mills JN and Marsden CA (1999) Presumed hereditary elliptocytosis in a dog. *Australian Veterinary Journal* **77**, 15–16

Suliman H, Logan-Henfrey L, Majiwa P, Ole-Moiyoi O and Feldman B (1999) Analysis of erythropoietin and erythropoietin receptor genes expression in cattle during acute infection with Trypanosoma congolense infection (abstract). *Veterinary Clinical Pathology* **28**, 118–119

Verneau W and Moore PF (1999) An immunophenotypic study of canine leukaemias and preliminary assessment of clonality by polymerase chain reaction. *Veterinary Immunology and Immunopathology* **69**, 145–164

Weiss DJ and Lulich J (1999) Myelodysplastic syndrome with sideroblastic differentiation in a dog. *Veterinary Clinical Pathology* **28**, 59–63

Polycythaemia

Elizabeth Villiers

INTRODUCTION

Polycythaemia is characterized by an increase in the packed cell volume, red blood cell count and haemoglobin concentration. It may be relative (owing to diminished plasma volume) or absolute. Absolute polycythaemia may result from increased concentrations of erythropoietin (secondary polycythaemia) or from the myeloproliferative disease, polycythaemia vera (primary polycythaemia). The term polycythaemia implies an increased number of several haemopoietic cell lines, and humans with polycythaemia vera have erythrocytosis accompanied by neutrophilia and thrombocytosis. However, dogs and cats with polycythaemia vera usually have normal neutrophil and platelet counts and so the term primary erythrocytosis may be more appropriate.

ERYTHROPOIESIS

In the bone marrow the pluripotent stem cell gives rise to the committed erythrocyte progenitor cell known as a burst-forming unit, which divides and differentiates into colony-forming units. These in turn divide and differentiate into erythroblasts, which continue to divide into early, intermediate and then late normoblasts. Reticulocytes are formed when the nucleus is extruded from late normoblasts and the red cells reach full maturation in the blood stream. The key regulator of erythropoiesis is erythropoietin (EPO). This hormone is produced in the kidneys and acts by stimulating the colony-forming units and, to a lesser extent, the burst-forming units (Giger, 1992). EPO also hastens the release of reticulocytes into the blood stream. The synthesis of EPO is not regulated by the number of circulating red cells but by the degree of renal hypoxia. Hypoxia triggers an increased rate of production of EPO, whereas high tissue oxygenation results in a reduced rate. Other hormones such as corticosteroids and thyroxine (T4) stimulate the production of EPO but have no intrinsic EPO activity.

RELATIVE POLYCYTHAEMIA

Relative polycythaemia arises when the plasma volume is decreased, usually as a result of fluid loss.

Thus the packed cell volume (PCV) is increased, but the total mass of circulating red blood cells (RBCs) is normal. Relative polycythaemia may arise in animals with acute diarrhoea, extensive burns, heat stroke or water deprivation, and clinical signs of dehydration are usually obvious. The PCV is mildly increased and there is an accompanying increase in plasma proteins (unless plasma protein has been lost, as in burn injuries). Occasionally, relative polycythaemia may result from splenic contraction after stress (e.g. severe pain) or excitement. Splenic contraction leads to the release of large numbers of red cells into the circulation. Relative polycythaemia resolves after rehydration or removal of the cause of splenic contraction.

SECONDARY POLYCYTHAEMIA

Secondary polycythaemia results from increased EPO production. This may be a physiologically appropriate response to systemic hypoxia or may occur in the absence of systemic hypoxia, known as physiologically inappropriate polycythaemia. This condition occurs most commonly in association with renal neoplasia. In animals with secondary polycythaemia, serum EPO concentrations are usually increased.

Physiologically appropriate secondary polycythaemia

Two of the most common causes of tissue hypoxia are chronic pulmonary disease (e.g. feline allergic bronchitis) and right-to-left shunting cardiovascular disease. Right-to-left shunting may occur in patent ductus arteriosus. Initially there is a left-to-right shunt leading to increased blood flow in the pulmonary artery. Pulmonary hypertension and compensatory right ventricular hypertrophy result in increased pulmonary artery pressure, and when this exceeds the aortic pressure the direction of blood flow in the patent ductus reverses. Thus deoxygenated blood is delivered into the descending aorta resulting in hypoxia in the caudal half of the body and a subsequent increase in EPO production. Right-to-left shunting may also occur in animals with a coexisting atrial septal defect and pulmonic stenosis; and in tetralogy of Fallot in which there is a large ventricular septal defect and pulmonic stenosis.

Physiologically appropriate polycythaemia may also occur in animals living at high altitude. In humans, polycythaemia may be caused by massive obesity and haemoglobinopathies. Obesity has not been recognized as a cause of polycythaemia in dogs and cats. Haemoglobinopathies such as methaemoglobin reductase deficiency may cause polycythaemia (Hasler and Giger, 1996), but these disorders are rare in dogs and cats.

Physiologically inappropriate secondary polycythaemia

The most common cause of physiologically inappropriate secondary polycythaemia is renal neoplasia. Polycythaemia has been reported in association with renal adenocarcinoma (also known as renal cell carcinoma) (Scott and Patnaik, 1972; Peterson and Zanjani, 1981; Waters and Prueter, 1986; Crow *et al.*, 1995). Polycythaemia has also been reported in association with renal lymphoma and renal fibrosarcoma (Nelson *et al.*, 1983; Gorse, 1988).

The mechanism of inappropriate EPO production is not fully understood. It may be due to increased production/secretion of EPO or an EPO-like substance from the tumour, or it may result from local tissue hypoxia in the kidney, which is caused by a disruption of the renal microvasculature by the tumour.

In humans, several extrarenal tumours have been associated with secondary polycythaemia, including hepatoma, uterine leiomyoma, ovarian carcinoma and phaeochromocytoma. Polycythaemia secondary to extrarenal neoplasia is uncommon in the dog and cat, but has been reported in a dog with a nasal fibrosarcoma (Couto *et al.*, 1989). In this case the tumour was found to have high EPO activity, suggesting that the tumour cells produced EPO. The polycythaemia resolved after resection of the tumour.

Non-neoplastic renal diseases such as renal cysts and hydronephrosis are well recognized causes of secondary polycythaemia in humans. However, in dogs and cats only small numbers of such cases have been documented. Hasler and Giger (1996) reported secondary polycythaemia in one cat with a renal capsular effusion and in a second cat with fatty infiltration of the kidney. EPO concentrations were noticeably increased in these two cats, confirming secondary polycythaemia. In a report by Waters and Prueter (1986), polycythaemia in a Labrador was thought to be associated with pyelonephritis due to *Cryptococcus neoformans* infection. However, in this case, EPO concentrations were not determined, and the polycythaemia could have been unrelated to the renal disease.

Mild polycythaemia may result from hyperadrenocorticism in dogs and hyperthyroidism in cats, since both cortisol and thyroid hormone stimulate increased production of EPO.

PRIMARY POLYCYTHAEMIA

Primary polycythaemia (polycythaemia vera, primary erythrocytosis) is a chronic myeloproliferative disease characterized by neoplastic proliferation of erythroid precursors, which mature into functionally and morphologically normal RBCs. The proliferation occurs independently of EPO and does not respond to normal feedback mechanisms. In animals with primary polycythaemia, serum EPO concentrations are normal or low.

In the dog, secondary polycythaemia is more common than primary polycythaemia. In the cat, primary polycythaemia is the more common form, and although infiltrative renal diseases such as lymphoma and feline infectious peritonitis are common in the cat, these diseases rarely result in polycythaemia.

CONSEQUENCES OF POLYCYTHAEMIA

An excessive number of RBCs results in increased blood volume and increased blood viscosity. The blood viscosity increases disproportionately with increases in the PCV above 50%. Blood capillaries and veins are distended to accommodate the increased blood volume, and this results in erythematous mucous membranes. Bleeding episodes such as epistaxis, haematuria and haematemesis may occur, and result from mechanical rupture of capillaries due to overdistension. Hyperviscosity leads to sludging of blood in small vessels, which leads to tissue hypoxia. The three organs most affected by increased blood viscosity are the central nervous system (CNS; in particular the cerebral cortex), the kidneys and the heart. Disorders of the CNS such as seizures, lethargy, weakness, ataxia, dementia, depression and coma may be seen. Glomerulonephropathy may result from glomerular and interstitial capillary hypoxia and lead to proteinuria and clinical signs of polydipsia and polyuria. Hyperviscosity and increased vascular resistance result in increased cardiac effort, and there may be an associated myocardial hypertrophy, which may progress to mild hypertrophic cardiomyopathy. Ocular abnormalities including distended tortuous blood vessels (Figure 4.1), and occasionally retinal haemorrhage may be present. The sluggish blood flow that results from hyperviscosity may predispose to thrombus formation. Iliac thrombosis has been reported in a dog with primary polycythaemia (McGrath, 1974). Figure 4.2 summarizes the clinical signs that may be seen in polycythaemic dogs and cats.

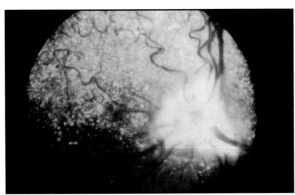

Figure 4.1: *Distended and tortuous retinal blood vessels resulting from hyperviscosity. (Photograph courtesy of N T Gorman.)*

Hyperaemic mucous membranes
Not always seen
Neurological signs
Disorientation Depression, stupor, coma Seizures Weakness Blindness Ataxia
Renal signs
Polydipsia/polyuria
Bleeding episodes
Epistaxis Haematemesis Haematuria Haemorrhagic diarrhoea
Ocular signs
Tortuous distended retinal vessels Retinal haemorrhage Distended scleral vessels Splenomegaly is occasionally seen in cats with primary erythrocytosis Paroxysmal sneezing is quite common in dogs (owing to increased blood viscosity in nasal mucosa)

Figure 4.2: *Clinical signs of polycythaemia.*

LABORATORY FINDINGS AND DIAGNOSIS

An increase in the packed cell volume (>55% in dogs and >45% in cats) indicates polycythaemia. In dogs and cats with absolute polycythaemia the PCV is often as high as 70–90%, whereas in relative polycythaemia the PCV is usually mildly increased (e.g. 60%). In absolute polycythaemia there may be a mild reticulocytosis, and microcytosis is sometimes seen in dogs, which occurs due to a relative iron deficiency in an active bone marrow. Primary polycythaemia is sometimes accompanied by a mild thrombocytosis.

Once polycythaemia is recognized, subsequent evaluation is aimed at determining whether the polycythaemia is relative, primary or secondary. Relative polycythaemia is identified when the PCV is increased but the red cell mass is normal. The red cell mass can be measured using an isotope dilution technique whereby RBCs are removed from the patient and labelled with radioactive chromium. The radioactivity of the labelled red cells is measured before they are reinjected into the patient, and the radioactivity of blood samples taken 20 and 30 minutes after injection is measured. In practice it is rarely necessary to measure the red cell mass, because animals with relative polycythaemia usually have obvious clinical signs of dehydration, and the PCV returns to normal when the patient is rehydrated. In addition, increased plasma protein concentration and a mild degree of polycythaemia both suggest relative polycythaemia.

Once relative polycythaemia has been excluded, investigations are aimed at distinguishing primary from secondary polycythaemia. This is achieved by searching for possible causes of secondary polycythaemia (e.g. cardiopulmonary disease or renal disease) and by evaluation of EPO concentrations.

Clinical signs of respiratory disease (e.g. coughing, dyspnoea) or cardiac disease (e.g. cardiac murmur, arrhythmia, cyanosis) point towards secondary appropriate polycythaemia. Thoracic radiography, echocardiography and electrocardiography are useful in diagnosing pulmonary or cardiac disease. If a blood gas machine is available (e.g. at the local hospital), the partial pressure of oxygen in arterial blood (PaO_2) should be measured. The femoral artery or the dorsal metatarsal artery are suitable sampling sites. The normal PaO_2 in a dog or cat breathing room air is 85–100 mmHg. In cases of physiologically appropriate polycythaemia the PaO_2 is usually noticeably reduced (e.g. <60 mmHg). A pulse oximeter may be used to measure the arterial haemoglobin saturation (SaO_2). The normal SaO_2 is 97%. As with the PaO_2, the SaO_2 is noticeably reduced in appropriate secondary polycythaemia. Animals with primary polycythaemia may have mildly reduced SaO_2 and PaO_2, which may be due to blood hyperviscosity resulting in poor tissue perfusion.

If systemic hypoxia has been ruled out, the investigation is aimed at searching for potential causes of inappropriate polycythaemia. This is most commonly due to renal neoplasia, although non-neoplastic renal disease should also be considered. A cranial abdominal mass or renomegaly may be obvious on clinical examination or may be detected on plain radiographs. An intravenous urogram and/or an ultrasound examination of the kidneys are used to identify neoplasia or other renal disease (Figure 4.3). Ultrasound examination is a convenient screening test. When renal abnormalities are detected, a fine needle aspirate or trucut biopsy may be obtained. Other tests such as biochemical screening and urine analysis are helpful. Serum urea and creatinine concentrations are usually normal in cases of renal neoplasia unless both kidneys are involved. In cases of renal neoplasia, urine analysis may reveal proteinuria, haematuria and an active sediment. Proteinuria may also be due to glomerulonephropathy, which may be secondary to polycythaemia.

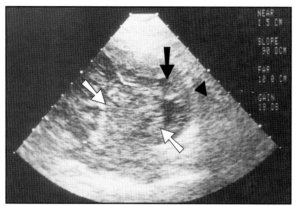

Figure 4.3: *Ultrasound examination of this kidney revealed a large tumour (open arrows) distorting the medulla (closed arrow) and cortex (arrowhead). (Photograph courtesy of M E Herrtage.)*

Glomerulonephropathy may be caused by polycythaemia as a result of renal hypoxia due to hyperviscosity (Page *et al.*, 1990; Quesnel and Kruth, 1992). Renal diseases such as pyelonephritis may cause secondary polycythaemia. Thus it may be difficult to determine if non-neoplastic renal disease is a consequence of primary polycythaemia or if it is the underlying cause of the polycythaemia, and in this situation serum EPO concentrations should always be evaluated.

A diagnosis of primary polycythaemia is made if causes of secondary polycythaemia have been excluded and if serum EPO concentrations are low or normal. As primary polycythaemia is largely a diagnosis of exclusion, the accuracy of this diagnosis depends on the extent of the clinicopathological investigation. Figure 4.4 summarizes the diagnostic approach to polycythaemia.

Serum EPO concentrations

Assessment of serum EPO concentrations is helpful in distinguishing primary from secondary polycythaemia, because high values point towards secondary polycythaemia and low or normal values are consistent

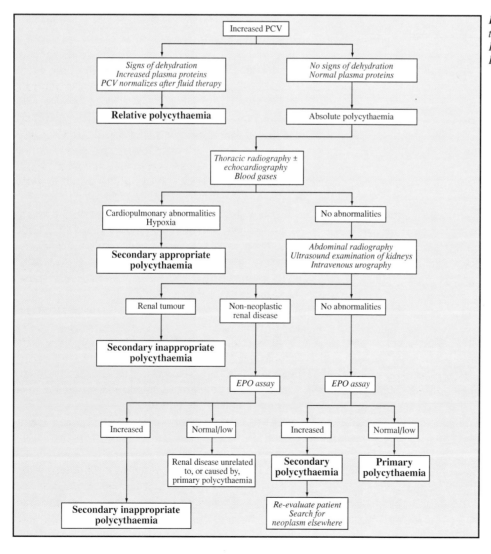

Figure 4.4: *Approach to the polycythaemic patient. PCV, packed cell volume; EPO, erythropoietin.*

with primary polycythaemia. EPO can be measured by using bioassays that detect the hormone's activity or by immunoassays that detect the EPO antigen (Giger, 1992). Bioassays are not sensitive enough to detect normal or reduced concentrations of EPO, and can only detect increased EPO activity. Another disadvantage of bioassays is that laboratory animals are used in the test. Two immunoassays that have been validated for use in dogs and cats are the EPO-Trac ^{125}I radioimmunoassay (Incstar Ltd) (Cook and Lothrop, 1994) and the Medac ELISA (Medac Diagnostics) (Hasler and Giger, 1996). Dogs and cats with primary polycythaemia have low or low–normal concentrations of EPO; and a low or normal serum EPO value in an animal with no signs of secondary polycythaemia supports a diagnosis of primary polycythaemia. High concentrations of serum EPO are only seen in secondary polycythaemia. A study using a radioimmunoassay in polycythaemic dogs found that serum EPO concentrations were slightly to moderately increased in dogs with congenital heart disease and pulmonary disorders and moderately to noticeably increased in dogs with renal tumours (Giger, 1991). However, not all cases of secondary polycythaemia are associated with high serum EPO concentrations. In two reports, cats with renal tumours had normal serum EPO concentrations (Cook and Lothrop, 1994; Hasler and Giger, 1996). Possible explanations for this are that the renal tumours may have produced an EPO-like substance that was not recognized by the assay or that EPO production was cyclic. EPO concentrations may also be normal in animals with polycythaemia secondary to chronic hypoxia (Cook and Lothrop, 1994; Hasler and Giger, 1996). The animal may in time adapt to hypoxia, resulting in a gradual decrease in EPO production. Hence EPO concentrations should always be interpreted in conjunction with the clinical findings and should never replace a thorough clinicopathological evaluation.

In the United Kingdom, EPO concentrations in the dog and cat may be assayed at Cambridge Specialist Laboratory Services Ltd (PO Box 967, Stapleford, Cambridge CB2 5XY). A serum sample or plasma collected in ethylenediamine tetra-acetic acid may be used.

Bone marrow cytology

Bone marrow aspirates are often obtained as part of the investigation of polycythaemic animals, but they do not help distinguish primary from secondary polycythaemia and are generally not useful. In both primary and secondary polycythaemia the bone marrow is usually hypercellular and the myeloid:erythroid ratio may be normal or decreased owing to hyperplasia of the erythroid series. Although primary polycythaemia is a myeloproliferative disease, the red cells and their precursors are morphologically normal and do not appear neoplastic (Figure 4.5).

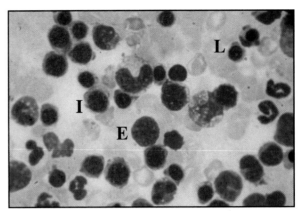

Figure 4.5: *Bone marrow aspirate from a dog with primary polycythaemia showing erythroid hyperplasia (E, early normoblast; I, intermediate normoblast; L, late normoblast). The erythroid cells are morphologically normal, and bone marrow cytology does not help to differentiate primary from secondary polycythaemia. (Photograph courtesy of J K Dunn.)*

TREATMENT

Polycythaemia

The treatment of polycythaemia depends on the underlying cause of the disease. Animals with relative polycythaemia should be treated with fluid therapy to correct dehydration. Initial treatment of absolute polycythaemia, irrespective of the cause, is aimed at reducing the blood viscosity by reducing the number of circulating red cells. This is achieved by performing a phlebotomy, removing 20 ml/kg of blood and replacing the removed blood volume with 0.9% saline. This results in a decrease in the PCV by about 15%. The jugular vein is usually used. In dogs, blood may be collected by using a blood transfusion collection set, whereas in cats a 60 ml syringe and a 19 gauge butterfly needle are useful. In animals with polycythaemia secondary to chronic hypoxia, a more cautious approach is recommended because sudden removal of a large amount of blood may exacerbate the hypoxia and may result in hypotension. Therefore 5 ml/kg of blood is removed at one time, and repeated as needed until the PCV has decreased to 55–60%.

In animals with polycythaemia secondary to surgically resectable renal tumours, it is important to carry out phlebotomy before surgery because hyperviscosity is associated with an increased risk of thrombosis and/or excessive haemorrhage. Renal adenocarcinomas may be contained within the renal capsule or may invade surrounding structures such as the vena cava and may not be amenable to surgical excision. Occasionally, both kidneys may be affected. In dogs with renal adenocarcinoma, metastases to regional lymph nodes, liver, lungs and bone are present in more than half the cases at the time of diagnosis (Baskin and DePaoli, 1977). In those cases where surgical excision is possible, mean survival times after surgery are 6–10 months (Klein *et al.*, 1988), although survival times of several years have been reported (Withrow, 1996). In three dogs with polycythaemia secondary to renal adenocarcinoma that underwent nephrectomy, poly-cythaemia did not adversely affect the prognosis (Scott and Patnaik, 1972; Peterson and Zanjani, 1981; Waters and Prueter, 1986).

Primary polycythaemia

Three treatment modalities have been used in the treatment of primary polycythaemia: repeated phle-botomy, chemotherapy in the form of hydroxyurea and radioactive phosphorus. Combinations of phlebotomy and hydroxyurea, or phlebotomy and radioactive phos-phorus, have also been used.

In humans, phlebotomy alone is usually used as the first line of treatment, except in elderly patients or those with thrombotic complications. The main disad-vantage of phlebotomy is an increased risk of thrombo-sis, which is unrelated to the platelet count and thought to be due to the poor stability of the haematocrit. Therapy with aspirin to try to prevent thrombosis has not been widely successful and may result in haemorrhagic complications (Tartaglia, 1986). An-other disadvantage of phlebotomy is a risk of early progression to myelofibrosis and myeloid spleno-megaly, which is sometimes seen as a late complica-tion of the disease in humans (Najean et al., 1994). Frequent phlebotomies may lead to iron deficiency, which in turn leads to the development of microcytic red cells. Since the red cells are smaller, the PCV remains in the normal range for a longer period, and iron supplements are not routinely given unless there are signs of severe iron deficiency. Both radioactive phosphorus and hydroxyurea chemotherapy are effec-tive and well tolerated, with a lower incidence of thrombotic complications. They are, however, associ-ated with an increased incidence of leukaemia and, in the case of radioactive phosphorus, other cancers (Weinfeld et al., 1994; Najean et al., 1996). Radio-active phosphorus is often used in elderly patients because leukaemia is unlikely to occur in their lifetime.

In dogs and cats there are few reported cases of primary polycythaemia treated by phlebotomy alone. In one report a cat survived more than 20 months (Foster and Lothrop, 1988), and in another report a dog survived a year and was generally free of clinical signs (Meyer et al., 1993). Providing that the procedure is well tolerated, this method of treatment is safe and effective, although the risk of thrombosis may be increased as it is in humans. In the report by Meyer et al. (1993) the dog died suddenly, and the authors postulated that this may have been due to thrombosis.

The frequency of phlebotomies is determined by the PCV, which, together with the clinical response, should be monitored frequently (e.g. monthly). If phlebotomy is required more frequently than every 4-6 weeks, myelosuppressive therapy is recommended, and this is usually in the form of chemotherapy.

Hydroxyurea is the cytotoxic drug of choice and is generally well tolerated by animals. It causes revers-ible bone marrow suppression by inhibiting DNA synthesis without affecting RNA or protein synthesis. After an initial phlebotomy, a loading dose of 30 mg/kg/day is given for 7-10 days, followed by a mainte-nance dose of 15 mg/kg/day. Haematology is moni-tored at 7-14 day intervals until the PCV is stable and within the normal range, and then every 6-8 weeks. If the PCV increases while the animal is on maintenance therapy, phlebotomy may be repeated and/or the dose of hydroxyurea may be increased for 7-10 days, after which time the dose is reduced to the maintenance dose again. Since the drug causes bone marrow suppression it has the potential to cause thrombocytopenia, which may result in spontaneous bleeding, and neutropenia, which may result in life-threatening sepsis. It is there-fore mandatory to monitor the patient's haematology regularly while on maintenance treatment. If thrombo-cytopenia or neutropenia occurs, hydroxyurea treat-ment should be temporarily suspended until the counts return to normal and then reintroduced at a lower dose. Antibiotics should be given while the patient is neutro-penic. Other potential side effects in the dog include anorexia, vomiting and sloughing of the claws (Peterson and Randolph, 1982). In practice, such side effects are rarely seen.

Hydroxyurea is supplied in 500 mg capsules. These capsules should not be broken open as this would expose the handler to a potentially mutagenic and teratogenic substance. Therefore the total number of milligrams required for a set period should be calcu-lated and the capsules spread evenly over that period. For example, a cat weighing 3.5 kg would require a daily maintenance dose of 52.5 mg, which is one 10th of a tablet. Therefore, one tablet should be given every 10 days. This bolus-type dosing may occasionally result in an adverse reaction in cats, leading to met-haemoglobinaemia and haemolytic anaemia with Heinz bodies (Watson et al., 1994). Early detection of such a reaction could be achieved by initially giving a low dose more frequently (which would entail splitting capsules). Watson et al. (1994) recommended giving cats 125 mg every other day for 2 weeks, then 250 mg twice a week for 2 weeks, then 500 mg once a week. The cat could be admitted to hospital before each dose increment. Blood taken at the time of the initial phle-botomy should be stored in case a severe methaemo-globinaemia develops.

Radioactive phosphorus (^{32}P) has been used in small numbers of dogs with polycythaemia. After administration, ^{32}P is taken up by bone where it decays, thereby irradiating the adjacent haemopoietic cells in the bone marrow. It is well tolerated and associated with minimal short-term side effects, although the potential carcinogenic effects seen in human patients presumably also affect the dog. In a report by Smith and Turrel (1989), a single treatment resulted in long-term control in about 40% of cases, although 25% of cases showed no response. The main disadvantage of this treatment is the requirement for isolation of the animal in purpose-built premises.

REFERENCES AND FURTHER READING

Baskin GB and DePaoli A (1977) Primary renal neoplasms of the dog. *Veterinary Pathology* **14**, 591-605

Campbell KC (1990) Diagnosis and management of polycythaemia in dogs. *Compendium on Continuing Education for the Practicing Veterinarian* **12**, 543-550

Cook SM and Lothrop CD (1994) Serum erythropoietin concentrations measured by radioimmunoassay in normal, polycythaemia and anaemic dogs and cats. *Journal of Veterinary Internal Medicine* **8**, 18-25

Couto CG, Boudrieau RJ and Zanjani ED (1989) Tumour associated erythrocytosis in a dog with nasal fibrosarcoma. *Journal of Veterinary Internal Medicine* **3**, 183-185

Crow SE, Allen DP, Murphy CJ and Culbertson R (1995) Concurrent renal adenocarcinoma and polycythaemia in a dog. *Journal of the American Animal Hospital Association* **31**, 29-33

Foster ES and Lothrop CD (1988) Polycythaemia in a cat with cardiac hypertrophy. *Journal of the American Veterinary Medical Association* **192**, 1736-1738

Giger U (1991) Serum erythropoietin concentrations in polycythaemic and anaemic dogs. *Proceedings of the 9th American College Veterinary Internal Medicine Forum*, pp. 143-145. New Orleans, Louisiana

Giger U (1992) Erythropoietin and its clinical use. *Compendium of Continuing Education for the Practicing Veterinarian* **14**, 25-34

Gorse M J (1988) Polycythaemia associated with renal fibrosarcoma in a dog. *Journal of the American Veterinary Medical Association* **192**, 793-794

Hasler AH and Giger U (1996) Serum erythropoietin values in polycythaemic cats. *Journal of the American Animal Hospital Association* **32**, 294-301

Klein MK, Cockrell GL and Withrow SJ (1988) Canine primary renal neoplasms: a retrospective review of 54 cases. *Journal of the American Animal Hospital Association* **24**, 443-452

McGrath CJ (1974) Polycythaemia vera in dogs. *Journal of the American Veterinary Medical Association* **164**, 1117-1121

Meyer HP, Slappendel RJ and Greydanaus-van de Putten SWM (1993) Polycythaemia vera in a dog treated by repeated phlebotomies. *Veterinary Quarterly* **14**, 108-111

Najean Y, Dresch C and Rain JD (1994) The very long term course of polycythaemia: a complement to the previously published data of the Polycythaemia Vera Study Group. *British Journal of Haematology* **86**, 233-235

Najean Y, Rain JD, Goguel A, Lejeune F, Echard M and Grange MJ (1996) Risk of leukaemia, carcinoma and myelofibrosis in [32]P- or chemotherapy-treated patients with polycythaemia vera: a prospective analysis of 682 cases. The French Co-operative Group for the Study of Polycythaemias. *Leukaemia and Lymphoma.* **22 (suppl 1),** 111-119

Nelson RW, Hager D and Zanjani ED (1983) Renal lymphosarcoma with inappropriate erythropoietin production in a dog. *Journal of the American Veterinary Medical Association* **182**, 1396-1397

Page RL, Stiff ME, McEntee MC and Walter LG (1990) Transient glomerulonephropathy associated with primary erythrocytosis in a dog. *Journal of the American Veterinary Medical Association* **196**, 620-622

Peterson ME and Randolph JF (1982) Diagnosis of canine primary polycythaemia and management with hydroxyurea. *Journal of the American Veterinary Medical Association* **180**, 415-418

Peterson ME and Zanjani ED (1981) Inappropriate erythropoietin production from a renal carcinoma in a dog with polycythaemia. *Journal of the American Veterinary Medical Association* **179**, 995-996

Quesnel AD and Kruth SA (1992) Polycythaemia vera and glomerulonephritis in a dog. *Canadian Veterinary Journal* **33**, 671-672

Scott RC and Patnaik AK (1972) Renal carcinoma with secondary polycythaemia in a dog. *Journal of the American Animal Hospital Association* **8**, 275-283

Smith M and Turrel JM (1989) Radiophosphorus treatment of bone marrow disorders in dogs: 11 cases (1970-1987). *Journal of the American Veterinary Medical Association* **194**, 98-102

Tartaglia AP (1986) Adverse effects of anti-aggregating platelet therapy in the treatment of polycythaemia vera. *Seminars in Haematology* **23**, 172-175

Waters DJ and Prueter JC (1986) Secondary polycythaemia associated with renal disease in the dog: two case reports and review of literature. *Journal of the American Animal Hospital Association* **31**, 29-33

Watson ADJ, Moore AS and Helfand SC (1994) Primary erythrocytosis in the cat: treatment with hydroxyurea. *Journal of Small Animal Practice* **35**, 320-325

Weinfeld A, Swolin B and Westlin J (1994) Acute leukaemia after hydroxyurea therapy in polycythaemia vera and allied disorders: a prospective study of efficacy and leukaemogenicity with therapeutic implications (1994). *European Journal of Haematology* **52**, 134-139

Withrow SJ (1996) Tumours of the urinary system. In: *Small Animal Clinical Oncology, 2nd edn*, ed. SJ Withrow and EG MacEwen. WB Saunders, London

Erythrocyte Disorders: Selected Topics

(i) Iron Deficiency Anaemia

Mike Stone

INTRODUCTION

Iron deficiency anaemia in small animal medicine is most commonly seen as a result of insufficient intake of dietary iron or chronic blood loss. The following case history is an example of iron deficiency anaemia in a dog. An 8-year-old mixed breed dog weighing 29 kg was evaluated for melaena and anaemia. Haematology revealed microcytic hypochromic non-regenerative anaemia (Figure 5.1, day 1). On physical examination the patient was tachypnoeic and had pale mucous membranes. On rectal examination there was black stool, which gave a positive test result for occult blood. Tachypnoea resolved after the dog received one unit of packed red cells, and the packed cell volume (PCV) increased from 14% to 21%. Radiographs taken after the oral administration of barium sulphate re-vealed an ovoid filling defect inside a dilated loop of small intestine (Figure 5.2). A second transfusion of packed red cells was given, and an ulcerated leio-myoma was surgically removed from the mid-jeju-num. The dog was discharged two days after surgery, with a PCV of 31%. On day 15 the PCV was 23%, but there were 10.8% reticulocytes in the blood. Although iron deficiency was suspected, iron was not given, on the assumption that the blood transfusions and diet would supply adequate iron for haematopoiesis. On day 29, however, the reticulocyte response had dropped to 0.7%, with a PCV of 22%. Ferrous sulphate was begun at 100 mg orally twice daily, and after 3 weeks the PCV had increased to 41%. Iron therapy was continued once daily for 4 months. The dog completely recovered and continued to do well after iron therapy was discontinued.

	Day 1	Day 3	Day 15	Day 29	Day 54	Reference values
Packed cell volume (%)	14	21	23	22	41	37–56
Mean corpuscular volume (fl)	44	64	–	–	–	55–77
Mean corpuscular concentration (g/l)	307	320	–	–	–	337–365
Reticulocytes (%)	0.8	5.1	10.8	0.7	–	<2
Red cell morphology	3+ polychromasia	3+ polychromasia, 2+ hypochromasia, 2+ anisocytosis, 11 nucleated red cells/100 white cells		1+ polychromasia		
Total protein (g/l)	57	62	63	68	72	50–80
Total nucleated cell count (x 10^9/l)	30.7	51.2	16.7	15.2	10.8	5–15
Segmented neutrophils (x 10^9/l)	24.3	39	13.4	10.6	8.4	3.9–12
Band neutrophils (x 10^9/l)	1.5	1.9	1.0	2.3	0.5	0–1.0
Lymphocytes (x 10^9/l)	4.9	1.4	1.5	0.9	0.8	0.8–3.6
Eosinophils (x 10^9/l)	0	4.2	0.3	0.8	0.5	0–1.8
Platelets (x 10^9/l)	Increased	520	–	Increased	–	200–500

Figure 5.1: Haematology of a dog with iron deficiency anaemia.

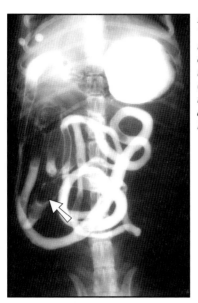

Figure 5.2: Ventrodorsal radiograph showing ovoid filling defect in small intestine (arrow) of a dog 30 minutes after oral administration of barium.

PATHOPHYSIOLOGY

Sixty five per cent of body iron occurs in haemoglobin, 3% in myoglobin, 2% in enzymes and 30% in the storage forms of haemosiderin and ferritin. During iron deficiency, iron stores are depleted first, while blood haemoglobin concentrations are relatively spared. Once iron deficiency has progressed to the point of causing anaemia, body stores of iron will have been completely depleted. With iron replacement therapy, haemoglobin concentrations increase before body stores are replenished. Therapy for iron deficiency must therefore be continued well beyond the time it takes to return the haematocrit to normal.

Dietary iron is absorbed primarily in the upper small intestine and is carried in the plasma bound to a carrier protein, transferrin. Transferrin is manufac-

tured in the liver, and liver iron stores may regulate production. As iron stores are increased, less transferrin is produced. Iron bound to transferrin circulates in the plasma and ultimately ends up in the bone marrow where iron is released into the developing red blood cell. Haemoglobin production controls red cell division and release from the marrow. In the normal state the red cell is released from the marrow when a critical concentration of haemoglobin is reached inside the cell (about 33%). With iron deficiency, insufficient haemoglobin production occurs and the red cells continue to divide in order to approach the necessary haemoglobin concentration. Although the 33% haemoglobin concentration point is never reached (resulting in hypochromic cells), the extra division produces smaller (microcytic) cells. Thus the typical red cells produced during periods of iron deficiency are hypochromic and microcytic.

Haemoglobin in red cells circulates until the red cell's life span is reached. Old red cells are phagocytosed by cells of the mononuclear phagocytic system (MPS), and the haemoglobin is degraded to yield iron. When there are abundant body stores, iron is stored intracellularly as ferritin or haemosiderin. Ferritin is the more labile of the two storage forms and can more readily release its iron when required. Water-soluble ferritin molecules will denature if not used and form large water insoluble aggregates called haemosiderin. Haemosiderin can be seen on examination of bone marrow and in histological biopsy samples with special staining. Because ferritin is water soluble, it is lost during the staining procedure and cannot be seen. Iron obtained from the breakdown of haemoglobin may be released from the MPS cell, bound to transferrin, taken back to the bone marrow and reutilized to produce haemoglobin. Figure 5.3 shows this route of iron conservation.

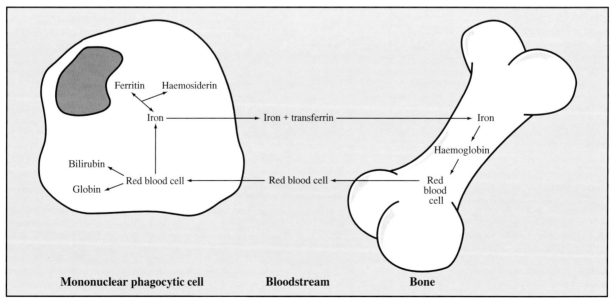

Figure 5.3: The body is able to reutilize iron from the breakdown of haemoglobin within mononuclear phagocytic cells. The iron binds to transferrin and is returned to the bone marrow and used to produce more haemoglobin.

The body is extremely efficient at iron conservation, and only small amounts of iron are lost in the urine, faeces, hair and squamous cells. The total daily iron loss is about 1 to 2 mg and intestinal absorption easily equals that amount. Blood is a rich source of iron, and chronic blood loss can therefore create iron deficiency. Blood contains about 0.5 mg of iron per millilitre. Thus a blood loss of 10 ml will create an iron deficit of 5 mg, which is greater than twice the body's normal daily loss.

CAUSES OF IRON DEFICIENCY

The major causes of iron deficiency in animals are summarized in Figure 5.4. Iron deficiency is quite common in young animals and is accepted as a normal phenomenon. Studies of normal blood values in kittens and puppies have established that the PCV is normal at birth but soon decreases, and a microcytic hypochromic anaemia develops. After animals are weaned, the PCV and red blood cell indices return to normal. The development of anaemia in kittens can be lessened by giving iron, suggesting iron deficiency as its cause (Weiser and Kociba, 1983).

Insufficient intake
Newborn animals
Blood loss
Internal parasitism (e.g. severe hookworm infestation)
External parasitism (e.g. severe flea infestation)
Bleeding gastrointestinal neoplasm or ulcer
Repeated phlebotomies from blood donors or polycythaemic patients
Rapid erythropoiesis
Erythropoietin therapy of anaemia

Figure 5.4: *Causes of iron deficiency.*

Iron deficiency in young animals is common because milk is low in iron. From birth until weaning, animals fed exclusively on a milk diet must rely upon their own stores of iron to create haemoglobin. In piglets, supplementation of iron at birth is economically important to increase growth rate, increase resistance to infection and decrease mortality, but this has not seemed necessary in other domestic species, even though iron deficiency is recognized (Mahaffey, 1986). In humans, iron deficiency in childhood may have damaging long-term consequences and should be prevented (Lozoff *et al.*, 1991; Oski, 1993). Further studies need to address the potential importance of neonatal iron deficiency in small animals.

Iron deficiency in older animals is most commonly caused by chronic blood loss. Parasites, bleeding neoplasms or ulcers and repeated phlebotomies are potential causes of iron deficiency (Comer, 1990). To create iron deficiency, blood loss must be chronic as body iron stores can correct a single bleeding episode. Blood loss must also be external to create iron deficiency. Bleeding into body cavities (haemoperitoneum, haemothorax, haematoma formation) or haemolysis will not cause iron depletion as the red cells will be phagocytosed and their iron reutilized.

Erythropoietin therapy may induce a profound erythropoiesis and increased demand for iron. Patients who have renal failure, borderline nutritional status and poor response to erythropoietin therapy may benefit from iron supplementation.

TESTS OF IRON METABOLISM

A common approach to the anaemic patient should include a complete blood count with reticulocyte and platelet counts, biochemical profile, urinalysis and faecal flotation. If the cause of anaemia is not readily apparent and iron deficiency is suspected, a radiographic barium study and testing for faecal occult blood should be considered, as the gastrointestinal system is the most common site of occult blood loss (Comer, 1990). Tests that are helpful to confirm the diagnosis of iron deficiency are listed below (Stone and Freden, 1990).

Haematology
With iron deficiency the development of a microcytic hypochromic anaemia is classic. The mean corpuscular volume (MCV) decreases more reliably than the mean corpuscular haemoglobin concentration (MCHC) (Weiser and O'Grady, 1983; Fulton *et al.*, 1988). A histogram graphically depicts the varying sizes of red cells and may be a more sensitive indicator of iron deficiency than a single MCV value. Iron deficiency is shown by an increase in the red cell distribution width (RDW), as shown in Figure 5.5. In humans, RDW is the first abnormal parameter to develop after depletion of bone marrow iron, occurring before serum iron concentration decreases (Oski, 1993). Red cells become less deformable during iron deficiency, and erythrocyte fragmentation may therefore be present. Thrombocytosis has frequently been observed with iron deficiency and may be associated with chronic blood loss (Schloesser *et al.*, 1965).

Serum iron concentration
Serum iron concentrations are expected to be low with iron deficiency. Serum iron will, however, also be low with acute or chronic inflammatory reactions, hypothyroidism and renal disease. Increased serum iron concentrations have been associated with glucocorti-

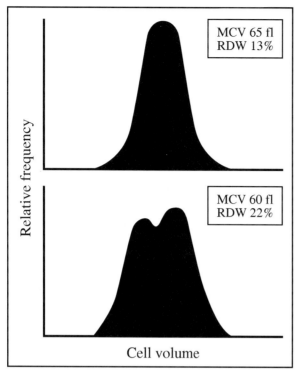

Figure 5.5: *Idealized histograms of normal (above) and iron deficient (below) canine erythrocytes. The widening of the curve in iron deficient erythrocytes represents a bipopulation of microcytic and normocytic red cells. MCV, mean corpuscular volume; RDW, red cell distribution width.*

coid administration, parenteral iron therapy and liver disease (Kaneko, 1980; Smith, 1992). Concentrations of serum iron also fluctuate on a daily basis.

Total iron binding capacity and transferrin saturation

Total iron binding capacity (TIBC) is the amount of iron that may potentially be held in the bound state in a given amount of blood. This value is an indirect measure of the amount of transferrin in the blood since transferrin is the major protein carrying iron. TIBC can be measured by flooding a blood sample with iron, removing the unbound portion, and determining the serum iron concentration. The per cent saturation of transferrin is calculated with TIBC and serum resting iron concentration. In the normal animal, serum iron concentration is about 100 µg/dl and TIBC is about 300 µg/dl, therefore the normal per cent saturation of transferrin is 100/300 or around 33%.

Iron deficiency causes serum iron concentration to decrease and transferrin saturation to fall. Less than 15% transferrin saturation is highly suggestive of iron deficiency (Weiser and O'Grady, 1983). Serum TIBC is higher than normal in humans with iron deficiency due to increased hepatic production of transferrin, but in the dog, transferrin production does not seem to increase with iron deficiency (Weeks *et al.*, 1990).

Erythrocyte protoporphyrin

Increased protoporphyrin concentrations are expected with iron deficiency. Protoporphyrin is an intermediate step in the production of haemoglobin, and when iron is limited, concentrations of this compound increase (Weeks *et al.*, 1990). Protoporphyrin concentrations may also be increased by lead poisoning and chronic inflammation.

Serum ferritin

Ferritin is a protein which stores iron. It is especially found in cells of the MPS in the liver, spleen and bone marrow. A small amount of circulating ferritin has been discovered and is believed to originate from the liver and spleen. The exact function of circulating ferritin is not known, but the serum concentration has been found to correlate well with total body iron stores (Weeks *et al.*, 1989). When iron stores are decreased the serum ferritin concentrations are low. Ferritin is an 'acute phase protein' and concentrations may be increased by an acute inflammatory insult. Increased concentrations have also been found in association with certain neoplasms (Newlands *et al.*, 1994).

Bone marrow iron

Bone marrow smears can be evaluated for iron stores with special staining. Bone marrow macrophages store iron if body stores are adequate. Bone marrow iron will be absent if iron depletion has progressed to the point of causing anaemia. This is the most accurate method of estimating body iron stores but has the disadvantage of being an invasive test. Bone marrow in the cat may not contain stainable iron in the normal state (Harvey, 1997).

In summary, the typical anaemia of iron deficiency is microcytic and hypochromic or normochromic with increased erythrocyte fragmentation, increased platelet numbers, low serum iron concentration, normal to increased TIBC, low transferrin saturation, increased erythrocyte protoporphyrin concentration, low serum ferritin concentration and iron absent from the bone marrow.

TREATMENT OF IRON DEFICIENCY

The therapeutic dose of iron is 2 to 10 mg/kg per day, based on the iron content of the preparation. Ferrous sulphate, ferrous fumarate and ferrous gluconate may all be effective, however ferrous sulphate has been recommended as the treatment of choice for iron deficiency (Harvey *et al.*, 1982). Food reduces absorption of iron in humans and it may be preferable to give iron in the fasting state, even if the dose must be reduced (Hillman, 1990). Side effects of giving iron orally are primarily gastrointestinal and may include abdominal pain, vomiting, diarrhoea or constipation.

Injectable iron dextran may be indicated in patients with malabsorptive disease or when intolerance to oral iron prevents effective therapy. Pain at the injection site may be prolonged and therefore intramuscular injection is discouraged unless specifically indicated. Iron dextran is given at 50 mg per cat i.m. for 18-day-old kittens (Weiser and Kociba, 1983) or 10 mg/kg i.m. as a single dose for adult dogs and cats (Mahaffey, 1986). Humans that are not compliant with oral therapy may be given iron dextran intravenously (Andrews, 1999) but the author has no experience with this method of administration in animals.

Response to therapy can be evaluated by increases in PCV and may be evident as early as 4 to 7 days after beginning iron therapy. The PCV should be normal or nearly so within 4 weeks of therapy. If the response is inadequate by this time, the diagnosis should be reconsidered.

Duration of therapy is governed by the need to replace iron stores. If iron therapy is stopped after the haematocrit has returned to normal, but before replenishment of iron stores, the animal is at risk of recurrence of iron deficiency should further bleeding occur. Iron supplementation is therefore recommended for 4-9 months to adequately replace body stores (Mahaffey, 1986). Iron stores could be evaluated by monitoring concentrations of serum ferritin or bone marrow iron if deemed necessary.

REFERENCES

Andrews NC (1999) Disorders of iron metabolism. *New England Journal of Medicine* **341**, 1986-1995

Comer KM (1990) Anemia as a feature of primary gastrointestinal neoplasia. *Compendium of Continuing Education for the Practicing Veterinarian* **12**, 13-19

Fulton R, Weiser MG, Freshman JL, Gasper PW, Fettman PW (1988) Electronic and morphologic characterization of erythrocytes of an adult cat with iron deficiency anemia. *Veterinary Pathology* **25**, 521-523

Harvey JW (1997) Bone marrow examination. In: *Proceedings of the 15th Annual College of Veterinary Internal Medicine Forum.* p. 12

Harvey JW, French TW, Meyer DJ (1982) Chronic iron deficiency anemia in dogs. *Journal of the American Animal Hospital Association* **18**, 946-960

Hillman RS (1990) Drugs effective in iron deficiency and other hypochromic anemias. In: *The Pharmacological Basis of Therapeutics, 8th edn*, ed. A Goodman Gilman *et al.*, pp. 1282-1292. Pergamon Press, New York

Kaneko JJ (1980) Iron metabolism. In: *Clinical Biochemistry of Domestic Animals, 3rd edn*, ed. JJ Kaneko, pp. 649-669. Academic Press, New York

Lozoff F, Jimenez E, Wolf AW (1991) Long-term developmental outcome of infants with iron deficiency. *New England Journal of Medicine* **325**, 687-694

Mahaffey EA (1986) Disorders of iron metabolism. In: *Current Veterinary Therapy, 9th edn*, ed. RW Kirk, pp. 521-524. WB Saunders, Philadelphia

Newlands CE, Houstoh DM, Vasconcelos DV (1994) Hyperferritinemia associated with malignant histiocytosis in a dog. *Journal of the American Veterinary Medical Association* **205**, 849-851

Oski FA (1993) Iron deficiency in infancy and childhood. *New England Journal of Medicine* **329**, 190-193

Schloesser LL, Kipp MA, Wenzel FJ (1965) Thrombocytosis in iron-deficiency anemia. *Journal of Laboratory and Clinical Medicine* **66**, 107-114

Smith JE (1992) Iron metabolism in dogs and cats. *Compendium of Continuing Education for the Practicing Veterinarian* **14**, 39-43

Stone MS, Freden GO (1990) Differentiation of anemia of inflammation from anemia of iron deficiency. *Compendium of Continuing Education for the Practicing Veterinarian* **12**, 963-967

Weeks BR, Smith JE, Northrop JK (1989) Relationship of serum ferritin and iron concentrations and serum total iron-binding capacity to nonheme iron stores in dogs. *American Journal of Veterinary Research* **50**, 198-200

Weeks BR, Smith JE, Stadler CK (1990) Effect of dietary iron content on hematologic and other measures of iron adequacy in dogs. *Journal of the American Veterinary Medical Association* **196**, 749-753

Weiser G, O'Grady M (1983) Erythrocyte volume distribution analysis and hematologic changes in dogs with iron deficiency anemia. *Veterinary Pathology* **20**, 230-241

Weiser MG, Kociba GJ (1983) Sequential changes in erythrocyte volume distribution and microcytosis associated with iron deficiency in kittens. *Veterinary Pathology* **20**, 1-12

(ii) Anaemia of Chronic Renal Disease

Andreas Hans Hasler

INTRODUCTION

Anaemia is a common problem of cats and dogs with chronic renal disease (CRD). As the condition progresses towards end-stage kidney disease, anaemia develops in virtually every patient (Cowgill, 1992). The severity of the anaemia correlates with the degree of renal disease as expressed by the creatinine and/or the urea concentration (King *et al.*, 1992). The signs and symptoms of anaemia in patients with chronic renal failure (CRF) do not differ from those seen in other patients with chronic anaemia, and include pallor of the mucous membranes and skin, tachycardia, tachypnoea, lethargy, weakness and anorexia.

PATHOPHYSIOLOGY

The pathophysiology of anaemia in animals with CRD is complex and may involve bone marrow failure, blood loss or haemolysis. Failure of erythropoiesis due to deficiency of erythropoietin (EPO) production by diseased kidneys is the major contributing factor in both human and veterinary patients (Cowgill, 1992).

Erythropoietin deficiency

A classic endocrine feedback system tightly regulates the red cell mass under normal circumstances (Erslev, 1990). EPO is the key factor in the regulation of red cell mass and erythrocyte production (Figure 5.6). It is a polypeptide hormone that belongs to the group of haematopoietic growth factors. It has a high degree of amino acid sequence homology among mammals, which explains the interspecies cross reactivity of hormone assays and the use of heterologous recombinant human EPO (rHuEPO) in replacement therapy. Renal tissue hypoxia, but not the number or mass of circulating red cells, stimulates the renal production of EPO and release of the hormone to the plasma. When the oxygen tension is sufficiently low, the oxygen sensor (believed to be a member of the haem protein family) is in the deoxy conformation and triggers the synthesis of EPO. The site of production of EPO in the kidney has been localized to the interstitial cells of the inner cortex laying adjacent to the proximal tubules. Cells that produce EPO may be active or inactive, and the number of active cells paral-

lels the degree of hypoxia. In non-uraemic patients, serum EPO concentrations are inversely correlated with the haematocrit, which means that EPO concentrations increase in proportion to the severity of anaemia (Figure 5.7). EPO acts in the bone marrow as both a growth factor and a differentiating factor for erythrocyte precursor cells. The stimulation of erythropoiesis results in an increase in circulating red cells, and as a consequence oxygen-carrying capacity is enhanced. The improved renal oxygenation is detected by the oxygen sensor in the kidney, and renal EPO production decreases.

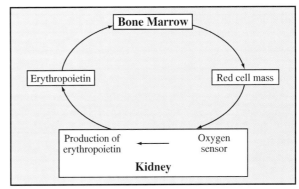

Figure 5.6: Synthesis and regulation of erythropoietin.

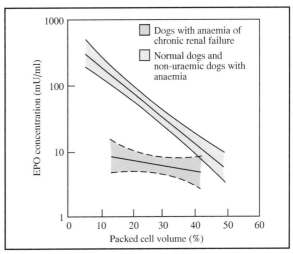

Figure 5.7: Serum erythropoietin (EPO) concentrations in healthy dogs and anaemic dogs compared with dogs with anaemia of chronic renal failure. Reproduced from Giger (1992) Erythropoietin and its clinical use. Compendium on Continuing Education for the Practicing Veterinarian *14, 25–35, with permission.*

By contrast, uraemic patients have an impaired regulatory loop and their ability to produce EPO in response to tissue hypoxia is abolished or decreased. Numerous studies in humans and animals have shown that serum EPO concentrations in uraemic patients are inappropriately low when compared with normal reference values (Figure 5.7). Anaemic dogs with CRF generally have low or normal plasma EPO concentrations. Mildly increased EPO concentrations may occasionally be found but are often inadequately increased in view of the degree of the anaemia (King *et al.*, 1992). In an experimental model of decreased renal mass, the EPO response paralleled the remaining functional renal mass (Oishi *et al.*, 1993). It has yet to be established whether the decrease in plasma EPO concentration is due to an impaired oxygen-sensing mechanism, a decreased synthesis of EPO or both.

Myelofibrosis and hyperparathyroidism

Secondary hyperparathyroidism is a common sequela to CRD. An increase in parathyroid hormone (PTH) concentration may lead to myelofibrosis (Rao *et al.*, 1993), and the fibrotic bone marrow has a decreased erythropoietic potential. Further, a direct inhibitory effect of PTH on erythropoiesis has been proposed. One study showed that anaemic dogs with CRD had significantly higher PTH values when compared with non-anaemic dogs with CRD (King *et al.*, 1992). PTH seems to influence erythrocyte survival time, as decreased survival time has been shown in dogs with surgically induced renal failure, which normalized after parathyroidectomy (King *et al.*, 1992). In addition to the role of PTH and myelofibrosis in the pathogenesis of the anaemia of CRD, there is much interest in the relationship between PTH, myelofibrosis and response to replacement therapy with exogenous EPO. Hyperparathyroidism and myelofibrosis are thought to be one reason for EPO resistance, and correction of hyperparathyroidism has been shown to improve the response to exogenous EPO (Rao *et al.*, 1993).

Increased osmotic fragility

Osmotic fragility of erythrocytes is increased in humans with CRD, however a single study of osmotic fragility in dogs with CRD did not find changes in this parameter (King *et al.*, 1992). These results suggest that altered osmotic fragility is not a major contributor to the anaemia of CRD in dogs.

Gastrointestinal and other bleeding

Bleeding into the gastrointestinal tract may be the most common cause of blood loss anaemia in uraemic patients and be manifest clinically as haematemesis, haematochezia or melaena. Gastrin has been implicated in the development of gastric ulcers. Gastrin concentration is increased as its metabolism in the diseased kidney is reduced. The resulting hypergastrinaemia increases

acid production leading to mucosal irritation, ulcers and consequently haemorrhage. Gastrointestinal bleeding may go undetected for a long time and, if persistent, can cause iron deficiency. Uraemia also has a direct effect on platelet function and hence may lead to haemorrhage.

Iron deficiency anaemia

Many dogs and cats with CRD have subnormal serum iron concentration and transferrin saturation below 15% (Cowgill, 1992). It is not clear whether this is related to decreased iron intake, diminished iron absorption or excessive iron loss.

CLINICAL EVALUATION

The minimal database for anaemia of CRD consists of history, physical examination, complete blood count (including red cell indices and reticulocyte count) and a complete serum chemistry panel including albumin, phosphate, blood urea nitrogen (BUN), creatinine, calcium and a complete urinalysis (Figure 5.8). Stool analysis for parasites and occult blood may be helpful to exclude gastrointestinal bleeding. The diagnosis of CRD should be based on findings consistent with the disease. It must be remembered that other diseases (e.g. hypoadrenocorticism) may cause concurrent azotaemia, isosthenuria and anaemia.

Complete blood count

Packed cell volume (PCV) is commonly used to assess anaemia in veterinary medicine. The RBC count or the haemoglobin concentration can also be used to document anaemia, but for simplicity only PCV is mentioned in the following discussion. The degree of anaemia should be re-evaluated once the animal is rehydrated. Patients with CRD are often dehydrated, and the 'haemoconcentration' may mask the full extent of the anaemia. As normal values for cats are lower than for dogs, the terms mild, moderate and severe anaemia imply different values in each species (Figure 5.9).

Red cell indices characterize the anaemia according to size and haemoglobin content of the erythrocytes. A normocytic–normochromic pattern occurs in the anaemia of erythropoietin deficiency. Any other pattern suggests a different form of anaemia (e.g. microcytic–hypochromic anaemia due to iron deficiency).

Reticulocyte count

The presence of a regenerative anaemia (Figure 5.9) rules out lack of EPO, and other causes of anaemia must be evaluated (e.g. haemolysis, gastrointestinal bleeding). Bone marrow examination is generally not indicated for primary evaluation of anaemia of CRD. The exception may be to document myelofibrosis or the presence of rHuEPO-antibodies.

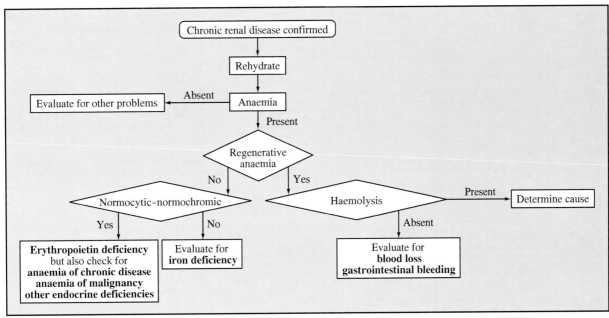

Figure 5.8: *Algorithm for diagnostic evaluation of anaemia of chronic renal disease.*

	PCV (normal range)	PCV with anaemia			Reticulocyte count in regenerative anaemia
		Mild	Moderate	Severe	
Dog	35–55%	30–35	25–30	<25	>60 x 10⁹/l
Cat	27–45%	23–27	18–23	<18	>50 x 10⁹/l

Figure 5.9: *Definition of the severity of anaemia in the dog and cat. PCV, packed cell volume.*

Blood loss

Any blood loss should be investigated. A concurrent hypoalbuminaemia may suggest blood loss, or a high BUN:creatinine ratio may suggest gastrointestinal bleeding. Although parasites (e.g. fleas, hookworms) in otherwise healthy animals rarely cause significant anaemia, they may contribute to anaemia in the patient with CRD.

Serum EPO concentration

It is not necessary to determine serum EPO concentrations to diagnose EPO-deficient anaemia of CRD. To the author's knowledge there is no study that suggests that EPO concentration is a useful prognostic indicator of the progress of the anaemia of CRD or the response to treatment. The finding of an appropriately increased EPO concentration in an anaemic animal may, however, direct the clinician to search for other causes of anaemia (e.g. blood loss).

PTH concentration

Determination of plasma PTH concentration may sometimes be helpful in cases of CRD, for example those animals that may be treated with calcitriol.

Hypertension

Arterial hypertension is a common complication of CRD, which may occur in up to 93% of cats or up to

69% of dogs with CRD (Polzin *et al.*, 1995). However, there is a transatlantic debate as to whether human values should be applied to dogs and whether hypertension in dogs with CRD is a substantial problem (Michell, 1996). Although overt clinical signs such as tortuous retinal vessels will alert the clinician, silent hypertension often goes unnoticed, as measuring blood pressure and interpretation of the results can be challenging in cats and dogs. Pre-existing hypertension is a relative contraindication for the administration of rHuEPO and if present should be controlled before such therapy.

TREATMENT

The anaemia of CRD is multifactorial, and treatment must therefore be tailored to the underlying disease. The approach should be practical and cost effective. The initial management should aim to minimize blood loss, whereas subsequent therapy should be directed towards increasing red cell mass.

Gastrointestinal and other blood loss

Patients with CRD require close monitoring and hence frequent blood sampling is needed for laboratory tests. Repeated blood collection may quickly render cats and small dogs anaemic. Testing should therefore be optimized and restricted where possible. Intestinal parasites (e.g. hookworms) and flea infestation should be addressed with proper therapy. Gastric ulceration may be alleviated with the use of H_2-blockers (e.g. cimetidine 5–10 mg/kg tid).

Iron deficiency is treated with oral iron sulphate. Starting doses of 100 to 300 mg/day for dogs and 50–100 mg/day for cats have been recommended. Side effects of oral iron supplementation include vomiting and diarrhoea. Therapy should be evaluated by monitoring plasma iron concentrations and transferrin saturation.

Blood transfusions

Prior to the availability of rHuEPO, the anaemia of CRD was treated by transfusion of whole blood or packed red blood cells. This approach remains the modality of choice in an acute situation where rapid improvement is a necessity. However, there are several inherent problems associated with such transfusions, which make this procedure unsuitable for long-term management:

- Even with careful crossmatching, incompatibilities may develop with repeated transfusions, and prohibit further use
- Few veterinary clinics have reliable access to blood products
- It is nearly impossible to restore the PCV to the normal range in animals with anaemia of CRD, thus the patient remains anaemic.

Recombinant human EPO

Following the discovery that the major determinant of uraemic anaemia is a relative or absolute deficiency of EPO, treatment has focused on replacement with exogenous EPO. Since the first trial in human medicine in 1985, using rHuEPO, a huge body of literature has shown the efficacy and benefits of treatment with EPO in humans and animals. rHuEPO has emerged as the mainstay for correction of uraemic anaemia in humans (Erslev and Besarab, 1997).

Benefits

Treatment with rHuEPO produces a dose-dependent increase in PCV in virtually every patient (Erslev and Besarab, 1997). It can be expected that the PCV will increase by 0.5–1% per day, and usually the red cell mass can be restored within a month (Cowgill et al., 1998). Thrombocytosis, but not leucocytosis, may accompany the increase in PCV. It is unclear whether this is a sign of iron deficiency or a direct effect of rHuEPO.

In addition to improvements in PCV, the most impressive benefits of effective rHuEPO therapy are significant subjective improvements in wellbeing, increased appetite and increased physical activity, documented in both humans and animals (Erslev and Besarab, 1997; Cowgill, 1995). The gain in appetite improves nutritional status, and resolution of hypokalaemia is reported in cats (Cowgill, 1995).

Indications

Treatment with rHuEPO is indicated in patients with moderate to severe anaemia caused by EPO deficiency and where clinical judgement suggests a possible benefit.

Contraindications

There are relative, but no absolute, contraindications to the use of rHuEPO in dogs and cats, one such case being animals with mild anaemia. Although these animals might benefit from an increased PCV and exhibit the same increase in wellbeing and quality of life, the potential for development of the major side effect (the possible development of antibodies) and the cost of therapy should be considered and discussed with the owner.

rHuEPO preparations

rHuEPO is available as epoietin alpha (Epogen®, Amgen Inc., USA; Eprex®, Cilag, Switzerland) or epoietin beta (Recormon®, Boehringer, Mannheim, Germany). The former preparation uses human albumin as a carrier whereas the latter does not. Some forms of rHuEPO require reconstitution with saline. All preparations must be stored refrigerated. Most treatments in animals have been with epoietin alpha (Epogen®). All commercial rHuEPO preparations are not licensed for use in animals, and it is advisable to receive written consent from the client.

Injection

The subcutaneous route is most often used in veterinary medicine as it is easy to use and can therefore be administered by owners at home. Owners should be instructed on how to inject rHuEPO (similar to insulin injections). It is conceivable that injection over the lateral chest and abdomen area leads to the most reliable absorption (similar to insulin injections).

Starting treatment

Replacement therapy can be divided into an initiation and maintenance phase. The initiation phase is characterized by an increase in PCV, and the dose is higher during this phase (Figure 5.10). The recommended dose is 100 U/kg three times a week. This has been shown to promote an erythropoietic response in most animals. In cases of hypertension or less severe anaemia, the smaller dose of 50 U/kg three times a week can be given. This dose is continued until the PCV has reached the lower end of the target value (30–40% for cats and 35–45% for dogs), which signals the end of the

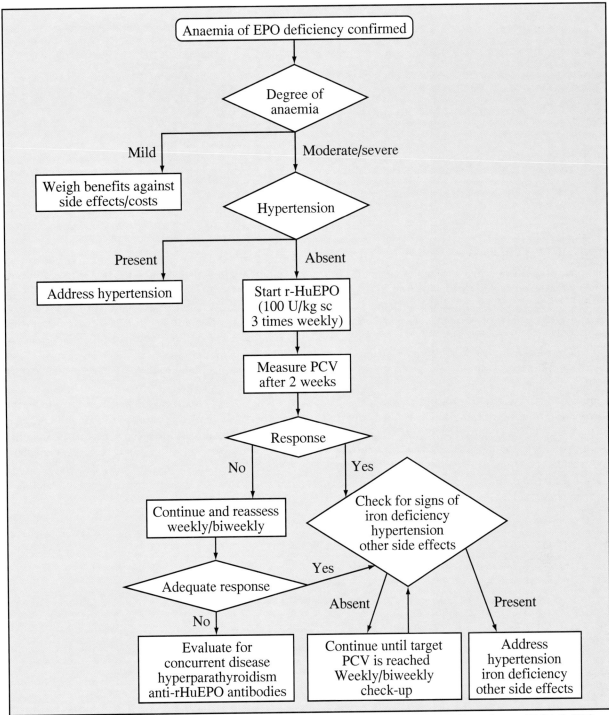

Figure 5.10: *Algorithm for treatment of anaemia of erythropoietin (EPO) deficiency with recombinant human EPO (rHuEPO. PCV, packed cell volume.*

initiating phase (usually within 4–8 weeks). At this point, the dose and interval is reduced and then titrated to effect (Figure 5.11). The reaction to changes in dose or interval is slow, and therefore it takes about 3 weeks to assess the impact of a different regimen. Hence, changes in rHuEPO dose or interval should not be made more than once every 3 weeks.

Once the lower end of the target interval is reached, the interval can be reduced to twice weekly, with the same dose (100 U/kg). If the PCV continues

to increase, the dose should be reduced to 75 U/kg once weekly. If the target PCV is not reached within 8–12 weeks, the dose can be titrated in steps of 25–50 U/kg. Besides increasing the dose, a thorough evaluation for resistance should be undertaken. The stimulated erythropoiesis puts a high demand on iron stores, which makes concurrent supplementation a necessity. Dosages of oral iron sulphate of 100–300 mg/day for dogs and 50–100 mg/day for cats have been recommended.

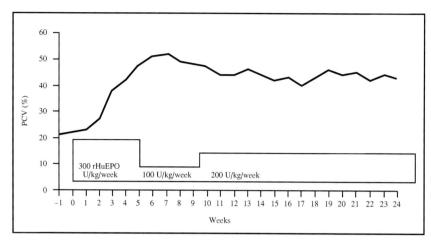

Figure 5.11: Response to treatment with recombinant human erythropoietin (rHuEPO). rHuEPO was given to a female American Cocker Spaniel with clinical and laboratory evidence of anaemia due to chronic renal disease. The starting dose was 300 U/kg/week divided three times weekly, and the packed cell volume (PCV) started to increase after one week and entered the normal range within 3 weeks. The PCV continued to increase above 50%, and the dose was reduced to 100 U/kg/week. A stable PCV in the normal range was reached, but the dose had to be increased to 200 U/kg/week.

Safety and side effects

There is no evidence that treatment with rHuEPO accelerates the progression of renal disease in humans (Jacobs, 1995). Local pain at the injection site of epoetin alpha (but not beta) is reported in human studies.

The most detrimental side effect of treatment is the development of antibodies against the rHuEPO molecule, which bind to both exogenous and endogenous EPO. Consequently, the body becomes resistant to rHuEPO with time, and a progressive decline of PCV will occur (Figure 5.12). Antibodies do not commonly appear until the fourth week of treatment, but may occur at any time thereafter. Whereas the overall incidence of anti-rHuEPO antibodies may only be 30%, such antibodies developed (along with refractory anaemia) in two of three dogs that were treated for more than 90 days and in five of seven cats that were treated for more than 180 days (Cowgill *et al.*, 1998; Cowgill, 1995). These results show that long-term treatment with rHuEPO is associated with a high degree of antibody stimulation. Although most authors claim that the antibodies disappear upon withdrawal, the memory immune response prohibits a second trial with rHuEPO. These patients will become dependent on blood transfusion. The major sign of antibodies is resistance to treatment after a preliminary response. Unfortunately, there is no commercial test for determining anti-rHuEPO antibody. Bone marrow examination with a myeloid:erythroid ratio of greater than eight is suggestive of resistance to EPO (Cowgill, 1995).

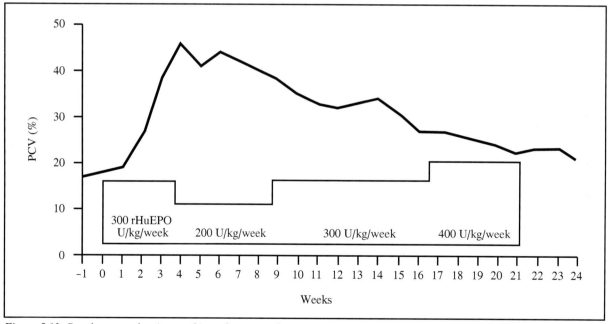

Figure 5.12: Development of anti-recombinant human erythropoietin (anti-rHuEPO) antibodies. Treatment with rHuEPO 300 U/kg/week was initiated in an 11 year old spayed Miniature Schnauzer with anaemia of chronic renal disease. After an initial response and normalization of anaemia (packed cell volume (PCV) of 47%), the dose of rHuEPO was reduced. The PCV decreased, and when a PCV of 38% was reached the dose of rHuEPO was increased to the initiation dose. No response was noted, and the rHuEPO was increased further to 400 U/kg/week. The PCV continued to decrease. As no other cause for rHuEPO resistance was found, antibody formation against rHuEPO was suspected and treatment discontinued.

Overshooting treatment (dose too high or intervals too frequent) may result in absolute polycythaemia. Treatment should be withheld, and phlebotomy may be necessary. This is one reason why incremental dose therapy is recommended.

Systemic hypertension can develop in patients with no prior record of blood pressure problems. The mechanisms by which rHuEPO therapy may increase blood pressure include increased blood viscosity, loss of hypoxic vasodilation and a direct vascular effect via increased synthesis of endothelin and other vasoactive substances (Mashio, 1995). Whether hypertension is responsible for the seizures seen in animals treated with rHuEPO is unclear.

Resistance to treatment

Some patients may require much higher doses of rHuEPO than others, creating the concept of EPO resistance, which parallels the insulin resistance that may occur in the therapy of diabetes mellitus (Figure 5.13).

Development of anti-rHuEPO antibodies
Iron deficiency
Neoplastic disease
Secondary hyperparathyroidism
Inflammatory states, infection
Malnutrition

Figure 5.13: Possible causes of resistance to human recombinant erythropoietin (rHuEPO).

FUTURE DIRECTIONS

Replacement therapy with rHuEPO has limitations owing to the heterologous nature of the molecule. Development of antibodies against rHuEPO is not a feature of replacement treatment in humans, and hence it is conceivable that use of a homologous product for dogs (recombinant canine EPO) and cats (recombinant feline EPO) would prevent the induction of antibodies against EPO. The EPO gene in dogs has been cloned, and its activity in vitro and in vivo has been proven in a mouse model (Macleod *et al.*, 1998). Clinical studies are presently under way at several veterinary institutions in the United States, however no information concerning the commercial release of rCaEPO is available. As long as heterologous EPO is used, a commercial assay for anti-rHuEPO antibodies would improve the assessment of antibody status and resistance.

The correction of anaemia might improve quality of life and alleviate some of the uraemic problems but it does not stop progression of renal disease, and other aspects of the uraemic syndrome may dictate euthanasia. Haemodialysis is not generally available for the management of renal disease in dogs and cats, but with more widespread use, life span and quality of life could be improved. Renal transplantation in cats and dogs is restricted to only a few places. The problems to overcome are initially of an ethical nature. Successful renal transplantation will, however, be a major advancement and will resolve the anaemia of CRD along with other uraemic problems.

REFERENCES

Cowgill LD (1992) Pathophysiology and management of anaemia in chronic progressive renal failure. *Seminars in Veterinary Medicine and Surgery Small Animal* **7**, 175-182

Cowgill LD (1995) CVT Update: Use of recombinant human erythropoietin. In: *Current Veterinary Therapy, 12th edn*, ed. JD Bonagura and RW Kirk, pp. 961-962. WB Saunders, Philadelphia

Cowgill LD, James KM *et al.* (1998) Use of recombinant-human-erythropoietin for management of anemia in dogs and cats with renal failure. *Journal of the American Veterinary Medical Association* **212**, 521-530

Erslev AJ (1990) Erythropoietin. *Leukemia Research* **14**, 683-688

Erslev AJ and Besarab A (1997) Erythropoietin in the pathogenesis and treatment of the anemia of chronic renal failure [editorial]. *Kidney International* **51**, 622-630

Jacobs C (1995) Starting r-HuEPO in chronic renal failure: when, why, and how? *Nephrology Dialysis Transplantation* **10(suppl 2)**, 43-47

King LG, Giger U *et al.* (1992) Anemia of chronic renal failure in dogs. *Journal of Veterinary Internal Medicine* **6**, 264-270

Macleod JN, Tetreault JW *et al.* (1998) Expression and bioactivity of recombinant canine erythropoietin. *American Journal of Veterinary Research* **59**, 1144-1148

Mashio G (1995) Erythropoietin and systemic hypertension. *Nephrology Dialysis Transplantation* **10(suppl 2)**, 74-79

Michell AR (1996) Renal insufficiency and hypertension in dogs. In: *Proceedings of the 6th Annual congress of the European Society of Veterinary Internal Medicine*, ed. NL Veldhofen, J Rothuizen *et al.* pp. 50-51

Oishi A, Sakamoto H *et al.* (1993) Evaluation of erythropoietin production in dogs with reduced functional renal tissue. *Journal of Veterinary Medical Science* **55**, 543-548

Polzin DJ, Osborne CA, *et al.* (1995) Chronic renal failure. In: *Textbook of Veterinary Internal Medicine, 4th edn*, ed. SJ Ettinger and EC Feldman, pp. 1734-1760. WB Saunders, Philadelphia

Rao DS, Shih M *et al.* (1993) Effect of serum parathyroid hormone and bone marrow fibrosis on the response to erythropoietin in uremia. *New England Journal of Medicine* **328**, 171-175

(iii) Immune-Mediated Haemolytic Anaemia

Andrew Mackin

INTRODUCTION

Immune-mediated haemolytic anaemia (IMHA) is one of the most common causes of anaemia in small animals and is also one of the most prevalent immune-mediated diseases. Although IMHA is often rewarding to treat, it is also often fatal if misdiagnosed or treated inappropriately, and practitioners are advised to develop a working familiarity with the clinical signs, diagnosis and treatment of the condition.

IMHA can be subdivided into two main types: primary, idiopathic or autoimmune haemolytic anaemia (AIHA) and secondary IMHA. AIHA is a classic autoimmune disorder with no recognized underlying cause. It is the most frequent form of IMHA in dogs and also occurs in cats, albeit less commonly. Although AIHA can occur in dogs of any age, breed and sex, the condition typically affects young adult and middle-aged animals and is particularly common in certain breeds of dog such as Cocker Spaniels, English Springer Spaniels, Poodles, Old English Sheepdogs and Collies (Day and Penhale, 1992; Klag *et al.*, 1993; Day, 1996; Reimer *et al.*, 1999). Most studies report that the condition is more common in bitches, although several studies report no sex predilection (Jackson and Kruth, 1985; Halliwell and Gorman, 1989; Klag *et al.*, 1993; Thompson, 1995; Reimer *et al.*, 1999).

IMHA can also occur secondary to a wide range of pathological processes, so called secondary IMHA. Many different infectious, allergic, inflammatory and neoplastic causes of secondary IMHA have been suspected in dogs and cats (Jackson and Kruth, 1985; Jones and Gruffydd-Jones, 1991; Cotter, 1992; Lifton, 1999; Noble and Armstrong, 1999), based predominantly on associations with disease and extrapolation from similar phenomena in humans, although complete proof of causation is usually lacking. Relatively well documented causes of secondary IMHA include feline leukaemia virus (FeLV) or infections with *Haemobartonella felis* in cats (Miller, 1999), and recent vaccination or haemolymphatic neoplasia (particularly lymphoma) in dogs. Certain drugs may also trigger IMHA in small animals. Figure 5.14 lists the potential causes of secondary IMHA.

Drugs
Trimethoprim/sulphonamide*
Penicillins
Cephalosporins
Levamisole (dogs)*
Propylthiouracil (cats)*
Non-steroidal anti-inflammatory drugs such as phenylbutazone
Dipyrone
Quinidine
Chlorpromazine

Infectious/parasitic
Feline leukaemia virus infection*
Haemobartonellosis (especially *H. felis* in cats)*
Babesiosis*
Ehrlichiosis
Leishmaniasis
Dirofilariasis

Neoplastic
Lymphoproliferative diseases (especially lymphoma, leukaemia)*
Haemangiosarcoma

Miscellaneous
Post vaccinal*
Bee sting envenomation

Immunological
Systemic lupus erythematosus*
Transfusion reactions*
Neonatal isoerythrolysis (especially in cats)*
Antilymphocyte globulin therapy (transplantation patients)*

*Figure 5.14: Potential causes of secondary immune-mediated haemolytic anaemia. *Underlying causes that are either well documented in the dog and cat or strongly suspected on the basis of compelling anecdotal evidence.*

Secondary IMHA affects animals of any age, breed or sex and should be strongly suspected in patients presenting with a signalment atypical for AIHA, such as geriatric animals. Unlike the dog, IMHA in the cat is most commonly secondary (Halliwell and Gorman, 1989).

Distinguishing between primary and secondary IMHA is important for treatment to be effective. Although both conditions can be similar clinically and diagnostically, secondary IMHA will not respond well to treatment unless the underlying cause is eliminated and will recur during remission unless repeat exposure to the cause is avoided. Practitioners, however, probably overdiagnose primary or idiopathic IMHA because, without meticulous attention to history, physical examination and diagnostic testing, the underlying causes of secondary IMHA may be missed.

Although transfusion reactions and neonatal isoerythrolysis are types of IMHA they are not covered in this chapter (see Chapters 15 and 16).

MECHANISMS OF RED CELL DESTRUCTION

The mechanism underlying typical cases of IMHA is antibody-mediated cytotoxic (type II hypersensitivity) destruction of circulating erythrocytes. Although most cases share this common mechanism, the disease is otherwise heterogeneous: in AIHA, the most studied form of IMHA, both the pattern of immunoglobulin and complement involvement in destruction of red blood cells (RBCs) and the site of antibody attachment to RBC membranes varies widely between patients. Although the most common immunoglobulin type involved in AIHA is IgG, less commonly IgM or (rarely) IgA may also be implicated, along with variable involvement of complement (Jackson and Kruth, 1985; Jones *et al.*, 1990; Barker *et al.*, 1992, 1993; Klag *et al.*, 1993; Day, 1996). Antibodies may attach to various components of the RBC membrane, particularly (but not exclusively) glycophorins (Barker *et al.*, 1991; Barker and Elson, 1995).

In IMHA, antibody attachment to the membranes of RBCs triggers their destruction by several different mechanisms (Cotter, 1992; Jain, 1993). In severe cases, with high levels of antibody attachment and complement fixation, membranes may be so damaged that extracellular water leaks into the cytoplasm, causing swelling and rupture of the RBC while it is still in the circulation, so called intravascular haemolysis (Figure 5.15). Since IgM is better than IgG at complement fixation, intravascular haemolysis is more likely in IgM-mediated IMHA. In less severe cases of IMHA, antibody attachment and subsequent cell membrane damage leads to an accelerated rate of destruction of affected erythrocytes by tissue macrophages within the mononuclear phagocytic system (MPS), a process that occurs outside the circulation (extravascular haemolysis). Destruction of erythrocytes by the MPS is mediated by Fc receptors on the macrophage surface, which bind the Fc component of the antibodies attached to the RBC membranes (Figure 5.16). Because the MPS is located throughout the body, extravascular haemolysis can occur in many organs but typically is most pronounced in the liver and, particularly, the spleen. In some patients with high levels of anti-RBC antibodies, many individual antibodies can each bind to two different erythrocytes, a process that causes the cells to clump together (agglutinate). Patients with significant RBC agglutination typically have an increased rate of extravascular haemolysis, since clumping of RBC facilitates their removal by the MPS.

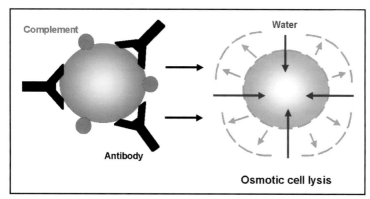

Figure 5.15: Mechanisms of intravascular haemolysis. High levels of antibody attachment and complement fixation can cause severe damage to circulating red blood cell (RBC) membranes. Because RBC contents such as haemoglobin are osmotically active, the resultant increase in membrane permeability allows extracellular water to leak across an osmotic gradient into the cell, leading to intravascular swelling and rupture of affected cells.

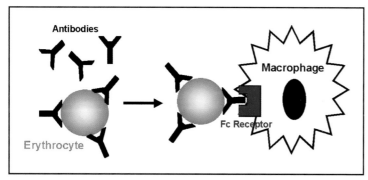

Figure 5.16: Mechanisms of extravascular haemolysis. The Fc component of anti-red blood cell (RBC) antibodies attached to RBC membranes is recognized and bound by Fc receptors located on the surface of tissue macrophages within the MPS. Although cell destruction by the MPS is part of the normal process by which the body removes ageing red cells from the circulation, high levels of antibody-mediated macrophage-RBC binding in patients with IMHA leads to a greatly increased rate of extravascular RBC damage and phagocytosis by tissue macrophages (erythrophagocytosis).

Typically, IMHA is caused by antibodies directed against circulating mature RBCs, with the bone marrow mounting a healthy regenerative response to the resultant anaemia (Jones and Gruffydd-Jones, 1991). In some patients, however, antibodies may also be directed against RBC precursors in the bone marrow at any stage in their development (Jonas *et al.*, 1987; Weiser, 1992). Haemolytic anaemia with an inappropriately poor regenerative response will develop if antibodies are directed against cell membrane components that are present both on mature RBCs and their marrow precursors. By contrast, if antibodies are directed against membrane components that are present only on RBC precursors in the bone marrow and not on mature RBCs, non-regenerative anaemia will develop without peripheral haemolysis. Pure red cell aplasia (PRCA), in which all stages of RBC precursor in the bone marrow are noticeably reduced or absent, is the most extreme form of this process (Jones and Gruffydd-Jones, 1991).

In AIHA, autoantibodies are directed against components of the membranes of the patient's own RBCs. Although the same process can occur with secondary IMHA, antibodies may alternatively be directed against a foreign antigen (such as a drug or virus) that is attached to the RBC membrane, against normal membrane components of the RBC that are antigenically similar to non-RBC antigens that are associated with the underlying disease process or against membrane components that are normally hidden but are exposed by the underlying disease.

CATEGORIES OF IMHA

Typical IMHA is caused by antibodies that exert their effects at body temperature, so called warm reactive antibodies. Some animals, however, have anti-RBC antibodies that are only reactive at much lower temperatures. Although such cold reactive antibodies usually cause minimal harmful effects, their presence may cause specific clinical syndromes. Classically, IMHA has been subdivided into five main categories (Halliwell and Gorman, 1989; Stewart and Feldman, 1993a; Thompson, 1995) based on the thermal reactivity of the anti-RBC antibodies and their major clinical effects at optimal temperature. These categories are:

- *Agglutination (warm antibody type):* high levels of antibody lead to detectable autoagglutination of RBCs (agglutination is usually associated with acute severe extravascular haemolysis)
- *Intravascular haemolysis (warm antibody type):* intravascular haemolysis, usually associated with high levels of antibody and complement fixation, causes an acute severe anaemia with detectable haemoglobinaemia and haemoglobinuria

- *Incomplete antibody (warm antibody type):* anti-RBC antibodies cause extravascular haemolysis, without detectable autoagglutination or haemoglobinaemia/haemoglobinuria (disease onset is often chronic or subacute, and resultant anaemia varies from mild to severe)
- *Agglutination (cold antibody type):* anti-RBC antibodies are only reactive at cold temperatures, and agglutination does not occur at body temperature. Agglutination can, however, occur within the vasculature of the extremities, particularly in colder weather. Obstruction of the blood supply to the peripheral vasculature due to agglutination and thrombus formation can lead to ischaemic necrosis of the ear or tail tips, the end of the nose, and the foot pads
- *Non-agglutinating haemolysis (cold antibody type):* antibodies are only reactive at cold temperatures, and haemolysis does not occur at body temperature (in cold weather, however, some degree of haemolysis may occur within the vasculature of the extremities, which manifests clinically as transient haemoglobinaemia and haemoglobinuria).

Although the above categorization system is derived by extrapolation from human medicine, all five categories of IMHA have been reported in small animals. Fortunately (since both cause severe, acute and life-threatening disease) the agglutinating and intravascular haemolysing warm antibody types of IMHA are relatively uncommon in small animals, and the comparatively milder incomplete warm antibody type predominates. Agglutinating and (especially) haemolysing cold antibody types of IMHA are rare in both dogs and cats (Halliwell and Gorman, 1989).

CLINICAL SIGNS

Clinical signs typically associated with most cases of IMHA reflect the presence of both moderate to severe anaemia (lethargy, weakness, pale mucous membranes, haemic heart murmur) and compensatory responses caused by tissue hypoxia and stimulation of the sympathetic nervous system (tachypnoea, tachycardia, bounding pulses) (Klag *et al.*, 1993; Reimer *et al.*, 1999). Some patients may also show clinical signs of an ongoing immunological or inflammatory process, such as pyrexia, anorexia and, uncommonly, lymphadenopathy (Klag *et al.*, 1993). Surprisingly, since the MPS within the spleen and liver is usually the main site of RBC destruction, splenomegaly and/or hepatomegaly are only variably present in animals with IMHA (Jackson and Kruth, 1985; Klag *et al.*, 1993; Reimer *et al.*, 1999).

Patients with IMHA of acute onset tend to be severely affected by their anaemia and are often depressed, weak or even collapsed. Transient hyperbilirubinaemia, bilirubinuria and tissue jaundice (Figure 5.17) may occasionally be seen during acute severe episodes of IMHA whereas, because intravascular haemolysis is uncommon, haemoglobinaemia and haemoglobinuria are observed infrequently. Patients with extravascular haemolysis due to subacute or chronic IMHA can compensate to some extent for their lack of erythrocytes and may be bright despite the presence of severe anaemia. In these patients, the liver can often cope with the extra bilirubin released by the breakdown of RBCs, and jaundice does not occur.

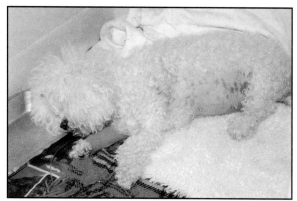

Figure 5.17: *Severe extravascular haemolysis in a dog that presented with severe IMHA. Acute extravascular haemolysis and resultant bilirubin production overwhelmed hepatic mechanisms of bilirubin uptake, conjugation and excretion, leading to profound tissue jaundice. The dog was severely anaemic, weak and depressed.*

Pulmonary thromboembolism is a well recognized complication of IMHA, and is particularly common in those animals with acute severe anaemia that are receiving high-dose glucocorticoids (Bunch *et al.*, 1989; Klag *et al.*, 1993; Day, 1996). Pulmonary thromboembolism should always be suspected in anaemic patients that suddenly develop severe and persistent dyspnoea. Disseminated intravascular coagulation (DIC) can also complicate severe cases of IMHA (Cotter, 1992; Klag *et al.*, 1993).

DIAGNOSIS OF IMHA

Haematology in patients with IMHA typically shows a moderate to severe anaemia, which is most commonly extremely regenerative, with anisocytosis, polychromasia, a high corrected reticulocyte count and, sometimes, increased numbers of nucleated RBCs. Reticulocyte counts can, however, sometimes be inappropriately low (Jones and Gruffydd-Jones, 1991; Klag *et al.*, 1993), either because anaemia is peracute (since it takes about 5 days for the marrow to mount a strong regenerative response) or because antibodies are also directed against RBC precursors. White cell and neutrophil counts are often moderately to profoundly increased, probably in response to both non-specific marrow stimulation and the inflammatory process associated with the break-

down of RBCs (Jackson and Kruth, 1985; Weiser, 1992; Jain, 1993; Day, 1996). Occasionally, white cell counts can be high enough to mimic myelogenous leukaemia, a reaction sometimes called a 'leukaemoid response'. Platelet counts are usually normal unless the animal also has immune-mediated thrombocytopenia (IMT). Concurrent IMHA and thrombocytopenia, a condition known as Evan's syndrome, may affect up to about 10% of dogs with IMHA (Klag *et al.*, 1993).

Haematology can often give clues that suggest a specific aetiological diagnosis, namely, spherocytosis, agglutination and other RBC abnormalities.

Spherocytosis

Spherocytes are small spherical erythrocytes that, when present in high numbers, strongly suggest a diagnosis of IMHA (Halliwell and Gorman, 1989; Weiser, 1992; Thompson, 1995). Spherocytes are formed when macrophages remove a piece of RBC membrane without cell destruction or a significant loss of cytoplasmic contents (Figure 5.18).

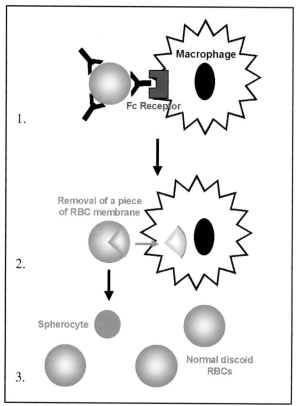

Figure 5.18: *Spherocyte formation. (1) Antibody-coated erythrocytes are recognized and bound by Fc receptors on macrophages. (2) Rather than phagocytose and destroy the erythrocyte completely, the macrophage then removes a piece of RBC membrane before releasing the cell back into the circulation. (3) Because the unchanged volume of RBC cytoplasm must now be contained within a lesser amount of membrane, the cell adopts a spherical shape. Spherocytes are recognized on a blood smear as a small dense RBC with a loss of central pallor and may be registered by automated haematology analysers as a decrease in mean corpuscular volume. Spherocytes are difficult to identify in the cat as normal RBCs tend to be much smaller and denser than those in the dog.*

Agglutination

Examination of blood smears may show microscopic autoagglutination (clumping) of erythrocytes. Such agglutination can form large rafts of RBCs that, on close inspection of a tube containing anticoagulated blood, are visible to the naked eye as multiple red speckles (Figure 5.19). Similar speckles can, however, be created by rouleaux formation, a phenomenon that

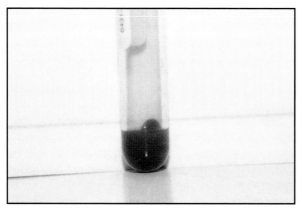

Figure 5.19: EDTA-anticoagulated blood sample from a dog with severe IMHA, showing the appearance of gross autoagglutination. Large clumps of agglutinated red cells are visible to the naked eye as red speckles lining the vacutainer tube.

can occur in normal animals, especially cats. Practitioners should therefore perform a slide agglutination test (Figures 5.20 and 5.21) to differentiate rouleaux from genuine autoagglutination (Halliwell and Gorman, 1989; Cotter, 1992; Thompson, 1995). A positive test result with slide agglutination is highly suggestive of IMHA and also suggests that the condition is likely to be acute and severe. A negative test result, however, is the most common result in patients with IMHA since most animals have non-agglutinating antibodies.

Automated haematology analysers sometimes register a clump of agglutinated erythrocytes as a single cell, often of a size too large to even be recorded as a RBC (Weiser, 1992). Resultant erroneous results may include an artifactually high mean corpuscular volume (MCV) or, if clumped cells are not recognized as erythrocytes, lowering of the calculated haematocrit (Cotter, 1992). Since the haemoglobin within all erythrocytes is still measured by the analyser, this leads to an erroneously high estimation of mean corpuscular haemoglobin concentration (MCHC). When agglutination is suspected to be the cause of a lower than expected haematocrit, packed cell volume (PCV), which is not affected by RBC clumping, should be monitored by microhaematocrit tube centrifugation rather than an automated analyser.

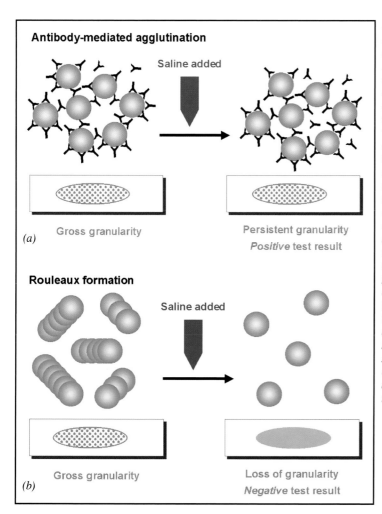

Figure 5.20: Agglutination is associated with a high level of anti-red blood cell (RBC) antibody and is caused by antibodies that attach to more than one RBC, thereby drawing the cells together into one large clump. (a) Large clumps are visible as speckling or granularity in a drop of anticoagulated blood placed on a microscope slide and viewed against a white background. Persistence of such visible granularity for 1 to 2 minutes after the blood has been mixed with a small amount of normal saline is considered to be a positive test result with slide agglutination. (b) Rouleaux, or stacked RBCs, can also appear as speckles to the naked eye, but the granularity clears within a few minutes of adding saline, at a ratio of one drop of saline to one drop of blood in dogs and two or three drops of saline to one drop of blood in cats. A negative test result with slide agglutination is indicated by either an absence of granularity or clearance of granularity after the addition of saline. Slide agglutination is best performed at room temperature or above. False positives can occur at lower temperatures, although a positive test result at 4°C in an animal with necrosis of extremities supports a diagnosis of cold agglutinating IMHA. After completion of a slide agglutination test, a coverslip may be placed over the blood/saline mix and the slide examined microscopically to confirm the presence of RBC agglutination.

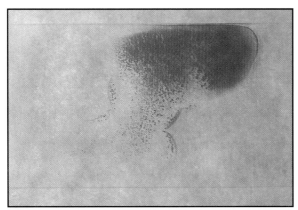

Figure 5.21: Typical appearance of a positive test result with slide agglutination.

Other red blood cell abnormalities

Careful examination of RBC morphology may suggest an underlying cause of either immunological or non-immunological haemolysis. Diagnostically useful RBC abnormalities include detection of parasites such as *Haemobartonella felis* (which may cause secondary IMHA), Heinz bodies (suggesting haemolysis secondary to oxidative damage) and schistocytosis (suggesting a microangiopathic haemolytic process such as DIC).

Serum biochemistry and urinalysis are often normal in dogs with IMHA. Potential abnormalities in some patients include mild to moderate increases in concentrations of liver enzymes (thought to indicate hepatic hypoxia secondary to severe anaemia) and variable hyperglobulinaemia (Klag *et al.*, 1993). Since serum albumin is usually normal, hypoalbuminaemia is an unexpected finding that may suggest anaemia is due to occult blood loss rather than haemolysis, or that the patient has a concurrent illness. Mild to moderate hyperbilirubinaemia and bilirubinuria may occur transiently in animals with acute severe anaemia. Since the liver is usually able to cope with all but the transient overwhelming loads of bilirubin produced by acute severe haemolysis, severe hyperbilirubinaemia or persistence

of jaundice for more than 3–5 days (even in profoundly anaemic animals) usually indicates concurrent hepatic disease or biliary obstruction. Haemoglobinaemia and haemoglobinuria are uncommon transient events that indicate severe intravascular haemolysis (Weiser, 1992).

Immunological testing

Specific immunological testing can be used to support a tentative diagnosis of IMHA. The most widely used test is the direct antiglobulin test (DAT) or Coombs' test (Halliwell and Gorman, 1989), which detects antibodies and/or complement bound to RBC membranes (Figure 5.22). A standard DAT as provided by most laboratories typically uses a mix of antibodies directed against IgG, IgM (to a variable extent) and complement, and is performed at body temperature (Jones *et al.*, 1990; Cotter, 1992; Thompson, 1995). Modifications of the routine screening DAT that may increase its diagnostic value include running the test at different temperatures, using individual antibodies against IgG, IgM, IgA and complement as well as the standard polyvalent antibody/complement mix and fully titrating these reagents (Jones *et al.*, 1990; Day, 1996). Positive DAT results at 4°C, however, are of minimal diagnostic significance unless the patient has clinical signs consistent with cold antibody type agglutination or intravascular haemolysis (Halliwell and Gorman, 1989; Cotter, 1992; Weiser, 1992).

Strictly interpreted, a positive DAT result supports a diagnosis of IMHA, whereas a negative test result suggests a non-immunological cause of haemolysis. Numerous studies, however, have shown that a DAT can often be of only mediocre diagnostic accuracy: although sensitivity and specificity improve with meticulous attention to test methodology, both false positive and false negative results do occur relatively commonly (Jones *et al.*, 1990; Cotter, 1992; Weiser, 1992; Stewart and Feldman, 1993b; Thompson, 1995; Miller, 1999). Practitioners should therefore be aware that since IMHA can occur in the presence of a negative DAT result and,

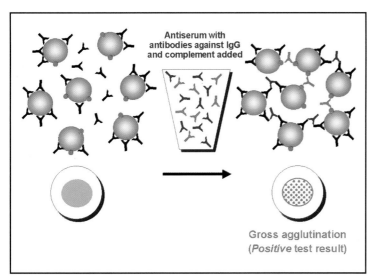

Antiserum with antibodies against IgG and complement added

Gross agglutination (*Positive* test result)

Figure 5.22: Direct antiglobulin (Coombs') test. Species-specific antiserum containing antibodies directed against either dog or cat immunoglobulin (IgG, IgM and, sometimes, IgA) and complement, either individually or as a polyvalent mixture, is added to a washed suspension of erythrocytes from the patient. When the patient's cells are coated with antibody and/or complement, the addition of antibodies directed against these particular components causes visible red blood cell (RBC) agglutination (a positive test result). In this example, illustrating a typical case of IMHA in a dog, the patient's cells are coated with both antibody (IgG) and complement. When a standard antiserum containing antibodies against dog IgG and complement is added to the washed red cells and the mixture is incubated, antibodies bind to IgG or complement attached to more than one RBC, thereby causing cell clumping and visible agglutination.

conversely, a positive test result does not absolutely prove the presence of IMHA, sometimes a diagnosis must be based on clinical judgement despite the presence of an apparently discrepant DAT result. Performing a DAT is, however, still recommended in all patients with suspected IMHA even if criteria such as spherocytosis or a positive test result with slide agglutination already strongly suggest a diagnosis, since a positive DAT result will add support to the diagnosis and characterize the disease further by determining the involvement of various immunoglobulin types and complement.

Various other immunological tests for detecting anti-RBC antibody have been reported, including an enzyme-linked immunosorbent assay (Campbell and George, 1984) and a direct enzyme-linked antiglobulin test (Barker *et al.*, 1992; 1993). Although some of these tests may arguably be more sensitive than the DAT, they are not commonly available. Regardless of whether a DAT or an alternative test for anti-RBC antibody is used, however, clinicians should be aware that a positive test result merely records the presence of antibody and does not determine whether IMHA is primary (AIHA) or secondary.

Uncommonly, IMHA (with or without IMT) will be merely one component of systemic lupus erythematosus, a multisystemic immunological disturbance. Measurement of serum antinuclear antibody (ANA) is therefore indicated in those patients displaying involvement of more than one body system, such as IMT, glomerulonephritis, polyarthritis, polymyositis or immune-mediated skin disease. By contrast, ANA is not indicated (and is usually negative) in those patients suspected of having uncomplicated IMHA.

Identification of underlying disease

Since IMHA is often secondary, particularly in cats and in dogs with atypical signalment, confirmation of IMHA is not necessarily the end of the diagnostic trail. Primary or AIHA can only be diagnosed with absolute certainty once potential hidden underlying causes have been thoroughly investigated. Unfortunately, this presents practitioners with a dilemma: although IMHA is unlikely to be treated effectively unless underlying causes have been identified and eliminated, a complete search for such causes can be time consuming, expensive, potentially invasive and, in the case of primary IMHA, ultimately fruitless. Standard and relatively inexpensive screening tests for underlying disease that ideally should be performed in all animals with IMHA include haematology (with careful examination of a blood smear), serum biochemistry, urinalysis, thoracic and abdominal radiography and, in cats, testing for retroviruses (particularly FeLV). Further tests that might be considered in some patients, particularly elderly animals in which underlying neoplasia (especially occult lymphoproliferative disease) is a real possibility, include abdominal ultrasonography, lymph node aspiration cytology and bone marrow analysis.

Bone marrow analysis

Bone marrow analysis (aspiration cytology and/or core biopsy histopathology) is also indicated in all patients with suspected non-regenerative forms of IMHA. PRCA is characterized by a relative or complete lack of RBC precursors within the bone marrow, whereas cytological or histopathological evidence of an erythroid 'maturation arrest' (preponderance of immature RBC precursors, with an absence of more mature RBC precursors) suggests that, rather than being directed against early stem cells, antibodies are directed against a later stage of RBC development in the bone marrow (Jonas *et al.*, 1987; Holloway and Meyer, 1990). Marrow cytology and/or histopathology may also reveal macrophages phagocytosing erythrocytes or RBC precursors (Holloway and Meyer, 1990). In such patients, techniques such as immunofluorescent or immunoperoxidase staining of bone marrow samples may confirm the presence of antibodies directed against RBC precursors (Stewart and Feldman, 1993b).

MANAGEMENT OF IMHA

The cornerstone of the management of IMHA is immunosuppressive therapy, particularly with glucocorticoids. The major mechanisms of immunosuppressive therapy in general are to decrease anti-RBC antibody synthesis, decrease the binding affinity between antibodies and erythrocytes and decrease destruction of antibody-coated cells by the MPS (Miller, 1992) (Figure 5.23). Even if new anti-RBC antibody synthesis by plasma cells is arrested immediately, pre-existing immunoglobulins may survive in the circulation for a week or more, therefore reduction of antibody synthesis is usually not an important part of the initial treatment of IMHA.

Initial immunosuppressive therapy

Initial immunosuppressive therapy for dogs and cats with IMHA usually consists of oral prednisolone (or prednisone; not licensed for veterinary use in the UK) at a starting dose of 2 to 4 mg/kg/day, given once daily or split twice daily (Stewart and Feldman, 1993b). Some authors recommend commencing treatment with an immediate intravenous dose of injectable glucocorticoids (most commonly dexamethasone at a dose of about 0.1 to 0.2 mg/kg) before commencing oral drugs (Thompson, 1995), but there is little evidence that this hastens response to therapy. The most important short-term effect of glucocorticoids is inhibition of the MPS, sometimes termed a 'medical splenectomy'. Treatment response is rarely immediate: when glucocorticoids alone are effective, an increase in PCV usually occurs 3–7 days after commencing therapy but can be delayed for as long as one month (Stewart and Feldman, 1993b).

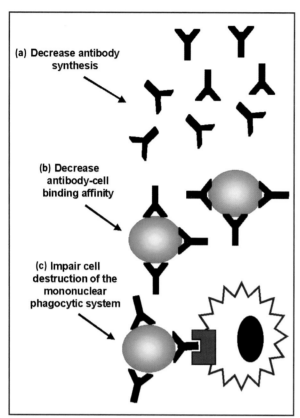

Figure 5.23: *Immunosuppressive agents can reduce immune-mediated destruction of red blood cells (RBCs) by several different mechanisms. (a) Many agents eventually reduce anti-RBC synthesis by plasma cells although, since immunoglobulins have a circulating half-life of more than a week, this effect is rarely immediately beneficial. Several other processes may be more rapidly effective: (b) some agents may reduce the binding affinity of anti-RBC antibodies to the erythrocyte surface membrane, (c) whereas many drugs will, by various mechanisms, impair RBC destruction of the mononuclear phagocytic system. Glucocorticoids, the most important immunosuppressive agents used to treat IMHA, exert their beneficial effects by all of the illustrated mechanisms.*

Many dogs with IMHA do not respond adequately to glucocorticoids alone and require additional immunosuppressive therapy. Commencing treatment with glucocorticoids and concurrent azathioprine (starting dose 2 mg/kg/day orally) or cyclophosphamide (starting dose 50 mg/m² every second day orally) is recommended at the time of diagnosis in those dogs with clinical evidence of severe IMHA (Cotter, 1992; Lifton, 1999) such as profound anaemia (PCV of less than 10%), signs of major clinical compromise (particularly weakness, stupor and collapse), a positive test result with slide agglutination and jaundice or haemoglobinaemia/haemoglobinuria.

Some authors prefer cyclophosphamide to azathioprine, primarily because cyclophosphamide may be a more potent and rapidly acting immunosuppressive agent. However, cyclophosphamide predisposes dogs to severe and refractory sterile haemorrhagic cystitis and is therefore not suitable for chronic therapy. Aza-

thioprine is a much safer drug for long-term use and, since there is minimal clinical evidence to support the contention that this drug is less efficacious or slower to effect than cyclophosphamide in dogs with IMHA (Cotter, 1992), it is probably the immunosuppressive agent of choice.

Even when not commenced during the initial therapy of canine IMHA, cyclophosphamide or azathioprine often needs to be added within a few weeks of starting treatment with corticosteroids (Stewart and Feldman, 1993b). Indications for concurrent immunosuppressive agents are a failure to respond to glucocorticoids alone or intolerable side effects to steroids, such as polydipsia, polyuria, polyphagia and tachypnoea. Addition of these agents often enables a more rapid reduction in corticosteroid doses.

Cats do not tolerate immunosuppressive agents as well as dogs, and it is often difficult to break standard tablets down to sizes small enough to safely dose cats. Cats are, however, tolerant of long-term high doses of glucocorticoids, and most cats with IMHA will respond to steroids alone. For this reason, azathioprine (at a reduced dose of 0.3 mg/kg/day) or cyclophosphamide (same dose as recommended for dogs) is rarely needed.

Supportive/ancillary therapy

Patients with severe anaemia have generalized tissue hypoxia and benefit from reducing oxygen demand by instituting strict cage rest until anaemia responds to therapy. Severely compromised patients can also be supported with oxygen supplementation. Haemoglobin oxygen saturation is, however, already near maximal, and supplementation with oxygen therefore increases saturation only minimally. Oxygen supplementation is also laborious and expensive. Because patients with haemolytic anaemia have a normal blood volume, fluid therapy is of little benefit and may contribute to volume overload.

Patients with IMHA are prone to pulmonary thromboembolism and DIC (Cotter, 1992; Lifton, 1999), particularly those with severe anaemia and/or a positive test result with slide agglutination and those requiring transfusion, therefore some clinicians recommend heparin be used prophylactically during the hospitalization of severely affected animals (Thompson, 1995). The true efficacy of such prophylactic therapy is, however, unknown (Miller, 1999). A safe low dose of heparin that does not cause spontaneous bleeding and does not require careful monitoring of coagulation parameters is 75 to 100 U/kg three to four times daily subcutaneously (Cotter, 1992; Stewart and Feldman, 1993b).

Transfusion

Cage rest and standard immunosuppressive drugs are successful in most dogs and cats with non-life-threatening IMHA. However, initial response to therapy can sometimes be sluggish (a week or more), particularly in those animals with poor bone marrow responsiveness due to either peracute anaemia or immune-mediated damage to RBC precursors. In the meantime, transfusion may be needed to support those patients with life-threatening acute and severe anaemia (PCV less than 10% or signs of severe compromise, such as collapse or stupor). Transfused red cells often have a very short lifespan (days or even hours) in patients with IMHA, and transfusions may actually increase the rate of haemolysis (Halliwell and Gorman, 1989). For this reason, transfusions should be avoided when possible in stable patients with IMHA (Thompson, 1995; Miller, 1999). In those patients that are severely compromised, however, transfusions are life-saving and should not be withheld (Klag *et al.*, 1993; Miller, 1999).

Whole blood may be safely transfused at a rate of up to 20 ml/kg/h, usually at a maximum daily volume of 20 ml/kg. Multiple transfusions as often as every one or two days may be needed in severely affected animals. Since patients with IMHA are normovolaemic, volume overload after transfusion can become a significant risk in animals that have already recently received high volumes of blood or other fluids. In these patients, blood transfusions should be given slowly (maximum rate of 4 ml/kg/h). When available, packed RBCs are preferable to whole blood. Since crossmatches are often positive in patients with IMHA (because the animal has antibodies against its own RBC and can even 'crossmatch' positive against its own and donor blood), compatible donors should be used if blood typing is available (see Chapters 15 and 16). Bovine polymerized haemoglobin has recently become available as a safe and effective (although often prohibitively expensive) alternative means of providing temporary oxygen-carrying support for severely anaemic patients.

Monitoring response to therapy

Haematocrit should be monitored daily until an appreciable response to immunosuppressive therapy is observed and the PCV increases above about 15% in cats and 20% in dogs, after which PCV should be monitored at least weekly until anaemia resolves completely. Given an adequate treatment response, drug therapy should be gradually tapered to an acceptable maintenance dose that can be given safely long term without significant side effects. In dogs, prednisolone and azathioprine can often both be tapered to 0.5 to 1 mg/kg every second day, a maintenance dose that is usually well tolerated. Similar maintenance doses of prednisolone may be achievable in cats although, as side effects from steroids are typically minimal, higher doses are also usually acceptable. Since cyclophosphamide therapy can eventually cause sterile cystitis (which can be irreversible) or even bladder neoplasia, there is no safe maintenance dose of this particular drug. Both cyclophosphamide and azathioprine can be

unpredictably myelosuppressive, therefore white cell counts should be regularly monitored throughout therapy (Cotter, 1992). Furthermore, as azathioprine can (rarely) cause an idiosyncratic hepatotoxicity, liver enzymes should also be monitored regularly for increases far beyond those expected with glucocorticoid therapy alone.

One simple approach to tapering therapy in stable patients with IMHA is to recheck PCV about every 2 weeks and then, if anaemia is still in remission, to reduce the dose of one drug by 50% after each visit. In animals receiving several immunosuppressive agents, the drug that is causing the most side effects is tapered first. In most instances this means that prednisolone is tapered first and, once steroid doses are low enough to cause no side effects, then the other drug is similarly tapered. Once a well tolerated maintenance dose of all drugs is attained, therapy should ideally be continued for at least a further 3 months, with monthly monitoring of PCV. Presuming that an underlying cause of IMHA has not been identified and eliminated, tapering therapy too rapidly increases the risk of a life-threatening relapse. Clinicians should be aware that chronic azathioprine therapy can cause a mild non-regenerative anaemia (PCV greater than 30%) in dogs. This causes no patient compromise, and persistence of a mild anaemia in patients on this drug is not a reflection of inadequate treatment.

Once anaemia has been in remission for 3 to 6 months, therapy can be cautiously withdrawn. Haematocrit should be monitored regularly over the months following cessation of therapy. Patients with a poor regenerative response, particularly those with severe immune-mediated marrow disease such as PRCA, can take many months to respond to therapy (Cotter, 1992). Such animals should be supported with an initial blood transfusion followed by standard immunosuppressive therapy (Jonas *et al.*, 1987). Because destruction of peripheral erythrocytes is often minimal in animals with immunological marrow disease, donated red cells may survive in the circulation for up to several months. Although immunosuppression may not cause an increase in PCV for up to 3 months, response to therapy can be detected earlier by careful monitoring of serial reticulocyte counts or bone marrow samples.

Advanced emergency therapy

Despite appropriate standard therapy and multiple transfusions, some patients with IMHA succumb to acute severe anaemia during the first week or two of treatment. Beneficial treatment options in an emergency include high-dose human intravenous gammaglobulin, plasmapheresis and splenectomy.

High-dose human intravenous gammaglobulin

High doses of intravenous gammaglobulin have been shown to occasionally cause rapid (and sometimes sustained) remission of various immunohaematological disorders in humans, including IMHA (Miller, 1992) (Figure 5.24). The product used in humans, as a 12 hour intravenous infusion at doses ranging from 0.5 to 1.5 g/kg, has been shown to have the same effect in some dogs, without apparent side effects (Kellerman and Bruyette, 1997; Scott-Moncrieff and Reagan, 1997). The product can, however, be prohibitively expensive, especially in large dogs.

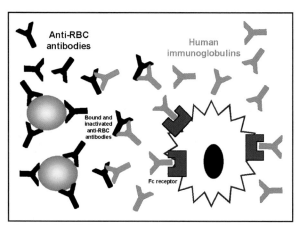

Figure 5.24: *High dose gammaglobulin is a blood product created by extracting, concentrating and pooling a 'soup' of many differing antibodies from numerous human donors. One proposed mechanism of action is that, since such a wide and heterogenous range of immunoglobulins are contained within high dose gammaglobulin, the product may actually contain antibodies that are specifically directed against the recipient's own anti-red blood cell (RBC) antibodies, thereby binding and inactivating them (black arrow). However, the main effect of high dose gammaglobulin is to saturate the Fc receptors of the mononuclear phagocytic system with excess donated antibodies, leaving few receptors available to bind to the patient's own anti-RBC antibodies attached to the RBC surface membrane.*

Plasmapheresis

Plasmapheresis is an effective method of rapidly removing unbound anti-RBC antibodies from the circulation, although antibodies that are already bound to RBC membranes will persist and may cause ongoing disease (Matus *et al.*, 1985; Miller, 1992).

Splenectomy

As the spleen is usually the major site of RBC destruction in IMHA and is often also an important site of antibody production, splenectomy can be effective at attaining rapid remissions in patients with life-threatening disease (Miller, 1992). The procedure is risky, especially in unstable patients, and response rates are highly unpredictable (Jackson and Kruth, 1985), probably because other organs in the MPS (particularly the liver) continue to destroy red cells. Furthermore, for the remainder of their lives splenectomized animals will have an increased susceptibility to systemic infection and blood-borne parasites such as *Haemobartonella* (Thompson, 1995).

Chronic refractory IMHA

An initial adequate response to standard immunosuppressive therapy does not necessarily guarantee that patients with IMHA will be simple to manage in the longer term. In some patients anaemia relapses as therapy is tapered. Persistence with higher than maintenance doses of glucocorticoids and other immunosuppressive agents is, however, not an acceptable alternative due to drug side effects. In these patients, additional treatments that may then permit an acceptable dose reduction of the standard drugs include danazol and cyclosporin.

Danazol

Danazol (an impeded androgen), in combination with other immunosuppressive therapy, has been reported to cause an eventual partial or complete remission of IMHA in some dogs (Stewart and Feldman, 1993b). Danazol may therefore be worth considering (at a dose of 5 mg/kg two to three times daily orally) in chronic cases that are refractory to standard treatment alone (Stewart and Feldman, 1993b). Results of a recent study, however, indicate that many dogs will not detectably respond to the drug (Miller, 1999). The most important mechanism of action of danazol is probably to reduce the MPS Fc receptor/antibody binding affinity. Side effects, which are uncommon, include masculinization of bitches and idiosyncratic hepatotoxicity. Danazol is expensive, however, and even when effective can take months to achieve maximum efficacy (Stewart and Feldman, 1993b).

Cyclosporin

Cyclosporin A, a selective T-cell immunosuppressant that blocks amplification of the immune response, has been used to treat dogs with refractory IMHA (Miller, 1992; Gregory, 1999). Initial oral daily doses of cyclosporin of either 10–25 mg/kg (olive oil-based suspension) or 4–15 mg/kg (microemulsion) are adjusted to attain trough whole blood concentrations of the drug of at least 500 ng/ml (Gregory, 1999). Cyclosporin A is expensive and can cause gastrointestinal disturbances, gingival hyperplasia and, uncommonly, nephrotoxicity or hepatotoxicity.

Sometimes, one of the emergency treatments for IMHA, such as splenectomy or intravenous gammaglobulin, may 'kick start' refractory chronic cases and render standard therapy more effective. Splenectomy, in particular, may on occasion permit subsequent significant reductions in immunosuppressive drug dosage. This beneficial effect is, however, inconsistent and unpredictable.

Secondary IMHA

Whenever an underlying cause of IMHA can be identified and eliminated, ongoing specific drug therapy is often not necessary. In contrast, drugs are unlikely to be able to be discontinued while the underlying disease process persists. Drugs or vaccines given over the 4–6 week period before onset of IMHA should be avoided in the future whenever possible. When IMHA is not associated with recent vaccination, however, there is probably no need to modify or avoid routine vaccinations in the future.

In the cat, IMHA is often secondary to infection with either FeLV or *Haemobartonella felis* (Halliwell and Gorman, 1989). Cats with IMHA should therefore always be tested for FeLV. Cats with IMHA that are positive for FeLV often initially respond well to standard immunosuppressive therapy, although long-term prognosis is poor. Cats with *H. felis* infection typically present with recurring episodes of haemolytic anaemia. During anaemic crises, organisms may not be apparent, as affected cells are either destroyed or sequestered in the spleen. Organisms reappear on red cells during remission of anaemia and are discovered by serial blood smears. Cats with IMHA should probably receive oral tetracycline or oxytetracycline at a dose rate of 20 mg/kg three times daily, even if organisms are not seen on initial smears. Concurrent immunosuppressive therapy in cats with *H. felis* infection is not contraindicated. In fact, as anaemia due to *H. felis* infection has an immune-mediated component, glucocorticoids are indicated during acute crises.

PROGNOSIS

Published mortality rates for IMHA are often high, ranging from about one-third to one-half of all presented cases (Jackson and Kruth, 1985; Halliwell and Gorman, 1989; Cotter, 1992; Klag *et al.*, 1993; Reimer *et al.*, 1999), with death/euthanasia usually attributable to either severe anaemia or pulmonary thromboembolism during the initial acute crisis, or persistent/recurrent disease or unacceptable drug side effects during chronic therapy. Negative prognostic indicators include the presence of profound jaundice or haemoglobinaemia/haemoglobinuria, a poor regenerative response, and a positive test result with slide agglutination (Klag *et al.*, 1993). As our understanding of IMHA increases and our treatment options expand, deaths due to this disease should become less frequent.

REFERENCES

Barker RN and Elson CJ (1995) Red blood cell glycophorins as B and T-cell antigens in canine autoimmune haemolytic anaemia. *Veterinary Immunology and Immunopathology* **47**, 225–238

Barker RN, Gruffydd-Jones TJ and Elson CJ (1993) Red cell-bound immunoglobulins and complement measured by an enzyme-linked antiglobulin test in dogs with autoimmune haemolysis or other anaemias. *Research in Veterinary Science* **54**, 170–178

Barker RN, Gruffydd-Jones TJ, Stokes CR and Elson CJ (1991) Identification of autoantigens in canine autoimmune haemolytic anaemia. *Clinical and Experimental Immunology* **85**, 33–40

Barker RN, Gruffydd-Jones TJ, Stokes CR and Elson CJ (1992) Autoimmune haemolysis in the dog: relationship between anaemia and the levels of red blood cell bound immunoglobulins and complement measured by an enzyme-linked antiglobulin test.

Veterinary Immunology and Immunopathology **34**, 1–20

Bunch SE, Metcalf MR, Crane SW and Cullen JM (1989) Idiopathic pleural effusion and pulmonary thromboembolism in a dog with autoimmune hemolytic anemia. *Journal of the American Veterinary Medical Association* **195**, 1748–1753

Campbell KL and George JW (1984) Application of the enzyme-linked immunosorbent assay to detect canine erythrocyte antibodies. *American Journal of Veterinary Research* **45**, 747–752

Cotter SM (1992) Autoimmune hemolytic anemia in dogs. *Compendium of Continuing Education for the Practicing Veterinarian* **14**, 53–59

Day MJ (1996) Serial monitoring of clinical haematological and immunological parameters in canine autoimmune haemolytic anaemia. *Journal of Small Animal Practice* **37**, 523–534

Day MJ and Penhale WJ (1992) Immune-mediated disease in the old English sheepdog. *Research in Veterinary Science* **53**, 87–92

Gregory, CR (1999) Immunosuppressive agents. In: *Current Veterinary Therapy XIII: Small Animal Practice*, ed. JD Bonagura, pp. 509–513. WB Saunders, Philadelphia

Halliwell REW and Gorman NT (1989) Autoimmune blood diseases. In: *Veterinary Clinical Immunology*, ed. REW Halliwell, pp. 308–336. WB Saunders, Philadelphia

Holloway SA and Meyer DJ (1990) Prednisolone and danazol for treatment of immune-mediated anemia thrombocytopenia and ineffective erythroid regeneration in a dog. *Journal of the American Veterinary Medical Association* **197**, 1045–1048

Jackson ML and Kruth SA (1985) Immune-mediated hemolytic anemia and thrombocytopenia in the dog: a retrospective study of 55 cases diagnosed from 1969 through 1983 at the Western College of Veterinary Medicine. *Canadian Veterinary Journal* **26**, 245–250

Jain NC (1993) Hemolytic anemias of noninfectious origin. In: *Essentials of Veterinary Hematology*, ed. NC Jain, pp, 193–209. Lea and Febiger, Philadelphia

Jonas LD, Thrall MA and Weiser MG (1987) Nonregenerative form of immune-mediated hemolytic anemia in dogs. *Journal of the American Animal Hospital Association* **23**, 201–204

Jones DRE and Gruffydd-Jones TJ (1991) The haematological consequences of immune-mediated anaemia in the dog. *Comparative Haematology International* **1**, 83–90

Jones DRE, Gruffydd-Jones TJ, Stokes CR and Bourne FJ (1990) Investigation into factors influencing performance of the canine antiglobulin test. *Research in Veterinary Science* **48**, 53–58

Kellerman DL and Bruyette DS (1997) Intravenous human immunoglobulin for the treatment of immune-mediated hemolytic anemia in 13 dogs. *Journal of Veterinary Internal Medicine* **11**, 327–332

Klag AR, Giger U and Shofer FS (1993) Idiopathic immune-mediated hemolytic anemia in dogs: 42 cases (1986-1990). *Journal of the American Veterinary Medical Association* **202**, 783–788

Lifton SJ (1999) Managing immune-mediated hemolytic anemia in dogs. *Veterinary Medicine* **94**, 532–545

Matus RE, Schrader LA, Leifer CE, Gordon BR and Hurvitz AI (1985) Plasmapheresis as adjuvant therapy for autoimmune hemolytic anemia in two dogs. *Journal of the American Veterinary Medical Association* **186**, 691–693

Miller E (1992) Immunosuppressive therapy in the treatment of immune-mediated disease. *Journal of Veterinary Internal Medicine* **6**, 206–213

Miller E (1999) Diagnosis and treatment of immune-mediated hemolytic anemia. In: *Current Veterinary Therapy XIII: Small Animal Practice*, ed. JD Bonagura, pp. 427–433. WB Saunders, Philadelphia

Noble SJ and Armstrong PJ (1999) Bee sting envenomation resulting in secondary immune-mediated hemolytic anemia in two dogs. *Journal of the American Veterinary Medical Association* **214**, 1026–1027

Reimer ME, Troy GC and Warnick LD (1999) Immune-mediated hemolytic anemia: 70 cases (1988-1996). *Journal of the American Animal Hospital Association* **35**, 384–391

Scott-Moncrieff JC and Reagan WJ (1997) Human intravenous immunoglobulin therapy. *Seminars in Veterinary Medicine and Surgery (Small Animal)* **12**, 178–185

Stewart AF and Feldman BF (1993a) Immune-mediated hemolytic anemia, part I. An overview. *Compendium of Continuing Education for the Practicing Veterinarian* **15**, 372–381

Stewart AF and Feldman BF (1993b) Immune-mediated hemolytic anemia, part II. Clinical entity diagnosis and treatment theory. *Compendium of Continuing Education for the Practicing Veterinarian* **15**, 1479–1491

Thompson JP (1995) Immunologic diseases. In: *Textbook of Veterinary Internal Medicine*, 4th edn, ed. SJ Ettinger and EC Feldman, pp. 2002–2029. WB Saunders, Philadelphia

Weiser MG (1992) Diagnosis of immunohemolytic disease. *Seminars in Veterinary Medicine and Surgery (Small Animal)* **7**, 311–314

(iv) *Haemobartonella felis*

Darren Foster

INTRODUCTION

Haemobartonella felis is a mycoplasma (previously classified as a rickettsia) that parasitizes the red blood cells (RBCs) of cats. It has a worldwide distribution. The clinical condition with variable signs, including regenerative anaemia, pyrexia and malaise, is referred to as haemobartonellosis or feline infectious anaemia (FIA). The prevalence of the disease is unknown owing to the lack of a serological test for the organism and because chronic carriers cannot be easily identified. The major mode of transmission is believed to involve blood-sucking insects (particularly the flea), transplacental and transmammary infection and iatrogenic inoculation via blood transfusions. Treatment generally involves the use of antibiotics and corticosteroids combined with supportive care. Primary haemobartonellosis carries a good prognosis.

THE ORGANISM

H. felis is an epicellular mycoplasma that parasitizes the RBCs of cats. It can cause disease as a primary pathogen or by opportunistic infection as a sequelae to other diseases, particularly those where immunosuppression is a feature. Three forms of the organism have been identified on the surface of RBCs: rods, cocci and rings. These may occur singly or in rows or clusters. All forms are firmly adherent to the surface of the RBC and are partially embedded in the membrane. These forms were previously thought to represent different stages in the life cycle of the parasite, although recently it has been shown by polymerase chain reaction (PCR) that these forms represent morphologically and genetically distinct strains of the organism (Foley *et al.*, 1998). Rarely, organisms are found free in the serum, probably representing accidental detachment.

EPIDEMIOLOGY

Prevalence
The reported prevalence of infection varies greatly. Several factors will influence the outcome of surveys. These include prevalence in a given area, types of cats selected, the cyclical nature of the parasitaemia, the existence of carrier states, the presence of ectoparasites, and the ability of a given laboratory to identify the organism. The recorded prevalence of the organism varies from 4.9% to 23.2% (Carney and England, 1993). All surveys undoubtedly underestimate the true prevalence.

Predisposing factors
No age, breed, or sex susceptibility has been shown with *H. felis* infections, although some authors believe young male cats (Hayes and Priester, 1973), especially those with high flea burdens, may be more at risk (Nash and Bobade, 1986). Cats with feline leukaemia virus (FeLV) infection have long been thought to be at increased risk of infection with *H. felis* (Nash and Bobade, 1986). Although FeLV may not actually predispose to infection itself, it may result in more severe parasitaemia, anaemia and clinical signs. Other risk factors include recent illness, lack of vaccinations, roaming outdoors, and a young age (Grindem *et al.*, 1990).

Incubation period
The reported incubation period (the time from inoculation to the first appearance of parasites in the peripheral circulation) ranges from 2 to 34 days (Harvey and Gaskin, 1977; Van Steenhouse *et al.*, 1993), although the average is 6 to 17 days (Maede and Hata, 1975).

Carrier status
It is generally believed that the carrier status can be as long as 2 years but may in fact be much longer. Some authors describe a relapse of the acute stage that may occur with immunosuppression or stress from disease, although later work failed to confirm this finding (Harvey and Gaskin, 1978). Stress does increase the number of parasites but not necessarily clinical disease (Harvey and Gaskin, 1978). Treatment of anaemia with antibiotics or corticosteroids does not prevent occurrence of the carrier state, and prior exposure to the organism does not induce immunity (Pedersen, 1987).

Spread between individuals
H. felis can be transmitted experimentally via the oral, intraperitoneal, subcutaneous or intravenous route by

using infected whole blood. Whether any or all of these modes of transmission are important in the field situation is debatable.

Inoculation
Subcutaneous inoculation via cat bites is considered unlikely as little blood is transferred between cats, even with the presence of severe gingivitis and stomatitis, and saliva is not considered infectious (Harvey and Gaskin, 1977). Oral transmission has been shown to occur experimentally, but considering the large volumes of blood required (2–5 ml), it is extremely doubtful that this represents a real risk in the normal spread of infection. Intraperitoneal inoculation with infected blood has been a common way of transmitting infection under experimental conditions (Harvey and Gaskin, 1977) but would be unimportant in naturally acquired infections. Iatrogenic infection via whole blood transfusion is a real risk.

Ectoparasites
Ectoparasites, particularly fleas, have long been implicated as a possible mode of transmission. Considering the widespread occurrence of this parasite and the difficulty in horizontal transmission by other means, the existence of an ectoparasite vector would seem likely.

Vertical transmission
Vertical transmission via transplacental infection has been shown by the fact that kittens as young as 3 hours have been found to be infected with the organism (Harbutt, 1963). Infection of kittens via suckling is also considered possible but there is no conclusive evidence for this.

Natural infection
Natural infection probably occurs mainly via insect vectors (particularly fleas), although iatrogenic infection after blood transfusion and vertical transmission in utero and via suckling, although less important, should be considered.

PATHOGENESIS

Movement within the cat

The acute phase
Once inside the cat, *H. felis* remains within the bloodstream and associated organs such as the spleen. The period from the first appearance of the parasite to the last parasitaemic episode is referred to as the acute phase of the infection. Clinical signs develop during this period and can be mild and inapparent or result in severe anaemia and even death. RBCs and associated parasites are held within the spleen until 'pitting' (the removal of organisms by splenic

macrophages and reticular cells) occurs. After removal of parasites, the RBCs are returned to the circulation in large numbers. For this reason, the packed cell volume (PCV) can decrease quickly and then return to within normal limits with the same rapidity. This process may occur within hours (Harvey and Gaskin, 1977). Although the PCV may return to normal, the lifespan of the RBC is considerably reduced owing to the development of a Coombs' positive anaemia (Zulty and Kociba, 1990) and increased fragility after loss of membrane and membrane phospholipids (Maede, 1980).

The recovery phase
The recovery phase follows the acute phase. In the recovery phase, parasite numbers decrease and the PCV increases. The PCV increases more slowly than the rapid decrease in the number of parasites. The PCV remains within normal limits during this phase. Most (if not all) cats become chronic carriers. These cats have normal PCVs, and parasites may be intermittently found in small numbers.

Mechanisms of anaemia
The mechanism of anaemia in haemobartonellosis is complex. An understanding of the processes involved will lead to a more rational treatment regimen. Anaemia occurs via four major mechanisms: sequestration of RBCs, antibody-mediated haemolysis, erythrophagia and a decreased lifespan due to haemolysis.

Sequestration of RBCs
RBCs are held within the spleen until parasites are removed via pitting by splenic macrophages and reticular cells (Maede, 1979). The removal of the parasite results in a quick return of the RBCs to the circulation. This process explains the rapid fluctuations in PCV that occur during the acute phase of infection.

Antibody-mediated haemolysis
A large proportion of the anaemic process is due to the occurrence of a Coombs' positive anaemia and autoagglutination. This may be the direct result of the parasite or reflect damage to the erythrocyte membrane during parasitism or pitting, resulting in exposure of hidden antigens to the immune system or changes in the antigen structure of the RBC membrane. Electron microscopical studies reveal permanent erosions in the RBC membrane after removal of the parasite (Jain and Keaton, 1973). Coombs' positive anaemia may also result from decreased cholesterol and phospholipids in the RBC membrane (Maede, 1980).

Erythrophagia
Erythrophagia within both the spleen by splenic macrophages and the blood from transformed monocytes has been shown (Maede, 1978, 1979). Splenic erythrophagia is more important than peri-

pheral phagocytosis. Spherocytes and RBCs that are attached to each other (autoagglutination) are less pliable than normal cells and will be removed by the complex reticular networks of the spleen.

Decreased lifespan due to haemolysis

Although the parasite is epicellular it seems that *H. felis* causes irreversible changes to RBCs that result in increased osmotic fragility (Maede, 1975, 1980; Maede and Hata, 1975). This is related to a decreased concentration of erythrocyte lipids, almost certainly due to the loss of membrane after removal of the parasite (Maede, 1980).

CLINICAL SIGNS

Clinical signs vary depending on the stage of parasitaemia and the existence of intercurrent diseases, which may contribute to the clinical signs or result in more severe parasitaemia and anaemia. Should the haemogram reveal anaemia and *H. felis* organisms without evidence of regeneration, the clinician should ask two important questions. Firstly, has there been adequate time for regeneration and, secondly, are there any underlying diseases present that are preventing regeneration (e.g. FeLV, myelofibrosis, myelophthisis or toxic insult)? Cats that develop acute anaemias will show more severe clinical signs than cats that have anaemia of gradual onset.

Three categories of clinical presentation have been reported (Carney and England, 1993), but not every cat will fall into one of these major categories:

- Kittens and some adult cats with peracute anaemia, with sudden weakness, pallor and hypothermia that were otherwise normal before the onset of clinical signs
- Other kittens and most adult cats that show sudden and significant fever, acute anaemia, weakness, pallor, cardiac murmur, splenomegaly, diffuse body tenderness, dyspnoea and tachypnoea
- Adult cats that are slightly anaemic, with mild fever, lethargy and weight loss.

The clinical state is generally divided into the acute, recovery and carrier phases.

Acute phase

The acute phase is the stage from the first to the last parasitaemic episode (Van Steenhouse *et al.*, 1993). Anaemia and other clinical signs occur during this period. The haematocrit will fall initially and then quickly rise as RBCs are returned to the circulation. Most cats show a varied mixture of signs, none of which are specific.

Figure 5.25 lists the acute clinical signs.

Acute	Chronic
Lethargy	Weight loss
Anaemia	Mild anaemia
Hepatomegaly	Intermittent pyrexia
Splenomegaly	
Whole body tenderness	
Tachypnoea	
Dyspnoea	
Pyrexia	
Jaundice	

Figure 5.25: Clinical signs of haemobartonellosis.

Recovery phase

Although the PCV returns to normal, parasites can be identified during the recovery phase. Most (if not all) cats then become carriers.

Chronic carrier phase

Parasites may be found during the chronic carrier phase, and the PCV may fluctuate from normal to slightly below normal. This may last for 2 or more years. Relapse of clinical signs is possible but should be considered rare, as it has been difficult to reproduce relapse under experimental conditions (Harvey and Gaskin, 1978). Figure 5.25 lists the signs of chronic haemobartonellosis.

DIAGNOSIS

The lack of a widely available specific serological test, the tedious nature of examining blood smears for the parasite and the high incidence of false positive and negative results make diagnosis difficult. Definitive diagnosis rests on identification of the organism (Figure 5.26). The clinician must pay attention to sampling techniques and the cyclic nature of the parasitaemia, which may increase the chance of a positive diagnosis.

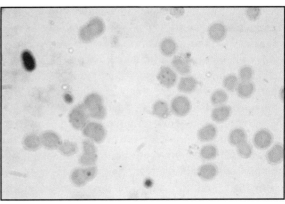

Figure 5.26: Haemobartonella felis *observed on the surface of red blood cells from a cat by using a Romanowsky staining method.*

The timing and frequency of sample taking is important. As the anaemia progresses the number of organisms decreases, making diagnosis more difficult. Organisms are said to disappear from the circulation quickly on beginning treatment, necessitating diagnosis before treatment is initiated.

Blood samples

Making smears of peripheral blood samples immediately after blood collection is the preferred method. Some authors favour the auricular vein as the site for venepuncture whereas others prefer the jugular. Anticoagulants (particularly ethylenediamine tetra-acetic acid) may dislodge the parasite from the surface of the RBC, which dramatically reduces the chance of finding the organism (Harvey and Gaskin, 1977). This is particularly true if the sample is left standing. Multiple smears taken over several days may be required to identify the organism, especially if the anaemia is severe.

Staining techniques

Staining techniques for identifying *H. felis* classically involve Romanowsky methods, although acridine orange is considered superior (Bobade and Nash, 1987). The disadvantages of staining with acridine orange are that it requires 24 hours for fixation and uses ultraviolet light microscopy, which is not always readily available. Therefore, not all veterinary laboratories use this method, and in cases with a high clinical suspicion it would be wise to find a laboratory that is experienced in looking for *H. felis*. False positives are commonly a result of protein precipitates, background debris or Howell–Jolly bodies. Stains should be freshly made and preferably filtered to prevent some of these problems. False negatives are common and may be as high as 50% in some cases (Carney and England, 1993) owing to the cyclical nature of the parasitaemia and inexperience of the investigator.

Haematology

Haematology generally reveals a regenerative anaemia with anisocytosis, macrocytosis and reticulocytosis. Many cats become Coombs' positive during the course of the infection. Spontaneous autoagglutination may also occur, and when it does a Coombs' test is not necessary. Autoagglutination must be differentiated from rouleaux formation, which is common in normal cats. The anaemia also waxes and wanes considerably during the course of infection and, whereas the number of circulating RBCs may decrease dramatically owing to sequestration in the spleen, RBC numbers can also quickly recover after removal of the parasite. The haemogram should be checked frequently for signs of recovery or deterioration. Monitoring the haemogram and the progression of clinical signs closely will enable the clinician to make more accurate judgements as to the need for blood transfusion or other changes in therapy.

Ancillary tests

Ancillary tests are of utmost importance in *H. felis* infections to rule out underlying diseases. Testing for FeLV and feline immunodeficiency virus (FIV) is useful. FeLV has previously been considered an important predisposing factor for the development of *H. felis* infection, and up to 46% of cats with *H. felis* have been reported to be positive for FeLV (Cotter *et al.*, 1975). These percentages are probably no longer correct.

Although alterations to the serum biochemical screen are non-specific, they may alert the clinician to the presence of underlying diseases that may influence the treatment or prognosis. In moribund cats, blood glucose concentration should be monitored, as *Haemobartonella* in other species (particularly mice) causes fatal hypoglycaemia by unknown mechanisms (Harvey and Gaskin, 1977). Severe life-threatening hypothermia is also common.

Recently, detection of the organism by PCR and western blot analysis has been described (Rikihisa *et al.*, 1997; Berent *et al.*, 1998; Foley *et al.*, 1998; Alleman *et al.*, 1999). The availability of this test may increase and allow an accurate way of identifying infected or carrier cats.

The aim of the diagnostic investigation should be to determine if *H. felis* is acting as a primary pathogen or a secondary opportunist, as the latter carries a worse prognosis, especially if the underlying disease is difficult to treat. Although this distinction may not always be possible, clinicians should do their best to differentiate primary from secondary haemobartonellosis.

TREATMENT

The need for and the type of treatment required will vary depending on the case. Treatment should not be considered as an all or nothing approach but as a custom-made plan depending on the severity of anaemia and related clinical signs and the presence of underlying disease.

As idiopathic haemolytic anaemia is rare in the cat, it may be prudent to treat for *Haemobartonella* even if organisms cannot be identified in cats with suspected immune-mediated RBC destruction.

Antibiotics

Antibiotics, particularly the tetracyclines, have been considered the drugs of choice by many authors, although others have found them to have little or no effect in eliminating or reducing the parasitaemic state (Harvey and Gaskin, 1978; Bobade *et al.*, 1988). No known treatment prevents the carrier status. Doxycycline, oxytetracycline and tetracycline are considered the drugs of choice.

Chloramphenicol is also reported as an effective treatment but can severely depress erythrogenesis, which is important in recovery from this condition. In addition, chloramphenicol can cause vomiting, anorexia, ataxia, neutropenia and sudden death in cats (Reid and Oehme, 1989).

Enrofloxacin has been anecdotally reported to be effective in the treatment of haemobartonellosis. The reported success of enrofloxacin comes from demonstrating cessation of parasitaemia. This may not be a true treatment success, but may reflect the cyclical nature of this infection. Enrofloxacin may be considered as a treatment choice either alone or in combination with tetracyclines and immunosuppressive therapy, especially in cats that do not respond to tetracycline antibiotics.

Thiacetarsemide sodium

Anecdotal evidence suggests that thiacetarsemide sodium can be used to treat haemobartonellosis. Although this may be true, detailed trials regarding the safety and efficacy of this drug are unavailable. Thiacetarsemide sodium is hepatotoxic, causes tissue necrosis if given perivascularly and is unlicensed for use in the cat.

Corticosteroids

As the pathogenesis of anaemia in *H. felis* infection is due to more than the parasite itself, and involves immune mechanisms, immune suppression with corticosteroids is considered valuable and perhaps the most important aspect of treatment. The exact timing for the withdrawal of corticosteroids is debatable and depends on the rapidity of recovery. Once the PCV returns to normal, therapy should be tapered within 1–2 weeks while monitoring closely for relapse. Figure 5.27 lists the treatment regimens.

Whole blood transfusions

Whole blood transfusions may be necessary in severely anaemic cats showing clinical signs of acute anaemia. Blood typing is imperative before undertaking transfusion.

PROGNOSIS

The prognosis for haemobartonellosis is generally regarded as fair to good, as 65% of affected cats recover from infection without treatment (Harvey and Gaskin, 1977) and 75% of cats survive if treatment is given (Bobade *et al.*, 1988). Prognosis depends on the presence of underlying disease and the ease with which it can be treated.

FURTHER CONSIDERATIONS

Immunosuppression and tumourigenesis

Some evidence suggests that 'anaemic stress' after *H. felis* infection can be oncogenic and result in an increased incidence of leukaemia and lymphoma (Priester and Hayes, 1973; Kociba *et al.*, 1983). Although association is not proof, anaemic stress leads to the development of myelogenous leukaemia in rats and mice (Priester and Hayes, 1973). Indeed, *H. felis* may itself lead to immunosuppression, as the incidence of FeLV infection after *H. felis* infection is reported to be increased (Kociba *et al.*, 1983). Although this was a small survey and it is possible that early FeLV infection may not have been detected, this is an interesting observation.

Blood donors

A potential source of infection with *H. felis* is via iatrogenic inoculation after blood transfusion. All cats that are blood donors should test negative for FeLV and FIV and have several blood smears examined for the presence of *H. felis*. Considerable controversy exists as to whether blood donors should be splenectomized to enhance detection of the parasite.

Drug	Dose
Doxycycline	1–3 mg/kg bid for 21 days
Oxytetracycline	25 mg/kg tid for 21 days
Tetracyclines	22 mg/kg tid for 21 days
Enrofloxacin	5 mg/kg sid for 21 days
Any of the above in combination with either prednisolone or dexamethasone:	
Prednisolone	2 mg/kg bid for 2–3 treatments then 1 mg/kg bid for 4–6 treatments and 1 mg/kg sid for 4–6 treatments
Dexamethasone	0.3 mg/kg sid for 2–3 days then 0.15 mg/kg sid for 2–3 days and 0.15 mg/kg sid for 2–3 days

Figure 5.27: *Drugs commonly used for the treatment of haemobartonellosis.*

REFERENCES

Alleman AR, Pate MG, Harvey JW, Gaskin JM and Barbet AF (1999) Western immunoblot analysis of the antigens of *Haemobartonella felis* with sera from experimentally infected cats. *Journal of Clinical Microbiology* **37**, 1474-1479

Berent LM, Messick JB and Cooper SK (1998) Detection of *Haemobartonella felis* in cats with experimentally induced acute and chronic infections, using a polymerase chain reaction. *American Journal of Veterinary Research* **59**, 1215-1220

Bobade PA and Nash AS (1987) A comparative study of the efficiency of acridine orange and some Romanowsky staining procedures in the demonstration of *Haemobartonella felis* in feline blood. *Veterinary Parasitology* **26**, 169-172

Bobade PA, Nash AS and Rogerson P (1988) Feline haemobartonellosis: clinical, haematological and pathological studies in natural infections and the relationship to infection with feline leukaemia virus. *Veterinary Record* **122**, 32-36

Carney HC and England JJ (1993) Feline haemobartonellosis. In: *Veterinary Clinics of North America: Feline Infectious Diseases*, eds. JD Hoskins and AS Loar, pp. 79-90. WB Saunders, Philadelphia

Cotter SUM, Hardy WE and Essex M (1975) Association of feline leukaemia virus with lymphosarcoma and other disorders in the cat. *Journal of the Veterinary Medical Association* **166**, 449-454

Foley JE, Harrus S, Poland A, Chomel B and Pederson NC (1998) Molecular, clinical, and pathologic comparison of two distinct strains of *Haemobartonella felis* in domestic cats. *American Journal of Veterinary Research* **59**, 1581-1588

Grindem CB, Corbett WT and Tomkins MT (1990) Risk factors for Haemobartonella felis infection in cats. *Journal of the Veterinary Medical Association* **196**, 96-99

Harbutt PR (1963) A clinical appraisal of feline infectious anaemia and its transmission under natural conditions. *Australian Veterinary Journal* **39**, 401-405

Harvey JW and Gaskin JK (1978) Feline haemobartonellosis: attempts to induce relapses of clinical disease in chronically infected cats. *Journal of the American Animal Hospital Association* **13**, 28-38

Harvey JW and Gaskin JM (1977) Experimental feline haemobartonellosis. *Journal of the American Animal Hospital Association* **13**, 28-38

Hayes HM and Priester WA (1973) Feline infectious anaemia. Risk by age, sex and breed; prior disease; seasonal occurrence; mortality. *Journal of Small Animal Practice* **14**, 797-804

Jain NC and Keeton KS (1973) Scanning electron microscopic features of Haemobartonella felis. *American Journal of Veterinary Research* **34**, 697-700

Kociba GJ, Glade Weiser M and Olsen RG (1983) Enhanced susceptibility to feline leukaemia virus in cats with Haemobartonella felis infection. *Leukaemia Reviews International* **1**, 88-89

Maede Y (1975) Studies on haemobartonellosis, IV. Lifespan of erythrocytes of cats infected with *Haemobartonella felis. Japanese Journal of Veterinary Science* **37**, 461-464

Maede Y (1978) Studies on haemobartonellosis, V. Role of the spleen in cats infected with *Haemobartonella felis. Japanese Journal of Veterinary Science*. **40**, 141-146

Maede Y (1979) Sequestration and phagocytosis of *Haemobartonella felis* in the spleen. *American Journal of Veterinary Research* **40**, 691-695

Maede Y (1980) Studies on haemobartonellosis, VI. Changes of erythrocyte lipids concentration and their relation to osmotic fragility. *Japanese Journal of Veterinary Science* **42**, 281-288

Maede Y and Hata R (1975) Studies on haemobartonellosis, II. The mechanism of anaemia produced by infection with *Haemobartonella felis. Japanese Journal of Veterinary Science* **37**, 49-54

Nash AS and Bobade PA (1986) Haemobartonella felis infection in cats from the Glasgow area. *Veterinary Record* **119**, 373-375

Pedersen NC (1987) Basic and clinical immunology In: *Diseases of the Cat: Medicine and Surgery, Vol 1*, ed. J Holzworth, pp.169-170. WB Saunders, Philadelphia

Priester WA and Hayes HM (1973) Brief communication: feline leukaemia after feline infectious anaemia. *Journal of the National Cancer Institute* **51**, 289-291

Reid FM and Oehme FW (1989) Toxicoses. In: *The Cat: Diseases and Clinical Management*, ed. RG Sherding, p. 203. Churchill Livingstone, New York

Rikihisa Y, Kawahara M, Wen B, Kociba G, Fuerst P, Kawamori F, Suto C, Shibata S and Futohashi M (1997) Western blot analysis of *Haemobartonella muris* and comparison of 16S rRNA gene sequence of *H. muris, H. felis*, and *Eperythrozoon suis. Journal of Clinical Microbiology* **35**, 823-829

Van Steenhouse JL, Millard JR and Taboada J (1993) Feline haemobartonellosis. *Compendium of Continuing Education for the Practising Veterinarian* **15**, 535-545

Zulty JC and Kociba GJ (1990) Cold agglutinins in cats with haemobartonellosis. *Journal of the Veterinary Medical Association* **6**, 907-911

(v) Canine Babesiosis

Remo Lobetti

INTRODUCTION

Canine babesiosis is a tick-borne disease of worldwide importance, which ranges in severity from relatively mild to fatal. Although haemolytic anaemia is the hallmark, several variations and complications can occur. The causative organism of canine babesiosis is either *Babesia canis* or *Babesia gibsoni*. Three subtypes or strains of *B. canis* are recognized, namely, *B. canis canis, B. canis vogeli* and *B. canis rossi*. *B. canis canis* and *B. canis vogeli* occur in Europe and North Africa respectively, whereas *B. canis rossi* occurs in southern Africa (Uilenberg *et al.*, 1989). *B. gibsoni* occurs in Asia, North America and North and East Africa (Taboada, 1998). The genus *Babesia* was named after Victor Babes, who in 1887 established the aetiology of the disease in cattle in Romania. The first report of canine babesiosis was in South Africa in 1885 by Hutcheon; however, the parasites were only recognized much later by Purvis in 1896 and Koch in 1897.

LIFE CYCLE

In the adult tick, schizogony occurs in the gut epithelial cells, resulting in the formation of large merozoites. These then undergo successive cycles of schizogony within a variety of cell types, including the oocytes. In the salivary glands, schizogony results in the formation of small infective merozoites. After the tick has attached to a dog (the host) and feeds, the merozoites in the tick's saliva enter the dog's erythrocytes with the aid of a specialized apical complex. Once inside the erythrocyte, the merozoite transforms into a trophozoite, from which further merozoites develop by a process of merogony. Once divided, they leave the cell to enter other erythrocytes. Trans-stadial and transovarial transmission can occur, and it is thought that a tick can remain infective for several generations.

EPIDEMIOLOGY

Babesiosis is solely a tick-borne disease, with *B. canis canis* being transmitted by *Dermacentor reticulatus*,

B. canis vogeli and *B. gibsoni* by *Rhipicephalus sanguineus* and *B. canis rossi* by *Haemophysalis leachi*. *B. canis* can affect dogs of all ages, although most cases are in young dogs. A seasonal variation occurs, with the highest incidence in the summer months. The source of infection is carrier ticks, or ticks feeding on dogs that are either ill or incubating the disease and then feeding on a susceptible dog (Lobetti, 1998). Other possible sources of infection are carrier dogs and blood transfusions.

PATHOGENESIS

The incubation period after exposure to a tick is 10–21 days. Intraerythrocytic parasitaemia causes both intravascular and extravascular haemolysis, resulting in regenerative anaemia, haemoglobinaemia, haemoglobinuria and bilirubinuria. Pyrexia also develops, which is attributed to the release of endogenous pyrogens after erythrolysis, destruction of the parasite and/or activation of inflammatory mediators. Splenomegaly occurs as a result of hyperplasia of the mononuclear phagocytic system. The haemolytic crisis that develops results in anaemic hypoxia, anaerobic metabolism and metabolic acidosis. Compounding the problem is the fact that the remaining haemoglobin is not functioning optimally, thereby exacerbating the anaemic hypoxia (Taylor *et al.*, 1993).

The many and varied clinical manifestations of canine babesiosis are difficult to relate to an organism that is solely restricted to the erythrocyte. Although the clinical manifestations are diverse, the mechanisms promoting them are probably more uniform. Multiple organ dysfunction syndrome (MODS) is now recognized as the end result of tissue inflammation initiated by several different conditions, including hypovolaemia, septic shock and infectious organisms. Babesiosis can cause severe tissue hypoxia, with consequent widespread tissue damage and probable release of inflammatory mediators. Widespread inflammation and multiple organ damage can thus occur (Jacobson and Clark, 1994). The systemic inflammatory response syndrome (SIRS) that precedes MODS is caused by excessive release of inflammatory mediators. This syndrome is broadly defined and considered to be present if two or more of the following occur: tachycardia, tachypnoea or respiratory alkalosis, hypothermia or hyperthermia and leucocytosis or leucopenia with a neutrophilic left shift (Cipolle *et al.*, 1993). By this definition, most cases of babesiosis have SIRS.

In one study, 87% of cases were positive for SIRS, 52% showed single organ damage and 48% had multiple organ damage (Welzl *et al.*, 1999). Although outcome was not affected by whether one or multiple organs showed evidence of damage, specific organ involvement significantly affected outcome: risk of death increased 57-fold and fivefold with involvement of the central nervous system and renal dysfunction, respectively. Liver or muscle damage did not affect outcome.

CLINICAL MANIFESTATIONS

Canine babesiosis can be clinically classified into uncomplicated and complicated forms. Uncomplicated cases typically present with signs relating to acute haemolysis, including fever, anorexia, depression, pale mucous membranes, splenomegaly and waterhammer pulse. This form is further divided into mild, moderate or severe disease, according to the severity of the anaemia. A case of mild uncomplicated babesiosis can progress to become severe uncomplicated, when anaemia becomes life threatening. The complicated form of babesiosis refers to clinical manifestations that are not easily explained by the haemolytic process alone. Rare complications include gastrointestinal disturbances, myalgia, ocular involvement, upper respiratory signs, cardiac involvement, necrosis of the extremities, fluid accumulation or disease with a chronic clinical course. Overlap between the different categories of the complications can also occur.

Acute renal failure
Evidence of renal damage is common in both complicated and uncomplicated cases but does not necessarily predict renal failure. A recent study showed celluria of the renal tubular epithelium, enzymuria, proteinuria and variable azotaemia in dogs with babesiosis without overt acute renal failure (ARF), although ARF was also documented in several dogs in the same study (Lobetti *et al.*, 1999). Acute renal failure in babesiosis typically presents with anuria or oliguria despite adequate rehydration but is an uncommon complication. An increased concentration of serum urea alone is an unreliable indicator of renal insufficiency in babesiosis, as a disproportionate increase in urea, compared with creatinine, concentration occurs, which has been related to the catabolism of lysed erythrocytes. Renal failure is diagnosed on the basis of ongoing evaluation of urine volume, urine analysis and degree of azotaemia.

Cerebral babesiosis
Cerebral babesiosis is defined as the presence of concurrent neurological signs in an animal with babesiosis. The presentation is typically peracute, with clinical signs being a combination of incoordination, hindquarter paresis, muscle tremors, nystagmus, anisocoria, intermittent loss of consciousness, seizures, stupor, coma, aggression, paddling or vocalization (Jacobson and Clark, 1994). Pathological changes in the brain are congestion (Figure 5.28), haemorrhage and/or necrosis (Figure 5.29) and sequestration/pavementing of parasitized erythrocytes in capillary beds (Figure 5.30).

Coagulopathy
The most consistent haemostatic abnormality in babesiosis is profound thrombocytopenia, which is a routine finding in both complicated and uncomplicated cases. Despite the degree of thrombocytopenia, clinically apparent haemorrhages are relatively rare. Although disseminated intravascular coagulation (DIC) has been reported in canine babesiosis, confirmation of DIC is difficult because of the nature of the underlying disease process and the reported unreliability of the human fibrin degradation product test (Jacobson and Clark, 1994). Clinical signs of DIC are difficult to recognize until haemorrhages develop in the hypocoagulable phase, where signs are related to organ dysfunction induced by microthrombi (Figure 5.31).

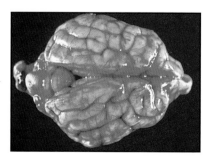

Figure 5.28: Brain of a dog that died from cerebral babesiosis, showing generalized congestion. (Courtesy of Dr Anne Pardini, Department of Pathology, Faculty of Veterinary Science, University of Pretoria.)

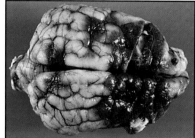

Figure 5.29: Brain of a dog that died from cerebral babesiosis, showing focal areas of necrosis. (Courtesy of Dr Anne Pardini, Department of Pathology, Faculty of Veterinary Science, University of Pretoria.)

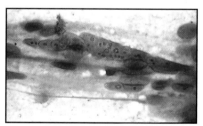

Figure 5.30: Histopathological section from a brain of a dog that died from cerebral babesiosis, showing capillary blood vessels containing sequestrated parasitized erythrocytes. (Courtesy of Dr Anne Pardini, Department of Pathology, Faculty of Veterinary Science, University of Pretoria.)

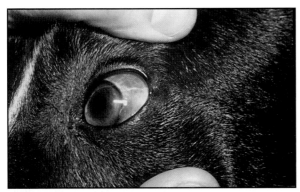

Figure 5.31: *Scleral haemorrhage in a dog with babesiosis complicated by disseminated intravascular coagulation.*

Icterus and hepatopathy

In some cases of babesiosis, icterus and increased concentrations of liver enzymes and bile acids occur, which are indicative of a liver insult (Miller, 1999). Whether the insult is due to inflammatory cytokines, hypoxic damage or a combination of these is not known. As the icterus (Figure 5.32) does not seem to be due to haemolysis alone, liver dysfunction seems to be, at least, contributory. Histopathological changes usually associated with icterus include both diffuse and periportal lesions, whereas icteric dogs with babesiosis show a centrilobular lesion. Hypoxic insults can cause diffuse hepatocellular swelling, and thus the hypoxia in severe babesiosis may be severe enough to cause a hepatopathy.

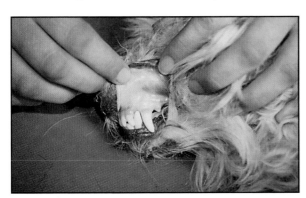

Figure 5.32: *Dog with severe icterus due to babesiosis.*

Immune-mediated haemolytic anaemia

Immune-mediated haemolytic anaemia (IMHA) is the increased destruction of erythrocytes due to antibodies against the erythrocyte membrane, which can be either primary (in which the membrane is normal) or secondary (in which the membrane is altered and recognized as 'foreign'). Secondary IMHA is assumed to be the case in babesiosis. The cardinal feature of babesiosis-associated IMHA is continuing haemolysis despite successful antibabesial treatment. Diagnosis is by the in-saline agglutination test and/or detection of spherocytosis. The Coombs' test is not diagnostic as both uncomplicated cases and cases complicated with IMHA give a positive Coombs' test result.

Acute respiratory distress syndrome

Acute respiratory distress syndrome (ARDS) is a severe and frequently catastrophic complication of babesiosis. Typical clinical signs are a sudden increase in respiratory rate (although this may be caused by other factors, such as pyrexia and acidosis), dyspnoea, moist cough and blood-tinged frothy nasal discharge. The diagnosis of ARDS is based on the presence of diffuse pulmonary infiltrates on thoracic radiographs, hypoxaemia due to ventilation–perfusion mismatch, normal pulmonary capillary wedge pressure and reduced pulmonary compliance (Frevert and Warner, 1992). In most clinical situations, pulmonary wedge pressure, blood gas analysis and compliance cannot be measured. Thus the diagnosis of ARDS depends on the recognition of risk factors for ARDS, thoracic radiographs (Figure 5.33) and the exclusion of other causes of pulmonary oedema, especially cardiogenic causes and fluid overload, the latter particularly where oliguric renal failure is present. Fluid loads that can be tolerated by normal dogs may fatally exacerbate pulmonary oedema in ARDS.

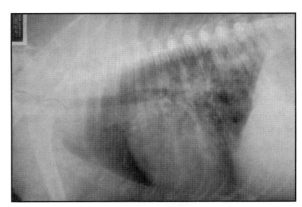

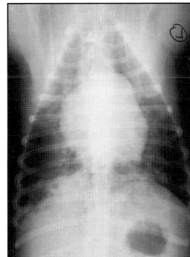

Figure 5.33: *Lateral and dorsoventral radiographs from a dog with babesiosis complicated by acute respiratory distress syndrome, showing severe pulmonary oedema.*

Haemoconcentration

The paradoxical phenomenon of severe intravascular haemolysis combined with haemoconcentration constitutes the syndrome known as 'red biliary'. Clinical features are congested mucous membranes, visible haemoglobinaemia and/or haemoglobinuria and high to normal or increased haematocrit (Jacobson and Clark, 1994). Haemoconcentration has been associated with other complications, such as cerebral babesiosis, DIC, ARF and ARDS. Haemoconcentration in babesiosis is thought to be due to reduction in blood volume, because of fluid shifts from the vascular to the extravascular compartment. As plasma protein concentrations are normal, plasma, rather than a filtrate of plasma, is shifted from the vasculature. The widespread increase in capillary permeability, which occurs in SIRS, may play an important role in the pathogenesis of 'red biliary'.

Hypotension

Dogs with severe and complicated babesiosis are frequently presented in a state of collapse and clinical shock, the latter resembling the hyperdynamic phase of septic shock. In one study, hypotension occurred frequently in babesiosis, and the presence and severity of hypotension increased with severity of the disease (Jacobson et al., 1999). The presence of hypotension in dogs with complicated babesiosis is consistent with the hypothesis that inflammatory mechanisms play a major role in this disease and can result in a sepsis-like state. It is likely that hypotension in babesiosis is a combination of vasodilation, reduced vascular volume due to increased vascular permeability and/or dehydration, and myocardial depression. Hypotension can play a role in the pathophysiology of the disease, as it has been hypothesized to facilitate parasite sequestration.

CLINICAL PATHOLOGY

The primary haematological abnormalities in canine babesiosis are anaemia, thrombocytopenia and leucocytosis (Figure 5.34). However, the haematological profile varies in different parts of the world: in France, mild anaemia and thrombocytopenia have been reported. In the Philippines, the only abnormality reported was mild anaemia. In Nigeria, peracute cases showed severe anaemia, neutrophilia, lymphocytosis and eosinopenia, acute and chronic cases showed only moderate anaemia, and only mild anaemia was present in the chronic cases. In South Africa, severe anaemia, neutrophilia, monocytosis, eosinopenia and thrombocytopenia have been reported (Reyers et al., 1998). The most remarkable differences observed between these reports were degree of anaemia, macrocytosis (representing reticulocytosis) and leucocytosis in general, but particularly neutrophilia.

Urine analysis may show hypersthenuria, bilirubinuria, haemoglobinuria, proteinuria, granular casts and epithelial cells of the renal tubule. Alterations in biochemical parameters varies depending on the severity of the case. Typically, uncomplicated cases can have no biochemical changes. However, an increased liver enzyme concentration, hypokalaemia (in more severely affected cases) and an increased serum urea concentration with a normal serum creatinine concentration may be evident. In complicated cases, biochemical changes reflect the underlying complication.

The most commonly reported acid–base disturbance in dogs with babesiosis and severe anaemia is metabolic acidosis. However, studies by Leisewitz et al. (1999) suggest that a mixed acid–base disturbance is present in many cases, which would reflect a more complex pathophysiology than previously assumed. Dogs with severe babesiosis can show a combination of abnormalities, including hyperchloraemic metabolic acidosis (low strong ion difference, SID), high anion gap metabolic acidosis (probably due to hyperlactataemia), hypoalbuminaemic alkalosis and hyperphosphataemic acidosis, dilutional acidosis and respiratory alkalosis. Respiratory alkalosis occurs as frequently as metabolic acidosis, and arterial blood pH is a poor indicator of the complexity of the pathology.

Parameter	Mean	Standard deviation	Range	Normal
Haematocrit	20.24	12.81	3–70	35–50%
Reticulocyte count	9.19	7.12	0.1–44.6	<1%
White cell count	20.09	15.82	0.4–109.6	6–15 x 10^9/l
Neutrophils	9.318	9.864	0–75.58	3–11.5 x 10^9/l
Band cells	3.453	4.839	0–49.32	0–0.3 x 10^9/l
Lymphocytes	2.439	2.022	0–23.07	1–4.8 x10^9/l
Monocytes	2.419	2.676	0–22.062	0.15–1.35 x 10^9/l
Eosinophils	0.143	0.354	0–4.088	0.1–1.25 x 10^9/l
Platelets	65.12	78.88	1–726	200–500 x 10^9/l

Figure 5.34: Haematological parameters from 921 cases of babesiosis due to Babesia canis evaluated at the Onderstepoort Veterinary Academic Hospital.

DIAGNOSIS

The diagnosis of babesiosis is made by demonstrating the presence of *Babesia* organisms within infected erythrocytes by using Romanowsky-type stains. Large (2 x 5 μm) pear-shaped organisms (usually present in pairs) are indicative of infection with *B. canis* (Figure 5.35), whereas *B. gibsoni* appears as smaller (1 x 3 μm) single round to oval organisms (Figure 5.36). Parasites can be detected in blood smears from peripheral blood as well as central blood. Serology is a more reliable method for detection of occult parasitaemias in less endemic areas. However, as there is serological crossreactivity between *B. canis* and *B. gibsoni*, identification of the parasite is still necessary.

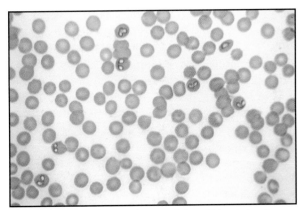

Figure 5.35: *Blood smear from peripheral blood showing multiple* Babesia canis *parasites. Diff-Quik® stain.*

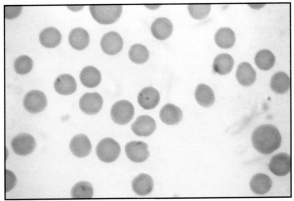

Figure 5.36: *Blood smear from peripheral blood showing multiple* Babesia gibsoni *parasites. Diff-Quik® stain.*

THERAPY

The primary therapeutic aim in the treatment of babesiosis is the reversal of life-threatening anaemia via blood transfusions, and elimination or suppression of the parasite with specific anti-babesial drugs. Mild to moderate uncomplicated cases require only antibabesial therapy, severe uncomplicated cases require antibabesial therapy and blood transfusions, and the complicated forms of the disease require additional therapy aimed at treating complications (Figure 5.37). In mild to moderate uncomplicated cases, noticeable signs of recovery can be expected within 24 hours of specific treatment.

Antibabesial therapy

The three recommended and recognized antibabesial drugs are diminazene aceturate, imidocarb and trypan blue. Other drugs that have been used are amicarbalide, euflavine, phenamidine, quinoronium sulphate and chloroquine. However, due to their poor efficacy and/or additional adverse effects, these drugs have been either discontinued or infrequently used (Swan, 1995).

Diminazene

Diminazene is the drug of choice and is given intramuscularly at a dosage of 3.5 mg/kg once only. The drug has a rapid action and a short-lived protective effect, making it unsuitable for chemoprophylaxis. Diminazene has a low therapeutic index, with toxicity resulting in depression or stupor, continuous vocalization, ataxia, opisthotonos, extensor rigidity, nystagmus and seizures. Nervous signs usually occur 24 to 48 hours after an overdose and are irreversible and potentially fatal.

Imidocarb

Imidocarb can be given either intramuscularly or subcutaneously at a dose of 6 mg/kg. Toxicity can cause severe renal tubular and hepatic necrosis.

Trypan blue

Trypan blue suppresses parasitaemia and alleviates clinical signs but does not eliminate infection. Consequently, it is often followed up with diminazene or imidocarb in an attempt to sterilize the infection. It is also used in repeated relapses after treatment with either diminazene or imidocarb. As the drug is irritant to tissues, it is given strictly intravenously as a 1% solution, at a dose of 10 mg/kg. Treatment can be repeated if necessary. Premunity may develop in some dogs, but relapses can occur at any stage owing to stress.

Blood transfusions

Transfusions are usually indicated in severe uncomplicated cases and in complicated cases that have a life-threatening anaemia. The decision to transfuse is based on clinical signs, history and haematological testing. Clinical signs that would indicate the need for transfusion are tachycardia, tachypnoea, waterhammer pulse, weakness and collapse. Although

Classification	Clinical signs	Therapeutic principles
Uncomplicated		
Mild to moderate	Acute haemolysis Mild/moderate anaemia	Antibabesial
Severe	Acute haemolytic crisis Life-threatening anaemia	Antibabesial Blood transfusion
Complicated		
Acute renal failure	Oliguria, anuria or polyuria	Antibabesial Fluids Diuretics Dopamine
Cerebral babesiosis	Collapsed Nystagmus Seizures Semi-coma, coma	Antibabesial Oxygen supplementation Barbiturate sedation Diuretics Elevation of the head
Coagulopathy	May be clinically silent Bleeding tendency Shock, organ dysfunction	Antibabesial Fresh frozen plasma Heparin

Icterus and hepatopathy	Profound bilirubinaemia and bilirubinuria
	Yellow discolouration of mucous
	  membranes
		Antibabesial
		Blood transfusion
		Fluids with potassium and
		  dextrose

Immune-mediated haemolytic
anaemia
	Persistent in-saline agglutination
	Worsening anaemia despite eradication
	  of parasites
		Antibabesial
		Blood transfusion
		Corticosteroids
		Azathioprine
		Cyclophosphamide
		Intravenous human
		  gammaglobulin

Acute respiratory distress syndrome (ARDS, 'shock lung')	Sudden onset tachypnoea Severe dyspnoea Cough Blood-tinged frothy nasal discharge	Antibabesial Oxygen supplementation Diuretics Pentoxifylline Colloids

Haemoconcentration ('red
biliary')
	Peracute onset
	Often collapsed
	Severe intravascular haemolysis with
	  normal or high haematocrit
		Antibabesial
		Fluids at double
		  maintenance rates
		Colloids

Hypotension	May not be 'classic' shock Congestion Bounding pulse may be present	Antibabesial Blood transfusion Fluids Colloids

Figure 5.37: *Clinical manifestations of babesiosis and therapeutic principles.*

the haematocrit is the most commonly used indicator of anaemia, erythrocyte count and haemoglobin concentration can also be used. There is no set haematocrit at which a transfusion should be given, as it must be evaluated in conjunction with the clinical signs and history. Generally, a transfusion is considered when the haematocrit is 15% or lower and always indicated when the haematocrit is 10% or lower. The degree of parasitaemia is not an important deciding factor, as it often bears little relation to the degree of anaemia.

Packed red blood cells are the component of choice for babesiosis. The administration of the plasma component of whole blood is unnecessary in most dogs with babesiosis and can place the patient at risk of volume overload. If rehydration is required, crystalloid replacement solutions are preferable. A blood transfusion not only has a favourable effect on oxygen status and acid–base balance in dogs with babesiosis but also replaces the subfunctional haemoglobin with functional haemoglobin.

Supportive therapy

Supportive therapy should be based on thorough patient assessment and ongoing monitoring, appropriate laboratory testing and accepted therapeutic principles for the complications that may be present: acute renal failure, immune-mediated haemolytic anaemia, DIC, hepatopathy, shock and pulmonary oedema.

PREVENTION

The primary means of disease prevention is the control of the vector tick by routinely dipping or spraying pets, by using tick collars or spot-on preparations and by environmental control by spraying the premises. The newer ectoparasitic agents (such as fipronil) are also effective.

A vaccine against a specific avirulent strain of canine babesia is available in France; however, cross immunity between the different strains of babesia seems not to occur. It has recently been shown that protective immunity to a virulent strain is possible, thus making vaccines from different parasite strains feasible (Lewis *et al.*, 1995).

Premunity has been recognized as important in controlling clinical signs of the virulent form of the disease in endemic areas. Therefore complete eradication of parasites from infected animals may not be advantageous in these areas, and thus the use of drugs to sterilize the infection may be undesirable (Penzhorn, 1994). The role that premunity plays in areas with less virulent strains is not known.

As babesial organisms can be transmitted by blood transfusions, it is important that all blood donors are negative for babesiosis.

REFERENCES AND FURTHER READING

Cipolle MD, Pasquale MD and Cerra FB (1993) Secondary organ dysfunction: from clinical perspectives to molecular mediators. *Critical Care Clinics* **9**, 261–298

Frevert CW and Warner AE (1992) Respiratory distress resulting from acute lung injury in the veterinary patient. *Journal of Veterinary Internal Medicine* **6**, 154–165

Jacobson LJ and Clark I (1994) The pathophysiology of canine babesiosis: new approaches to an old puzzle. *Journal of the South African Veterinary Association* **65**, 134–145

Jacobson L, Lobetti R and Vaughan-Scott T (1999) Hypotension: a common event in canine babesiosis. In: *Proceedings of a Canine Babesiosis and Ehrlichiosis Symposium*, Faculty of Veterinary Science, University of Pretoria, pp. 50–54

Leisewitz A, Jacobson L, De Morais H and Reyers F (1999) The mixed acid-base disturbances of severe canine babesiosis. In: *Proceedings of a Canine Babesiosis and Ehrlichiosis Symposium*, Faculty of Veterinary Science, University of Pretoria, pp. 37–44

Lewis BD, Penzhorn BL and Lopez-Rebollar LM (1995) Immune responses to South African *Babesia canis* and the development of a preliminary vaccine. *Journal of the South African Veterinary Association* **66**, 61–65

Lobetti RG (1998) Canine babesiosis. *Compendium on Continuing Education for the Practicing Veterinarian* **20**, 418–431

Lobetti R, Jacobson L and Vaughan-Scott T (1999) The effect of canine babesiosis on renal function. In: *Proceedings of a Canine Babesiosis and Ehrlichiosis Symposium*, Faculty of Veterinary Science, University of Pretoria, pp. 55–61

Miller D (1999) The yellow patient. In: *Proceedings of a Canine Babesiosis and Ehrlichiosis Symposium*, Faculty of Veterinary Science, University of Pretoria, pp. 81–83

Penzhorn BC (1994) Drug sterilisation of *Babesia canis* infection in dogs. *Journal of the South African Veterinary Association* **65**, 346–352

Reyers F, Leisewitz AL, Lobetti RG, Milner RJ, Jacobson LS and Van Zyl M (1998) Canine babesiosis in South Africa: more than one disease. Does this serve a model for falciparum malaria? *Annals of Tropical Medicine and Parasitology* **92**, 503–511

Swan GE (1995) Antibabesial drugs for use in dogs and cats. In: *Proceedings of a Canine Babesiosis Symposium*, Faculty of Veterinary Science, University of Pretoria, pp. 64–68

Taboada J (1998) Babesiosis. In: *Infectious Diseases of the Dog and Cat, 2nd edn*, ed. CG Greene, pp. 473–481. WB Saunders, Philadelphia

Taylor JH, Guthrie AJ, van der Walt JG and Leisewitz A (1993) The effect of *Babesia canis* induced haemolysis on the canine haemoglobin oxygen dissociation curve. *Journal of the South African Veterinary Association* **64**, 141–143

Uilenberg G, Franssen F, Perie NM and Spanger A (1989) Three groups of *Babesia canis* distinguished and a proposal for nomenclature. *Veterinary Quarterly* **11**, 33–40

Welzl C, Leisewitz A, Jacobson L, Myburgh E and Vaughan-Scott T (1999) The systemic inflammatory response and multiple organ dysfunction syndromes in canine babesiosis. In: *Proceedings of a Canine Babesiosis and Ehrlichiosis Symposium*, Faculty of Veterinary Science, University of Pretoria, pp. 27–31

Disorders of Leucocyte Number

John Dunn

INTRODUCTION

Total and differential white blood cell (WBC) counts can be helpful in assessing the cause, severity, duration and prognosis of a disease process. Abnormalities in leucocyte number should always be interpreted in association with the history, clinical examination, other components of the routine haemogram (red cell parameters, reticulocyte and platelet counts) and results of additional diagnostic tests.

Accurate interpretation of WBC counts requires a basic knowledge of leucocyte kinetics, pathophysiology of disease, normal cellular morphology and the effects of species and other non-disease variables on various leucocyte parameters. Interpretation should be based on absolute numbers rather than the relative percentage of each cell type.

TOTAL WHITE BLOOD CELL COUNT

Variations in leucocyte number may involve alterations in the rate of production, release, distribution and circulating lifespan of cells. Leucocytosis is the term used to describe an increase in the total number of circulating WBCs. In most cases leucocytosis is caused by an increase in the total number of neutrophils (neutrophilia). Leucopenia (decreased total WBC count) is less common than leucocytosis and is usually caused by neutropenia.

Total WBC counts are generally higher in young animals owing to an absolute increase in the number of lymphocytes. The number of lymphocytes gradually declines to adult values by 6–9 months of age.

GRANULOCYTES

Granulocytes are WBCs that possess specific (secondary) granules in their cytoplasm. These granules form at the myelocyte stage of maturation and their distinctive colour identifies the cell as a neutrophil, eosinophil or basophil. In addition, the mature granulocyte is characterized by the presence of a segmented nucleus with clumped nuclear chromatin.

Granulopoiesis

Granulopoiesis involves the production of neutrophils, eosinophils and basophils (Figure 6.1). Granulocyte life span has three phases: an intramedullary phase, an intravascular phase and a tissue phase. The intramedullary phase consists of a stem cell pool, a proliferating pool (myeloblasts, promyelocytes and myelocytes) and a maturation or storage pool (metamyelocytes, band and segmented granulocytes). The stem cell pool consists of a population of pluripotent stem cells, which give rise to committed progenitor cells known as colony-forming units (CFU). Neutrophils and monocytes originate from the same progenitor cell, the colony-forming unit – granulocyte–macrophage (CFU-GM), which differentiates into unipotent CFU (CFU-G and CFU-M) which produce neutrophilic and monocytic precursors, respectively (Figure 6.2). There are separate progenitor cells for eosinophils (CFU-Eos) and basophils (CFU-Bas).

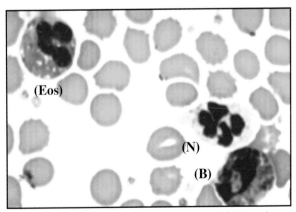

Figure 6.1: Canine eosinophil (Eos), neutrophil (N) and basophil (B). (© AXIOM Veterinary Laboratories.)

Neutrophils

Neutrophil production

Intramedullary phase: The maturation or storage pool in the bone marrow provides a buffer between supply and demand and prevents marrow depletion of neutrophils in situations when there is a sudden in-

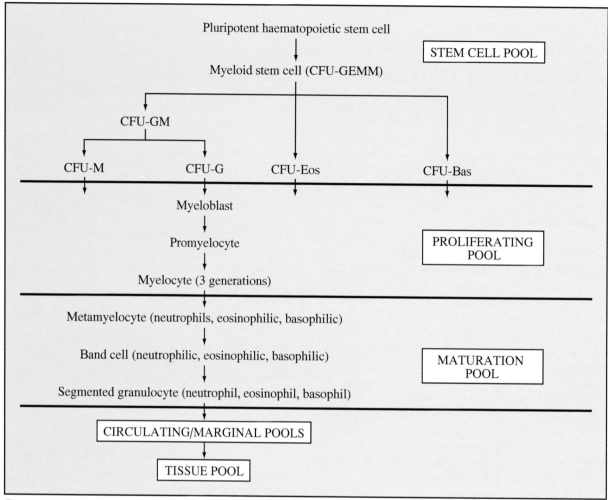

Figure 6.2: *Phases of granulocyte differentiation and maturation. Colony-forming unit (CFU) precursors are committed progenitor cells; GEMM, granulocyte–erythroid–monocyte–megakaryocyte; GM, granulocyte–macrophage ; M, monocyte; G, granulocyte; Eos, eosinophil; Bas, basophil.*

creased rate of utilization. This reserve pool contains about a 5-day supply of cells. Neutrophils move rapidly from the bone marrow to sites of acute inflammation. In response to a sudden increased demand for neutrophils, there is a lag phase of 3–4 days before increased granulopoiesis occurs.

Intravascular phase: Neutrophils leave the bone marrow after 3–5 days' maturation. Once in the blood vessel they may enter one of two functional compartments: they either remain in the circulation (circulatory pool) or adhere to the walls of small vessels primarily in the spleen, lungs and splanchnic region (marginal pool). Neutrophils in the marginal pool can be mobilized quickly in response to physiological stimuli (stress, exercise, excitement) and pathological stimuli (infection, inflammation). The marginal and circulating pools are approximately equal in the dog. In the cat, the marginal pool is about two to three times larger than the circulating pool. There is continual exchange of cells between the two compartments. The total blood pool of neutrophils is replaced approxi-

mately twice daily, and the average circulating cell lifespan varies from 6–14 hours. The circulating lifespan is shortened during acute infections as neutrophils pass rapidly into tissues. Neutrophils are normally lost in the lungs, saliva and urine and into the gastrointestinal tract. They are also phagocytosed by macrophages in the spleen, liver and bone marrow.

The absolute neutrophil count obtained at any one time does not reflect the dynamics of production and release of the cells. The absolute neutrophil count is influenced by the rate of granulopoiesis, the rate at which cells leave the bone marrow and enter the circulation, the shift of cells between the marginal and circulating pools and the rate at which cells leave the circulation and enter the tissues.

Tissue phase: Neutrophils randomly leave the circulation and enter the tissues and body cavities. In healthy animals there is no major tissue pool. Once in the tissues, neutrophils cannot re-enter the circulation, i.e. there is no exchange of cells between the tissue and circulating pools.

Neutrophil function

The primary function of neutrophils is the phagocytosis and killing of microorganisms. Neutrophils also have cytotoxic, parasiticidal and tumouricidal properties and may have a role in the coagulation and fibrinolytic pathways. Accumulation of neutrophils and the release of their various bioactive products, together with activation of complement components, results in increased vascular permeability and enhanced tissue damage at sites of acute inflammation.

Neutrophilia

Neutrophilia may result from increased movement of neutrophils from the marginal to the circulating pool, increased release of neutrophils from the storage pool into the circulation or decreased efflux from the circulation into the tissues. Increased numbers of circulating neutrophils may occur in response to physiological and pathological stimuli (see section on common white blood cell responses and Figure 6.3). Neutrophilia is a common physiological response to stress (resulting in increased circulating levels of cortisol) and exercise, fear or excitement (resulting in increased release of adrenaline).

Physiological:
    Adrenaline release
    Stress (endogenous or exogenous
      corticosteroids)
Reactive:
    Acute or chronic inflammation
Infectious (localized/systemic)
Non-infectious:
    Immune-mediated disease
    Surgery (tissue damage/stress)
    Tissue necrosis
    Haemorrhage or haemolysis
    Early stage of oestrogen toxicity
    Acute pancreatitis
Neoplasia:
    Large necrotic tumours
    Myeloproliferative disorders (e.g. acute or
      chronic myeloid leukaemia)*

---

*Figure 6.3: Causes of neutrophilia. *Some myeloproliferative disorders may present with a normal leucocyte profile.*

Neutrophilia is also a feature of most acute and chronic inflammatory disease processes. Haematological evidence of inflammation does not, however, necessarily imply an infectious aetiology as many non-septic disorders, for example, acute pancreatitis, immune-mediated polyarthritis and lesions resulting in a significant degree of tissue necrosis, frequently elicit similar neutrophilic responses. The magnitude of the neutrophilia caused by an acute inflammatory lesion is generally greater than that caused by chronic inflammation or a

physiological stimulus. The neutrophilia is also more likely to be associated with a significant left shift if an infectious agent is involved (some chronic inflammatory lesions may have normal neutrophil counts). Other causes of reactive neutrophilia, usually with a less pronounced left shift, include haemorrhage (especially into a body cavity), haemolysis, malignancy and recent surgery (resulting in tissue damage). Certain myeloproliferative disorders, for example, acute or chronic myeloid leukaemia, may result in the release of increased numbers of mature and/or immature neutrophils into the circulation.

Neutropenia

Neutropenia is the most common cause of leucopenia in small animals. It may occur as a result of decreased neutrophil survival or reduced or ineffective granulopoiesis (Figure 6.4).

Decreased neutrophil survival:
    Peracute bacterial infections especially those
      resulting in septicaemia or endotoxaemia
        Pyometra
        Peritonitis
        Aspiration pneumonia
        Acute salmonellosis
Ineffective or reduced granulopoiesis:
    Acute viral infections (canine parvovirus,
      feline panleucopenia, feline
      immunodeficiency virus, infectious canine
      hepatitis)
    Bone marrow suppression (e.g. later stages
      of oestrogen toxicity)
    Myelodysplasia (often associated with feline
      leukaemia virus infection)
    Myelophthisis (e.g. myeloproliferative and
      lymphoproliferative disorders)
    Drug-induced (e.g. cyclophosphamide,
      adriamycin)
    Radiation
    Canine cyclic haematopoiesis (grey collies)

Figure 6.4: Causes of neutropenia.

Decreased neutrophil survival: Peracute bacterial infections, particularly those associated with Gram-negative sepsis and endotoxaemia, result in an overwhelming demand for neutrophils and a marked decrease in their circulatory lifespan. The neutropenia is usually associated with a severe degenerative left shift. Animals that are endotoxaemic may also be thrombocytopenic. If the animal survives the peracute phase, the neutropenia usually gives way to a neutrophilic leucocytosis after 72–96 hours. Possible infectious causes of neutropenia include peritonitis, pyometra, aspiration pneumonia and acute salmonellosis.

Reduced or ineffective granulopoiesis: The peracute phase of certain viral infections such as canine parvovirus, feline panleucopenia and infectious canine hepatitis is associated with depressed myelopoiesis and severe neutropenia. Affected animals, in addition to being neutropenic, are also frequently lymphopenic. Aplastic anaemia is characterized by generalized bone marrow suppression; anaemia is therefore usually associated with severe neutropenia and thrombocytopenia.

Aplastic anaemia may occur as an idiopathic disease entity or may be associated with hyperoestrogenism (e.g. functional Sertoli cell tumours or administration of exogenous oestrogens) and chronic *Ehrlichia canis* infection. Neutropenia may also be caused by disorders that disrupt normal granulocytic maturation, for example, myeloproliferative or lymphoproliferative diseases (particularly acute myeloid or lymphoid leukaemia), myelodysplasia (often induced by feline leukaemia virus in the cat) and the administration of certain cytotoxic agents, most notably cyclophosphamide and adriamycin. In cats, neutropenia may also be associated with feline immunodeficiency virus infection. A less common cause of neutropenia is canine cyclic haematopoiesis, which occurs in grey collies.

Morphological abnormalities of neutrophils

Toxic changes: The release of bacterial toxins may result in morphological changes in circulating neutrophils (Figures 6.5 to 6.7). Non-bacterial toxins (e.g. cytotoxic agents) and other toxic products of tissue necrosis may result in similar toxic changes. These changes are often subtle and reflect abnormal maturation and differentiation of neutrophil precursors in the bone marrow. These toxic changes can be described as follows:

- Toxic granulation: reddish or metachromatic granules appear in the cytoplasm
- Diffuse cytoplasmic basophilia
- Vacuolated foamy cytoplasm
- Presence of Doehle bodies (remnants of reticuloendoplasmic reticulum); these large bluish intracytoplasmic inclusions are more common in the cat
- Giant neutrophils with bizarre nuclear morphology.

The severity of these toxic changes is usually graded by using a scale from 1 to 4.

Abnormalities of cytoplasmic granulation: Abnormally large granules can be seen in the cytoplasm of cats (particularly blue smoke Persians) with the rare inherited disorder known as Chediak–Higashi syndrome (Latimer and Robertson, 1994). These granules are reddish pink in colour.

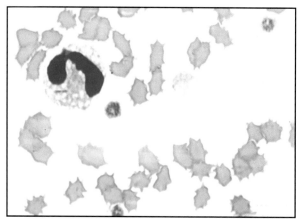

Figure 6.5: *Canine neutrophil showing cytoplasmic basophilia and vacuolation. Note the ingested bacterial rod. (© AXIOM Veterinary Laboratories.)*

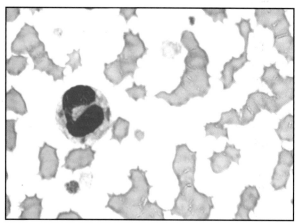

Figure 6.6: *Canine band neutrophil showing toxic changes. Note the Doehle bodies and cytoplasmic vacuolation. (© AXIOM Veterinary Laboratories.)*

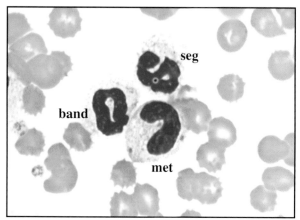

Figure 6.7: *Canine metamyelocyte (met), plus band and segmented (seg) neutrophils showing toxic changes. Note the small red cytoplasmic granules. Doehle bodies can be seen in the metamyelocyte. (© AXIOM Veterinary Laboratories.)*

Abnormalities of nuclear morphology: Hypersegmentation of polymorphogranulocyte nuclei indicates prolonged survival time in the circulation (Figure 6.8). Hypersegmented neutrophils may be found with corticosteroid therapy, hyperadrenocorticism and during the later stages of certain chronic inflammatory disorders.

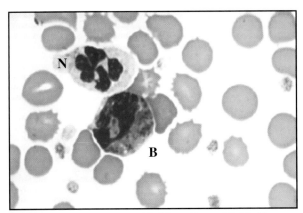

Figure 6.8: *Canine neutrophil (N) and basophil (B). The nucleus of the neutrophil is hypersegmented, indicating prolonged circulating survival time. Note the characteristic purple cytoplasmic granules and convoluted nucleus of the basophil. (© AXIOM Veterinary Laboratories.)*

Hyposegmentation of neutrophil nuclei is seen with Pelger–Huet anomaly, a rare inherited disorder of dogs and cats (Latimer, 1995). The neutrophils assume the appearance of bands or metamyelocytes (Figure 6.9); the leucogram may therefore be misinterpreted as evidence of a severe degenerative left shift. Neutrophil function is normal. Acquired nuclear hyposegmentation (pseudo Pelger–Huet anomaly) can be associated with bacterial infection, drug therapy, granulocytic leukaemia or feline leukaemia virus infections (Latimer and Tvedten, 1999).

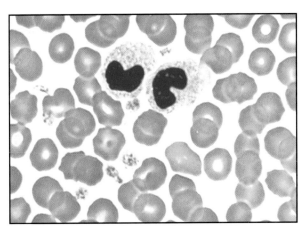

Figure 6.9: *Pelger–Huet anomaly. The nuclei of these two canine neutrophils are hyposegmented and the cells have the appearance of metamyelocytes. (© AXIOM Veterinary Laboratories.)*

Eosinophils

Eosinophil production

Eosinophils and basophils may share a common progenitor cell. The production and maturation of both cell types occur under the influence of interleukin 5 (IL-5). The storage pool of eosinophils in the marrow is minimal. Accelerated production and release of eosinophils occur in response to parasitic infections and allergic conditions. Eosinophil half-life in the circulation is extremely short (about 30 minutes in the dog). On leaving the circulation, eosinophils randomly enter the tissues where they may survive for several days.

Eosinophil function

Eosinophils are mobilized to sites of antigen–antibody complex deposition via activated complement components and a range of chemotactic molecules of the chemokine group (e.g. eotaxins 1 and 2). They are important regulators of hypersensitivity/immune-mediated and inflammatory reactions. Eosinophils contain histaminase and it has been proposed that they combat the effects of histamine released from IgE-sensitized mast cells in immediate type 1 hypersensitivity responses. They also have a parasiticidal function, which is antibody or complement dependent, but have limited phagocytic and bactericidal properties.

Eosinophilia

In most cases eosinophilia is associated with the increased production and release of eosinophils from the bone marrow (Figure 6.10). Other mechanisms that may contribute to increased numbers of circulating eosinophils are the preferential redistribution of cells from the marginal pool and prolonged intravascular survival. Causes of eosinophilia are given in Figure 6.11. Eosinophilia is a feature of many hypersensitivity reactions and parasitic infections. Eosinophilia in response to parasitism represents a hypersensitivity response to protein products released by the parasite.

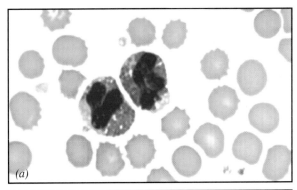

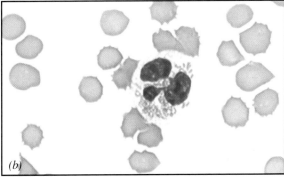

Figure 6.10: *(a) Canine band and segmented eosinophils. Note the typical round pink cytoplasmic granules. (b) Feline eosinophil. Note that the granules are more rod-shaped compared to those in canine eosinophils. (© AXIOM Veterinary Laboratories.)*

Hypersensitivity/immune-mediated reactions:
Atopic dermatitis
Feline bronchial asthma
Pulmonary infiltrate with eosinophils
Food allergies
Flea allergy dermatitis
Pemphigus foliaceus
Parasitism:
Ancylostoma spp.
Oslerus osleri
Angiostrongylus vasorum
Dirofilaria immitis
Eosinophilic gastroenteritis
Eosinophilic myositis
Eosinophilic granuloma complex
Canine panosteitis (common in German Shepherd Dogs)
Feline hypereosinophilic syndrome
Eosinophilic leukaemia or eosinophilic variant of chronic granulocytic leukaemia (rare)
Adrenocortical insufficiency
Oestrus in some bitches (?response to histamine release)
Tumour-associated eosinophilia in cats can be associated with myeloproliferative disease, lymphoma, mast cell tumour and transitional cell carcinoma

Figure 6.11: *Causes of eosinophilia.*

Eosinopenia

Eosinopenia is most frequently associated with acute physical or emotional stress and is mediated by the release of endogenous glucocorticoids. As such, eosinopenia may be a feature of many acute infectious, inflammatory or metabolic disorders. Causes of eosinopenia are given in Figure 6.12.

Stress (release of endogenous cortisol)
Hyperadrenocorticism
Glucocorticoid therapy
Acute infection or inflammation (stress)

Figure 6.12: *Causes of eosinopenia.*

Basophils

Basophil production

It is unclear whether basophils and tissue mast cells share a common progenitor cell (Meyer and Harvey, 1998a). Bone marrow storage of basophils is minimal. Basophil and eosinophil kinetics are closely related. Basophil granules contain histamine and after antigenic stimulation the cells synthesize eosinophil chemotactic factor of anaphylaxis (ECF-A). Both histamine and ECF-A when released into tissues result in the local accumulation of eosinophils. Conversely, eosinophils also infiltrate tissues in which there is a high concentration of mast cells (Jain, 1993a).

Basophil function

The biological functions of basophils are thought to be similar to those of mast cells. In addition to histamine and ECF-A, basophils contain other substances such as heparin, platelet activating factor, thromboxane A_2 (TxA_2) and leukotrienes, which are important mediators of allergic and inflammatory reactions. Basophils, like mast cells, degranulate after the interaction of antigen with specific cell-bound IgE. Heparin, released in response to postprandial lipaemia, promotes the release of lipoprotein lipase from vascular endothelial cells, which facilitates triglyceride metabolism and clearing of chylomicrons from the circulation.

Basophilia

Basophils are rarely present in the blood of healthy dogs and cats (hence basopenia is of no clinical significance). Basophilia (see Figures 6.1 and 6.8) is therefore nearly always important. Conditions that cause basophilia tend to be associated with increased numbers of circulating eosinophils. Basophilia is one of the more consistent haematological features of dirofilariasis. Rarer causes include the basophilic variant of chronic granulocytic leukaemia and hyperlipoproteinaemia.

Mast cells

Mast cells are not normally present in the blood of healthy dogs and cats. In cats the presence of circulating mast cells (Figure 6.13) is most frequently associated with mast cell tumours involving the spleen or the intestinal tract. Other causes of mastocythaemia include disseminated mast cell neoplasia (systemic mastocytosis involving the spleen, liver, lymph nodes and bone marrow), mast cell leukaemia and severe inflammatory disorders (Latimer and Tvedten, 1999).

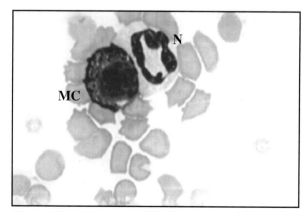

Figure 6.13: *Feline mast cell (MC) and neutrophil (N). The mast cell contains purple cytoplasmic granules. The nucleus is round, unlike the convoluted nucleus of the basophil.* (© *AXIOM Veterinary Laboratories.*)

MONOCYTES

Monocyte production

Monocytes are produced from committed stem cells common to granulocytes (CFU-GM). Monoblasts and promonocytes are the earliest recognizable monocyte progenitor cells in the bone marrow. Maturation to monocytes occurs under the influence of numerous growth factors, most notably granulocyte–monocyte colony stimulating factor (GM-CSF), M-CSF and IL-6. The production of monocytes increases in response to increased demand. There is no bone marrow storage pool of monocytes.

Monocyte function

Monocytes are released into the circulation as soon as they are produced. Like neutrophils, they are distributed in the circulation between circulating and marginal pools. After a short period in the circulation, monocytes migrate into tissues to become macrophages. Circulating monocytes (and their precursors in the bone marrow) and tissue macrophages comprise the mononuclear phagocytic system (MPS). The primary function of tissue macrophages is the phagocytosis of dead cells and foreign particulate material. They phagocytose intracellular organisms, particularly those that elicit a granulomatous inflammatory response (e.g. *Actinomyces* spp., *Nocardia* spp., Mycobacteriaceae and fungi), and secrete numerous biologically active substances such as IL-1, IL-6, tumour necrosis factor, complement components and proteolytic enzymes. Macrophages possess receptors for immunoglobulin and complement and therefore have the potential to phagocytose antibody-coated and/or complement-coated red cells and platelets.

Monocytosis

Mononuclear phagocytes accumulate at sites of acute and, particularly, chronic inflammation. Monocytosis is typically a feature of the subacute or chronic inflammatory response (Figure 6.14). Causes of monocytosis are given in Figure 6.15.

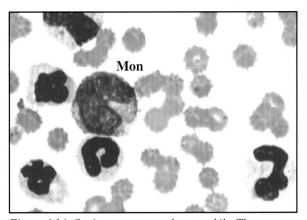

Figure 6.14: *Canine monocyte and neutrophils. The monocyte (Mon) is larger compared to the band neutrophil immediately below it. Note also the blue/grey cytoplasm. (© AXIOM Veterinary Laboratories.)*

Inflammatory conditions:
> Subacute or chronic inflammatory conditions particularly those characterized by suppuration, tissue necrosis or pyogranulomatous or granulomatous inflammation.
>
> The monocytosis is frequently accompanied by a mild to moderate neutrophilia with or without a left shift (e.g. subacute bacterial endocarditis or chronic pyelonephritis).
>
> Circulating monocytes may show reactive or 'toxic' changes in dogs with severe bacterial infections and/or endotoxaemia.
>
> Reactive monocytes have more cytoplasm, the nuclei become more lobulated and convoluted, and pinkish granules may appear in the cytoplasm

Feline immunodeficiency virus infection: Monocytosis is one of the more common haematological abnormalities in cats with feline immunodeficiency virus infection

Immune-mediated disease, e.g. autoimmune haemolytic anaemia or immune-mediated polyarthritis

Glucocorticoid therapy, hyperadrenocorticism and acute stress, especially in the dog

Malignant tumours, especially large tumours with necrotic centres

Monocytic or myelomonocytic leukaemia: Persistent and marked monocytosis, particularly if associated with the presence of immature monocytic precursors in the circulation or decreased numbers of other blood cell types, is highly suggestive of acute or chronic monocytic or myelomonocytic leukaemia

Figure 6.15: *Causes of monocytosis.*

Monocytopenia

Monocytopenia occasionally occurs in response to acute infection or inflammation but is usually of little clinical importance.

LYMPHOCYTES

Lymphocytes can be classified morphologically as small (Figure 6.16), medium or large. On a functional basis they are classified as T lymphocytes, B lymphocytes or null cells (non-T, non-B lymphocytes).

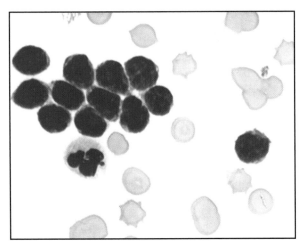

Figure 6.16: Small lymphocytes in feline blood. These cells have a narrow rim of cytoplasm and round nuclei which are notched or slightly indented. (© AXIOM Veterinary Laboratories.)

Lymphocyte production

All lymphocytes arise from a common bone marrow precursor. Immature T lymphocytes are exported to the thymus where they undergo maturation before being released to populate the secondary lymphoid tissues (e.g. lymph nodes, spleen and mucosal lymphoid aggregates). It is believed that one subpopulation of T cells may undergo development in the gut. B lymphocyte development occurs in the bone marrow, but in some species (including the dog) some B-cell maturation may occur within the gut. Mature B cells are released from these sites of primary development to populate secondary lymphoid tissues. Anatomically, T cells predominate in the thymus, lymph nodes and thoracic duct lymph whereas the spleen and bone marrow contain a higher percentage of B cells. The distribution of lymphocytes in peripheral blood is about 70% T cells, 20% B cells and 10% null cells. Most circulating lymphocytes are therefore T cells, which are either antigenically naïve (previously unexposed to antigen) or of the 'memory' subset (retaining memory of previous exposure to antigen). Both T and B lymphocytes recirculate between lymphoid and non-lymphoid tissues of the body by utilizing both vascular and lymphatic pathways.

Lymphocyte function

Antigenic stimulation of B cells results in their blastic transformation to plasma cells, which are capable of synthesizing and releasing immunoglobulin. Antibody production occurs primarily in secondary lymphoid tissues. Plasma cells are not normally present in the circulation; plasma cell leukaemia is an uncommon manifestation of multiple myeloma. Reactive lymphocytes (immunocytes) (Figure 6.17) can be present in low numbers in both healthy and ill animals. Increased numbers can be seen in young animals and in response to chronic antigenic stimulation or after vaccination. A small number of lymphocytes containing purple cytoplasmic granules may be present in the blood of normal animals (Figure 6.18). Increased numbers of these large granular lymphocytes (which are thought to be natural killer, NK, cells) can be seen in both non-neoplastic and neoplastic conditions (Meyer and Harvey, 1998b; Reagan *et al.*, 1998). Large granular lymphocytic leukaemia is a relatively rare lymphoproliferative disorder of both dogs and cats.

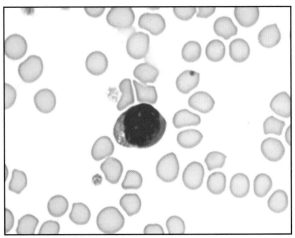

Figure 6.17: Reactive lymphocyte in canine blood. Note the increased amount of dark basophilic cytoplasm. These cells are sometimes called 'immunocytes'. Increased numbers can be seen in response to antigenic stimulation such as follows vaccination. (© AXIOM Veterinary Laboratories.)

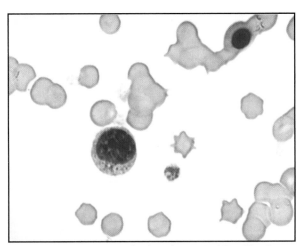

Figure 6.18: Large granular lymphocyte in feline blood. Note the reddish/purple cytoplasmic granules. Low numbers of these cells may be seen in normal cats and dogs. (© AXIOM Veterinary Laboratories.)

T cells play an important role in cell-mediated immunity. They also modulate the humoral immune response; disturbances of T-cell function have been associated with immune-mediated diseases such as haemolytic anaemia and thrombocytopenia. Cytotoxic T cells can kill tumour cells or cells infected with virus. NK cells are considered to be the dominant form of null cell and are important in immune surveillance. Antigenic stimulation of T cells, and to a lesser extent B cells, results in the production of cytokines, which play an important role in the pathogenesis of immunological and inflammatory responses. There are several families of cytokines that have numerous roles in leucocyte development, activation, chemoattraction and function.

The number of lymphocytes in the circulation depends on their rate of production, utilization and destruction. Since lymphocytes are continually recirculating, an increase or decrease in the number of circulating lymphocytes may not necessarily reflect altered lymphopoiesis.

Lymphocytosis

Lymphocytosis refers to an absolute increase in the number of circulating lymphocytes. Causes of lymphocytosis are given in Figure 6.19.

Lymphopenia

Causes of lymphopenia are given in Figure 6.20.

Physiological lymphocytosis:
>   With a concomitant neutrophilia this occurs in healthy animals in response to exercise, excitement and forceful handling.
>   This type of response is induced by adrenaline and is particularly common in fractious cats

Age:
>   Young animals have higher lymphocyte counts than adults. An increased number of reactive lymphocytes (immunocytes) may be present, especially after vaccination

Chronic infections, particularly those which elicit an antibody response. An increased number of reactive lymphocytes may be present

Hypoadrenocorticism: the lymphocytosis may be accompanied by an eosinophilia

Lymphocytic leukaemia:
>   Malignant proliferation of lymphoid cells in the bone marrow occurs with acute lymphoblastic leukaemia and chronic lymphocytic leukaemia, and in some cases of lymphoma.
>   It is worth remembering, however, that the presence of neoplastic lymphoid cells in the bone marrow may not necessarily result in the presence of similar cells in the peripheral blood and that some affected animals may have normal or even low lymphocyte counts

Figure 6.19: Causes of lymphocytosis.

Systemic stress:
>   Physiological lymphopenia is a feature of the stress leucogram and is typically associated with a neutrophilia and eosinopenia

Endogenous or exogenous glucocorticoids:
>   Hyperadrenocorticism and glucocorticoid administration result in haematological changes similar to those described above for the stress leucogram

Viral infections:
>   Lymphopenia is associated with the acute phase of most viral infections (e.g. canine distemper virus, infectious canine hepatitis).
>   Neutropenia may also occur in cats infected with feline leukaemia virus or feline immunodeficiency virus

Chylothorax: results in the loss of efferent lymph

Lymphangiectasia: results in the loss of afferent lymph

Immunosuppressive therapy or irradiation

Hereditary or acquired immunodeficiency syndromes, e.g. acquired feline leukaemia virus-related immunodeficiency or feline immunodeficiency virus infection

Figure 6.20: Causes of lymphopenia.

COMMON WHITE BLOOD CELL RESPONSES

Physiological responses

Age-related changes in leucocyte number
Total leucocyte counts tend to be higher in young animals of less than 3 months of age, primarily as a result of an absolute increase in the number of lymphocytes. Young animals therefore have a greater tendency to develop physiological lymphocytosis than adults. The total number of lymphocytes decreases gradually reaching normal adult values by 3–6 months of age.

Adrenaline-induced physiological leucocytosis
Physiological leucocytosis, mediated by the release of adrenaline, occurs in response to exercise, excitement and fear. This type of response occurs more frequently in cats than in dogs and is more commonly seen in young animals. Increased blood flow results in a shift of cells from the marginal to the circulating pool, and the development of a mild neutrophilia without a left shift. Alterations in WBC number occur rapidly but the response is transient, with WBC numbers returning to normal within 30 minutes of removal of the stimulus. In cats particularly, the neutrophilia is often accompanied

by a lymphocytosis (absolute lymphocyte count may be as high as 10.0 x 10⁹/l). Eosinophil and monocyte numbers are usually within normal limits but occasionally may be slightly increased.

Leucocyte response to stress or glucocorticoids (stress leucogram)

Stressful stimuli, in the form of pain, trauma, surgical procedures, extremes of body temperature and severe debilitating disorders such as sepsis, toxaemia, severe anaemia or metabolic disease, cause the release of endogenous glucocorticoids from the adrenal cortex. A similar stress response may also occur during late pregnancy in bitches. The WBC changes that occur in response to stress mimic those that occur with spontaneous hyperadrenocorticism or following the administration of exogenous glucocorticoid preparations. The 'stress' leucogram is characterized by mild neutrophilia, usually with no left shift, in association with eosinopenia, lymphopenia and occasionally monocytosis (lymphopenia and eosinopenia are the most consistent indicators of 'stress' or hypercortisolaemia and may occur in the absence of a neutrophilia). Neutrophilia is caused by a shift of marginated neutrophils into the circulating pool, increased release from bone marrow, increased circulating life span (neutrophils may appear hypersegmented) and decreased diapedesis of cells into the tissues. This type of physiological response is more 'chronic' than the adrenaline-induced response. After the administration of exogenous glucocorticoid preparations, alterations to WBC numbers can be expected within hours. The duration of this response depends on whether the glucocorticoid preparation is short or long acting. Although the magnitude of the neutrophilia may decrease with time, eosinopenia and lymphopenia persist for as long as the circulating level of glucocorticoid remains increased.

Physiological leucocytosis should be differentiated from reactive leucocytosis, which occurs in response to disease (see below).

Physiological leucopenia

Reduced blood flow in the anaesthetized animal may result in margination of circulating neutrophils and a physiological leucopenia.

Inflammatory responses

Inflammatory WBC responses may be initiated by infectious or non-infectious disease processes that result in an increased demand for leucocytes in tissues. The production and release of neutrophils from bone marrow increases to compensate for increased tissue demand, causing a neutrophilia. As the storage pool of neutrophils becomes depleted, band neutrophils or earlier precursor stages are released into the circulation (left shift). Depending on the type of antigenic stimulus, monocytes and eosinophils may also be produced and released in increased numbers into the circulation.

Regenerative left shift

A regenerative left shift is defined as an absolute increase in the total number of mature segmented neutrophils, which is accompanied by the appearance of immature neutrophil precursors in the circulation (the number of immature forms is usually less than 10% of the total number of segmented neutrophils). A reactive neutrophilia with a left shift (Figure 6.21) can be observed in various inflammatory disease states that result in an increased tissue demand for neutrophils. The left shift that accompanies a reactive neutrophilia is usually orderly and pyramidal. In contrast, the neutrophilic left shift that may occur in cases of acute or chronic myeloid (or myelomonocytic) leukaemia often seems less orderly, reflecting abnormal cellular maturation and differentiation. The extent of the left shift generally reflects the severity of the inflammatory response (or leukaemic process), whereas the magnitude of the total cell count reflects the ability of the marrow to meet the increased demand for cells.

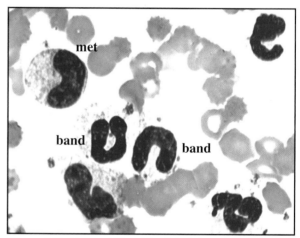

Figure 6.21: *Neutrophilia with a left shift in canine blood. Band neutrophils and a metamyelocyte (met) can be seen. Note also that these cells are showing toxic changes. (© AXIOM Veterinary Laboratories.)*

The left shift can be graded depending on the relative numbers of band neutrophils and younger stages present in the blood: mild (bands only present), moderate (bands and metamyelocytes present) or severe (bands, metamyelocytes, myelocytes and occasionally promyelocytes and myeloblasts present; leukaemoid response).

Degenerative left shift

A degenerative left shift occurs when the number of immature neutrophils exceeds or is greater than 10% of the total number of mature neutrophils. The total number of mature neutrophils may be decreased, normal or slightly increased. A degenerative left shift indicates depletion of the bone marrow reserve of segmented neutrophils. In contrast to a regenerative left shift, a degenerative left shift constitutes a less favourable prognostic sign.

Peracute inflammatory response

The peracute inflammatory response is usually a consequence of severe overwhelming infection, particularly Gram-negative sepsis associated with endotoxaemia (e.g. a bitch with coliform septicaemia and endotoxaemia resulting from a closed pyometra). Neutrophil production and release is unable to meet the sudden increased demand for neutrophils, resulting in neutropenia and a degenerative left shift, which may be accompanied by stress-induced lymphopenia and eosinopenia. If the animal survives this peracute phase, the total WBC count should return to normal and then start to increase within 24–48 hours so that the WBC picture resembles that of the acute inflammatory response.

Acute inflammatory response

The classic WBC response to an acute inflammatory focus is characterized by a neutrophilia with a left shift. A similar type of WBC picture can occur postoperatively in response to tissue damage and stress. A more pronounced neutrophilia occurs with localized infections. The production and release of neutrophils increase to compensate for increased tissue demand. As the marrow storage pool becomes depleted, band neutrophils or earlier maturation stages are released into the circulation.

Leukaemoid response: A leukaemoid response is characterized by an intense neutrophilia accompanied by a pronounced regenerative left shift. In some cases the total leucocyte count may exceed $80 \times 10^9/l$, and the left shift frequently includes metamyelocytes and myelocytes. Most leukaemoid responses are associated with localized infections (e.g. closed pyometra, pyothorax or peritonitis) and must be differentiated from chronic myelogenous (granulocytic) leukaemia. In some cases a leukaemoid response may involve other leucocyte types such as lymphocytes or eosinophils.

Leucoerythroblastic reaction: A leucoerythroblastic reaction typically occurs in response to acute blood loss or haemolysis. Nucleated red blood cells (normoblasts) and immature granulocyte precursors appear simultaneously in increased numbers in the circulation. Other causes include disseminated haemangiosarcoma and myeloproliferative disorders such as erythroleukaemia.

Chronic inflammatory response

Progression of an acute inflammatory response depends on the ability of the bone marrow to meet the continued tissue demand for neutrophils. If the marrow production of neutrophils equilibrates with tissue demand a steady state situation occurs. The neutrophilia may be relatively mild and may be associated with a variable left shift and absolute monocytosis (the latter is more indicative of ongoing tissue necrosis). These haematological features are typical of the classic chronic inflammatory response that occurs, for example, in dogs with subacute bacterial endocarditis or pyelonephritis.

In some cases, however, the continued excessive demand for neutrophils results in exhaustion of the storage pool and the development of leucopenia (neutropenia) and a degenerative left shift (i.e. a haematological picture resembling a peracute inflammatory response). The prognosis in such cases is usually more guarded (see below).

Prognostic indicators

The following haematological abnormalities occurring singly or in combination may be regarded as less favourable prognostic indicators:

- Normal or low total leucocyte count with a degenerative left shift
- Persistent neutropenia
- Persistent lymphopenia and/or eosinopenia
- Leukaemoid response
- Toxic changes present in neutrophils.

HAEMATOPOIETIC NEOPLASIA INVOLVING WHITE BLOOD CELLS

The term leukaemia describes the neoplastic proliferation of one or more haematopoietic cell lines in the bone marrow. The neoplastic cells usually enter the circulation and may also infiltrate other organs, most notably, the spleen, liver and lymph nodes. Therefore most leukaemias, including myeloproliferative disorders involving the granulocytic, monocytic, erythroid or megakaryocytic cell lines, either singly or in combination, and some lymphoproliferative disorders (primary lymphoid leukaemias and cases of lymphoma that involve the bone marrow) are characterized by an increased total WBC count.

Leukaemias are classified as acute or chronic depending on the degree of cellular differentiation and maturation (see Chapter 8). Acute leukaemias are generally characterized by a large number of abnormal circulating blast cells and, in addition to a mild to moderate leucocytosis, affected animals are often concurrently anaemic and/or thrombocytopenic. Some acute leukaemias, particularly acute lymphoblastic leukaemia, may present with normal or even low total WBC counts (a situation paradoxically referred to as aleukaemic leukaemia) or there may be only a few blast cells present in the circulation (subleukaemia).

In comparison, chronic leukaemias are characterized by the production of well differentiated cells. They almost invariably present with a pronounced leucocytosis (the predominant cell type depends on the particular cell line involved) and other cytopenias, if present, are usually less severe. Diagnosis of chronic myeloid (granulocytic) leukaemia is often difficult because granulocytic maturation remains orderly and usually progresses to completion. Affected animals have a pronounced leucocytosis with a left shift involving myelocytes and, in some cases, promyelocytes, which must be differentiated from an inflammatory leukaemoid response.

REFERENCES AND FURTHER READING

Coles EH (1986) Leukocytes. In: *Veterinary Clinical Pathology, 4th edn*, pp. 43-79. WB Saunders, Philadelphia

Duncan JR, Prasse KW and Mahaffey EA (1994) Leukocytes. In: *Veterinary Laboratory Medicine, 3rd edn*, pp. 37-62. Iowa State University Press, Ames

Jain NC (1993a) The basophils and mast cells. In: *Essentials of Veterinary Haematology*, pp. 258-265. Lea and Febiger, Philadelphia

Jain NC (1993b) Interpretation of leukocyte parameters. In: *Essentials of Veterinary Haematology*, pp. 295-306. Lea and Febiger, Philadelphia

Latimer KS (1995) Leukocytes in health and disease. In: *Textbook of Veterinary Internal Medicine: Diseases of the Dog and Cat, 4th edn*, ed. SJ Ettinger and EC Feldman, pp. 1892-1929. WB Saunders, Philadelphia

Latimer KS and Robertson SL (1994) Inherited leukocyte disorders. In: *Consultations in Feline Internal Medicine 2*, ed. JR August, pp. 503-507. WB Saunders, Philadelphia

Latimer KS and Tvedten H (1999) Leukocyte disorders. In: *Small Animal Clinical Diagnosis by Laboratory Methods, 3rd edn*, ed. MD Willard, H Tvedten and GH Turnwald, pp. 52-74. WB Saunders, Philadelphia

Meyer DJ and Harvey JW (1998a) Haematopoiesis and evaluating bone marrow. In: *Veterinary Laboratory Medicine: Interpretation and Diagnosis*, pp. 23-42. WB Saunders, Philadelphia

Meyer DJ and Harvey JW (1998b) Evaluation of leukocyte disorders. In: *Veterinary Laboratory Medicine: Interpretation and Diagnosis*, pp. 83-109. WB Saunders, Philadelphia

Reagan WJ, Sanders TG and DeNicola DB (1998) Lymphoproliferative and myeloproliferative disorders. In: *Veterinary Haematology: Atlas of Common Domestic Species*, pp. 49-57. Manson, London

Disorders of Leucocyte Function

Michael J. Day

INTRODUCTION

The present chapter considers disorders in which an animal may have persistent inflammatory or infectious disease associated with functionally defective peripheral blood leucocytes. Such disorders of leucocyte function may be broadly divided into those that are acquired in adult animals and those that are congenital diseases of younger animals, which are likely to have an inherited basis. The former group are relatively more common and occur as part of a wide spectrum of metabolic or infectious diseases, or secondary to drug therapy. By contrast, well documented examples of congenital defects in leucocyte function in small animals are rarely encountered.

The apparent rarity of such diseases may in part reflect the lack of widely available means to diagnose them. Tests of leucocyte function are generally only available in a research context and, as such, access to them by veterinary surgeons in general practice is restricted. Despite this poor availability, it is generally inadvisable to submit samples from such animals to laboratories that deal primarily with diagnosis in humans. There are specific requirements for the isolation of animal leucocytes and the performance of in vitro testing, and the interpretation of such assays is best performed by an experienced veterinary immunologist. The preferred sample for testing of leucocyte function is blood in preservative-free heparin, and a minimum volume of 10 ml is generally required. In most instances the laboratory will require control samples from one or two clinically normal, age-matched animals, which will be run in parallel with the test samples.

This chapter considers the range of in vitro assays that have been established for the assessment of the function of neutrophils, monocyte–macrophages and lymphocytes in small animals. The situations in which abnormal function may reflect an acquired problem are reviewed and the documented instances of primary congenital defects of leucocyte function discussed.

TESTS OF LEUCOCYTE FUNCTION

Figure 7.1 summarizes the range of tests available for assessing leucocyte function.

Neutrophil function
Neutrophil chemotaxis
Neutrophil phagocytosis and killing
Neutrophil respiratory burst after phagocytosis

Monocyte–macrophage function
Macrophage phagocytosis and killing

Lymphocyte function
Mitogen-driven lymphocyte proliferation
Antigen-driven lymphocyte proliferation
Cytokine protein or mRNA production by stimulated lymphocyte cultures
Antibody production by stimulated lymphocyte cultures
Cytotoxic killing of labelled target cells

Figure 7.1: Tests of leucocyte function.

Tests of neutrophil function

The neutrophil undertakes a variety of activities while participating in the inflammatory response in vivo. These cells must be mobilized from the bloodstream into extravascular tissue via molecular interactions mediated by adhesion molecules and are attracted along chemotactic gradients to sites of inflammation. Here they phagocytose appropriately opsonized particles or microorganisms and perform intracellular killing of such organisms via metabolic pathways involving oxygen-dependent and independent mechanisms. Each of these major functions of the neutrophil can be assessed by in vitro assay.

Isolation of neutrophils from peripheral blood

Several methods have been described for the isolation of neutrophils from peripheral blood. A study by our laboratory has compared the viability and yield of neutrophils obtained after percoll gradient centrifugation, dextran sedimentation followed by centrifugation over ficoll or centrifugation through commercially available medium for isolating neutrophils (Shearer and Day, 1997). The optimum protocol was that involving dextran sedimentation followed by ficoll centrifugation, which yielded about 65% of the total number of neutrophils in the whole blood sample, with a viability of 98% and neutrophil purity of 99%.

Neutrophil chemotaxis

Isolated neutrophils can migrate along chemotactic gradients established in vitro by the use of various chemical agents, serum, cytokines, complement components or other inflammatory mediators (Nagahata *et al.*, 1991; Thomsen *et al.*, 1991). The Boyden chamber or the under agarose assay is the most commonly used means of assessing chemotaxis. In the former, neutrophils are placed into one side of a chamber separated from the chemotactic agent by a millipore filter through which the agent will diffuse. Neutrophils migrate towards, and are trapped within, the filter, which can be stained and examined microscopically. In the under agarose assay, neutrophils placed into one well in an agarose gel will migrate towards a chemoattractant placed in a second well by moving underneath the gel. This movement is again assessed microscopically (Nagahata *et al.*, 1991).

Neutrophil phagocytosis and killing assays

In neutrophil phagocytosis and killing assays, isolated neutrophils are incubated under specific conditions with a known number of particles (e.g. latex beads, yeast, bacteria), which have been previously opsonized with serum antibody and/or complement. Autologous serum from the same animal should be used in parallel with normal serum to detect any deficiency in the presence of opsonins. After a set period of incubation, phagocytosis can be assessed by stopping the reaction and examining a stained preparation of cytocentrifuged cells. The number of neutrophils containing ingested particles or the number of particles per neutrophil can be measured. Studies in our laboratory have addressed the effect of opsonization on the phagocytosis of *Staphylococcus intermedius* by neutrophils in the dog (Figure 7.2; Shearer and Day, 1997).

In vitro assays for the intracellular killing ability of neutrophils in the dog have also been reported. We have developed a microplate assay in which purified canine neutrophils are incubated with a known number of opsonized *S. intermedius* over a 90-minute period. After phagocytosis has occurred (10 minutes), extracellular bacteria are lysed by the addition of specific enzyme (lysostaphin), and at various time points thereafter (0, 30, 60 and 90 minutes using quadruplicate samples) intracellular bacteria are released by osmotic lysis of the neutrophils. Serial dilutions of the viable intracellular bacteria are then plated on nutrient agar and the number of colonies determined. The number of viable intracellular organisms at each time point is defined by a fraction of the original number of phagocytosed organisms (100%), allowing a curve of intracellular killing kinetics to be produced (Figure 7.3).

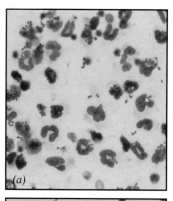

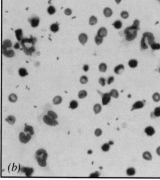

Figure 7.2: Neutrophils isolated from the peripheral blood of a normal dog were incubated with (a) Staphylococcus intermedius opsonized by fresh dog serum or (b) S. intermedius without prior serum opsonization. After 10 minutes the reactions were stopped by the addition of formal saline, and the preparations were cytocentrifuged. The neutrophils effectively phagocytosed large numbers of opsonized organisms in (a), with a high proportion of neutrophils containing staphylococci and a significant number of staphylococci per neutrophil. By contrast, the unopsonized staphylococci in (b) were poorly phagocytosed.

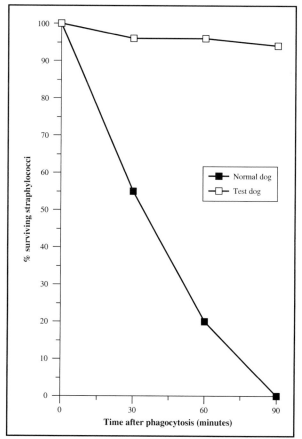

Figure 7.3: Assessment of in vitro neutrophil killing of Staphylococcus intermedius. *Opsonized S. intermedius were incubated with neutrophils from a normal dog and a dog with a suspected defect of neutrophil function (test dog). Phagocytosed organisms were progressively killed by the neutrophils from the normal dog over 90 minutes, but defective neutrophils were unable to kill the phagocytosed staphylococci.*

Assessment of neutrophil respiratory burst

The respiratory burst of neutrophils after phagocytosis of particles can be assessed using the nitroblue tetrazolium (NBT) test or chemiluminescence assay. In the former, there is reduction of the colourless NBT dye to dark blue formazan, which can be assessed spectrophotometrically, and in the latter the release of light during the oxidative burst is measured by a chemiluminometer or scintillation counter.

Tests of monocyte–macrophage function

Peripheral blood monocytes differentiate to become adherent macrophages during in vitro culture. The ability of these macrophages to phagocytose and kill organisms can be examined in a similar manner to the neutrophil assays described above. An in vitro assay for the ability of canine macrophages to phagocytose and kill the spores of *Aspergillus* was described by Day (1987). Peripheral blood mononuclear cells were obtained by density gradient centrifugation and plated on glass in culture medium. After 5–10 days of culture the adherent population were pure macrophages. Equal numbers of fungal spores and macrophages were cocultured for 2 hours, after which extracellular spores were removed by aspiration, and osmotic lysis of macrophages was performed to release adherent and phagocytosed spores. The percentage killing was then calculated. A similar phagocytic assay using *Candida albicans* has also been described for canine macrophages (DeBowes and Anderson, 1991).

Tests of lymphocyte function

Isolation of lymphocytes from peripheral blood

Mononuclear cells can be readily isolated from peripheral blood by the process of density gradient centrifugation, which involves layering diluted blood on to medium such as ficoll–hypaque (Figure 7.4). The cells collected from the resulting interface are a mixture of T and B lymphocytes and monocytes, and the relative proportions of each can be assessed by flow cytometry after labelling with monoclonal antibodies specific for unique surface markers of these cells (Cobbold and Metcalfe, 1994). These populations can also be used for in vitro functional studies. In the first instance it is normal to perform preliminary assays on whole unfractionated mononuclear cell preparations, and some assays have also been adapted for whole blood culture (Angus and Yang, 1978) eliminating the need for prior mononuclear cell enrichment. For more refined assays, it is possible to selectively purify T and B lymphocytes or subsets of these cells by methods such as panning, passage through nylon wool or immunoglobulin anti-immunoglobulin columns, erythrocyte rosetting, magnetic bead separation, cytotoxic depletion or cell sorting using the flow cytometer (reviewed by Mason *et al.*, 1987).

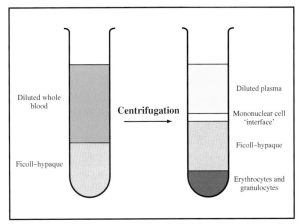

Figure 7.4: *Isolation of peripheral blood mononuclear cells by separation over ficoll–hypaque. A diluted blood sample is overlaid on to density gradient medium (ficoll–hypaque, typical specific gravity 1.077). After centrifugation, separation occurs and the mononuclear cells at the interface can be aspirated with a Pasteur pipette.*

Lymphocyte proliferation assays

Lymphocyte proliferation assays assess the ability of lymphocytes to respond to in vitro stimulation by mitogens or antigens by measuring the incorporation of radiolabelled thymidine (^{3}H-thymidine) into the DNA of dividing cells. Mitogens are substances (often plant derived) that non-specifically stimulate multiple clones of lymphocytes by binding to surface carbohydrate molecules. Some mitogens seem to preferentially activate T lymphocytes (concanavalin A, phytohaemagglutinin) whereas others will have an effect primarily on B lymphocytes (pokeweed mitogen, bacterial lipopolysaccharide, staphylococcal protein A). Lymphocytes are cultured with mitogen for 48–72 hours and ^{3}H-thymidine is added to the cultures during the final 18 hours. The cells are harvested and the proportion of radiolabel taken up by dividing cells determined, to give an index of stimulation relative to control cultures of mononuclear cells from clinically normal animals (Kristensen *et al.*, 1982).

In recent years such assays have been extended to enable in vitro stimulation using specific antigens that selectively activate antigen-specific lymphocyte clones through recognition of peptide antigen presented by accessory cells to the T-cell receptor. The kinetics of such cultures can be examined to determine whether a primary or secondary (memory) immune response has been made (Bishop, 1995). An alternative method of stimulating peripheral blood mononuclear cells relies on the response to recombinant interleukin 2 (IL-2) included in the culture (Helfand *et al.*, 1992; Lawrence *et al.*, 1995). Other indicators of cellular activation may be assessed by phenotypic analysis of the stimulated cells after culture. For example, activated T lymphocytes have greater expression of the IL-2 receptor (IL-2R) (Helfand *et al.*, 1992).

Release of cytokines or immunoglobulins by stimulated lymphocytes

When T lymphocytes are stimulated in culture, they will release soluble factors (cytokines) to the culture medium, which can be harvested by collection of the culture supernatant and quantified by enzyme-linked immunosorbant assay (ELISA) or bioassay. The latter involves the ability of the supernatant to support the growth of a cytokine-dependent cell line (Lawrence *et al.*, 1995). Cytokines such as IL-1, IL-2, IL-6, tumour necrosis factor (TNF) and interferon gamma (IFNγ) have been measured in the cat (Lawrence *et al.*, 1995; Rottman *et al.*, 1995) and dog (Mizuno *et al.*, 1993; Yamahita *et al.*, 1994; Rivas *et al.*, 1995). Alternatively, the cells can be collected from culture after stimulation and the presence of cytokine-specific mRNA within the cytoplasm determined by polymerase chain reaction (PCR) (Rottman *et al.*, 1995). There is not necessarily correlation between the identification of cytokine mRNA and secretion of the mature protein product. Such information provides accurate assessment of the normal functioning of lymphocytes in vitro and whether there is preferential activation of particular lymphocyte subsets upon challenge with a specific antigen (Pinelli *et al.*, 1994).

In the case of B lymphocytes, in vitro stimulation may lead to differentiation to plasma cells and release of immunoglobulin into the culture medium. Such antibody production can be detected by examination of the culture supernatant by ELISA (Rivas *et al.*, 1995).

Assessment of cytotoxic function

The function of cytotoxic lymphocytes or natural killer (NK) cells can be assessed in vitro by culturing peripheral blood lymphoid cells with specific radiolabelled (^{51}chromium is often used) target cell populations, which may include long-term cell lines of known susceptibility to NK cells, virally infected, histoincompatible or tumour cells. Specific ratios of target cells to cytotoxic cells are used and the release of radioisotope by damaged targets measured after a period of culture (Brown *et al.*, 1995; Nakada *et al.*, 1995).

ACQUIRED DEFECTS OF LEUCOCYTE FUNCTION

Figure 7.5 summarizes the acquired defects of leucocyte function recognized in small animals.

Physiological

Tests of leucocyte function should be interpreted in light of the age, breed and sex of the animal and with a view to temporal factors. It has been shown that mitogen-driven lymphocyte proliferation varies with the age of dogs (Gerber and Brown, 1974) and the season (Shifrine *et al.*, 1980), and that there is apparent diurnal variation in the responsiveness of lymphoid

Physiological
Age of animal
Diurnal variation
Dietary factors
Hormonal factors (e.g. endogenous corticosteroid, pregnancy hormones)
Drug therapy
Immunosuppressive drugs
Chronic disease
Demodicosis
Deep pyoderma
Anal furunculosis
Viral infection
Neoplasia
Deficiency of opsonins (e.g. immunoglobulin, complement)

Figure 7.5: *Acquired defects of leucocyte function.*

cells (Angus and Yang, 1978). Dietary factors, particularly vitamin intake, may affect lymphocyte responses to mitogens (Degen and Breitschwerdt, 1986a). The hormonal effects of pregnancy on leucocyte function have not been well characterized in small animals.

Drug therapy

Immunosuppressive and immunomodulatory drugs have pronounced effects on the immune system and these may be mirrored in the results of in vitro functional testing of leucocytes. For this reason, it is optimal to have withdrawn such treatment for several weeks before taking samples for functional studies. Corticosteroids have wide ranging effects on the function of granulocytes, monocytes and lymphocytes (Degen and Breitschwerdt, 1986a; Cohn, 1991; DeBowes and Anderson, 1991; Weiss, 1991), and it has recently been shown that cyclosporin can have potent suppressive effects on lymphocyte proliferation, even after absorption following topical administration for keratoconjunctivitis sicca (Gilger *et al.*, 1995).

CD4+ T lymphocyte balance

Recent work with experimental animal models has found that polarization of immune responses towards humoral (antibody-mediated) or cell-mediated activity is regulated by the preferential activation of subsets of the CD4+ T-cell population (Th2 and Th1, respectively). This phenomenon of 'immune deviation' may also hold for particular disease states in domestic animals. For example, dogs that are susceptible to visceral leishmaniasis make high concentrations of antibody but weak cell-mediated responses, with reduced in vitro production of cytokines such as IL-2 and TNF. Dogs resistant to the disease have the reverse profile of immunological activity (Pinelli *et al.*, 1994). Such preferential activation of specific facets of the immune response may be driven by numerous factors including the nature, dose and route of antigen exposure and the local tissue milieu (hormones and cytokines) at the site of exposure.

Chronic disease

Animals with chronic infectious, inflammatory or neoplastic disease often show reduced leucocyte function in vitro. In the past this has sometimes been attributed to a primary leucocyte defect that predisposes the animal to expression of the disease, but it is now considered more likely that the inflammatory and immune responses active in chronic disease themselves cause depression of leucocyte function. There are numerous examples of such observations throughout the literature, some of which have been misinterpreted as primary immunodeficiency.

Dogs with demodicosis often have depressed lymphocyte proliferation, and early studies suggested that this was related to a suppressive factor found in autologous serum (Scott *et al.*, 1974; Hirsch *et al.*, 1975). This serum factor may in turn be associated with concurrent bacterial pyoderma (Barta and Turnwald, 1983), and it has been proposed that serum immune complexes of antibody and staphylococcal antigen may act in this manner (DeBoer, 1994). More recent work has extended these observations by showing decreased production of IL-2 and decreased expression of IL-2R by stimulated lymphocytes from dogs with demodicosis (Lemarie *et al.*, 1994). Similarly, decreased neutrophil chemotaxis has been shown when neutrophils from normal dogs were incubated with serum from dogs with demodicosis (Latimer *et al.*, 1983). Serum factors able to suppress proliferative responses of autologous lymphocytes have also been identified in Basenji dogs with immunoproliferative small intestinal disease (Barta *et al.*, 1983) and a range of other disorders (Barta and Oyekan, 1981).

Some breeds of dog are susceptible to deep pyoderma, and immunodeficiency has been proposed as an underlying cause. Such animals do often have decreased lymphocyte proliferation (Miller, 1991) but this is unlikely to be a primary event. Recent studies have suggested that more subtle leucocyte abnormalities, such as failure of homing of cutaneous T lymphocytes (Day, 1994) or an imbalance of CD4:CD8 T cells (Chabanne *et al.*, 1995), may occur in susceptible dogs. Decreased chemotaxis of neutrophils has been found as a secondary event in dogs with pyoderma (Latimer *et al.*, 1982).

Similarly, dogs with anal furunculosis may have depression of mitogen-induced lymphocyte proliferation, but these responses return to normal after recovery from the disease (Killingsworth *et al.*, 1988). German Shepherd Dogs with nasal or disseminated aspergillosis are recorded as having depression of lymphocyte proliferation (Barrett *et al.*, 1977; Day *et al.*, 1986; Day, 1987) and neutrophil NBT reduction (Day *et al.*, 1986) but these observations are again likely to be due to chronic depression of cell-mediated immunity (Figures 7.6 and 7.7).

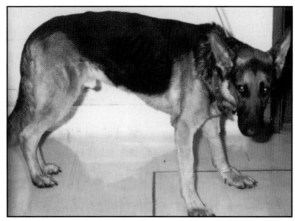

Figure 7.6: *German Shepherd Dog with late stage disseminated aspergillosis. Such animals may have depression of function of lymphocytes and neutrophils in vitro, however these findings are likely to be secondary to chronically high concentrations of inflammatory mediators and cytokines or to the release of fungal immunosuppressive metabolites (Day, 1987).*

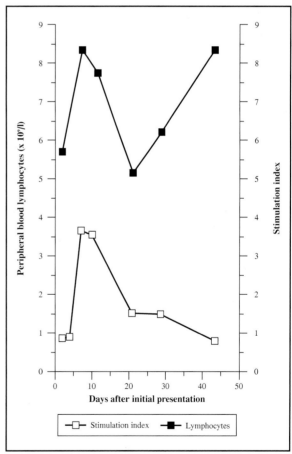

Figure 7.7: *Data from a German Shepherd Dog with disseminated aspergillosis showing serial monitoring of blood lymphocyte count and response to stimulation of purified mononuclear cells with phytohaemagglutinin in vitro. There is persistent lymphocytosis, with the total lymphocyte count fluctuating between 5.0 and 8.5 x 10⁹/l (normal range 1.0–4.8 x 10⁹/l). The stimulation index relative to cultures of lymphocytes from a control dog is initially normal but decreases terminally, despite increasing numbers of peripheral blood lymphocytes. This terminally depressed lymphocyte function is likely to reflect the presence of chronic multisystemic inflammation.*

Miniature Dachshunds seem to be predisposed to respiratory disease caused by *Pneumocystis carinii,* and an underlying immunodeficiency has been postulated to explain this association (Farrow *et al.,* 1972; Copland, 1974; Botha and van Rensburg, 1979; McCully *et al.,* 1979). Despite this, few published studies have been performed. Two cases dealt with by this author had no evidence of depressed lymphocyte response to mitogen.

Viral infection may cause acquired abnormalities of leucocyte function. Cats with feline immunodeficiency virus infection have depressed response of peripheral blood mononuclear cells to T- and B-cell mitogens (Bishop, 1995; Callanan, 1995) associated with reduced production of IL-2 (Lawrence *et al.,* 1995), and there is reduced ability of these cells to respond to primary or secondary stimulation with antigens in vitro (Bishop, 1995). Canine distemper virus, canine parvovirus and feline leukaemia virus infections may also suppress lymphocyte proliferative responses to mitogens (Krakowka *et al.,* 1975; Degen and Breitschwerdt, 1986a).

In the case of neutrophils and macrophages, apparent dysfunction of chemotaxis or phagocytosis may be attributable to underlying deficiency of opsonins such as serum immunoglobulin or complement. Serum from dogs with deficiency of the third component of complement (C3) was inefficient at opsonizing *Pneumococcus* for phagocytosis by neutrophils from normal dogs and failed to effectively attract such neutrophils after zymosan activation (Winkelstein *et al.,* 1982). In the dog, the adherence of neutrophils to nylon wool has been shown to be decreased in those with poorly controlled diabetes mellitus (Latimer and Mahaffey, 1984) and this may have a role in the occurrence of secondary infections in this disease. A deficiency of granulocyte myeloperoxidase has been documented in lead-intoxicated dogs (Caldwell *et al.,* 1979).

CONGENITAL DISORDERS OF LEUCOCYTE FUNCTION

Figure 7.8 summarizes the congenital disorders of leucocyte function recognized in small animals.

Immunodeficiency of Weimaraners
Granulocytopathy of Irish Setters (CLAD)
Neutrophil defects in Dobermann Pinschers
Canine cyclic haematopoiesis
Pelger–Huet anomaly
Chediak–Higashi syndrome
X-linked combined immunodeficiency
Immunodeficiency syndrome of Irish Wolfhounds
Lethal acrodermatitis of Bull Terriers

Figure 7.8: Congenital defects of leucocyte function.

Immunodeficiency of Weimaraners

In 1980 a colony of Weimaraners was described with growth hormone deficiency, thymic aplasia and failure of peripheral blood lymphocytes to respond to T-cell mitogens (Roth *et al.,* 1980). Affected dogs had a wasting syndrome and increased susceptibility to infection. Since 1984, an apparently separate syndrome of chronic recurrent infection in young Weimaraners has been recognized in Australia (Studdert *et al.,* 1984; MJ Day, unpublished observations), the United States (Couto *et al.,* 1989), Belgium (Hansen *et al.,* 1995) and the United Kingdom (Day *et al.,* 1997). These dogs had a left shift neutrophilia, with neutrophil dominated inflammatory lesions at postmortem examination. A range of immunological tests has been performed on these populations. In the initial series of dogs there was no apparent abnormality in neutrophil or lymphocyte function (Studdert *et al.,* 1984), but subsequent studies by Couto *et al.* (1989) suggested that a primary defect in neutrophil function (chemiluminescence), in the face of normal function of lymphocytes, monocytes and NK cells, was present in these dogs. A single case reported by Hansen *et al.* (1995) showed defective neutrophil phagocytosis in vitro despite normal responses to chemotactic agents. More consistently, reduced concentrations of serum IgG have been documented in these animals (Couto *et al.,* 1989; Hansen *et al.,* 1995; Day *et al.,* 1997), but there is debate as to whether this is a primary event or secondary to immune complex formation. The syndrome of hypertrophic osteodystrophy that is recognized in Weimaraner puppies may have some overlap with this immunodeficiency disorder, and one group of dogs with methaphyseal lesions were reported to have concurrent systemic disease and hypogammaglobulinaemia (Abeles *et al.,* 1999).

Granulocytopathy of Irish Setters (CLAD)

In 1975 an Irish Setter with chronic recurrent infection associated with pyrexia and neutrophilia was investigated for suspected immunodeficiency. Abnormalities in the bactericidal activity of neutrophils following normal phagocytosis were discovered, and the disease was reported to be inherited in an autosomal recessive manner (Renshaw *et al.,* 1975, 1977). The disorder was termed canine granulocytopathy syndrome. Subsequent studies showed that neutrophils from the affected dog had reduced glucose oxidation by the hexose monophosphate shunt but an increased ability to reduce NBT (Renshaw and Davis, 1979). Some years later, an Irish Setter with severe bacterial infections and lack of tissue pus formation in the face of peripheral blood neutrophilia was reported by Giger *et al.* (1987). The dog had inherited a deficiency in the expression of surface integrin molecules (CD11b and CD18), which manifested as an inability of neutrophils to adhere to various surfaces in vitro and, by extrapolation, to vascular endothelium in vivo. Neutrophil chemotaxis and aggregation were also impaired. The defect was thought to be inherited in an autosomal recessive manner but a relationship to the canine granulocytopathy syndrome was not definitively established. A deficiency in leucocyte adhesion molecules, now known as canine leucocyte adhesion deficiency (CLAD), is also recognized in Irish Setters in Sweden (Trowald-Wigh *et al.*, 1992, 2000) and the United Kingdom. A molecular diagnostic test for this disorder has recently been reported by the Swedish group (Kijas *et al.*, 1999).

Neutrophil defects in Dobermann Pinschers

In 1987 a series of related Dobermann Pinschers with chronic rhinitis and pneumonia was reported. These dogs showed defective killing by neutrophils of phagocytosed *Staphylococcus* and had a reduced ability to reduce NBT and produce superoxide after stimulation by opsonized zymosan (Breitschwerdt *et al.*, 1987). The relationship of this syndrome to the granulocytopathy of Irish Setters has not been determined.

Canine cyclic haematopoiesis

Canine cyclic haematopoiesis (also called cyclic neutropenia or Grey Collie syndrome) is characterized by cyclic neutropenia (every 12 days) in addition to myeloperoxidase deficiency of neutrophils (Chusid *et al.*, 1975). The dogs have diluted coat colour and display a range of clinical signs during the neutropenic episodes. Cycling of monocytes, reticulocytes and platelets also occurs (Trail *et al.*, 1984). There is no genetic mutation of haemopoietic stem cell factor (Dale *et al.*, 1995). The disease is inherited in an autosomal recessive manner.

Pelger–Huet anomaly

The Pelger-Huet anomaly has been documented in several dog breeds including the American Foxhound and Basenji. There is decreased segmentation of granulocyte nuclei, and defective neutrophil chemotaxis in affected dogs has been described (Bowles *et al.*, 1979) but not confirmed by later studies (Latimer *et al.*, 1989). These functional defects appear not to predispose to infection (Hoskins and Taboada, 1992). The anomaly also occurs in the cat where there is additional abnormality of monocytes and megakaryocytes (Weiss, 1991).

Chediak–Higashi syndrome

The Chediak-Higashi syndrome is recognized in the Persian and is characterized by abnormal lysosomes and granules within the cytoplasm of granulocytes. This abnormality may be associated with defective neutrophil chemotaxis, degranulation and bactericidal activity (Weiss, 1991). It is accompanied by abnormalities of coat and ocular fundic pigmentation and increased susceptibility to infection (Guilford, 1987).

X-linked combined immunodeficiency

Severe combined immunodeficiency (SCID) is recognized as an inherited, X-linked recessive trait in Basset Hounds and Corgis, which succumb to severe bacterial and viral infections after loss of maternally derived immunity by 8–16 weeks of age. The dogs have thymic hypoplasia and lymphopenia. Isolated lymphocytes fail to respond to the mitogens phytohaemagglutinin and concanavalin A or to recombinant IL-2, but IgM synthesis can be detected after exposure to PWM. Recent studies have shown that these findings are secondary to mutations in the common γ chain of the receptors for IL-2, IL-4, IL-7, IL-9 and IL-15 and that the mutations in Bassets and Corgis are different (Somberg *et al.*, 1994, 1995; Felsburg *et al.*, 1999).

Immunodeficiency syndrome of Irish Wolfhounds

Chronic recurrent respiratory disease has been recognized in related Irish Wolfhounds in several geographical areas, and an underlying immunodeficiency has been proposed. One reported study of three cases has identified subnormal mitogen-driven lymphocyte proliferation in affected dogs, which might be interpreted as an underlying defect of cell-mediated immunity (Leiswitz *et al.*, 1997). By contrast, other research has identified serum IgA deficiency in affected pedigrees (Day, 1998) and these investigations are ongoing.

Lethal acrodermatitis of Bull Terriers

Lethal acrodermatitis is an inherited syndrome of Bull Terriers characterized by retarded growth, cutaneous hyperkeratosis and infections of the skin and respiratory tract (Jezyk *et al.*, 1986). These dogs have subnormal plasma zinc concentrations and show depletion of T lymphocytes from tissue and depressed lymphocyte proliferative responses to mitogens, in the face of normal phagocytosis and killing by neutrophils.

DIAGNOSTIC APPROACH TO SUSPECTED DISORDERS OF LEUCOCYTE FUNCTION

Animals with suspected disorders of leucocyte function are likely to fall into two major groups as defined by an acquired or congenital pathogenesis. Acquired defects of leucocyte function occur as secondary phenomena in adult animals, and the diagnostic approach should focus on characterization of the underlying disease state. Inherited defects of leucocyte function should be considered when young littermates present with chronic recurrent infections (often involving the skin or respiratory tract) that do not respond to standard antimicrobial therapy or recur after cessation of therapy. The differential diagnoses include other primary immunodeficiency disorders such as immunoglobulin or complement deficiency, or aplasia of lymphoid tissue with leucopenia. A diagnostic approach to such disease should include:

- A haematology profile, specifically a differential leucocyte count and morphology
- Serum protein analysis, specifically the determination of globulin concentrations
- Characterization of any infectious agent by culture
- A full postmortem examination of any dead littermates, with histological examination of lymphoid and haemopoietic organs.

Where available, appropriate immunodiagnostic tests would include:

- Quantification of serum immunoglobulins and complement
- The ability of peripheral blood lymphocytes to respond to mitogens
- Neutrophil and macrophage function.

Such tests are not widely available to veterinary surgeons in the United Kingdom, although quantification of serum immunoglobulins (IgG, IgM, IgA for dogs; IgG for cats) is performed by the Clinical Immunology Diagnostic Laboratory at the University of Bristol.

THERAPY FOR DISORDERS OF LEUCOCYTE FUNCTION

Appropriate antimicrobial therapy for many of the diseases described will result in clinical improvement but in the case of the primary congenital leucocyte defects this will only be a temporary effect as such diseases are often lethal. Although a variety of therapeutic approaches has been used in primary and secondary leucocyte disorders, the effects have been poorly characterized, and many such treatments are still considered experimental. Genetic counselling should be given to breeders when inherited defects of leucocyte function are diagnosed.

Immunomodulatory agents
A range of immunomodulatory agents has been used in therapeutic trials in the dog, but their immunological effects are poorly defined. These include products such as staphage lysate (DeBoer *et al.*, 1990), staphoid A-B (Pukay, 1985), killed *Propionibacterium* (Becker *et al.*, 1989) and levamisole (Degen and Breitschwerdt, 1986b; Guilford, 1987). The potential for development of side effects after administration of levamisole is considered to outweigh the usefulness of this agent.

Hormones
Some of the Weimaraner puppies with immunodeficient dwarfism reported by Roth *et al.* (1984) were treated with growth hormone and fractions of the thymic hormone thymosin. Although there was clinical improvement, the defective proliferative response of the lymphocytes in these dogs was not normalized.

Bone marrow transplantation and recombinant cytokines
Cytokines have profound influences on the development and function of leucocytes, and there is potential for therapeutic exploitation of this fact. For example, recombinant canine granulocyte-colony stimulating factor and recombinant canine stem cell factor have been used successfully in the treatment of cyclic haematopoiesis (Mishu *et al.*, 1992; Dale *et al.*, 1995). Bone marrow transplantation has also been successfully attempted in dogs with cyclic haematopoiesis (Dale and Graw, 1974; Dale *et al.*, 1995)

Genetic approaches
When defects of leucocyte function are attributed to specific genetic abnormalities, the therapeutic use of gene replacement therapy may in future be possible. Irish Setters with genetic deficiency of leucocyte adhesion molecules (CLAD) may be a candidate group for such an approach (Giger *et al.*, 1987), and experimental gene transfer has already been undertaken in haemopoietic progenitor cells of normal dogs and dogs with cyclic haematopoiesis (Karlsson, 1991).

REFERENCES

Abeles V, Harrus S, Angles JM, Shalev G, Aizenberg I, Peres Y and Aroch I (1999) Hypertrophic osteodystrophy in six weimaraner puppies associated with systemic signs. *Veterinary Record* **145**, 130-134

Angus K and Yang TJ (1978) Lymphocyte response to phytohemagglutinin: temporal variation in normal dogs. *Journal of Immunological Methods* **21**, 261-269

Barrett RE, Hoffer RE and Schultz RD (1977) Treatment and immunological evaluation of three cases of canine aspergillosis. *Journal of the American Animal Hospital Association* **13**, 328-334

Barta O and Oyekan P (1981) Lymphocyte transformation test in veterinary clinical immunology. *Comparative Immunology, Microbiology and Infectious Disease* **4**, 209-221

Barta O, Breitschwerdt EB, Shaffer LM and Pourciau SS (1983) Lymphocyte transformation and humoral immune factors in basenji dogs with immunoproliferative small intestinal disease. *American Journal of Veterinary Research* **44**, 1954-1959

Barta O and Turnwald GH (1983) Demodicosis, pyoderma, and other skin diseases of young dogs, and their associations with immunologic dysfunctions. *Compendium of Continuing Education for the Practicing Veterinarian* **5**, 995-1002

Becker AM, Janik TA, Smith EK, Sousa CA and Peters BA (1989) *Propionibacterium acnes* immunotherapy in chronic recurrent pyoderma. *Journal of Veterinary Internal Medicine* **3**, 26-30

Bishop S (1995) Functional abnormalities in the immune system of FIV-infected cats. In: *Feline Immunology and Immunodeficiency*, ed. BJ Willett and O Jarrett, pp. 150-169. Oxford Science, Oxford

Botha WS and van Rensburg IBJ (1979) Pneumocystosis: a chronic respiratory distress syndrome in the dog. *Journal of the South African Veterinary Association* **50**, 173-179

Bowles CA, Alasker RD and Wolfle TL (1979) Studies of the Pelger-Huet anomaly in foxhounds. *American Journal of Pathology* **96**, 237-248

Breitschwerdt EB, Brown TT, DeBuyssscher EV, Andersen BR, Thrall DE, Hager E, Ananaba G, Degen MA and Ward MDW (1987) Rhinitis, pneumonia, and defective neutrophil function in the Doberman Pinscher. *American Journal of Veterinary Research* **48**, 1054-1062

Brown WC, Collisson EW and Song W (1995) Cytotoxic T lymphocyte responses to feline immunodeficiency virus. In: *Feline Immunology and Immunodeficiency*, ed. BJ Willett and O Jarrett, pp. 306-317. Oxford Scientific, Oxford

Caldwell KC, Taddeini L, Woodburn RL, Anderson GL and Lobell A (1979) Induction of myeloperoxidase deficiency in granulocytes in lead-intoxicated dogs. *Blood* **46**, 921-930

Callanan JJ (1995) Feline immunodeficiency virus infection: a clinical and pathological perspective. In: *Feline Immunology and Immunodeficiency*, ed. BJ Willett and O Jarrett, pp. 111-130. Oxford Scientific, Oxford

Chabanne L, Marchal T, Denerolle P, Magnol JP, Fournel C, Monier JC and Rigal D (1995) Lymphocyte subset abnormalities in German shepherd dog pyoderma (GSP). *Veterinary Immunology and Immunopathology* **49**, 189-198

Chusid MJ, Bujak JS and Dale DC (1975) Defective polymorphonuclear leukocyte metabolism and function in canine cyclic neutropenia. *Blood* **46**, 921-930

Cobbold S and Metcalfe S (1994) Monoclonal antibodies that define canine homologues of human CD antigens: summary of the first international canine leukocyte antigen workshop (CLAW). *Tissue Antigens* **43**, 137-154

Cohn LA (1991) The influence of corticosteroids on host defense mechanisms. *Journal of Veterinary Internal Medicine* **5**, 95-104

Copland JW (1974) Canine pneumonia caused by *Pneumocystis carinii*. *Australian Veterinary Journal* **50**, 515-518

Couto CG, Krakowka S, Johnson G, Ciekot P, Hill R, Lafrado L and Kociba G (1989) In vitro immunologic features of weimaraner dogs with neutrophil abnormalities and recurrent infections. *Veterinary Immunology and Immunopathology* **23**, 103-112

Dale DC and Graw RG (1974) Transplantation of allogeneic bone marrow in canine cyclic neutropenia. *Science* **183**, 83

Dale DC, Rodger E, Cebon J, Ramesh N, Hammond WP and Zsebo KM (1995) Long-term treatment of canine cyclic hematopoiesis with recombinant canine stem cell factor. *Blood* **85**, 74-79

Day MJ (1987) A study of the immune response in canine disseminated aspergillosis. PhD Thesis, Murdoch University, Western Australia

Day MJ (1994) An immunopathological study of deep pyoderma in the dog. *Research in Veterinary Science* **56**, 18-23

Day MJ (1998) Mechanisms of immune-mediated diseases in small animals. *In Practice* **20**, 75-86

Day MJ, Penhale WJ, Eger CE, Shaw SE, Kabay MJ, Robinson WF, Huxtable CRR, Mills JN and Wyburn RS (1986) Disseminated aspergillosis in dogs. *Australian Veterinary Journal* **63**, 55-59

Day MJ, Power C, Oleshko J and Rose M (1997) Low serum immunoglobulin concentrations in related weimaraner dogs. *Journal of Small Animal Practice* **38**, 311-315

DeBoer DJ (1994) Immunomodulatory effects of staphylococcal antigen and antigen-antibody complexes on canine mononuclear and polymorphonuclear leukocytes. *American Journal of Veterinary Research* **55**, 1690-1696

DeBoer DJ, Moriello KA, Thomas CB and Schultz KT (1990) Evaluation of a commercial staphylococcal bacterin for the management of idiopathic recurrent superficial pyoderma in dogs. *American Journal of Veterinary Research* **51**, 636-639

DeBowes LJ and Anderson NV (1991) Phagocytosis and erythrocyte antibody-rosette formation by three populations of mononuclear phagocytes obtained from dogs treated with glucocorticoids. *American Journal of Veterinary Research* **52**, 869-872

Degen MA and Breitschwerdt EB (1986a) Canine and feline immunodeficiency, part I. *Compendium of Continuing Education for the Practicing Veterinarian* **8**, 313-323

Degen MA and Breitschwerdt EB (1986b) Canine and feline immunodeficiency, part II. *Compendium of Continuing Education for the Practicing Veterinarian* **8**, 379-386

Farrow BRH, Watson ADJ, Hartley WJ and Huxtable CRR (1972) Pneumocystis pneumonia in the dog. *Journal of Comparative Pathology* **82**, 447-453

Felsburg PJ, Hartnett BJ, Henthorn PS, Moore PF, Krakowka S and Ochs HD (1999) Canine X-linked severe combined immunodeficiency. *Veterinary Immunology and Immunopathology* **69**, 127-135

Gerber JD and Brown AL (1974) Effect of development and ageing on the response of canine lymphocytes to phytohemagglutinin. *Infection and Immunity* **10**, 695-699

Giger U, Boxer LA, Simpson PJ, Lucchesi BR and Todd RF (1987) Deficiency of leukocyte surface glycoproteins Mo1, LFA-1, and Leu M5 in a dog with recurrent bacterial infections: an animal model. *Blood* **69**, 1622-1630

Gilger BC, Andrews J, Wilkie DA, Wyman M and Lairmore MD (1995) Cellular immunity in dogs with keratoconjunctivitis sicca before and after treatment with topical 2% cyclosporine. *Veterinary Immunology and Immunopathology* **49**, 199-208

Guilford WG (1987) Primary immunodeficiency diseases of dogs and cats. *Compendium of Continuing Education for the Practicing Veterinarian* **9**, 641-650

Hansen P, Clercx C, Henroteaux M, Rutten VPMG and Bernadina WE (1995) Neutrophil phagocyte dysfunction in a weimaraner with recurrent infections. *Journal of Small Animal Practice* **36**, 128-131

Helfand SC, Modiano JF and Nowell PC (1992) Immunophysiological studies of interleukin-2 and canine lymphocytes. *Veterinary Immunology and Immunopathology* **33**, 1-16

Hirsch DC, Baker BB, Wiger N, Yaskulski SG and Osburn BI (1975) Suppression of in vitro lymphocyte transformation by serum from dogs with generalised demodicosis. *American Journal of Veterinary Research* **36**, 1591-1595

Hoskins JD and Taboada J (1992) Congenital defects of the dog. *Compendium of Continuing Education for the Practicing Veterinarian* **14**, 873

Jezyk PF, Haskins ME, MacKay-Smith WE and Patterson DF (1986) Lethal acrodermatitis in bull terriers. *Journal of the American Veterinary Medical Association* **188**, 833-839

Karlsson S (1991) Treatment of genetic defects in hemopoietic cell function by gene transfer. *Blood* **78**, 2481-2492

Kijas JMH, Bauer TR, Gafvert S, Marklund S, Trowald-Wigh G, Johannisson A, Hedhammar Å, Binns M, Juneja RK, Hickstein DD and Andersson L (1999) A missense mutation in the β-2 integrin gene (ITGB2) causes canine leukocyte adhesion deficiency. *Genomics* **61**, 101-107

Killingsworth CR, Walshaw R, Reimann KA and Rosser EJ (1988) Thyroid and immunologic status of dogs with perianal fistula. *American Journal of Veterinary Research* **49**, 1742-1745

Krakowka S, Cockerell G and Koestner A (1975) Effects of canine distemper virus infection on lymphoid function *in vitro* and *in vivo*. *Infection and Immunity* **11**, 1069-1078

Kristensen F, Kristensen B and Lazary S (1982) The lymphocyte stimulation test in veterinary immunology. *Veterinary Immunology and Immunopathology* **3**, 203-277

Latimer KS, Kircher IM, Lendl PA, Dawe DL and Brown J (1989) Leukocyte function in Pelger-Huet anomaly of dogs. *Journal of Leukocyte Biology* **45**, 301-310

Latimer KS and Mahaffey EA (1984) Neutrophil adherence and movement in poorly and well-controlled diabetic dogs. *American Journal of Veterinary Research* **45**, 1498-1500

Latimer KS, Prasse KW and Dawe DL (1982) A transient deficit in neutrophilic chemotaxis in a dog with recurrent staphylococcal pyoderma. *Veterinary Pathology* **19**, 223-229

Latimer KS, Prasse KW, Mahaffey EA, Dawe DL, Lorenz MD and Duncan JR (1983) Neutrophil movement in selected canine skin diseases. *American Journal of Veterinary Research* **44**, 601-605

Lawrence CE, Callanan JJ, Willett BJ and Jarrett O (1995) Cytokine production by cats infected with feline immunodeficiency virus: a longitudinal study. *Immunology* **85**, 568-574

Leiswitz AL, Spencer JA, Jacobson LS and Schroeder H (1997) Suspected primary immunodeficiency syndrome in three related Irish wolfhounds. *Journal of Small Animal Practice* **38**, 209-212

Lemarie SL, Foil CS and Horohov DW (1994) Evaluation of interleukin-2 production and interleukin-2 receptor expression in dogs with generalised demodicosis. *Proceedings of the American Academy of Veterinary Dermatology* p. 26

Mason DW, Penhale WJ and Sedgwick JD (1987) Preparation of lymphocyte subpopulations. In: *Lymphocytes, a Practical Approach*, ed. GGB Klaus, pp. 35-54. IRL Press, Oxford

McCully RM, Lloyd J, Kuys D and Schneider DJ (1979) Canine pneumocystis pneumonia. *Journal of the South African Veterinary Association* **50**, 207-213

Miller WH (1991) Deep pyoderma in two German shepherd dogs associated with a cell-mediated immunodeficiency. *Journal of the American Animal Hospital Association* **27**, 513-517

Mishu L, Callahan G, Allebban Z, Maddux JM, Boone TC, Souza LM and Lothrop CD (1992) Effects of recombinant canine granulocyte colony-stimulating factor on white blood cell production in clinically normal and neutropenic dogs. *Journal of the American Veterinary Medical Association* **200**, 1957-1964

Mizuno S, Fujinaga T and Hagio M (1993) Characterization of dog interleukin-2 activity. *Journal of Veterinary Medical Science* **55**, 925-930

Nagahata H, Kociba GJ, Reiter JA and Couto CG (1991) Analysis of selected variables in the under-agarose assay for chemotactic responses of canine neutrophils. *American Journal of Veterinary Research* **52**, 965-969

Nakada Y, Tokumitu K, Kosaka T, Kuwabara M, Tanaka S and Koide F (1995) Correlation between canine NK cell mediated cytotoxicity and radical production. *Veterinary Immunology and Immunopathology* **45**, 285-295

Pinelli E, Killick-Kendrick R, Wagenaar J, Bernadina W, Del Real G and Ruitenberg J (1994) Cellular and humoral immune response in dogs experimentally and naturally infected with *Leishmania infantum*. *Infection and Immunity* **62**, 229-235

Pukay BP (1985) Treatment of canine bacterial hypersensitivity by hyposensitization with *Staphylococcus aureus* bacterin-toxoid. *Journal of the American Animal Hospital Association* **21**, 479-483

Renshaw HW, Chatburn C, Bryan GM, Bartsch RC and Davis WC (1975) Canine granulocytopathy syndrome: neutrophil dysfunction in a dog with recurrent infections. *Journal of the American Veterinary Medical Association* **166**, 443-447

Renshaw HW, Davis WC and Renshaw SJ (1977) Canine granulocytopathy syndrome: defective bactericidal capacity of neutrophils from a dog with recurrent infections. *Clinical Immunology and Immunopathology* **8**, 385-395

Renshaw HW and Davis WC (1979) Canine granulocytopathy syndrome: an inherited disorder of leukocyte function. *American Journal of Pathology* **95**, 731-744

Rivas AL, Kimball ES, Quimby FW and Gebhard D (1995) Functional and phenotypic analysis of in vitro stimulated canine peripheral blood mononuclear cells. *Veterinary Immunology and Immunopathology* **45**, 55-71

Roth JA, Kaeberle ML, Grier RL, Hopper JG, Spiegel HE and McAllister HA (1984) Improvement in clinical condition and thymus morphological features associated with growth hormone treatment of immunodeficient dwarf dogs. *American Journal of Veterinary Research* **45**, 1151-1155

Roth JA, Lomax LG, Altszuler N, Hampshire J, Kaeberle ML, Shelton M, Draper DD and Ledet AE (1980) Thymic abnormalities and growth hormone deficiency in dogs. *American Journal of Veterinary Research* **41**, 1256-1262

Rottman JB, Freeman EB, Tonkonogy S and Tompkins MB (1995) A reverse transcription-polymerase chain reaction technique to detect feline cytokine genes. *Veterinary Immunology and Immunopathology* **45**, 1-18

Scott DW, Farrow BRH and Shultz RD (1974) Studies on the therapeutic and immunologic aspects of generalised demodectic mange in the dog. *Journal of the American Animal Hospital Association* **10**, 233-243

Shearer DH and Day MJ (1997) An investigation of phagocytosis and intracellular killing of *Staphylococcus intermedius* by canine neutrophils in vitro. *Veterinary Immunology and Immunopathology* **58**, 219-230

Shifrine M, Taylor N, Rosenblatt LS and Wilson F (1980) Seasonal variation in cell mediated immunity of clinically normal dogs. *Experimental Haematology* **8**, 318-326

Somberg RL, Pullen RP, Casal ML, Patterson DF, Felsburg PJ and Henthorn PS (1995) A single nucleotide insertion in the canine interleukin-2 receptor gamma chain results in X-linked severe combined immunodeficiency disease. *Veterinary Immunology and Immunopathology* **47**, 203-213

Somberg RL, Robinson JP and Felsburg PJ (1994) T lymphocyte development and function in dogs with X-linked severe combined immunodeficiency. *Journal of Immunology* **153**, 4006-4015

Studdert VP, Phillips WA, Studdert MJ and Hosking CS (1984) Recurrent and persistent infections in related weimaraner dogs. *Australian Veterinary Journal* **61**, 261-263

Thomsen MK, Larsen CG, Thomsen HK, Kirstein D, Skak-Nielsen T, Ahnfelt-Ronne I and Thestrup-Pedersen K (1991) Recombinant human interleukin-8 is a potent activator of canine neutrophil aggregation, migration and leukotrienne B$_4$ biosynthesis. *Journal of Investigative Dermatology* **96**, 260-266

Trail PA, Yang TJ and Cameron JA (1984) Increase in the haemolytic complement activity of dogs affected with cyclic haematopoiesis. *Veterinary Immunology and Immunopathology* **7**, 359-368

Trowald-Wigh G, Ekman S, Hansson K, Hedhammer Å and Hard af Segerstad C (2000) Clinical, radiological and pathological features of 12 Irish setters with canine leucocyte adhesion deficiency. *Journal of Small Animal Practice* **41**, 211-217

Trowald-Wigh G, Hakansson L, Johannisson A, Norrgren L and Hard af Segerstad C (1992) Leucocyte adhesion protein deficiency in Irish setter dogs. *Veterinary Immunology and Immunopathology* **32**, 261-280

Weiss DJ (1991) White cells. *Advances in Veterinary Science and Comparative Medicine* **36**, 57-86

Winkelstein JA, Johnson JP, Swift AJ, Ferry F, Yolken R and Cork LC (1982) Genetically determined deficiency of the third component of complement in the dog: *in vitro* studies on the complement system and complement-mediated serum activities. *Journal of Immunology* **129**, 2598-2602

Yamahita K, Fujinaga T, Hagio M, Miyamoto T, Izumisawa Y and Kotani T (1994) Bioassay for interleukin-1, interleukin-6, and tumour necrosis factor-like activities in canine sera. *Journal of Veterinary Medical Science* **56**, 103-107

Leucocyte Disorders: Selected Topics

(i) Neutropenia

Anthony Abrams-Ogg

INTRODUCTION

Neutropenia may be an incidental laboratory finding, but more commonly it is discovered in the work-up of a sick animal. When a septic neutropenic animal is presented, there are three possible scenarios:

- Primary bacterial sepsis, where tissue demands overwhelm marrow granulocyte reserve and production, as in bacterial peritonitis. Prior to illness the marrow was normal
- Primary impairment of granulopoiesis, as in feline leukaemia virus infection, and therefore an increase in susceptibility to infection. Secondary sepsis occurs, which in turn exacerbates neutropenia. Impairment of granulopoiesis is usually a facet of acquired generalized impairment of haematopoiesis, but neutropenia is the first peripheral blood abnormality to appear because of the neutrophil's short life span
- Concurrent tissue injury promoting sepsis and impaired granulopoiesis, as in parvoviral infections and cytotoxic chemotherapy.

Specific causes of neutropenia in the dog and cat are listed in Figure 8.1.

Inherited	Cyclic haematopoiesis in grey Collies Chediak–Higashi syndrome (cats)
Infectious	Canine parvovirus-2 Feline parvovirus Feline leukaemia virus Feline immunodeficiency virus (FIV) Ehrlichiosis Overwhelming sepsis Systemic mycosis Toxoplasmosis (cats)
Neoplastic	Lymphocytic leukaemia, leukaemic lymphoma Multiple myeloma Myelogenous leukaemia, myelodysplasia Metastatic cancer (myelophthisis) Oestrogen-secreting (Sertoli cell) tumour (dog)

Therapeutics	Anticancer and immunosuppressive therapy causing predictable myelosuppression
	        Cytotoxic chemotherapeutic agents
	        Large-field radiation therapy
	
	Drugs with known risk for causing myelosuppression
	        Dog: oestrogens, phenylbutazone
	        Cat: chloramphenicol, griseofulvin (especially in FIV infected cats),
	                propylthiouracil, methimazole, carbimazole
	
	Drugs with reported idiosyncratic reactions causing neutropenia (any drug has potential to
	cause neutropenia by immune or direct myelotoxic mechanisms)
	        Dog: cephalosporins, sulphonamides, metronidazole, angiotensin-converting
	                enzyme inhibitors, phenobarbital, streptozotocin (mild neutropenia)
	        Cat: cephalosporins, amitriptyline

Miscellaneous	Idiopathic (may be inherited) Granulocyte colony-stimulating factor deficiency Immune-mediated neutropenia Myelofibrosis Disseminated intravascular coagulation (dog) Hypoadrenocorticism (neutropenia is mild and is not associated with secondary infection)
Normal	Mild neutropenia may be a normal finding in some breeds, e.g. Belgian Tervuren, Greyhound

Figure 8.1: *Aetiology of neutropenia in the dog and cat.*

DIAGNOSIS OF NEUTROPENIA

Neutropenia is diagnosed with routine haematology. If the haemogram is obtained by use of an automated haematology analyser, it is recommended that a blood smear be examined to complete the haematological evaluation. Whether manual or automated methods are used, clots in the sample may result in artificial neutropenia. Haemodilution from aggressive fluid therapy may result in mild depression of leucocyte counts.

There are no clinical signs associated with neutropenia in itself. Signs are due to the underlying disease and infection. When secondary infection occurs, most neutropenic animals will develop a fever. Occasionally only lethargy, inappetence and tachycardia occur. This is most likely in elderly animals and in animals treated with anti-inflammatory drugs, which may have blunted febrile responses. Septic animals may also present with vomiting and/or diarrhoea or may be in shock. If granulopoiesis is impaired, the signs of local inflammation are subtle, and the site of infection may be difficult to identify.

Diagnosis of the specific cause of neutropenia is often possible on the basis of history, physical examination and routine laboratory and serological tests. On a haemogram, a minimal left shift and pancytopenia suggest that granulopoietic failure is contributing to neutropenia. However, many pathophysiological processes affect haematology results and, with the exception of the presence of neoplastic cells or certain infectious organisms, there are no pathognomonic patterns for any given cause of neutropenia. Serial evaluation of haemograms may be necessary in some cases to explain abnormalities. Bone marrow biopsy should be considered if there is evidence of impaired granulopoiesis.

INFECTIOUS COMPLICATIONS OF NEUTROPENIA

Risk factors
Several different factors in humans determine the risk, severity and outcome of secondary infection during neutropenia (Feld, 1989). These factors include:

- Severity and duration of neutropenia
- Disruption of natural barriers and immunosuppression
- Tumour type and biological stage in patients with cancer
- Microbial organisms involved and site of infection.

These factors seem to be applicable to dogs and cats and will be discussed in turn.

Severity and duration of neutropenia
Severity of neutropenia is the most important risk factor for developing an infection. The risk increases exponentially with increasing severity of neutropenia (Figure 8.2). As the neutrophil count decreases, duration of neutropenia becomes an increasingly important factor as well.

Neutrophil count	Definition and risk of infection
Less than lower limit of normal range	Marginal neutropenia with minimal risk of infection
$<2.0 \times 10^9/l$	Mild neutropenia with mild risk of infection
$<1.0 \times 10^9/l$	Moderate neutropenia with moderate risk of infection
$<0.5 \times 10^9/l$	Severe neutropenia with high risk of infection
$<0.2 \times 10^9/l$	Severe neutropenia with very high risk of infection

Figure 8.2: *Risk of secondary infection during neutropenia. For a given degree of neutropenia, a higher risk of infection is associated with a decreasing, rather than a stable, neutrophil count.*

Duration of neutropenia is the most important risk factor in determining outcome of an infection. When neutropenia is of short duration (<7 days), most infections can be controlled with appropriate antimicrobial therapy. Infections complicating neutropenia of moderate duration (7-14 days) are more difficult to treat. Infections in patients with prolonged neutropenia (>14 days) are even more difficult to treat, especially if the neutrophil count is less than $0.2 \times 10^9/l$. The likelihood of clearing an established infection with antimicrobial therapy decreases in neutropenia because antimicrobial agents act in synergy with host defences to kill invading organisms.

Cats seem to tolerate better lower neutrophil counts and neutropenia of longer duration than do dogs. They are at less risk of developing infections, and their infections are more easily treated.

Disruption of natural barriers and immunosuppression
Disruption of natural physical barriers and suppression of humoral and cell-mediated immunity increases the risk of infection during neutropenia. Natural barriers are disrupted, with gastrointestinal damage during parvoviral infections and anticancer chemotherapy, facilitating invasion by enteric bacteria. Intravenous catheterization increases the risk of infection with cutaneous organisms. Immunosuppression may be present concurrently with

myelosuppression, either because of the primary disease (e.g. multiple myeloma), as a result of therapy (e.g. cyclophosphamide), or because of malnutrition secondary to inappetence. The risk of infection in neutropenic humans is greater with concurrent lymphopenia and monocytopenia.

Tumour type and biological stage in patients with cancer

Infections secondary to neutropenia are likely to be more severe in humans with acute compared with chronic haematological malignancies, haematological malignancies in relapse compared with malignancies in remission and haematological malignancies compared with solid tumours.

Microbiology

Infections in neutropenic animals may occur with environmental and hospital-acquired organisms or be acquired from other animals. However, the greatest source of infection is the animal's own flora, especially of the intestinal tract, which translocate to other sites. The most frequently isolated organisms are Gram-negative enteric bacilli (*Escherichia coli*, *Klebsiella* spp., *Enterobacter* spp.), followed by Gram-positive cocci (*Staphylococcus* spp., *Streptococcus* spp.) (Kowall, 1974; Dow *et al.*, 1989; Couto, 1990; Turk *et al.*, 1990). *Pseudomonas* spp. are less frequently isolated but are feared because of antimicrobial resistance. Despite being present in large numbers in the intestinal tract, anaerobic bacteria are not commonly the first invaders in opportunistic infection during neutropenia. It is possible, however, that anaerobic bacteria contribute to sepsis during parvoviral infections since intestinal proliferation of *Clostridium perfringens* in canine parvovirus-2 infection has been documented (Turk *et al.*, 1992).

The most common sites of infection are the bloodstream (bacteraemia) and the lung. Infections at these sites are more difficult to treat than infections at other sites (Feld, 1989). Pneumonia may occur as an opportunistic infection by upper respiratory flora or more commonly from translocation of intestinal bacteria. Local cellulitis may occur, manifested as oedema of one or more limbs. Other possible sites of infection include the oral cavity, gastrointestinal tract, urinary tract, heart and central nervous system.

Invasive fungal infections with *Candida* spp. and *Aspergillus* spp. have been reported as complications of cytotoxic therapy and parvoviral infections, but prevalence seems to be low (Kowall, 1974; Anderson and Pidgeon, 1987; Rosenthal, 1988). The risk of fungal infection increases with the duration of neutropenia, duration of antibacterial therapy and concurrent immunosuppressive therapy (e.g. with cyclosporin).

PATIENT MANAGEMENT

In small animal medicine, neutropenia is most commonly of short duration (<7 days) and/or of mild to moderate severity. Animals with neutropenia of prolonged duration usually have only mildly depressed neutrophil counts. This is in part due to use of only moderately aggressive anticancer chemotherapy and to euthanasia of severely neutropenic animals with a poor prognosis for prompt recovery. The discussion that follows concerns the management of infection. Underlying diseases should be treated in accordance with standard recommendations, and any drugs that are suspected of causing neutropenia should be withdrawn. Treatment options to control infections are:

- Isolation (reduce risk of increased neutrophil demand)
- Antimicrobial therapy: prophylactic therapy (reduce risk of increased neutrophil demand) and empirical treatment of febrile neutropenic patients and therapy of documented infections (assist existing neutrophils)
- Granulocyte transfusions (replace neutrophils)
- Haematopoietic cytokine therapy (stimulate neutrophil production and function)
- Removal of the focus of infection (reduce existing increased neutrophil demand).

Isolation

Isolation reduces the risk of acquiring infections from the environment and other animals. Neutropenic animals that do not require critical care should be maintained at home and confined to the house and garden or yard. In the veterinary hospital, contact with the general patient population should be avoided. Hands should be washed thoroughly and laboratory coats changed before handling neutropenic animals. The use of gloves and isolation gowns should be considered for severely neutropenic cases. Body temperature should be measured with a thermometer restricted to use in a particular patient. Table scraps should be avoided and only canned foods offered to dogs and cats with severe neutropenia.

Antimicrobial therapy

Antimicrobial therapy is the cornerstone of management of neutropenia. It may be divided into three categories:

- Prophylactic therapy
- Empirical treatment during febrile episodes
- Treatment of documented infections (where the sites of infection and/or infecting organisms are known).

Prophylactic therapy

Antimicrobial prophylaxis in the asymptomatic patient should be considered whenever a neutrophil count of less than 0.5 x 10^9/l is present or anticipated. Antimicrobial therapy is directed at intestinal flora, with the principal objective of reducing the Gram-negative and Gram-positive organisms most often responsible for infections. This objective is known as 'selective intestinal decontamination.' The intestinal anaerobic population is left relatively undisturbed since it contributes to resistance to fungal overgrowth and colonization by contagious organisms. A second objective of prophylactic therapy is to provide sufficient tissue drug levels to contain an incipient bacterial infection. Drug choices for prophylactic therapy are presented in Figure 8.3.

Antimicrobial prophylaxis is controversial. The benefits are not clear with respect to reducing infection and mortality. Prophylactic therapy in humans seems to be more beneficial in reducing infection rates during severe and prolonged neutropenia than during mild to moderate neutropenia (Wade, 1994). In one study of veterinary cancer patients receiving vincristine-doxorubicin-cyclophosphamide chemotherapy, which resulted in neutropenic episodes of short duration with a median neutrophil count of 0.8 x 10^9/l, trimethoprim–sulphonamide prophylaxis reduced the number of antibiotic-responsive febrile episodes from 40% to 20% (Couto, 1990). The potential advantages of prophylactic therapy include reductions in infection rate, time to onset of infection and speed at which an incipient infection develops into overwhelming sepsis. These benefits facilitate home management of neutropenic animals and improve quality of life. Potential disadvantages of prophylactic therapy include drug-induced inappetence and vomiting and development of resistant organisms (Wade, 1994). Antimicrobial prophylaxis may also be an unnecessary expense. However, in most cases treating sepsis is more expensive than preventing it.

Antimicrobial prophylaxis is recommended if severe and prolonged neutropenia is anticipated, such as with pancytopenia caused by oestrogen toxicosis in dogs. Routine prophylactic therapy during anticancer chemotherapy is not recommended if the owner can closely observe the animal for signs of infection and if the anticipated neutropenia is of short duration, such as occurs with many commonly used chemotherapeutic protocols. Prophylactic therapy is discouraged in cats, which are at less risk of infection secondary to neutropenia than are dogs but are at more risk of antibiotic-induced gastrointestinal disorders (Kunkle et al., 1995). The author currently uses prophylactic therapy in dogs during the more aggressive chemotherapy protocols involving weekly treatments with doxorubicin, cyclophosphamide and vincristine. Furthermore, for animals not receiving prophylaxis, antimicrobial therapy is begun in the asymptomatic animal when a neutrophil count below 0.5-1.0 x 10^9/l is noted on, or anticipated from, a pretreatment haemogram. The chemotherapy is not given, and antimicrobial therapy is continued until the animal is returned for its next chemotherapy treatment 4-7 days later, by which time the neutrophil count has usually recovered. In the event that chemotherapy is delayed again because the neutrophil count has not sufficiently recovered, antimicrobial prophylaxis is discontinued if the neutrophil count is above 1.0-2.0 x 10^9/l.

The author does not routinely use antimicrobial prophylaxis with protocols involving single agents (e.g. doxorubicin or carboplatin) being given every 3 weeks. However, if there has been a previous episode of chemotherapy-induced sepsis and/or neutropenia, then antimicrobial prophylaxis is given after the next treatment with the offending drug (the dose of which may also be reduced), but prophylaxis may be restricted to 5-10 days after treatment, which is the period during which most post-chemotherapy neutrophil nadirs occur.

Empirical treatment of febrile neutropenic patients

Asymptomatic animals with neutropenia and animals at risk of developing neutropenia should have body temperature monitored. Depending on anticipated risk, this may vary from measuring temperature when there are signs of lethargy or inappetence to routine monitoring 2-4 times a day. Axillary temperature measurements facilitate home monitoring and are 0.5-1°C lower than rectal temperature measurements. A rectal temperature above 39.0°C in dogs and above 39.2°C in cats should be regarded with suspicion. A temperature above 39.5°C in most cases represents a true fever.

Fever and/or unexplained depression and inappetence in a neutropenic animal should be considered infectious in origin until proven otherwise, and antimicrobial therapy should be initiated promptly. In most cases of infection secondary to transient myelosuppression, early therapy with familiar antibiotics and good supportive care will result in a successful outcome. The animal should be closely examined for any subtle signs of inflammation and an appropriate culture obtained. If there is no obvious site of infection, blood cultures should be considered before beginning therapy. The author currently obtains two simultaneous blood cultures of 5-10 ml each from different veins (Reller, 1994). Blood cultures are, however, expensive. Furthermore, results take 2-7 days to become available and often are either negative or do not alter initial therapy. For these reasons, the author does not always obtain blood cultures during anticancer chemotherapy when the anticipated duration of neutropenia is short and does not routinely obtain them for animals with parvoviral infections. Urine culture should also be considered, especially if the animal is polyuric, has signs of lower urinary tract inflammation or has faecal soiling of external genitalia. However, therapy should not be delayed while awaiting adequate urine production for collection. Cystocentesis should not be performed if the platelet count is less than 50 x 10^9/l; a free catch sample

Antimicrobial agent	Doses	Comment
Sulphonamides		
Trimethoprim–sulphamethoxazole	**15 mg/kg (combined dose) every 12 hours** 30 mg/kg (combined dose) every 12–24 hours	Inexpensive No prophylaxis against *Pseudomonas* spp. Risk of keratoconjunctivitis sicca with prolonged use May retard marrow recovery after severe myelosuppression
Trimethoprim-sulphadiazine	15 mg/kg (combined dose) every 12 hours 30 mg/kg (combined dose) every 12–24 hours	As for trimethoprim-sulphamethoxazole but more expensive
Ormetoprim-sulphadimethoxine	55 mg/kg on first day, then 27.5 mg/kg every 24 hours	As for trimethoprim-sulphamethoxazole but more expensive
Fluoroquinolones		
Enrofloxacin	**5-10 mg/kg every 12 hours (dog)** 10-20 mg/kg every 24 hours (dog) 2.5 mg/kg every 12 hours (cat) 5 mg/kg every 24 hours (cat)	Expensive Lower doses effective for 'selective intestinal decontamination' Doses >10 mg/kg needed to achieve tissue levels effective against *Pseudomonas* spp. Increased inappetence and vomiting at higher doses Risk of blindness in cats (uncommon)
Ciprofloxacin	**5-15 mg/kg every 12 hours** 10-30 mg/kg every 24 hours	As for enrofloxacin Smaller tablets with higher strength than enrofloxacin; tablet strength restricts use to dogs
Orbifloxacin	5 mg/kg every 12–24 hours	Expensive Less well evaluated than enrofloxacin or ciprofloxacin
Marbofloxacin	2-4 mg/kg every 12–24 hours	As for orbifloxacin
Difloxacin	5-10 mg/kg every 24 hours (dog)	As for orbifloxacin
β-lactam antibiotics		
Cephalexin	**30 mg/kg every 12 hours**	Expensive No prophylaxis against *Pseudomonas* spp. ?Better bioavailability of capsule formulation compared with tablets
Amoxicillin	10-20 mg/kg every 12 hours	Inexpensive No prophylaxis against *Pseudomonas* spp. Not first choice, but acceptable for cats not tolerating other choices Ampicillin causes diarrhoea more often than does amoxicillin
Amoxicillin-clavulanate	12.5-25 mg/kg every 12 hours	As for amoxicillin Increased activity against *Staphylococcus* spp., *Klebsiella* spp., *Escherichia coli* and *Bacteroides* spp. compared with amoxicillin
Combinations		
Fluoroquinolone + β-lactam antibiotic	As above	Reserved for animals with severe prolonged neutropenia

Figure 8.3: Drug choices for prophylactic oral antimicrobial therapy for the neutropenic dog and cat. Modified from Abrams-Ogg and Kruth (2000). Doses adapted from Allen (1998) and Greene and Watson (1998). Drugs and dosages presented in bold text are those most often used by the author. Use of certain drugs for prophylaxis during neutropenia may represent extra-label usage. Flexible dose labelling specifies once to twice daily use of most fluoroquinolones in dogs and cats depending on the clinical situation. Once daily use of fluoroquinolones in the lower dose range probably results in selective intestinal decontamination, although this has not been established for all drugs. Flexible dosing specifies twice daily use of most fluoroquinolones for treating systemic infections and is more appropriate than once daily use if the goal of antimicrobial prophylaxis is also to provide adequate tissue drug levels to treat incipient bacterial infections. Antifungal prophylaxis, with itraconazole for example, is used in humans but does not seem to be necessary for dogs and cats.

may be substituted and submitted for quantitative culture. Urethral catheterization should be avoided because of the risk of introducing infection. Faecal culture should be considered if the animal has diarrhoea. Thoracic radiographs should be obtained if there are any respiratory signs and may be considered as part of the minimum database. A normal thoracic radiograph, however, does not rule out pneumonia. Culture of tracheal or bronchoalveolar lavage fluid should be performed if there are clinical or radiographic signs of pneumonia. A serum biochemical profile and abdominal imaging should be obtained if there is vomiting, abdominal distension or abdominal pain. All the above tests should be considered for any febrile animal presenting with neutropenia of undetermined cause with no obvious site of infection and for any neutropenic animal that is severely ill.

It is likely that pyrexia or unexplained depression in a neutropenic animal is due to infection. Because untreated infection may be rapidly fatal and because neutropenic animals have died of sepsis despite negative antemortem culture results, the recommendation is to initiate empirical antibiotic therapy while awaiting culture results, and, in most cases, to continue therapy in spite of negative culture results (Hughes et al., 1997). Previous culture results, localizing signs, Gram-stain of body fluid and the antimicrobial susceptibility pattern of a suspected nosocomial pathogen may assist in antimicrobial selection. If there is a history of prophylactic therapy with a fluoroquinolone, a febrile episode is most likely due to a Gram-positive organism.

In most cases the choice of antimicrobial therapy must be empirical. The antibiotics chosen should be bactericidal, have limited marrow toxicity and be active against Gram-negative enteric bacilli, Pseudomonas spp. and Gram-positive cocci. Standard recommended drug doses are employed. A representative selection of antibiotics and doses are presented in Figures 8.4 and 8.5.

Drug	Comment
Combination therapy	
Aminoglycoside + first-generation cephalosporin	Commonly used in veterinary medicine Relatively inexpensive Spectrum may not cover *Pseudomonas* spp. ?Cephalosporin increases risk of aminoglycoside nephrotoxicity
Aminoglycoside + aminopenicillin	Commonly used for treatment of parvoviral infections Relatively inexpensive Spectrum may not cover *Pseudomonas* or *Staphylococcus* spp. Aminopenicillin is more likely to disturb gastrointestinal flora than first-generation cephalosporin Can prevent β-lactamase activity by using ampicillin–sulbactam (parenteral substitute for amoxicillin-clavulanate), but it is expensive
Aminoglycoside + antipseudomonal penicillin or ceftazidime	Not as commonly used in veterinary medicine Expensive Synergy against *Pseudomonas* spp. and Enterobacteriaceae Less activity against Gram-positive organisms Can prevent β-lactamase activity by using ticarcillin–clavulanate or piperacillin-tazobactam
Fluoroquinolone substituted for aminoglycoside in above combinations	May be more expensive than aminoglycoside Combinations more likely to be additive than synergistic Avoids aminoglycoside nephrotoxicity
Combination of two β-lactam antibiotics*	?Resistance more likely to develop Potential for antagonism Avoids aminoglycoside nephrotoxicity ?Prolongation of neutropenia
Monotherapy	
Cephalosporins	
Cefoxitin (second generation [cefamycin])	Substitute for aminoglycoside + aminopenicillin Not effective against *Pseudomonas* spp. Effective against anaerobes More likely to disturb gastrointestinal flora
Ceftazidime (third generation)	Expensive Less activity against Gram-positive organisms than combinations
Carbapenems	
Imipenem–cilastatin	Expensive Active against complete microbial spectrum

Figure 8.4: Drug choices for empirical parenteral antimicrobial therapy for the febrile neutropenic dog and cat. Modified from Abrams-Ogg and Kruth (2000).
For example: first-generation cephalosporin plus antipseudomonal penicillin, first-generation cephalosporin plus third-generation cephalosporin and third-generation cephalosporin + antipseudomonal penicillin.

Antimicrobial agent	Dose
Aminoglycosides	
Netilmycin	2–3 mg/kg i.v. tid
	or 6 mg/kg i.v. once daily
Amikacin	5–10 mg/kg i.v., i.m., s.c. tid
	or 15–20 mg/kg i.v., i.m., s.c. once daily
Tobramycin	2 mg/kg i.v., i.m., s.c. tid
	or 6 mg/kg i.v., i.m., s.c. once daily
Gentamicin	2–3 mg/kg i.v., i.m., s.c. tid
	or 6–10 mg/kg i.v., i.m., s.c. once daily
Comment: these drugs are listed in order of increasing nephrotoxicity. To reduce the risks of nephrotoxicity due to aminoglycoside antibiotics: use doses at the lower end of the dose range, use once daily administration, avoid their use in dehydrated animals and avoid their use in animals receiving frusemide.	
Cephalosporins	
Cephazolin	20–30 mg/kg i.v., i.m., tid–qid
Cephalothin	25–40 mg/kg i.v., i.m., tid–qid
Cefoxitin	20–30 mg/kg i.v., i.m., s.c. tid–qid
Ceftazidime	25–30 mg/kg i.v., i.m., s.c. tid–qid or
	4.4 mg/kg i.v. loading dose, followed by 4.1 mg/kg/h i.v. (constant rate infusion) (Moore *et al.*, 1999)
Comment: the author initially uses these cephalosporins at 30 mg/kg i.v. tid	
Fluoroquinolones	
Ciprofloxacin	5–10 mg/kg i.v.(1-hour infusion) once to twice daily
Enrofloxacin	5–10 mg/kg i.v., i.m. once to twice daily
Comment: the author initially uses enrofloxacin at 5 mg/kg i.v. twice daily in dogs and once daily in cats. The 10 mg/kg bid dose is only used if *Pseudomonas* spp. are isolated or suspected. Enrofloxacin is approved for i.m. use only, but the solution is irritating to tissues and the author prefers i.v. administration. For i.v. injection, the solution should be injected over 20–60 mins; it may be diluted (1 part parenteral solution with 9 parts sterile water for injection) if desired. The parenteral solution should not be given s.c. It may be necessary to reduce the dose and/or dosing interval in animals at risk for seizures.	
The author has given enrofloxacin intravenously to cats without adverse effects. However, the injectable solution is not approved for use in cats, and there are anecdotal reports of acute loss of vision following s.c. injection and acute death following i.v. injection in cats.	
Aminopenicillins	
Ampicillin	20–40 mg/kg i.v., i.m., s.c. tid–qid
Ampicillin–sulbactam	20–50 mg/kg i.v., i.m. tid–qid
Antipseudomonal penicillins	
Piperacillin	25–50 mg/kg i.v., i.m. tid–qid
Piperacillin–tazobactam	25–50 mg/kg i.v., i.m. tid–qid
Ticarcillin	40–75 mg/kg i.v., i.m. tid–qid
Ticarcillin–clavulanate	30–50 mg/kg i.v., i.m. tid–qid
Carbapenems	
Imipenem–cilastatin	2–10 mg/kg i.v. (1-hour infusion), i.m. (reconstitute with 1% lignocaine without adrenaline) tid–qid
Comment: the author initially uses 5 mg/kg i.v. tid	

Figure 8.5: *Drug doses for empirical parenteral antimicrobial therapy for the febrile neutropenic dog and cat. Modified from Abrams-Ogg and Kruth (2000). Doses adapted from Allen (1998) and Greene and Watson (1998). Optimal doses in recommended dose ranges are not known. Intravenous routes of administration are preferred. All intravenous injections are given over 15–20 minutes unless otherwise indicated.*

Combination therapy has historically been preferred over monotherapy to increase the antibacterial spectrum, take advantage of additive and synergistic effects while minimizing toxicity and to reduce the development of resistance. Most approaches have combined an aminoglycoside antibiotic with a β-lactam antibiotic, although other approaches have also been developed to avoid aminoglycoside nephrotoxicity and to improve efficacy. When fluoroquinolones are used it should be noted that they seem to have a limited activity against Gram-positive organisms in neutropenic patients. For infections complicating the episodes of neutropenia most commonly encountered by veterinarians, the various protocols are probably of equivalent efficacy. The author currently uses enrofloxacin plus cephazolin in cancer patients, ampicillin plus gentamicin or cefoxitin alone in animals with parvoviral diseases and imipenem–cilastatin for initial therapy in animals with overwhelming sepsis associated with severe neutropenia of undetermined cause.

The intravenous route of antibiotic administration is preferred. Intravenous catheterization is preferable to repetitive venepuncture for drug injection and is often necessary for fluid therapy. However, there must be strict adherence to asepsis during catheter placement and use (Figure 8.6). Although a conventional recommendation is that intravenous catheters should be changed every 2–3 days, longer dwell times are possible with proper catheter care (Mathews *et al.*, 1996). The catheter should definitely be changed if there are signs of phlebitis or infection of the insertion site. If duration of catheterization is anticipated to be more than a few days or if frequent blood sampling is necessary, a jugular catheter is preferred.

Drug toxicity should be considered. Animals receiving aminoglycosides should be monitored for evidence of nephrotoxicity such as casts in the urine, glucosuria and azotaemia, especially when the duration of therapy is longer than 5 days. Fluoroquinolones should be avoided in immature animals because of the possibility of inducing cartilage defects. Fluoroquinolones may cause seizures and other neurological signs in geriatric animals, animals with hypoalbuminaemia and animals with a history of seizures. Numerous antibiotics inhibit platelet function (Catalfamo and Dodds, 1988). This effect is most important with penicillins, and an animal so treated should be observed for haemorrhage if there is concurrent thrombocytopenia, especially if the platelet count is less than $20 \times 10^9/l$. Fluoroquinolones have minimal effect on platelet function, and cephazolin does not alter platelet function in normal dogs (Wilkens *et al.*, 1995).

After starting antibiotic therapy, reduction of fever is expected within 72 hours and the animal should appear more alert. Increased depression accompanying a decreasing temperature may be a sign of impending septic shock. Therapy should continue for 1–7 days after the animal's neutrophil count increases to more than $1.0–2.0 \times 10^9/l$ and fever resolves. If the fever has resolved but prolonged neutropenia is anticipated, then consideration may be given to changing to oral therapy with the same agents as used for antimicrobial prophylaxis (see Figure 8.3).

Pyrexia may not resolve promptly if:

- It is not bacterial in origin (and this should be reconsidered)
- The organism is not sensitive to the antimicrobial agents
- Drug doses are too low (uncommon)
- Host defences are so severely compromised that the infection and associated fever will not resolve with any antimicrobial agent until defences are repaired.

Initial culture results may assist therapeutic decision making with unresponsive fever. If a resistant organism is documented, antimicrobial therapy may be changed on the basis of susceptibility testing. However, the organism involved may be reported as sensitive to the current medication, or an infectious cause of the fever may not be documented, in which case another empirical judgement will be necessary. If the animal is clinically stable the current medication may be continued until the fever resolves and the neutrophil count improves as previously discussed. This situation is encountered occasionally in treating parvoviral infections. If the animal's clinical status is deteriorating, however, new antimicrobial agents should be employed. In most cases it is preferable to use new drugs in addition to, rather than as a substitute for, existing therapy. The choice of additional drugs depends on which antibiotics were used for initial therapy. Failure of response to empirical therapy with cefoxitin or an aminoglycoside plus a first-generation cephalosporin would prompt additional therapy against *Pseudomonas* spp. with ticarcillin, piperacillin, ceftazidime or imipenem–cilastatin. If a resistant Gram-negative enteric organism is suspected (e.g. with signs of intestinal injury or pneumonia), choices for additional therapy include an aminoglycoside, fluoroquinolone, second- or third-generation cephalosporin and imipenem–cilastatin. If a resistant Gram-positive cutaneous organism is suspected (e.g. with catheter-associated phlebitis or pneumonia), the animal should be treated with clindamycin 10 mg/kg i.v., i.m. or s.c. bid. Vancomycin and teicoplanin are the drugs of choice for resistant Gram-positive infections in humans, but there is limited veterinary experience with these drugs. The recommended dose for vancomycin in the dog and cat is 15 mg/kg i.v. tid. A non-responding fever may also be due to infection with an anaerobic organism. Additional therapy could include metronidazole (10–15 mg/kg i.v., 1-hour infusion, tid), clindamycin, cefoxitin or imipenem–cilastatin.

1. The hair over and surrounding the venepuncture site is liberally clipped, including the clipping of long hairs in the vicinity of the site that could contaminate the catheter.
2. The operator's hands are thoroughly washed.
3. The skin over and surrounding the venepuncture site is surgically prepared.
4. A sterile gauze square, or alternatively a gauze square soaked in the solution used for final skin preparation with the excess solution squeezed out, is placed immediately distal to the venepuncture site. This gauze square protects the needle and catheter from skin contamination during venepuncture (a).

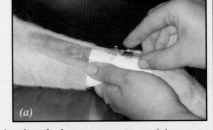

5. If it is necessary to palpate the venepuncture site, the operator's fingers are cleansed with the final skin preparation solution before palpation and the venepuncture site is similarly cleansed after palpation.
6. After catheter insertion, an injection cap is locked on to the catheter hub.
7. The catheter is secured by placing the end of a strip of half-inch wide tape, adhesive side up, under the wings of the catheter, and then folding the tape over the catheter and wrapping it around the leg.
8. The catheter is flushed with 3 ml heparinized saline (1 IU heparin/ml saline).
9. Povidone–iodine ointment is applied to the catheter insertion site, which is then covered with a sterile plaster or similar adhesive bandage as illustrated (b).

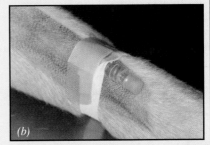

10. The centre of a second strip of half-inch wide tape, adhesive side down, is placed under the hub of the catheter.
11. The ends of the tape are wrapped around the leg while applying traction in a proximal direction, criss-crossing under the leg and coming up over the plaster and/or catheter hub – this prevents distal migration of the catheter.
12. A strip of one-inch tape is wrapped around the leg, covering the plaster and catheter hub.
13. A second strip of one-inch tape is placed under the hub of the catheter and wrapped around the leg in a similar fashion to the second strip of half-inch tape, covering the plaster. Additional strips of one-inch tape may be wrapped around the catheter and leg to provide extra security.
14. The leg is bandaged from the toes to a level above the catheter insertion site, with gauze wrap and self-adherent wrap. The wraps are passed underneath and over the catheter hub to expose the hub and provide additional security.
15. The leg is palpated two to three times a day over, above and below the insertion site. The bandage should be changed a minimum of every 4 days, or sooner if it is wet, soiled or displaced distally, if there is pain or swelling on palpation of the leg, if there is pain on injection through the catheter, or if the animal is more depressed or has a worsening fever.
16. When the bandage is changed the insertion site and leg should be examined for signs of inflammation. The catheter should be removed if such signs are present. If there is no indication for catheter removal and the catheter is left in place, the insertion site should be gently cleansed with 3% hydrogen peroxide and then 10% povidone–iodine solution, and a fresh plaster with povidone–iodine ointment applied.
17. If the animal is not receiving intravenous fluid therapy, the catheter should be flushed with heparinized saline every 4 hours.
18. For intravenous fluid therapy, an extension set with a luer-lock is attached to the catheter hub as illustrated (c), and the intravenous delivery set is attached to the extension set and secured to the outside of the bandage. This technique minimizes disconnection of the intravenous fluid line from the catheter, facilitates recognition that disconnection has occurred and permits changing of the intravenous fluid line without changing the bandage.
19. Injection ports should be cleaned with alcohol and allowed to dry before injection, as illustrated.

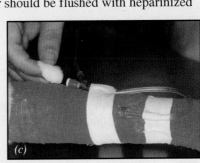

20. The intravenous fluid line should be changed a minimum of every 3 days because damaged injection ports are a potential portal of entry for bacteria, or whenever blood has permanently backed-up into the line.

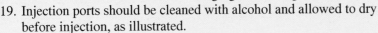

Figure 8.6: *Aseptic placement and use of an over-the-needle catheter in the cephalic vein (Mathews et al., 1996). A polyurethane catheter is recommended.*

Although imipenem–cilastatin is expensive, it is less expensive than triple coverage with enrofloxacin, cephazolin and metronidazole and may therefore be substituted for the latter. If initial therapy is with enrofloxacin plus cephazolin, the author currently intensifies therapy with ceftazidime or metronidazole or changes to imipenem–cilastatin.

The preceding recommendations are appropriate for most cases but may not be feasible due to cost restrictions or inability of the owner to return the animal to the hospital. In such cases, initial therapy with oral antimicrobial therapy may be warranted. In addition, oral antimicrobial agents may be sufficient for initial treatment of neutropenic animals that have been febrile and clinically stable for several days. A fluoroquinolone plus a first-generation cephalosporin or aminopenicillin will provide broad-spectrum antibacterial activity similar to the injectable combinations discussed previously and is recommended for oral therapy in animals with moderate to severe neutropenia. For clinically stable animals with mild neutropenia and mild pyrexia, treatment as described in Figure 8.3 may suffice. Treatment for *Ehrlichia canis* infection with oral tetracyclines may also control infection secondary to neutropenia. Doxycycline is preferred when a dog with ehrlichiosis is neutropenic as it causes less disturbance of intestinal colonization resistance than do tetracycline and oxytetracycline. In all cases the animal should be closely observed for deterioration, and arrangements made to initiate parenteral therapy. Oral antimicrobial therapy is not appropriate when the animal is dehydrated or vomiting, or when there is disruption of the intestinal mucosa.

Empirical antifungal therapy is used in humans but is not recommended in the dog or cat unless a fungal infection is documented. If neutropenia and antibacterial therapy persist beyond 10 days, then faeces should be monitored by cytology or culture for *Candida* spp. overgrowth, especially if antibacterial agents are being used that disturb intestinal flora (e.g. amoxicillin, cefoxitin, metronidazole).

Treatment of documented infections
Treatment of documented bacterial infections should consist of bactericidal antibiotics, probably initially in combination, with the choices based upon susceptibility testing. Initial therapy should be parenteral in most cases, and a change to oral therapy may be considered if the animal is stable and the infection is responding. Treatment of bacteraemia without evidence of other organ involvement should continue for 1 to 7 days after the animal's neutrophil count increases above 1.0–2.0 x 10^9/l and fever resolves. Treatment of pneumonia and urinary tract and soft tissue infections should continue for at least 7 days after the animal's neutrophil count increases above 1.0–2.0 x 10^9/l and clinical and radiographic signs resolve. Pneumonia is

typically treated for at least 6 weeks. The infection may transiently seem to become worse as the neutrophil count increases, but fever should be decreasing if antimicrobial therapy is appropriate.

Amphotericin B is the drug of choice for aspergillosis. Amphotericin B can also be used to treat systemic candidiasis, but treatment with ketoconazole or itraconazole therapy may be sufficient (Weber *et al.,* 1985). Intestinal candidiasis can be treated with nystatin, ketoconazole or itraconazole, whereas fluconazole is the drug of choice for urinary candidiasis.

GRANULOCYTE TRANSFUSIONS

Neutrophils normally have short circulating and tissue residence times. These times are further reduced in sepsis, and any transfused neutrophils are rapidly consumed. However, even a transient increase in total body neutrophil numbers above a critical level may permit survival in some cases of severe sepsis. Neutrophils are usually transfused in humans by using granulocyte concentrates. Donors are treated with granulocyte colony-stimulating factor (see Haematopoietic cytokine therapy) with or without corticosteroids to increase blood neutrophil levels, and then neutrophils are collected by leucapheresis. Neutrophils may also be transfused via exchange transfusion.

Neutrophil transfusion in humans is most beneficial in the treatment of severe prolonged neutropenia and in neonatal sepsis. Granulocyte transfusion has been largely unexplored in small animal medicine because of the expense of treating such cases and technical difficulties, although dogs have been transfused in research facilities (Christensen *et al.,* 1982; Weiss, 1991). Large volumes of blood must be processed to procure sufficient neutrophils to treat a mature animal. Furthermore, granulocyte crossmatching is necessary to minimize loss of effectiveness from alloimmunization during long-term transfusion support, and irradiation of granulocyte concentrate is recommended to minimize transfusion-associated graft-versus-host disease in patients with severe immunosuppression. However, preparation of granulocyte concentrates for short-term transfusion support of septic puppies and kittens is feasible in some veterinary clinics. For dogs, 6% hetastarch is added in a 1:8 ratio to a unit of fresh whole blood to promote red cell sedimentation. The bag is stored vertically at room temperature for 1 hour, at which point the plasma and buffy coat are expressed into a satellite bag, which is then centrifuged at 5000 *g* for 5 minutes at room temperature (see Chapter 15). The supernatant plasma is expressed, leaving the granulocytes in 20 ml of plasma. For cats, the collecting syringe containing a unit of fresh blood is stored vertically at room temperature for 1 hour. The plasma is expressed into a storage bag followed by expression of the buffy coat into a second storage bag or syringe. The resulting granulocyte concentrates may be stored at room temperature for 8 hours. The dose is 1 x 10^9 granulocytes/kg in a volume of 15 ml/kg i.v. once to twice daily. The volume of fresh whole blood needed to provide the neutrophils may be calculated by using the formula:

Volume of donor blood (l) =

$$\frac{\text{Recipient weight (kg) x granulocyte dose } (1 \times 10^9 \text{granulocytes/kg})}{\text{Donor neutrophil count } (x\ 10^9 \text{ granulocytes/l}) \times 0.75}$$

In this formula 0.75 represents the proportion of granulocytes in the unit of fresh whole blood that will be extracted. The transfusion is given through a standard 170 µm filter over 1 to 2 hours. The most likely transfusion reaction is a fever.

If granulocyte concentrate transfusion for a septic neonate is not feasible, fresh whole blood transfusion (22 ml/kg) should be considered, as this is anecdotally beneficial in treating severe parvovirus infection in kittens (Kowall, 1974). This benefit may be in part owing to transfused neutrophils.

HAEMATOPOIETIC CYTOKINE THERAPY

Recombinant human granulocyte colony-stimulating factor (rHuG-CSF) or filgrastim (Neupogen, Amgen) and recombinant human granulocyte–macrophage colony-stimulating factor (rHuGM-CSF) or sargramostim (Leukine, Immunex) stimulate granulocyte progenitor cells and mature neutrophils, thereby enhancing neutrophil production, differentiation, marrow release and function. The rHuGM-CSF also has several effects on macrophages and other haematopoietic cells. The drugs are most useful in humans when given prophylactically after cytotoxic chemotherapy and large field irradiation to reduce the duration and severity of neutropenia. They are less useful in established neutropenia due to cytotoxic therapy with or without secondary infection, because progenitor cells may be exhausted and/or endogenous cytokine levels are already increased. They are of limited utility in aplastic anaemia (immune-mediated pancytopenia) as endogenous cytokine levels are often markedly increased. Utility of cytokine therapy with neutropenia due to a drug reaction varies with the mechanism of toxicosis. Cytokine therapy reduces severity of cyclic neutropenia and certain other idiopathic neutropenic conditions and may be beneficial in humans with acquired immunodeficiency syndrome. Prophylactic cytokine therapy is beneficial in experimental models of overwhelming sepsis, but the role of cytokine therapy in established sepsis is not clear – it is potentially beneficial, of no benefit or detrimental

depending on circumstances. Prophylactic therapy and therapy of established neonatal sepsis are also being investigated. Side effects of rHuG-CSF and rHuGM-CSF in humans include bone pain and rarely side effects from overproduction of neutrophils. Side effects of rHuGM-CSF also include influenza-like syndromes and capillary leak syndrome.

Recombinant canine G-CSF and GM-CSF have been produced but are not commercially available. However, rHuG-CSF has been given to dogs and cats. The drug is a potent stimulator of granulopoiesis, but the effect is transient in normal animals because of neutralizing antibody formation. Increased neutrophil counts begin to decline after 17–23 days of rHuG-CSF treatment, and neutropenia will occur if treatment is continued (Fulton et al., 1991; Hammond et al., 1991). Veterinarians have successfully used rHuG-CSF to ameliorate myelosuppression in dogs and cats receiving anticancer chemotherapy. Typically the drug is given at a dose of 5 µg/kg s.c. once daily to febrile neutropenic animals or prophylactically when the neutrophil count decreases below 0.5–1.0 x 10^9/l, and is continued until the neutrophil count increases above 1.0–2.0 x 10^9/l. (Neupogen is supplied as a 300 µg/ml preservative-free solution in a single-use vial. Because of the cost of the product, veterinarians typically use the vial for multiple doses. It is essential that the vial be penetrated aseptically and stored under refrigeration. To facilitate small dose measurements, it has been recommended to dilute rHuG-CSF to a concentration of 100 µg/ml in a 5% dextrose solution that contains 1% autologous patient serum that has been heat-inactivated in a 56°C water bath for 30 minutes. The diluted rHuG-CSF is stored under refrigeration for four weeks (Henry et al., 1998).) The short courses of therapy and possibly concurrent immunosuppression from cytotoxic chemotherapy reduce the antibody effect and permit repeated use (Henry et al., 1995).

Prophylactic use of rHuG-CSF beginning 5 days after a chemotherapy treatment has also been used (Henry et al., 1998). This is later than is typically used in humans, where rHuG-CSF is given 1 to 2 days after chemotherapy. The drug should not be given within 24 hours before or after chemotherapy as this will increase cytotoxic progenitor cell injury. When rHuG-CSF is used, stimulation of granulopoiesis can result in a left shift and toxic changes in the neutrophils that may be confused with a response to infection. Side effects other than antibody formation are minimal. The use of rHuG-CSF is expensive and the cost benefit compared with the risk of developing and cost of treating sepsis in dogs and cats is not known. Similarly, although the use of rHuG-CSF prevents dose reduction and may permit dose escalation of anticancer drugs in dogs and cats, the benefits on improved tumour control and patient survival are not known.

The use of rHuG-CSF for treating parvoviral infections in dogs and cats has also been recommended. In one study, treatment of dogs with 5 µg/kg bid–tid increased neutrophil counts (Kraft and Kuffer, 1995), whereas in another study treatment of dogs with 5 µg/kg once daily did not, nor did it affect survival or duration of hospitalization (Rewerts *et al.*, 1998). In the former study there was no apparent benefit to cats. The use of rHuG-CSF may be of limited utility in parvoviral infections because of increased endogenous cytokine levels, viral replication in stimulated progenitor cells or exhaustion of progenitor cells and mature neutrophils at the time of treatment (Cohn *et al.*, 1999; London, 2000). Therapy with rHuG-CSF has been reportedly or anecdotally beneficial with myelosuppression due to oestrogen and phenobarbital toxicosis in dogs and griseofulvin toxicosis in cats. The role of rHuG-CSF therapy for neutropenia due to FeLV and FIV infections has yet to be defined.

Dogs have also been treated with rHuGM-CSF. Stimulation of granulopoiesis is less compared with rHuG-CSF. Given the lower efficacy and greater potential for side effects, the use of rHuGM-CSF is in general not recommended for the treatment of neutropenia in dogs and cats.

REMOVAL OF THE FOCUS OF INFECTION

Excision or debridement of the site of infection should be considered in animals with neutropenia due to overwhelming sepsis or in animals with primary neutropenia where a secondary infection has localized in soft tissue and is not responding to antimicrobial therapy alone. Other therapeutic strategies in the management of sepsis have recently been reviewed (Hardie, 2000).

REFERENCES AND FURTHER READING

Abrams-Ogg ACG and Kruth SA (2000) Infections associated with neutropenia in the dog and cat. In: *Antimicrobial Therapy in Veterinary Medicine, 3ʳᵈ edn*, ed. J Prescott and D Baggot. Iowa State University Press, Ames

Allen DG (1998) *Handbook of Veterinary Drugs, 2ⁿᵈ edn*. Lippincott-Raven, Philadelphia

Anderson PG and Pidgeon G (1987) Candidiasis in a dog with parvoviral enteritis. *Journal of the American Animal Hospital Association* **23,** 27–30

Catalfamo JL and Dodds WJ (1988) Hereditary and acquired thrombopathias. *Veterinary Clinics of North America: Small Animal Practice* **18,** 185–194

Christensen RD, Anstall HB and Rothstein G (1982) Use of whole blood exchange transfusion to supply neutrophils to septic, neutropenic neonates. *Transfusion* **22,** 504–506

Cohn LA, Rewerts JM, McCaw DL, Boon GD, Wagner-Mann C and Lothrop CD (1999) Plasma granulocyte colony-stimulating factor concentrations in neutropenic, parvoviral enteritis-infected puppies. *Journal of Veterinary Internal Medicine* **13,** 581–586

Couto CG (1990) Management of complications of cancer chemotherapy. *Veterinary Clinics of North America: Small Animal Practice* **20,** 1037–1053

Dow SW, Curtis CR, Jones RL and Wingfield WE (1989) Bacterial culture of blood from critically ill dogs and cats. *Journal of the American Veterinary Medical Association* **195,** 113–117

Feld R (1989) The compromised host. *European Journal of Cancer and Clinical Oncology* **25(Suppl 2),** S1–S7

Fulton R, Gasper PW, Ogilvie GK, Boone TC, and Dornsife RE (1991) Effect of recombinant human granulocyte colony-stimulating factor on hematopoiesis in normal cats. *Experimental Hematology* **19,** 759–767

Greene CE and Watson ADJ (1998) Antimicrobial drug formulary. In: *Infectious Diseases of the Dog and Cat, 2ⁿᵈ edn*, ed. CE Greene, pp. 790–919. WB Saunders, Philadelphia

Hammond WP, Csiba E, Canin A, Hockman H, Souza LM, Layton JE and DC Dale (1991) Chronic neutropenia: a new canine model induced by human granulocyte colony-stimulating factor. *Journal of Clinical Investigation* **87,** 704–710

Hardie EM (2000) Therapeutic management of sepsis. In: *Kirk's Current Veterinary Therapy XIII Small Animal Practice,* ed. JD Bonagura, pp. 272–275. WB Saunders, Philadelphia

Henry CJ, Buss MS and Lothrop CD (1998) Veterinary uses of recombinant human granulocyte colony-stimulating factor. Part I. Oncology. *Compendium on Continuing Education for the Practising Veterinarian* **20,** 728–734

Henry CJ, Lothrop CD and Goodman S (1995) Dogs receiving mitoxantrone and cyclophosphamide do not produce clinically significant antibody titers to rhG-CSF. *Proceedings of the 13ᵗʰ Annual Veterinary Medical Forum of the American College of Veterinary Internal Medicine* p. 1020

Hughes WT, Armstrong D, Bodey GP, Brown AE, Edwards JE, Feld R, Pizzo P, Rolston KV, Shenep JL and Young LS (1997) 1997 guidelines for the use of antimicrobial agents in neutropenic patients with unexplained fever. *Clinical Infectious Diseases* **25,** 551–573

Kowall NL (1974) Feline panleukopenia. In: *Current Veterinary Therapy V Small Animal Practice,* ed. RW Kirk, pp. 957–959. WB Saunders, Philadelphia

Kraft W and Kuffer M (1995) Behandlung schwerer neutropenien bei hund und katze mit filgrastim. *Tierarztliche Praxis* **23,** 609–613

Kunkle GA, Sundlof S and Keisling K (1995) Adverse effects of oral antibacterial therapy in dogs and cats: an epidemiologic study of pet owners' observations. *Journal of the American Animal Hospital Association* **31,** 46–55

London C (2000) Hematopoietic cytokines: the myelopoietic factors. In: *Kirk's Current Veterinary Therapy XIII Small Animal Practice,* ed. JD Bonagura, pp 403–408. WB Saunders, Philadelphia

Mathews KA, Brooks MJ and Valliant AE (1996) A prospective study of intravenous catheter contamination. *Journal of Veterinary Emergency Medicine and Critical Care* **6,** 33–43

Moore K, Lautzenhiser S, Fialkowski J and Rosin E (1999) Continuous infusion versus subcutaneous administration of ceftazidime in the treatment of *Pseudomonas aeruginosa* infection in dogs. *Journal of Veterinary Internal Medicine* **13,** 237

Ogilvie GK and Moore AS (1995) *Managing the Veterinary Cancer Patient.* pp. 149–155. Veterinary Learning Systems, Trenton

Reller LB (1994) What the practicing physician should know about blood cultures. In: *Blood Culture Controversies – Revisited,* ed. F Koontz, pp. 1–8. ASM Audioconference, Iowa City

Rewerts JM, McCaw DL, Cohn LA, Wagner-Mann C and Harrington D (1998) Recombinant human granulocyte colony-stimulating factor for treatment of puppies with neutropenia secondary to parvovirus infection. *Journal of the American Veterinary Medical Association* **213,** 991–992

Rosenthal RC (1988) Autologous bone marrow transplantation for lymphoma. *Proceedings of the 6ᵗʰ Annual Veterinary Medical Forum of the American College of Veterinary Internal Medicine* pp. 397–399

Rubin RH and Young LS (1994) *Clinical Approach to Infection in the Compromised Host, 3ʳᵈ ed,* ed. RH Rubin and LS Young. Plenum, New York

Turk J, Fales W, Miller M, Pace L, Fischer J, Johnson G, Kreeger J, Turnquist S, Pittman L, Rottinghaus A and Gosser H (1992) Enteric *Clostridium perfringens* infection associated with parvoviral enteritis in dogs: 74 cases (1987–1990). *Journal of the American Veterinary Medical Association* **200,** 991–994

Turk J, Miller M, Brown T, Fales W, Fischer J, Gosser H, Nelson S, Shaw D and Solorzano R (1990) Coliform septicemia and pulmonary disease associated with canine parvoviral enteritis: 88 cases (1987–1988). *Journal of the American Veterinary Medical Association* **196,** 771–773

Wade JC (1994) Epidemiology and prevention of infection in the compromised host. In: *Clinical Approach to Infection in the Compromised Host, 3rd edn,* ed. RH Rubin and LS Young, pp. 5–31. Plenum, New York

Weber MJ, Keppen M, Gawith KE and Epstein RB (1985) Treatment of systemic candidiasis in neutropenic dogs with ketoconazole. *Experimental Hematology* **13,** 791–795

Weiss DJ (1991) White cells. In: *Advances in Veterinary Science and Comparative Medicine, Vol 36: Comparative Transfusion Medicine,* ed. SM Cotter, pp. 57–86. Academic Press, San Diego

Weiss DJ (1995) Leukocyte disorders and their treatment. In: *Kirk's Current Veterinary Therapy XII Small Animal Practice,* ed. JD Bonagura, pp. 452–457. WB Saunders, Philadelphia

Wilkens B, Sullivan P, McDonald TP and Krahwinkel DJ (1995) Effects of cephalothin, cefazolin, and cefmetazole on the hemostatic mechanism in normal dogs: implications for the surgical patient. *Veterinary Surgery* **24,** 25

(ii) Eosinophilia

Krystyna Grodecki

INTRODUCTION

In normal dogs and cats, only a small percentage of the white blood cell differential is comprised of eosinophils. The bone marrow is the site of eosinophil production, maturation and storage. Activated T lymphocytes and macrophages produce various cytokines (e.g. interleukin-5), which control the production of eosinophils (McEwen, 1992; Jain, 1993). The total bone marrow transit time for eosinophils is about 3 days in humans (Latimer, 1995) and 5.5 days in rats (McEwen, 1992), although eosinophil production and release has been shown to be faster in parasitized rats (McEwen, 1992). The bone marrow transit times in the dog and cat are not known. The half-life of eosinophils in the circulation in humans ranges from 2 to 12 hours (Latimer, 1995) and is presumed to be similar in dogs and cats (Latimer and Rakich, 1989). A marginal pool of eosinophils is also present. Eosinophils enter tissues randomly and may function there for several days, after which they are removed by the mononuclear phagocytic system, degenerate within tissues or are lost via epithelial transmigration (McEwen, 1992). They do not usually re-enter the blood (Jain, 1993). Eosinophils are essentially tissue cells and are found in high numbers (relative to numbers in the circulation) in subepithelial sites in the skin and respiratory, gastrointestinal and urogenital tracts. Diseases of these tissues are more likely to be associated with tissue eosinophilia with or without blood eosinophilia than are diseases of other tissues. The fact that these tissues interact with an environment with constant antigenic exposure and that they contain large numbers of mast cells, may offer a partial explanation for this observation (McEwen, 1992).

Eosinophils are widely known for their parasiticidal abilities; however, they also possess phagocytic and bactericidal capabilities, are mediators of tissue injury and have been incriminated as regulators of allergic (hypersensitivity) and inflammatory responses. Parasiticidal activity occurs via interaction of eosinophils with T and B lymphocytes and mast cells and is enhanced in the presence of antibody and/or complement (Jain, 1993). Eosinophils can phagocytose foreign particles such as bacteria, yeasts, protozoans, mycoplasmata, mast cell granules, immune complexes, antibody-coated red blood cells and inert particles, although the phagocytic as well as bactericidal capabilities of eosinophils are far less effective than those of neutrophils (McEwen, 1992; Jain, 1993). Eosinophils are potent inflammatory cells, which may be present in a variety of inflammatory processes and may induce tissue damage. The role of eosinophils as regulators of allergic and inflammatory responses has not been proved (McEwen, 1992), although evidence exists to suggest this function (McEwen, 1992; Jain, 1993). Eosinophils also take part in coagulation and fibrinolysis (Jain, 1993).

EOSINOPHILIA

Latimer (1995) has defined eosinophilia as an absolute eosinophil count of greater than $0.75 \times 10^9/l$ in the cat and greater than $1.3 \times 10^9/l$ in the dog. Veterinary clinical pathology laboratories often provide haematological reference ranges derived from local animal populations, so these reference ranges are likely to vary regionally.

The fact that eosinophils in the circulation are simply 'in transit' between their site of production and site of function suggests that the number of blood eosinophils is only a crude indicator of the dynamic state of eosinophils (McEwen, 1992). Eosinophilia, therefore, should be considered significant only if persistent and reproducible (McEwen, 1992). It is important to note that localized lesions that contain large numbers of eosinophils (tissue eosinophilia) frequently may not be accompanied by blood eosinophilia (Duncan *et al.*, 1994). Also, animals with eosinophilic disorders may have a blood response that is diminished by a concurrent stress effect mediated by corticosteroids (eosinopenic effect) (Duncan *et al.*, 1994).

Mechanistically, blood eosinophilia may be the result of increased production of eosinophils, increased release from the bone marrow storage compartment, redistribution from the marginal pool or increased intravascular survival (Jain, 1993). Most eosinophilias are due to the first two mechanisms (Jain, 1993).

Eosinophilia is known for its association with parasitism and hypersensitivity, although it has also been associated with many other diverse conditions (Tvedten, 1994). Only a few surveys determining the frequency of conditions associated with eosinophilia in the dog and cat have been conducted. One large retrospective study (Center *et al.*, 1990) of 312 cats (which constituted about 5% of cats having a complete blood count (CBC) performed in this hospital setting) with eosinophilia (defined as an absolute eosinophil count of greater than 1.5 x 10⁹/l) found that eosinophilia was indeed associated with a variety of diagnoses (see Figures 8.7 to 8.9). However, the most common diagnoses (over half of the reported cases) consisted of flea allergy dermatitis (FAD), eosinophilic granuloma complex, asthma, chronic upper respiratory tract inflammation and gastrointestinal disease associated with diarrhoea and endoparasites. One flaw in these data was the fact that some of the cats with these different diagnoses had concomitant flea infestation or endoparasitism and that not all cats had faecal examinations or heartworm tests performed.

Jain (1993) conducted a survey of 72 cats with eosinophilia but did not provide specific diagnoses or information regarding association with parasitism. In this study, 15% of cats with eosinophilia had respiratory disease, 32% had skin disease, 18% had gastrointestinal disease, 17% had suppurative disease and 18% had miscellaneous conditions. Two surveys of eosinophilia in the dog have been reported. In the study described by Jain (1993), of a total of 337 dogs with eosinophilia, 43% had respiratory disease, 8% had skin disease, 8% had miscellaneous conditions, 7% had involvement of the female genital tract, 7% had bone and joint disease, 7% had neurological conditions, 6% had gastrointestinal disease, 4% had urinary tract involvement, 4% had neoplasia, 2% had ocular involvement, 2% had suppurative disease and 2% had cardiac disease. These findings were broadly corroborated in a study of 105 dogs with eosinophilia (Lilliehook *et al.*, 2000) where inflammatory diseases of the gut, skin or lungs comprised 36% of the test population.

Parasitism

Parasitism is the most frequent cause of eosinophilia in the dog and cat (Latimer and Rakich, 1989), although parasitism does not consistently result in eosinophilia (Bush, 1991). Figure 8.7 lists some of the parasites that may be associated with eosinophilia in dogs and cats. The discovery of ectoparasites or endoparasites should not necessarily mark the end of an investigation of eosinophilia, as their presence does not necessarily imply a causative role (Tvedten, 1994). Eosinophilia is more likely to develop when parasites migrate through body tissues, providing prolonged contact between the parasite and host tissue (migrating stages of ascarids, hookworms or heartworms, for example), or attach to or disrupt mucosal surfaces (Center, 1985), whereas parasites living free in the gastrointestinal tract are less likely to stimulate an eosinophilia (Center, 1985; Bush, 1991; Duncan *et al.*, 1994). In the case of migrating larvae, eosinophilia may develop before detection of ova in the faeces, and migrating larvae cannot therefore be completely ruled out as a cause for eosinophilia. Some parasites may not stimulate an eosinophilia until they die and expose previously

Dog	Cat
Angiostrongylus vasorum (Prestwood *et al.*, 1981; Patteson *et al.*, 1993)	*Aelurostrongylus abstrusus* (Center *et al.*, 1990; Hawkins, 1995)
Crenosoma vulpis (Cobb and Fisher, 1992; Peterson *et al.*, 1993; Shaw *et al.*, 1996)	Coccidiosis (Center *et al.*, 1990)
Filaroides hirthi (Hirth and Hottendorf, 1973; Torgerson *et al.*, 1997)	Fleas (Prasse *et al.*, 1987; Center and Randolph, 1991)
Fleas (Latimer, 1995)	Giardiasis (Center *et al.*, 1990)
Oslerus (Filaroides) osleri (Barsanti and Prestwood, 1983; Levitan *et al.*, 1996)	*Ollulanus tricuspis* (Latimer, 1995)
Pneumocystis carinii (Greene and Chandler, 1984; Ramsay *et al.*, 1997)	*Toxocara cati* (Parsons, 1987; Center *et al.*, 1990)
Strongyloides spp. (Gibbons *et al.*, 1988; Duncan *et al.*, 1994)	*Toxocara canis* (Parsons *et al.*, 1989)
Toxocara canis (Parsons, 1987)	Toxoplasmosis (Center *et al.*, 1990)
Trichuris vulpis (Hendrix *et al.*, 1987; Leib and Matz, 1995)	Trombiculid mites (Latimer, 1995)
Uncinaria stenocephala (Bowman, 1992)	

Figure 8.7: *Parasites that may be associated with eosinophilia in the dog and cat in the United Kingdom. Parasites associated with eosinophilia but not indigenous to the United Kingdom include: in the dog,* Ancylostoma *spp. (Burrows* et al.*, 1995), Dipetalonema reconditum (Rawlings and Calvert, 1995), Dirofilaria immitis (Rawlings and Calvert, 1995), Hepatozoon canis (Craig, 1984), Heterobilharzia americana (Slaughter* et al.*, 1988), Paragonimus kellicotti (Hawkins, 1995), Spirocerca lupi (Latimer, 1995), Trichinella spiralis (Campbell, 1991); in the cat,* Ancylostoma *spp. (Bush, 1991), Dirofilaria immitis (Rawlings and Calvert, 1995), Paragonimus kellicotti (Hawkins, 1995), Platynosomum concinnum (Hitt, 1997), Strongyloides* spp. *(Duncan* et al.*, 1994), Trichinella spiralis (Burrows* et al.*, 1995).*

unexposed antigens (Tvedten, 1994). Ectoparasites such as fleas and ticks may promote eosinophilia (Latimer and Rakich, 1989). Center and Randolph (1991) observed that cats with a 'generous' flea infestation, in the absence of obvious dermal hypersensitivity, developed eosinophilia of up to 7.0 x 10^9/l. The same authors also observed ear mite infestations associated with eosinophilia, which resolved with miticidal treatment.

Hypersensitivity and inflammation

Figure 8.8 lists hypersensitivity and inflammatory conditions that may be associated with eosinophilia in the dog and cat. As with parasitic infections these conditions do not invariably result in eosinophilia.

In the study by Center *et al.* (1990), cats with flea allergy dermatitis comprised the largest proportion (20.5%) of cats with eosinophilia (range 1.5-23.5 x

10^9/l). Cats with either FAD or eosinophilic granuloma complex (range 1.5-46.2 x 10^9/l) had the highest median eosinophil counts (3.3 x 10^9/l for both). Eosinophilic plaque was most commonly associated with eosinophilia and was associated with the highest eosinophil counts of all cats with the eosinophilic granuloma complex. Eosinophilia has been associated with atopy and food hypersensitivity in the cat (Center *et al.*, 1990; Roudebush, 1995; Scott *et al.*, 1995a) whereas in dogs with these conditions, eosinophilia is rare (Willemse, 1984).

Of respiratory disorders noted in the study by Center *et al.* (1990), the highest eosinophil counts were associated with feline asthma/allergic bronchitis (range 1.6-20.7 x 10^9/l) and septic pneumonia (range 1.6-11.7 x 10^9/l), although cats with pneumonia were believed to have had underlying allergic

Dog	Cat
Alimentary tract	
Oral eosinophilic granuloma (Madewell *et al.,* 1980) Eosinophilic gastritis/enteritis/colitis (Johnson, 1992; Burrows *et al.*, 1995; Leib and Matz, 1995) Gastrointestinal eosinophilic granuloma (Burrows *et al,.* 1995; Leib and Matz, 1995)	Eosinophilic enteritis (Leib and Matz, 1995; Guilford, 1996) Lymphoplasmacytic gastroenteritis (Dennis *et al.*, 1992; Hart *et al.*, 1994)
Genitourinary tract	
Pyometra (Latimer, 1995)	Pyometra (Prasse *et al.*, 1987; Center *et al.*, 1990) Lower urinary tract disease (Center *et al.*, 1990)
Musculoskeletal system	
Eosinophilic myositis/atrophic myositis/masticatory muscle myositis (Smith, 1989; Gilmour *et al.*, 1992) Panosteitis/endostosis (Johnson *et al.*, 1995)	
Respiratory tract	
Pulmonary infiltrates with eosinophils (Calvert, 1987; Taboada, 1991) Pulmonary eosinophilic granuloma (Taboada, 1991)	Allergic bronchitis/asthma (Center *et al.*, 1990; Hawkins, 1995) Chronic upper respiratory tract inflammation (Center *et al.*, 1990)
Skin	
Eosinophilic granuloma (Scott *et al.*, 1995b) Flea allergy dermatitis (Scott *et al.*, 1995a) Sterile eosinophilic pustulosis (Scott *et al.*, 1995b)	Eosinophilic granuloma complex (Center *et al.*, 1990; Scott *et al.*, 1995b) Flea allergy dermatitis (Center *et al.*, 1990; Scott *et al.*, 1995a) Atopy (Center *et al.*, 1990; Scott *et al.*, 1995a) Food hypersensitivity (Center *et al.*, 1990; Roudebush, 1995)
Other	
	Eosinophilic keratitis (Glaze, 1982; Collins *et al.*, 1986; Carrington *et al.*, 1992) Chronic focal infection or inflammation, e.g. abscess, gingivitis/stomatitis, soft tissue trauma (Center *et al.*, 1990) Steatitis (O'Donnell and Hayes, 1987)

Figure 8.8: Hypersensitivity and inflammatory conditions that may be associated with eosinophilia in the dog and cat. (Modified from Latimer (1995) with permission).

bronchitis. Previous studies (reviewed by Taboada, 1991) documented eosinophilia in 50–75% of cats with asthma, although one study (Corcoron *et al.*, 1995) reported eosinophilia in only 5 of 23 cats with asthma. Mild to moderate eosinophilia associated with chronic inflammation of the upper respiratory tract was an unexpected finding by Center *et al.* (1990). The authors speculated that the presence of eosinophilia may have been a reflection of localization of inflammation to mucous membranes exposed to the environment.

Pulmonary infiltrates with eosinophils (PIE), more commonly seen in dogs than cats, is an all inclusive phrase for any disease process with radiographic evidence of infiltrative lung disease and blood eosinophilia and/or eosinophilic inflammation found on cytological assessment of a transtracheal wash or bronchoalveolar lavage fluid. Blood eosinophilia is not always present in PIE. Underlying causes include environmental allergens, drugs, parasites, bacterial and fungal infections, neoplasia and idiopathic causes. Heartworm infection is the most common cause in endemic areas (Calvert, 1987; Taboada, 1991). Pulmonary eosinophilic granulomatosis, a PIE syndrome, is a rare condition of unknown aetiology, although it has been reported in dogs with heartworm disease (Confer *et al.*, 1983; Calvert, 1987).

Center *et al.* (1990) found that chronic soft tissue inflammation involving a variety of tissues also seemed to cause a mild to moderate eosinophilia in cats, and that cats with lower urinary tract inflammation unexpectedly had eosinophilia of similar magnitude. Pyometra in both dogs and cats has been cited as a cause of eosinophilia by many authors (Prasse *et al.*, 1987; Bush, 1991; Young, 1997), although eosinophilia is not expected to be the primary or only change in the leucogram.

Miscellaneous conditions

Figure 8.9 lists neoplasia-related and miscellaneous conditions associated with eosinophilia. Eosinophilia associated with tumours, hypereosinophilic syndrome and eosinophilic leukaemia is rarely seen, however the magnitude of the eosinophilia may be striking.

Dog	Cat
One case: fibrosarcoma (Couto, 1984)	One case each: basal cell tumour, gastric carcinoma, myxosarcoma, osteosarcoma, pilomatrixoma, renal carcinoma, salivary carcinoma, two poorly defined tumours (Center *et al.*, 1990)
One case: mammary carcinoma (Losco, 1986)	One case each: squamous cell carcinoma, sweat gland adenocarcinoma (Couto, 1985)
	One case: transitional cell carcinoma (Sellon *et al.*, 1992)
Disseminated mast cell neoplasia (Klausner and Perman, 1981; O'Keefe *et al.*, 1987; Pollack *et al.*, 1991)	Mast cell neoplasia; disseminated and visceral (Center *et al.*, 1990; Bortnowski and Rosenthal, 1992; Peaston and Griffey, 1994)
	Lymphoma (Prasse *et al.*, 1987; Center *et al.*, 1990)
Myeloid leukaemia (Latimer, 1995)	Two cases: myeloproliferative disease (Center *et al.*, 1990)
Suspected eosinophilic leukaemia (Moulton and Harvey, 1990; Ndikuwera *et al.*, 1992; Jensen and Nielsen, 1992)	Eosinophilic leukaemia (Swenson *et al.*, 1993; Huibregste and Turner, 1994)
Suspected hypereosinophilic syndrome (Goto *et al.*, 1983; Balmer-Rusca and Hauser, 1993)	Hypereosinophilic syndrome (Hendrick, 1981; Huibregste and Turner, 1994; Plotnick, 1994; Wilson *et al.*, 1996)
Lymphomatoid granulomatosis (Lucke *et al.*, 1979; Postorino *et al.*, 1989; Berry *et al.*, 1990)	Experimental feline leukaemia virus associated-leukaemoid reaction/leukaemia (Lewis *et al.*, 1985)
	?Hyperthyroidism (Center *et al.*, 1990; Thoday and Mooney, 1992)
Hypoadrenocorticism (Hardy, 1995; Peterson *et al.*, 1996)	Hypoadrenocorticism (Peterson *et al.*, 1989; Hardy, 1995)
Experimental rhIL-2 administration (Latimer, (1995)	Experimental rhIL-2 administration (Latimer,1995)
?Oestrus (Schalm *et al.*, 1975)	
German Shepherd Dog (Bush, 1991; Lilliehook, 1997)	Pemphigus foliaceus, cutaneous lupus erythematosus, chronic renal failure, cardiac disorders, panleucopenia, feline infectious peritonitis, immune haemolytic anaemia (Center *et al.*, 1990)
	Methimazole (and potentially carbimazole) therapy (Peterson *et al.*, 1988; Feldman and Nelson, 1996)

Figure 8.9: *Neoplastic and miscellaneous conditions that have been associated with eosinophilia in the dog and cat. (Modified from Latimer (1995) with permission).*

A retrospective study of 16 dogs with systemic (disseminated) mastocytosis documented only two dogs with eosinophilia (O'Keefe *et al.*, 1987). Disseminated mast cell neoplasia was associated with mild to moderate eosinophilia in the study by Center *et al.* (1990). Cutaneous mast cell tumours were not associated with eosinophilia in this study of cats and have not previously been reported to be associated with eosinophilia (Buerger and Scott, 1987). Profound eosinophilia was present in two cats (11.5 and 88.3 x 10^9/l at presentation) with gastrointestinal mast cell tumours (Bortnowski and Rosenthal, 1992). Another case report (Peaston and Griffey, 1994) reported profound eosinophilia (45.6 x 10^9/l) in a cat with a visceral mast cell tumour. Six cats with eosinophilia (range 1.6–3.2 x 10^9/l) in the study by Center *et al.* (1990) had lymphoma, and two cats with alimentary lymphoma in another report had profound eosinophilia (>60 x 10^9/l) (Prasse *et al.*, 1987). In all of these cases (as well as the miscellaneous tumours from the study by Center *et al.* listed in Figure 8ii.3) it is possible that the observed eosinophilia represented a paraneoplastic syndrome, but there was no conclusive proof of this hypothesis.

Hypereosinophilic syndrome (HES) in cats and humans is characterized by a persistent and profound eosinophilia of prolonged duration and unknown aetiology, bone marrow hyperplasia of eosinophil precursors and multiple organ infiltration by mature eosinophils (Huibregste and Turner, 1994). Some authors speculate that eosinophilic enteritis, HES and eosinophilic leukaemia in the cat are parts of a spectrum of the same disease (Hendrick, 1981). HES is a diagnosis of exclusion, and differentiation from eosinophilic leukaemia is controversial. HES has not been adequately documented in the dog (Goto *et al.*, 1983; Balmer-Rusca and Hauser, 1993).

In the few reports of eosinophilic leukaemia in the cat, one cat was naturally infected with feline leukaemia virus (FeLV) (Swenson *et al.*, 1993) and the remainder were negative for FeLV or had not been tested. Only rare cases of suspected eosinophilic leukaemia in the dog have been reported (Moulton and Harvey, 1990; Ndikuwera *et al.*, 1992). Jensen and Neilsen (1992) reported an 'eosinophilic leukaemoid reaction' of unknown aetiology in a dog. Although eosinophilic leukaemia was suspected, the lack of diagnostic criteria for eosinophilic leukaemia in the dog precluded a definitive diagnosis in this case.

The study by Center *et al.* (1990) included three hyperthyroid cats with mild eosinophilia. This was an unexpected finding, particularly as previous reports have stated that 15% of cats with hyperthyroidism exhibit eosinopenia (Feldman and Nelson, 1996). However, a report describing features of 126 hyperthyroid cats in the United Kingdom found that 12 of 57 (21.1%) cats in which a CBC was performed exhibited eosinophilia (Thoday and Mooney, 1992). The authors did not, however, indicate whether other causes of eosinophilia had been ruled out.

Eosinophilia has been reported in 4–30% of dogs with hypoadrenocorticism (Hardy, 1995). Stressed dogs with adequate adrenocortical function usually exhibit a stress leucogram (mature neutrophilia, lymphopenia and eosinopenia) as a result of glucocorticoid action. Eosinophilia or normal numbers of eosinophils in a stressed patient (a reverse 'stress leucogram') suggests the possibility of hypoadrenocorticism. Peterson *et al.* (1996) reported that 56.5% of 225 dogs with hypoadrenocorticism had eosinophil counts within the reference range. Only 1 of 10 cats with primary hypoadrenocorticism exhibited an eosinophilia in one study (Peterson *et al.*, 1989).

Many authors have suggested that oestrus is a cause of eosinophilia in the dog (Schalm *et al.*, 1975; Jain, 1993; Bush, 1991; Young, 1997) but the evidence for this association seems to be purely anecdotal. In the rat, uterine (but not blood) eosinophilia may be induced by oestrogen (Bustos *et al.*, 1995). Oestrogen also causes accumulation of eosinophils in the uterus of other species (mice, cows, hamsters, humans) (Tchernitchin *et al.*, 1989), although to the author's knowledge no similar investigations have been conducted in the dog.

A few authors, including Bush (1991), have noted that some large breed dogs (especially German Shepherd Dogs) exhibit eosinophilia, a finding which has been regarded as a normal breed characteristic. Bush (1991) suggests that there may be a breed predisposition to eosinophilic disorders in the German Shepherd Dog given the higher incidence of eosinophilic enteritis, myositis and panosteitis, and has proposed that the finding of eosinophilia in apparently normal dogs could reflect subclinical disease. Lilliehook (1997) documented significant differences in the numbers of eosinophils in the blood of normal German Shepherd Dogs (mean of 0.85 x 10^9/l) versus normal Beagles (0.36 x 10^9/l). Although this finding may be associated with breed, in an individual animal other causes of eosinophilia should be considered.

APPROACH TO THE INVESTIGATION OF EOSINOPHILIA

Eosinophilia may be detected either on profiles performed on sick animals as part of a diagnostic investigation or on apparently healthy animals undergoing routine health screening. Eosinophilia may or may not be the main or most significant change present. It is assumed that before taking a blood sample, the clinician has already obtained a history and conducted a thorough physical examination. Information derived from the history and physical examination may provide evidence for the cause of the eosinophilia or may direct the clinician along a specific path of further investigation. If, however, no obvious abnormalities that might explain the eosinophilia are detected, an organized search for the most common disorders associated with eosinophilia is warranted.

As diseases of the skin or gastrointestinal or respiratory tracts are most commonly associated with eosinophilia, it seems logical to initially investigate these body systems and to rule out common parasitic and allergic processes. The skin is easily evaluated for the presence of ectoparasites (fleas), signs of hypersensitivity (FAD, atopy, food allergy, eosinophilic granuloma complex) and masses. Fine needle aspirates of skin masses should be examined cytologically. Histopathological assessment of biopsies of skin lesions may also be required (Figure 8.10). The gastrointestinal tract may be evaluated initially by repeated faecal examinations. If endoparasites or ectoparasites are present, the haemogram should be repeated after appropriate therapy to assess for the persistence of eosinophilia. As stated, parasitism may not necessarily be the cause of the eosinophilia. Biopsies of the gastrointestinal tract may be necessary to confirm or exclude eosinophilic inflammatory diseases of the gastrointestinal tract. The respiratory tract may be assessed radiographically, via cytological assessment of a transtracheal wash (Figure 8.11) or bronchoalveolar lavage fluid as well as a Baermann faecal examination. Testing for heartworm should be performed in areas endemic for this parasite.

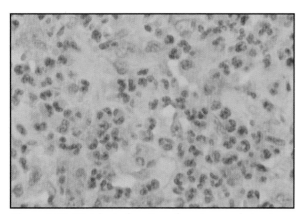

Figure 8.10: *Histological section of a cutaneous lesion in a cat with eosinophilic plaque (eosinophilic collagenolytic granuloma). Large numbers of eosinophils are present in the dermis. Haematoxylin and eosin. (Courtesy of Dr M. Gains.)*

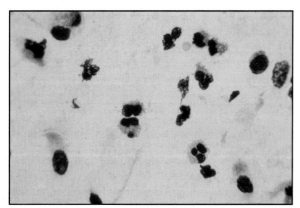

Figure 8.11: *Cytological preparation of a transtracheal wash showing increased numbers of eosinophils. Wright–Giemsa. (Courtesy of Dr C. Belford.)*

Suspected hypoadrenocorticism may be confirmed by performing an adrenocorticotrophin stimulation test. If these procedures do not prove fruitful, a search for the less common neoplastic, inflammatory and infectious diseases is in order (Center *et al.*, 1990; Tvedten, 1994).

There are no well established 'rules' to indicate when it is necessary to assess a bone marrow aspirate or core biopsy in the investigation of eosinophilia. Common sense, however, would suggest that the assessment of bone marrow is most useful as part of a complete diagnostic investigation of a persistent unexplained eosinophilia, in helping to distinguish between rare causes of eosinophilia (HES, eosinophilic leukaemia, eosinophilia associated with neoplasia), and in further assessing a profound eosinophilia. As stated, the diagnoses of both HES and eosinophilic leukaemia are diagnoses of exclusion. Differentiation of the two conditions is controversial in humans, as it is in cats. A review by Huibregste and Turner (1994) suggests several differentiating criteria in the cat. Differentiation, however, may be an academic pursuit as both diseases hold a grave prognosis.

The clinician must always take into consideration the effect of corticosteroid therapy on eosinophil numbers. A single dose of corticosteroid in an animal with an eosinophil count within the reference range produces an eosinopenia within 1 to 6 hours, depending on dose and route of administration (Latimer, 1995). Eosinophil concentrations return to normal within 24 hours of a single treatment with most corticosteroid preparations (Duncan *et al.*, 1994; Tvedten, 1994; Latimer, 1995) and 2 to 3 days after ending long term (10 days or more) corticosteroid therapy (Duncan *et al.*, 1994). An animal with a condition associated with eosinophilia that is concurrently stressed or being treated with corticosteroids exhibits an eosinophil count which is a reflection of the process that has the greater effect at the time.

REFERENCES

Balmer-Rusca E and Hauser B (1993) Case report: persistent eosinophilia in a dog. Hypereosinophilic syndrome? *Kleintierpraxis* **38,** 137–138

Barsanti JR and Prestwood AK (1983) Parasitic disease of the respiratory tract. In: *Current Veterinary Therapy VIII, Small Animal Practice*, ed. RW Kirk, pp. 241–246. WB Saunders, Philadelphia

Berry CR, Moore PF, Thomas WP, Sisson D and Koblik PD (1990) Lymphomatoid granulomatosis in seven dogs (1976–1987). *Journal of Veterinary Internal Medicine* **4,** 157–166

Bortnowski HB and Rosenthal RC (1992) Gastrointestinal mast cell tumours and eosinophilia in two cats. *Journal of the American Animal Hospital Association* **28,** 271–275

Bowman DD (1992) Hookworm parasites of the dog and cat. *Compendium of Continuing Education for the Practicing Veterinarian* **14,** 585–596

Buerger RG and Scott DW (1987) Cutaneous mast cell neoplasia in cats: 14 cases (1975–1985). *Journal of the American Veterinary Medical Association* **190,** 1440–1444

Burrows CF, Batt RM and Sherding RG (1995) Diseases of the small intestine. In: *Textbook of Veterinary Internal Medicine, 4th edn*, ed. SJ Ettinger and EC Feldman, pp. 1169–1231. WB Saunders, Philadelphia

Bush BM (1991) White blood cells. In: *Interpretation of Laboratory Results for Small Animal Clinicians,* ed. BM Bush, pp. 132-195. Blackwell Scientific, Oxford

Bustos S, Soto J, Bruzzone N, Vasquez V and Tchernitchin AN (1995) Effect of *p,p'*-DDT and estrogen on the presence in the circulation and degranulation of blood eosinophil leukocytes. *Bulletin of Environmental Contamination and Toxicology* **55,** 309-315

Calvert CA (1987) Selected complications and sequelae of canine heartworm disease. *Seminars in Veterinary Medicine and Surgery (Small Animal)* **2,** 56-63

Campbell BG (1991) *Trichuris* and other trichellinoid nematodes of dogs and cats in the United States. *Compendium of Continuing Education for the Practicing Veterinarian* **13,** 769-778

Carrington SP, Crispin SM and Williams D (1992) Characteristic conditions of the feline cornea. *Veterinary Annual* **32,** 83-96

Center SA (1985) Feline diseases, part II. *Proceedings of the 52nd Annual Meeting of the American Animal Hospital Association.* pp. 199-207

Center SA and Randolph JF (1991) Eosinophilia. In: *Consultations in Feline Internal Medicine,* ed. JR August, pp. 349-358. WB Saunders, Philadelphia

Center SA, Randolph JF, Erb HN and Reiter S (1990) Eosinophilia in the cat: a retrospective study of 312 cases (1975-1986). *Journal of the American Animal Hospital Association* **26,** 349-358

Cobb MA and Fisher MA (1992) *Crenosoma vulpis* infection in a dog. *Veterinary Record* **130,** 452

Collins BK, Swanson JF and MacWilliams PS (1986) Eosinophilic keratitis and keratoconjunctivitis in a cat. *Modern Veterinary Practice* **67,** 32-35

Confer AW, Qualls CW Jr., MacWilliams PS and Root CR (1983) Four cases of pulmonary nodular eosinophilic granulomatosis in dogs. *Cornell Veterinarian* **73,** 41-51

Corcoran BM, Foster DJ and Luis Fuentes V (1995) Feline asthma 'syndrome': a retrospective study of the clinical presentation in 29 cats. *Journal of Small Animal Practice* **36,** 481-488

Couto CG (1984) Tumour associated eosinophilia in a dog. *Journal of the American Veterinary Medical Association* **184,** 837

Couto CG (1985) Hematologic abnormalities in small animal cancer patients, part II. White blood cell, platelet and combined abnormalities. *Compendium of Continuing Education for the Practicing Veterinarian* **7,** 21-27

Craig TM (1984) Hepatozoonosis. In: *Clinical Microbiology and Infectious Diseases of the Dog and Cat,* ed. CE Greene, pp. 771-780. WB Saunders, Philadelphia

Dennis JS, Kruger JM and Mullaney TP (1992) Lymphoplasmacytic gastroenteritis in cats: 14 cases (1985-1990). *Journal of the American Veterinary Medical Association* **200,** 1712-1718

Duncan JR, Prasse KW and Mahaffey EA (1994) Leukocytes. In: *Veterinary Laboratory Medicine, 3rd edn,* eds. JR Duncan, KW Prasse and EA Mahaffey, pp. 37-62. Iowa State University Press, Ames, Iowa

Feldman EC and Nelson RW (1996) Feline hyperthyroidism (thyrotoxicosis). In: *Canine and Feline Endocrinology and Reproduction, 2nd edn,* ed. EC Feldman and RW Nelson, pp. 118-166. WB Saunders, Philadelphia

Gibbons LM, Jacobs DE and Pilkington JG (1988) Strongyloides in British greyhounds. *Veterinary Record* **122,** 114

Gilmour MA, Morgan RV and Moore FM (1992) Masticatory myopathy in the dog: a retrospective study of 18 cases. *Journal of the American Animal Hospital Association* **28,** 300-306

Glaze MB (1982) Feline eosinophilic keratitis. *Southwestern Veterinarian* **35,** 35-37

Goto N, Kawamura M, Inoue M and Sato A (1983) Pathology of two cases of canine disseminated hypereosinophilic disease. *Japanese Journal of Veterinary Science* **45,** 305-312

Greene CE and Chandler FW (1984) Pneumocystosis. In: *Clinical Microbiology and Infectious Diseases of the Dog and Cat,* ed. CE Greene, p. 859. WB Saunders, Philadelphia

Guilford WG (1996) Idiopathic inflammatory bowel diseases. In: *Strombeck's Small Animal Gastroenterology, 3rd edn,* ed. DR Strombeck, DA Williams and DJ Meyer, pp. 451-486. WB Saunders, Philadelphia

Hardy RM (1995) Hypoadrenal gland disease. In: *Textbook of Veterinary Internal Medicine, 4th edn,* ed. SJ Ettinger and EC Feldman, pp. 1579-1592. WB Saunders, Philadelphia

Hart JR, Shaker E, Patnaik AK and Garvey MS (1994) Lymphocytic-plasmacytic enterocolitis in cats: 60 cases (1988-1990). *Journal of the American Animal Hospital Association* **30,** 505-514

Hawkins E (1995) Diseases of the lower respiratory system. In: *Textbook of Veterinary Internal Medicine, 4th edn,* ed. SJ Ettinger and EC Feldman, pp. 767-811. WB Saunders, Philadelphia

Hendrick M (1981) A spectrum of hypereosinophilic syndromes exemplified by six cats with eosinophilic enteritis. *Veterinary Pathology* **18,** 188-200

Hendrix CM, Blagburn BL and Lindsay DS (1987) Whipworms and intestinal threadworms. *Veterinary Clinics of North America* **17,** 1355-1375

Hirth RS and Hottendorf GH (1973) Lesions produced by a new lungworm in beagle dogs. *Veterinary Pathology* **10,** 385-407

Hitt ME (1997) Flukes, liver and pancreatic. In: *The 5 Minute Veterinary Consult-Canine and Feline,* eds. LP Tilley and FWK Smith, p. 604. Williams and Wilkins, Baltimore

Huibregste BA and Turner JL (1994) Hypereosinophilic syndrome and eosinophilic leukemia: a comparison of 22 hypereosinophilic cats. *Journal of the American Animal Hospital Association* **30,** 591-599

Jain NC (1993) The eosinophils. In: *Essentials of Veterinary Hematology,* ed. NC Jain, pp. 247-257. Lea and Febiger, Philadelphia

Jensen AL and Nielsen OL (1992) Eosinophilic leukemoid reaction in a dog. *Journal of Small Animal Practice* **33,** 337-340

Johnson SE (1992) Canine eosinophilic gastroenterocolitis. *Seminars in Veterinary Medicine and Surgery (Small Animal)* **7,** 145-152

Johnson KA, Watson ADJ and Page RC (1995) Skeletal diseases. In: *Textbook of Veterinary Internal Medicine, 4th edn,* ed. SJ Ettinger and EC Feldman, pp. 2077-2103. WB Saunders, Philadelphia

Klausner JS and Perman V (1981) Non-cutaneous systemic mastocytosis and mast cell leukemia in a dog-case report and literature review. *Journal of the American Animal Hospital Association* **17,** 361-368

Latimer KS (1995) Leukocytes in health and disease. In: *Textbook of Veterinary Internal Medicine, 4th edn,* ed. SJ Ettinger and EC Feldman, pp. 1892-1929. WB Saunders, Philadelphia

Latimer KS and Rakich PM (1989) Clinical interpretation of leukocyte responses. *Veterinary Clinics of North America (Small Animal Practice)* **19,** 637-668

Leib MS and Matz ME (1995) Diseases of the large intestine. In: *Textbook of Veterinary Internal Medicine, 4th edn,* ed. SJ Ettinger and EC Feldman, pp. 1232-1260. WB Saunders, Philadelphia

Levitan DM, Matx ME, Findlen CS and Fister RD (1996) Treatment of *Oslerus osleri* infestation in a dog-case report and literature review. *Journal of the American Animal Hospital Association* **32,** 435-438

Lewis MG, Kociba GJ, Rojko JL, Stiff MI, Haberman AB, Velicer LV and Olsen RG (1985) Retroviral-associated eosinophilic leukemia in the cat. *American Journal of Veterinary Research* **46,** 1066-1070

Lilliehook I (1997) Diurnal variations of canine blood leukocyte counts. *Veterinary Clinical Pathology* **26,** 113-117

Lilliehook I, Gunnarsson L, Zakrisson G and Tvedten H (2000) Diseases associated with pronounced eosinophilia: a study of 105 dogs in Sweden. *Journal of Small Animal Practice* **41,** 248-253

Losco PE (1986) Local and peripheral eosinophilia in a dog with anaplastic mammary carcinoma. *Veterinary Pathology* **23,** 536-538

Lucke VM, Kelly DF, Harrington GA, Gibbs C and Gaskell CJ (1979) Lymphomatoid granulomatosis of the lungs in young dogs. *Veterinary Pathology* **16,** 405

Madewell BR, Stannard AH, Pulley LT and Nelson VG (1980) Oral eosinophilic granuloma in Siberian Husky dogs. *Journal of the American Veterinary Medical Association* **177,** 701-703

McEwen BJ (1992) Eosinophils: a review. *Veterinary Research Communications* **16,** 11-44

Moulton JE and Harvey JW (1990) Tumors of the lymphoid and hematopoietic tissues. In: *Tumors of Domestic Animals, 3rd edn,* ed. JE Moulton and JW Harvey, pp. 231-307. University of California Press, Berkeley

Ndikuwera J, Smith DA, Obwelo MJ and Masvingwe C (1992) Chronic granulocytic leukemia/eosinophilic leukemia in a dog? *Journal of Small Animal Practice* **33,** 553-557

O'Donnell JA II and Hayes KC (1987) Nutrition and nutritional disorders. In: *Diseases of the Cat, Medicine and Surgery,* ed. J Holzworth, pp 15-39. WB Saunders, Philadelphia

O'Keefe DA, Couto CG, Binke-Schwark C and Jacobs RM (1987) Systemic mastocytosis in 16 dogs. *Journal of Veterinary Internal Medicine* **1,** 75-80

Parsons JC (1987) Ascarid infections of cats and dogs. *Veterinary Clinics of North America* **17,** 1307-1399

Parsons JC, Bowman DP and Grieve RB (1989) Pathological and haematological response of cats experimentally infected with *Toxocara canis* larvae. *International Journal for Parasitology* **19,** 479-488

Patteson MW, Gibbs C, Wotton PR and Day MJ (1993) *Angiostrongylus vasorum* infection in seven dogs. *Veterinary Record* **133,** 565-570

Peaston AE and Griffey SM (1994) Visceral mast cell tumour with eosinophilia and eosinophilic peritoneal and pleural effusion in a cat. *Australian Veterinary Journal* **71,** 215-217

Peterson EW, Bar SC, Gould WJ III, Beck KA and Bowman DD (1993) Use of fenbendazole for treatment of *Crenosoma vulpis* infection in a dog. *Journal of the American Veterinary Medical Association* **202**, 1483-1484

Peterson ME (1995) Hyperthyroid diseases. In: *Textbook of Veterinary Internal Medicine, 4th edn*, ed. SJ Ettinger and EC Feldman, pp. 1466-1486. WB Saunders, Philadelphia

Peterson ME, Greco DS and Orth DN (1989) Primary hypoadrenocorticism in ten cats. *Journal of Veterinary Internal Medicine* **3**, 55-58

Peterson ME, Kintzer PP and Hurvitz AI (1988) Methimazole treatment of 262 cats with hyperthyroidism. *Journal of Veterinary Internal Medicine* **2**, 150-157

Peterson ME, Kurtzer PP and Kass PH (1996) Pre-treatment clinical and laboratory findings in dogs with hypoadrenocorticism. 225 cases (1979-1993). *Journal of the American Veterinary Medical Association* **208**, 85-91

Plotnick A (1994) A case report: hypereosinophilic syndrome in a cat. *Feline Practice* **22**, 28-31

Pollack MJ, Flanders JA and Johnson RC (1991) Disseminated malignant mastocytoma in a dog. *Journal of the American Animal Hospital Association* **27**, 435-440

Postorino NC, Wheeler SL, Park RD, Powers BE and Withrow SJ (1989) A syndrome resembling lymphomatoid granulomatosis in the dog. *Journal of Veterinary Internal Medicine* **3**, 15-19

Prasse KW, Mahaffey EA, Cotter SM and Holzworth J (1987) Hematology of normal cats and characteristic responses to disease. In: *Diseases of the Cat: Medicine and surgery,* ed. J Holzworth, pp. 739-807. WB Saunders, Philadelphia

Prestwood AK, Greene CE, Mahaffey EH and Burgess DE (1981) Experimental canine angiostrongylosis I. Pathologic manifestations. *Journal of the American Animal Hospital Association* **17**, 491-497

Ramsay IK, Foster A, McKay J and Herrtage MC (1997) *Pneumocystis carinii* pneumonia in two Cavalier King Charles spaniels. *Veterinary Record* **140**, 372-373

Rawlings CA and Calvert CA (1995) Heartworm disease. In: *Textbook of Veterinary Internal Medicine, 4th edn*, ed. SJ Ettinger and EC Feldman, pp. 1046-1067. WB Saunders, Philadelphia

Roudebush P (1995) Adverse reactions to foods: allergies. In: *Textbook of Veterinary Internal Medicine, 4th edn*, ed. SJ Ettinger and EC Feldman, pp. 258-262. WB Saunders, Philadelphia

Schalm OW, Jain NC and Carroll EJ (1975) The leukocytes: structure, kinetics, function and clinical interpretation. In: *Veterinary Hematology, 3rd edn*, ed. OW Schalm, NC Jain and EJ Carroll, pp. 471-536. Lea and Febiger, Philadelphia

Scott DW, Miller WH and Griffin CE (1995a) Immunologic skin disease. In: *Small Animal Dermatology, 5th edn*, ed. DW Scott, WH Miller and CE Griffin, pp. 484-626. WB Saunders, Philadelphia

Scott DW, Miller WH and Griffin CE (1995b) Miscellaneous skin disease. In: *Small Animal Dermatology, 5th edn*, ed. DW Scott, WH Miller and GE Griffin, pp. 902-955. WB Saunders, Philadelphia

Sellon RK, Rottman JB, Jordan HL, Wells MR, Simpson PM, Nelson P and Keene BW (1992) Hypereosinophilia associated with transitional cell carcinoma in a cat. *Journal of the American Veterinary Medical Association* **201**, 591-593

Shaw DH, Conley GA, Hogan DM and Horney BS (1996) Eosinophilic bronchitis caused by *Crenosoma vulpis* infection in dogs. *Canadian Veterinary Journal* **37**, 361-363

Slaughter JB, Billups LH and Acor GK (1988) Canine heterobilharziasis. *Compendium for Continuing Education for the Practicing Veterinarian* **10**, 606-612

Smith MO (1989) Idiopathic myositides in dogs. *Seminars in Veterinary Medicine and Surgery (Small Animal)* **4**, 156-160

Swenson CL, Carothers MA, Wellman ML and Kociba GJ (1993) Eosinophilic leukemia in a cat with naturally acquired feline leukemia virus infection. *Journal of the American Animal Hospital Association* **29**, 497-501

Taboada J (1991) Pulmonary diseases of potential allergic origin. *Seminars in Veterinary Medicine and Surgery (Small Animal)* **6**, 278-285

Tchernitchin AN, Mena MA, Soto J and Unda C (1989) The role of eosinophils in the action of estrogens and other hormones. *Medical Science Research* **17**, 5-10

Thoday KL and Mooney CD (1992) Historical, clinical and laboratory features of 126 hyperthyroid cats. *Veterinary Record* **131**, 257-264

Torgerson PR, McCarthy G and Donnelly WJC (1997) *Filaroides hirthi* verminous pneumonia in a West Highland White terrier bred in Ireland. *Journal of Small Animal Practice* **38**, 217-219

Tvedten H (1994) Leukocyte disorders. In: *Small Animal Clinical Diagnosis by Laboratory Methods, 2nd edn*, ed. MD Willard, H Tvedten and GH Turnwald, pp. 53-70. WB Saunders, Philadelphia

Willemse A (1984) Canine atopic disease-investigation of eosinophilia and the nasal mucosa. *American Journal of Veterinary Research* **45**, 1867-1869

Wilson SC, Thomson-Kerr K and Houston DM (1996) Hypereosinophilic syndrome in a cat. *Canadian Veterinary Journal* **37**, 679-680

Young KM (1997) Eosinophilia and basophilia. In: *The 5 Minute Veterinary Consult-Canine and Feline*, ed. LP Tilley and FWK Smith, pp. 222-223. Williams and Wilkins, Baltimore

(iii) Leukaemia

Joanna Morris and Jane Dobson

INTRODUCTION

This chapter is concerned with the diagnosis and management of neoplastic conditions of the haematopoietic system (leukaemia). Leukaemia is not a common diagnosis in small animal practice, however, increasing use of haematological evaluation of the sick patient has led to an appreciation that leukaemia is a significant cause of morbidity and mortality in cats and dogs. Leukaemia encompasses a complex group of diseases, some of which are not well characterized or understood in veterinary medicine. This chapter addresses principally those neoplastic conditions of white blood cells, since those of red blood cells (e.g. polycythaemia vera) are covered elsewhere.

Leukaemia

Leukaemia is a progressive malignant disease of the bone marrow, characterized by abnormal proliferation and development of haematopoietic cells and their precursors. In most instances, excessive numbers of abnormal neoplastic cells are present in both the peripheral blood and the bone marrow. This may be accompanied by a reduction in the number of normal blood cells (cytopenia), as the bone marrow becomes overwhelmed by the neoplastic cells.

Aleukaemic leukaemia (smouldering leukaemia)

On occasion, the neoplastic process is contained within the bone marrow and is not accompanied by excessive numbers of abnormal circulating cells. The haemogram will reflect the ongoing disease process in the marrow in the form of non-regenerative cytopenias.

THE HAEMATOPOIETIC SYSTEM

The principal organ that forms blood in the adult animal is the red bone marrow. Liver, spleen and peripheral lymphoid tissues play a role in haematopoiesis in fetal development and act as sites of extramedullary haematopoiesis in the adult in times of excessive demand. An understanding of leukaemia requires an appreciation of the structure and function of bone marrow (Figures 8.12 and 8.13).

It is generally accepted that all haematopoietic cell lineages are derived from pluripotent stem cells sited in the bone marrow. These give rise to differentiating progenitor cells, which divide and differentiate into functional mature blood cells. In the early stages of haematopoiesis the stem and progenitor cells remain relatively undifferentiated and retain the capacity for cell division and multiplication. As the cells become more differentiated and committed to a certain cell lineage, the capacity for replication is progressively diminished and ultimately is lost in the mature cell lines seen in the peripheral blood. Hence for each cell lineage there is a pyramidal arrangement of cells within the bone marrow with dividing undifferentiated cells at the apex and non-dividing mature cells at the base (Figure 8.14). It is not fully understood whether the pluripotent haematopoietic stem cells give rise to lymphoid precursors or whether lymphoid cells have a separate stem cell to the granulocyte/monocyte lines. Lymphocytes released from the bone marrow may require processing by other lymphoid tissues before they are capable of assuming the functions of mature T and B cells.

The proliferation and differentiation of haematopoietic cells is controlled by numerous growth factors (Figure 8.15). The erythroid compartment is controlled by the circulating glycoprotein hormone, erythropoietin, which is produced in the kidney in response to changes in oxygen tension but acts on target cells in the bone marrow. The myeloid compartment is controlled by locally produced regulatory molecules called colony-stimulating factors (CSFs), which are produced by a variety of cell types including lymphocytes, monocytes, macrophages, fibroblasts and endothelial cells. These act at the level of the committed progenitor cells but can also affect the function and survival of mature cells. Interleukin-3 (IL-3) and granulocyte–macrophage colony-stimulating factor (GM-CSF) have a broad spectrum of

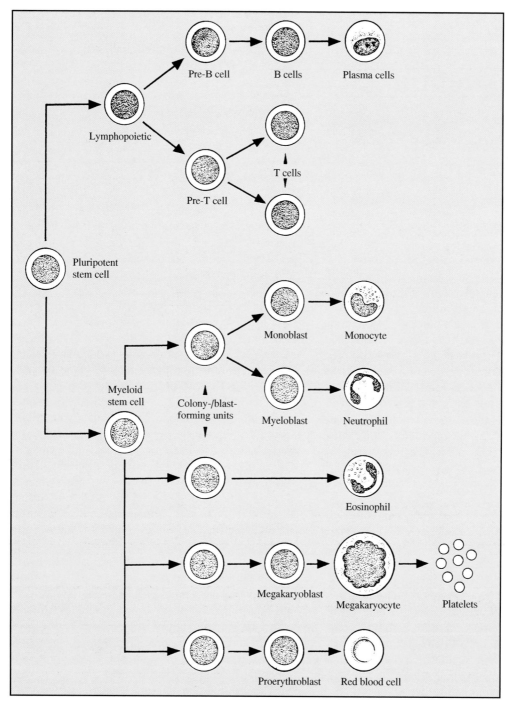

Figure 8.12:
Schematic diagram
depicting the
structure of bone
marrow and
haematopoiesis.
The different cell
lineages recognized
in peripheral blood
are progeny of
pluripotent stem
cells.

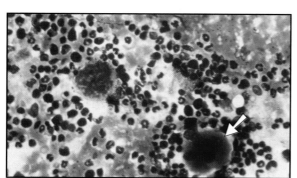

Figure 8.13: Photomicrograph of normal canine bone marrow showing different cell lines at various stages of differentiation. A megakaryocyte (arrowed) is notable in the lower right quadrant of the picture.

activity, whereas granulocyte colony-stimulating factor (G-CSF) and macrophage colony-stimulating factor (M-CSF) are lineage restricted. Megakaryocyte differentiation and platelet production are controlled by thrombopoietin, also known as megakaryocyte growth and development factor (MGDF).

Neoplastic transformation may occur at several levels of this proliferative/maturation process. Transformation of stem cells or early precursors causes a massive proliferation of undifferentiated cells that are incapable of maturation, resulting in acute leukaemia. Transformation of late precursor cells causes an overproduction of mature differentiated cells, resulting in chronic leukaemia (Figure 8.16).

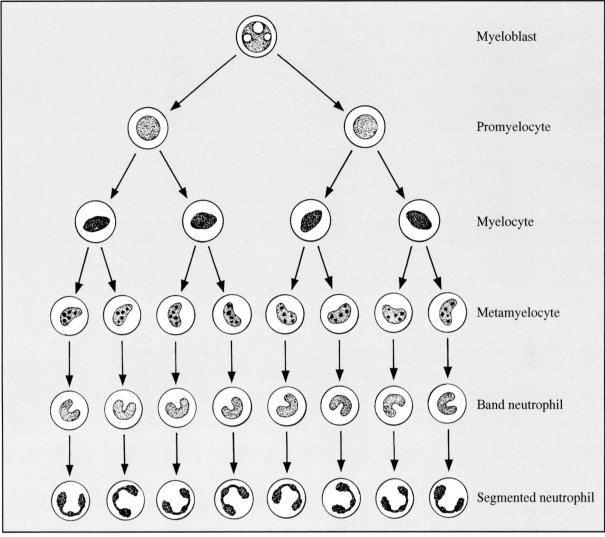

Figure 8.14: *Schematic diagram of normal maturation process of bone marrow showing pyramidal arrangement, with the dividing undifferentiated cells at the apex and non-dividing mature cells at the base.*

Haematopoietic growth factor	Target cells
Interleukin-3	Haematopoietic stem cells Progenitors of all cell lineages (except lymphoid) Mature mast cells, megakaryocytes, macrophages, eosinophils, basophils
Interleukin-5	B and T lymphocytes Eosinophil progenitors
Granulocyte–macrophage colony-stimulating factor	Progenitor and mature neutrophils, eosinophils and macrophages Erythroid and megakaryocyte progenitors Antigen-presenting dendritic cells
Granulocyte colony-stimulating factor	Progenitor and mature neutrophils
Macrophage colony-stimulating factor	Progenitor and mature macrophages Progenitor osteoclasts Microglial cells Cells of female reproductive tract
Erythropoietin	Erythroid progenitors and early erythroblasts
Thrombopoietin (megakaryocyte growth and development factor)	Megakaryocyte progenitors

Figure 8.15: *Haematopoietic growth factors.*

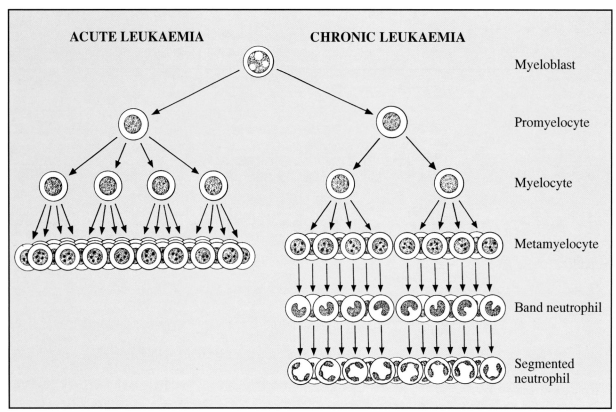

ACUTE LEUKAEMIA   **CHRONIC LEUKAEMIA**

Myeloblast

Promyelocyte

Myelocyte

Metamyelocyte

Band neutrophil

Segmented
neutrophil

*Figure 8.16: Schematic diagram of bone marrow depicting the difference between acute and chronic leukaemia in level of
transformation and outcome. In acute leukaemia, transformation of early precursors results in a massive proliferation of
undifferentiated cells. In chronic leukaemia, transformation at a later stage results in an overproduction of mature
differentiated cells.*

Acute leukaemias

Acute leukaemias are aggressive, rapidly
progressing, conditions characterized by excessive numbers of abnormal undifferentiated or
'blast' cells in both the bone marrow and peripheral blood, and accompanied by severe non-
regenerative cytopenias.

Chronic leukaemias

Chronic leukaemias tend to be less aggressive than
acute leukaemias and are slowly progressing conditions characterized by excessive numbers of mature
differentiated cells in the bone marrow and peripheral blood. This may or may not be accompanied
by cytopenia in other cell lines. If cytopenia is
present it is usually less severe than that seen in
acute leukaemia.

It is important clinically to distinguish between
these two forms of leukaemia as each carries a very
different prognosis. However, the division between
acute and chronic leukaemia is not always absolute,
and on occasion cases are encountered that share some
features of each. Furthermore, there are recorded instances of chronic leukaemia progressing to a more
acute disease (see below).

CLASSIFICATION OF LEUKAEMIA

Different types of leukaemia are recognized according to the cell lineage involved. The most common
types of leukaemia are listed in Figure 8.17. Other
extremely rare forms of leukaemia include eosinophilic and basophilic leukaemia (variants of
chronic granulocytic leukaemia), megakaryocytic
leukaemia and mast cell leukaemia. Another rare
malignant disease of the monocyte lineage, malignant histiocytosis, is sometimes included as a type
of leukaemia.

Myeloproliferative disease

Myeloproliferative disease (MPD) is a general term
used to describe all the non-lymphoid neoplastic and
dysplastic conditions of haematopoietic cells. The
term was introduced because the myeloid leukaemias
represent a constantly changing spectrum of diseases,
which may progress from dysplastic marrow conditions to aleukaemic leukaemias and finally to overt
leukaemia. In addition, although one particular cell
lineage may predominate at any time, a second cell
lineage is often affected and, as the disease progresses,
transitions to other cell lineages may occur. Thus,
depending on the time of sampling, the diagnosis of the
specific cell line involved may differ.

Myeloid	
Granulocytic	Acute myeloid leukaemia (AML)
	Chronic myeloid/granulocytic leukaemia (CML/CGL)
Monocytic	Acute monocytic leukaemia (AMoL)
Mixed	Acute myelomonocytic leukaemia (AMML)
Lymphoid	
	Acute lymphoblastic leukaemia (ALL)
	Chronic lymphocytic leukaemia (CLL)
Erythroid	
Erythroid only	Erythremic myelosis (acute) Polycythaemia vera (chronic)
Mixed	Erythroleukaemia

Figure 8.17: Classification of the more common types of leukaemia.

Lymphoproliferative disease

Lymphoproliferative disease (LPD) is the term used to describe all the neoplastic (and dysplastic) conditions arising from lymphoid cells. Because only one cell lineage is involved there is not the same spectrum of disease as seen with the myeloid leukaemias, and dysplastic conditions occur rarely, if at all. In addition to acute lymphoblastic leukaemia (ALL) and chronic lymphocytic leukaemia (CLL), LPD includes lymphoma and multiple myeloma. In the past, the veterinary literature has applied the terms leukaemia, leukosis and lymphoma very loosely, without any distinction between the different diseases. Strictly speaking, neoplastic transformation of lymphoid cells in the bone marrow results in lymphoid leukaemia, whereas the more familiar form of lymphoid neoplasia, that is, lymphoma, arises from the solid organs of the lymphoid system (lymph nodes, thymus) and organs through which lymphocytes normally traffic (gut, skin). Confusion arises because lymphoma may progress to involve the bone marrow (stage V lymphoma), and these cases should be defined as 'leukaemic lymphomas.' In the dog, only around 10% of cases of lymphoma will show bone marrow abnormalities, but in the cat the association between lymphoma and feline leukaemia virus (FeLV) means that bone marrow abnormalities (especially of the erythroid series) are relatively common, and it can be difficult to distinguish between those that result from lymphoma and those that result from the virus.

AETIOLOGY

Both genetic and environmental factors are implicated in the cause of leukaemia in dogs and cats. Although genetic changes can occur spontaneously throughout the lifetime of the animal, various environmental agents can contribute to DNA damage and accelerate the neoplastic progression. Experimentally, exposure to ionizing radiation induces DNA damage and causes myeloproliferative disease in dogs. There is little strong evidence to suggest that viruses play a role in the development of leukaemia in dogs, despite the demonstration of the presence of virus-like particles in a dog with granulocytic leukaemia and the isolation of a novel retrovirus from a dog with lymphoblastic leukaemia (Sykes *et al.*, 1985; Safran *et al.*, 1992). In the cat, however, the oncogenic retrovirus, FeLV, is known to play a major part in the development of both LPD and MPD by insertion of the provirus into the cat's genome and consequent alteration of gene function (see Chapter 8). Between 60% and 90% of cats with LPD or MPD are reported in the literature to be FeLV positive, although in recent years the percentage of FeLV-positive cats with lymphoma has been much lower. Feline immunodeficiency virus (FIV) may also be involved in the development of LPD and MPD (Gardner, 1991; Hutson *et al.*, 1991).

In humans, many leukaemias arise when the genome is disrupted by structural rearrangements of chromosomes, for example, translocations and insertions. In many cases, a single chromosome rearrangement is identified consistently with a particular type of leukaemia. In chronic myeloid leukaemia (CML), a translocation between chromosomes 9 and 22 leads to a shortened chromosome 22, which is readily identified cytogenetically and called the 'Philadelphia chromosome.' Many translocations occurring in lymphoid leukaemias involve the loci encoding immunoglobulins and T-cell receptors, and are thought to originate during normal maturation of B and T cells, as the various receptor subunits on different chromosomes rearrange. Cytogenetic studies of leukaemia in the dog and cat are limited, and although translocations have been identified, no consistent changes have been detected as yet (Goh *et al.*, 1981; Grindem and Buoen, 1989; Carter *et al.*, 1990; Nolte *et al.*, 1993). In the cat, translocations occur in both FeLV positive and FeLV negative cats, suggesting that the virus itself is not responsible for the chromosome alterations (Gulino, 1992).

GENERAL APPROACH TO THE LEUKAEMIC PATIENT

The diagnosis and management of the different types of leukaemia are considered in detail below. However, there are several features of these diseases that are common to all, and a discussion of clinical presentation, general principles of diagnosis and management is pertinent.

Presenting signs	Underlying cause	
Non-specific	Lethargy	See text
	Weakness	See text
	Anorexia	See text
	Weight loss	See text
Specific		
Haemostatic	Swollen joints, gingival or gastrointestinal bleeding, bruising, epistaxis	Thrombocytopenia, bleeding diathesis, disseminated intravascular coagulation or hyperviscosity syndrome
Metabolic	Polydipsia, polyuria, vomiting	Hypercalcaemia or liver or gastrointestinal infiltration
Neurological	Disorientation, cerebral dysfunction, ataxia	Hyperviscosity syndrome, infiltration of nervous system or intracranial haemorrhage
Ocular	Ocular lesions, sudden blindness	Hyperviscosity syndrome or ocular infiltration
Musculoskeletal	Lameness, paresis	Bone lesions (multiple myeloma) or infiltration of nerves

Figure 8.18: Presenting signs of leukaemia.

Clinical presentation

The clinical presentation of leukaemia is variable because although the neoplastic cells arise in the bone marrow, the disease is essentially systemic, with neoplastic cells circulating in the blood and infiltrating other organs such as the lymph nodes, liver and spleen. Presenting signs result either from the effects of the expanding neoplastic cell population within infiltrated organs or from tumour-related complications and paraneoplastic syndromes. The majority of cases show non-specific signs such as lethargy, weakness, anorexia and weight loss, but some may have additional signs relating to the following complications (Figure 8.18).

Haematological complications

Direct infiltration of the bone marrow by neoplastic cells (myelophthisis) suppresses normal haematopoiesis and results in anaemia, thrombocytopenia and neutropenia, whereas alteration of cell surface antigens and aberrant production of antibodies from neoplastic lymphoid cells can lead to immune-mediated haemolytic anaemia and/or thrombocytopenia. Excessive numbers of cells in the circulation can result in hyperviscosity and formation of microthrombi. Disseminated intravascular coagulation (DIC) secondary to the above haematological complications is a common terminal event in leukaemia.

Metabolic complications

Infiltration of organs such as the liver may disrupt normal metabolic function and produce various associated signs such as vomiting, anorexia and clotting defects. In addition, other clinical signs relating to metabolic upsets may result from accompanying paraneoplastic syndromes (Figures 8.19 and 8.20).

Clinical signs	
Renal	Polydipsia, polyuria
Cardiovascular	Arrhythmias (bradycardia), cardiac arrest
Gastrointestinal	Vomiting, anorexia, constipation
Neuromuscular	Muscle weakness, sluggish reflexes
Central nervous system	Depression, stupor, coma

Figure 8.19: Clinical signs of hypercalcaemia.

Hypercalcaemia: Neoplastic lymphoid cells may produce humoral factors/cytokines other than parathyroid hormone (PTH)-related protein (e.g. interleukin-1, tumour necrosis factor and transforming growth factors), which stimulate osteoclastic resorption of bone and result in hypercalcaemia of malignancy (Rosol *et al.*, 1992). Hypercalcaemia occurs in about 10-20% of cases of lymphoid leukaemia and myeloma in the dog but is much less common in the cat. Hypercalcaemia has serious systemic effects, by reducing neuromuscular conduction and depressing the excitability of cell membranes. Hypercalcaemia also has a direct effect on the kidney tubules, initially through inhibition of antidiuretic hormone, causing inability to concentrate urine. Hypercalcaemia thus causes diuresis leading to hyposthenuria and severe polyuria. Dehydration rapidly ensues if the animal is not able to compensate through polydipsia. Calcium can also cause direct damage to the renal tubules, and the combined effects of ongoing tubular damage and decreased glomerular filtration rate due to hypovolaemia may cause irreversible renal failure.

Clinical signs	
Hyperviscosity	
Neurological/ocular	Depression, disorientation, coma, ocular changes, sudden blindness
Cardiac	Congestive heart failure
Haemostatic	Bleeding diathesis
Haematological	Epistaxis, gastrointestinal bleeding, bruising, haemolysis, petechiation
Renal	Polyuria, polydipsia
Other	Pyrexia

Figure 8.20: *Clinical signs of hypergammaglobulinaemia.*

Hyperproteinaemia: Hyperproteinaemia is usually due to hypergammaglobulinaemia resulting from aberrant production of immunoglobulins by neoplastic lymphoid cells, as occurs in cases of multiple myeloma and chronic lymphocytic leukaemia (CLL). Complications associated with excess plasma protein concentrations are hyperviscosity of the blood, interference with clotting factors leading to a tendency to bleed and renal damage caused by breakdown and excretion of immunoglobulins.

Hyperviscosity: Hyperviscosity of the blood causes sluggish circulation leading to poor oxygen transport in critical capillary beds within organs such as the kidney and brain. Hyperviscosity may be exacerbated by formation of aggregates or microthrombi of tumour cells in cases with extremely high blood cell counts.

Diagnosis

In most cases, the clinical findings on physical examination of the animal will not specifically suggest a diagnosis of leukaemia (Figure 8.21). Invariably a series of laboratory-based investigations are required to reach a definitive diagnosis of leukaemia and to assess the presence and severity of disease-related complications.

Haematology

Routine haematological assessment of the patient usually provides the first indication of leukaemia. Haematological abnormalities may include:

- Cytopenia
  - Anaemia (usually non-regenerative)
  - Neutropenia
  - Thrombocytopenia
- Increased cell numbers
  - Disproportionate increase of one cell lineage
- Abnormal cells
  - Early immature blood cells in the peripheral circulation.

Clinical findings	Underlying cause
Weight loss	Cancer cachexia, gastrointestinal upsets
Pyrexia	Neutropenia, hypergammaglobulinaemia, pyrogen release
Cardiac arrhythmias	Hypercalcaemia
Pale mucous membranes	Anaemia
Petechial haemorrhages	Thrombocytopenia
Ecchymotic haemorrhages, other evidence of bleeding	Bleeding diathesis, disseminated intravascular coagulation
Ocular lesions (retinal detachment, tortuous retinal vessels, hypopyon, iris infiltration)	Hyperviscosity syndrome, tumour infiltration
Neurological signs/abnormal cerebral function (disorientation, depression, stupor, paresis)	Hyperviscosity syndrome, infiltration of nerves/central nervous system, intracranial haemorrhage, hypercalcaemia
Lymphadenopathy	Infiltration of lymph nodes
Hepatosplenomegaly	Infiltration of abdominal organs, extramedullary haematopoiesis
Lameness, skeletal pain, muscle weakness	Infiltration of joints, multiple myeloma bone lesions, hypercalcaemia

Figure 8.21: *Clinical findings of leukaemia.*

Bone marrow evaluation

Assessment of bone marrow is essential to confirm the diagnosis of leukaemia and provide information upon which the prognosis and treatment strategy can be defined, depending on the degree of disruption of normal marrow elements.

Bone marrow may be sampled and evaluated in one of two ways (see Chapter 2):

- Bone marrow aspirate (examined by cytology)
- Bone marrow biopsy (examined by histology).

Biochemistry

- Electrolytes, especially calcium
- Urea and creatinine concentrations for renal function, especially if the animal is hypercalcaemic
- Hepatic enzymes (such as alkaline phosphatase and alanine aminotransferase)
- Protein (both albumin and globulin concentration, in order to detect hypergammaglobulinaemia).

Urinalysis

Urinalysis is especially indicated in cases with hypercalcaemia or hypergammaglobulinaemia.

Specific evaluations

- Serum protein electrophoresis, to determine nature of hypergammaglobulinaemia (may be monoclonal or polyclonal gammopathy)
- Haemostatic profile, including clotting time, coagulation assays (one-stage prothrombin time, OSPT; activated partial thromboplastin time, APTT) and tests for fibrin degradation products (FDPs) if DIC is suspected.

Diagnostic imaging

- Radiography and/or ultrasonography, to assess possible neoplastic infiltration of internal organs especially the liver, spleen and lung
- Skeletal radiography if animal presents with lameness or if myeloma is suspected.

GENERAL PRINCIPLES OF MANAGEMENT

Whereas some types of leukaemia present with acute and life-threatening complications requiring emergency medical management, others may not require treatment at all. Specific treatments are detailed in the following sections, but there are some general principles of management that apply to all cases.

Treatment of the leukaemic animal usually requires a dual approach: supportive treatment of disease-related complications (often necessitating emergency care) and specific treatment of the underlying disease.

Supportive treatment

Several supportive measures may be required to correct the haematological and metabolic complications of leukaemia.

Antibiotic therapy

Broad spectrum bactericidal antibiotic treatment is essential in the management of neutropenic patients where overwhelming sepsis poses a serious life-threatening risk (Figure 8.22).

Fluid therapy

Fluids are indicated for maintenance of the anorectic patient and correction of fluid losses and electrolyte

Management of neutropenia	Specific details
Stop/reduce chemotherapy	If neutropenia <2 x 10^9/l, stop treatment If neutropenia 2–3 x 10^9/l, reduce treatment by at least 50%, or stop treatment if pyrexic
Set up blood cultures and antibiotic sensitivity tests	Modify antibiotic therapy if antibiotic resistance detected
Start broad-spectrum bactericidal antibiotics immediately	Intravenous route essential, and continue for at least 7 days. Can use: cephalosporin or β-lactamase-resistant penicillin in combination with gentamycin or amikacin; fluoroquinolone derivatives such as enrofloxacin; trimethoprim–sulphamethoxazole
Supportive treatment	Intravenous fluid therapy, warmth
Prevent infection with strict asepsis	Use aseptic technique for all interventions such as blood samples

Figure 8.22: Management of neutropenia.

and acid–base disturbances, especially in the management of hypercalcaemia (Figure 8.23).

Blood transfusion and/or blood component therapy

Blood and blood products are indicated in the management of patients that are severely anaemic or actively bleeding.

Plasmapheresis

This may be indicated in the management of hyperviscosity (Figure 8.24) and polycythaemia (see Chapter 4).

Specific treatment

Chemotherapy

Anticancer cytotoxic drugs are traditionally used to treat leukaemia. Because of the diffuse infiltrative nature of the disease, radiation and surgery are rarely indicated (although bone marrow irradiation is sometimes used before bone marrow transplantation in human patients).

A large array of cytotoxic drugs is available from human medicine, and although none of these agents are licensed for veterinary use, there is considerable experience of the effects and actions of these agents in the cat and dog. Most forms of leukaemia are at least potentially susceptible to several cytotoxic drugs, especially the alkylating agents, the antimetabolites and the anti-tumour antibiotics. Cytotoxic drugs are given usually in combinations rather than as single agents in order to achieve an additive tumouricidal effect and minimize toxicity.

Numerous protocols that combine drugs of different actions and with different toxicities have been used to treat leukaemias in the cat and dog, and some of these are set out in detail in the following sections. For a more detailed consideration of the principles and practice of cancer chemotherapy, see the reading list at the end of this chapter.

Three phases of treatment are usually defined:

- Induction: aggressive and intensive treatment, aimed at eradication of as much tumour as possible in order to achieve clinical remission (no detectable disease)
- Maintenance: less aggressive and less frequent treatment, aimed at keeping the tumour in remission (drug therapy is tapered over a long period but is rarely stopped altogether)
- Rescue: recourse to aggressive treatment in the face of tumour recurrence (relapse of the disease).

The patient must be monitored throughout chemotherapy, not only to assess response to therapy but to be sure of detecting any drug-related complications at an early stage and therefore preventing serious side effects. Although each drug has its own specific toxicities, most chemotherapeutic agents are myelosuppressive, and frequent haematological evaluation is vital to check that serious cytopenias do not develop. Many leukaemic patients have severe haematological abnormalities before commencing therapy, and the risk of drug-induced complications is therefore increased. In some cases, especially for acute leukaemias, it may be advisable not to start chemotherapy at all.

Management of hypercalcaemia	Specific details
Restore circulating volume	Intravenous fluid therapy with normal saline (0.9%) to replace fluid losses
Aid calciuresis	Intravenous fluid therapy with normal (0.9%) saline at 2–3 times maintenance Administration of frusemide at 2 mg/kg bid or tid (only after circulating volume restored) Administration of prednisolone at 2 mg/kg daily (only after a diagnosis has been obtained as steroid therapy will lyse lymphoid cells and may prevent the correct diagnosis being made)
Treat underlying disease	Specific chemotherapy

Figure 8.23: Management of hypercalcaemia.

Management of hyperviscosity	Specific details
Plasmapheresis (if hyperviscosity severe)	Remove 20 ml/kg body weight of whole blood and replace with either centrifuged blood cells from the patient, which have been resuspended in crystalloid fluid or cells from a suitable donor
Treat underlying disease	Specific chemotherapy

Figure 8.24: Management of hyperviscosity.

Neutropenia (neutrophil count less than 3×10^9/l) is the most serious haematological concern because of the risk of sepsis. Gram-negative bacteria that enter the circulation from the gastrointestinal tract are the most common source of infection, although intravenous catheters, urinary catheters or skin wounds may also introduce bacteria. Without neutrophils no pus is produced to indicate infection, and so pyrexia remains the only consistent indicator of infection. Any animal that becomes pyrexic while receiving chemotherapy should be admitted immediately, have a haematological evaluation and be treated accordingly (see Figure 8.22).

Haematopoietic growth factors are potentially useful to promote normal marrow function in animals at risk of neutropenia while receiving chemotherapy. This type of treatment (biological therapy) is currently undergoing veterinary trials in the United States (Ogilvie, 1993a). The human recombinant molecules G-CSF and GM-CSF are commercially available but their use in normal dogs stimulates neutralizing antibody production against the foreign protein, resulting in leucopenia. In dogs receiving chemotherapy, however, antibodies do not develop and the human recombinant growth factors are beneficial (Henry *et al.*, 1998). The canine recombinant equivalents, although effective in increasing the numbers of granulocytes and monocytes in dogs and cats (Nash *et al.*, 1991; Obradovich *et al.*, 1991, 1993; Ogilvie *et al.*, 1992), are not yet commercially available.

ACUTE LEUKAEMIA

Epidemiology
Acute leukaemias account for less than 10% of all haematopoietic neoplasms in the dog and 15-35% in the cat, although it is difficult to obtain an accurate estimate because of the failure to distinguish lymphoma from leukaemia in many cases. Similarly, the true proportion of myeloid and lymphoid leukaemias is unclear. Although the majority of acute leukaemias are lymphoid when classified morphologically by con-

ventional staining, the use of cytochemical stains (Figure 8.25), immunocytochemical stains and flow cytometry now indicate that myeloid leukaemias may account for up to 75% of acute leukaemias in both the dog and the cat (Couto, 1992; Vernau and Moore, 1999). Affected animals are young to middle aged, but the affected age range is broad (1-12 years). There may be a slight sex predisposition to acute leukaemia in the dog (male:female ratio of 3:2) but there is no breed predisposition in dogs or cats.

Clinical features
Acute leukaemias are characterized by aggressive behaviour and rapid progression. Affected animals often present with non-specific vague signs, but signs specific for leukaemia-associated complications are also common. Pallor, pyrexia, mild lymphadenopathy and pronounced hepatosplenomegaly are frequent clinical findings. Although lymphoid and myeloid leukaemias cannot be reliably distinguished on the basis of physical examination, subtle differences do exist. For example, pyrexia, shifting lameness (due to bone pain), ocular lesions and DIC are more common in acute myeloid leukaemia (AML) whereas neurological signs and mild lymphadenopathies are more common with acute lymphoblastic leukaemia (ALL).

Diagnostic investigations

Haematology
Haematology usually shows noticeable abnormalities in acute leukaemias. Neoplastic blast cells are observed in the circulation for both myeloid and lymphoid leukaemias (although blast cells are occasionally absent in AML) and often result in leucocytosis (Figures 8.26 and 8.27). White blood cell counts are usually highest in ALL ($100-600 \times 10^9$/l). Cytopenias (non-regenerative anaemia, thrombocytopenia and neutropenia) are present in all cases, although anaemia and thrombocytopenia may be less severe in acute monocytic leukaemia (AMoL). Evaluation of coagulation profiles and FDPs may indicate DIC.

Type of leukaemia	Marker				
	Monocyte	Granulocyte			
	α-naphthyl butyrate esterase	Chloroacetate esterase	Myeloperoxidase	Lipase	Alkaline phosphatase
Acute myeloid leukaemia	–	+	+	–	+
Acute monocytic leukaemia	+	–	–	+	–
Acute myelomonocytic leukaemia	±	±	±	±	±
Acute lymphoblastic leukaemia	–(+)	–	–	–	–(+)

***Figure 8.25:** Cytochemical staining reactions for acute leukaemias.*

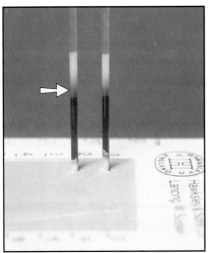

Figure 8.26: *Haematocrit of dog with leucocytosis showing thick buffy coat (arrowed).*

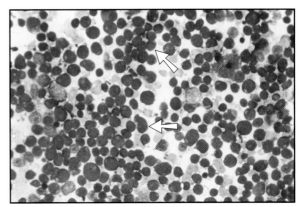

Figure 8.29. *Photomicrograph of bone marrow from dog with acute lymphoblastic leukaemia. The bone marrow is dominated by large and intermediate lymphoid cells (arrowed).*

Specific diagnosis

The specific diagnosis of acute leukaemia is based on the predominance (40–50%) of blast cells in the bone marrow, usually accompanied by similar cells in peripheral blood. ALL is best differentiated from AML and AMoL by cytochemical staining (Jain *et al.*, 1981; Couto, 1985; Facklam and Kociba, 1985, 1986; Grindem *et al.*, 1985a and b, 1986), immunocyto-chemical labelling or flow cytometric analysis (Vernau and Moore, 1999), as morphological appearance alone may not be diagnostic (Figure 8.30). However, commercial veterinary diagnostic laboratories in the United Kingdom do not often use such stains, and ALL is therefore overdiagnosed.

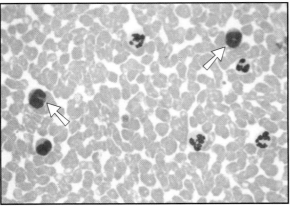

Figure 8.27: *Photomicrograph of blood film from dog with acute myeloid leukaemia containing abnormal immature myeloid cells (arrowed).*

Biochemistry

Biochemistry may indicate hypercalcaemia, or hepatic or renal dysfunction.

Bone marrow

Bone marrow usually appears hypercellular, with a predominance of blast cells and a consequent reduction in other cell lineages (Figures 8.28 and 8.29).

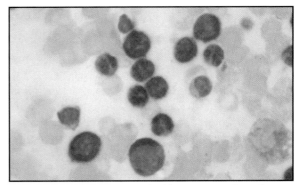

Figure 8.30: *Photomicrograph of bone marrow from dog, stained with chloroacetate esterase. The stain is taken up by normal neutrophils and by their precursors. (Picture courtesy of John Dunn.)*

In some cases the distinction of ALL from lymphoma is difficult because animals with either disease may have lymphadenopathy, haematological abnormalities and lymphoblasts in the bone marrow. In general, cases of ALL have a milder lymphadenopathy but more severe bone marrow changes and cytopenias, and therefore appear systemically ill (Leifer and Matus, 1985; Morris *et al.*, 1993), whereas cases of lymphoma are generally not systemically unwell and have less severely affected bone marrow but present with a massive lymphadenopathy.

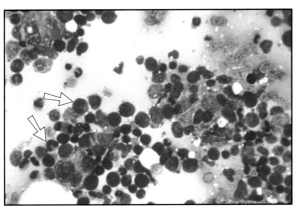

Figure 8.28: *Photomicrograph of bone marrow from dog with acute myeloid leukaemia showing a predominance of early myeloid cells (arrowed).*

Management

Supportive treatment

Supportive measures for acute leukaemia include fluid therapy for dehydration, anorexia or hypercalcaemia, blood transfusion for severe loss of red cells or platelets and antibiotic therapy for secondary infections.

Specific treatment

The aim of specific therapy for acute leukaemia is to destroy the leukaemic cells by using chemotherapy, and thereby allow resumption of normal haematopoiesis (Figure 8.31). These aims are, however, rarely achieved in veterinary medicine (see below), and treatment of acute leukaemia in dogs is not usually successful. Euthanasia is an option that should be considered at the time of diagnosis.

Schedules for chemotherapy have been described:

- Drugs recommended for the treatment of ALL are similar to those recommended for lymphoma, that is, vincristine and prednisolone plus an alkylating agent
- Drugs recommended for the treatment of AML include prednisolone, mercaptopurine or thioguanine in combination with cytosine arabinoside; the last agent is used because it may encourage differentiation of blast cells (Castaigne *et al.*, 1983).

Induction protocols for acute leukaemia are used until the white blood cell count returns to the normal range and blast cells are no longer seen in peripheral blood. In theory, drug doses and frequencies can then be reduced to maintenance levels, but in practice this is rarely achieved.

In veterinary medicine, the use of chemotherapy for the treatment of acute leukaemia is severely restricted by the degree of myelosuppression caused by the disease. The inability to preserve sufficient levels of normal blood cells during treatment is a constant problem. Furthermore, the toxicity of cytotoxic agents may be exacerbated by compromised hepatic and renal function. Most animal patients succumb to either overwhelming sepsis secondary to neutropenia, organ failure secondary to infiltration with neoplastic cells or DIC. Intensive medical care, bone marrow transplants and extracorporeal treatment of bone marrow are used in human medicine but are not routinely available for veterinary use. The development of canine recombinant G-CSF and GM-CSF may lead to significant improvements in the treatment of acute leukaemias.

Prognosis

The prognosis is poor for all acute leukaemias owing to failure to induce and maintain remission, organ failure (which enhances the cytotoxic effects of chemotherapeutic drugs) and septicaemia secondary to either the disease or the treatment.

Acute lymphoblastic leukaemia	
Induction	
Vincristine	0.5 mg/m^2 i.v. every 7 days
and prednisolone	40 mg/m^2 by mouth daily for 7 days then 20 mg/m^2 every 48 hours
Additional agents (if not neutropenic)	
Cyclophosphamide	50 mg/m^2 by mouth every 48 hours
or Cyclophosphamide and cytosine arabinoside	50 mg/m^2 by mouth every 48 hours 100 mg/m^2 s.c. or i.v. daily for 2–4 days (use divided doses if given i.v.)
or L-asparaginase	10,000–20,000 IU/m^2 i.m. every 2–3 weeks
Acute myeloid leukaemia	
Induction	
Cytosine arabinoside	100 mg/m^2 s.c. or i.v. daily for 2–6 days **or** 5–10 mg/m^2 s.c. twice daily for 2–3 weeks, then on alternate weeks
Additional agents (to increase response)	
Prednisolone	40 mg/m^2 by mouth daily for 7 days then 20 mg/m^2 every 48 hours
or 6-Thioguanine	50 mg/m^2 by mouth daily or every 48 hours
or 6-Thioguanine and doxorubicin	50 mg/m^2 by mouth daily or every 48 hours 10 mg/m^2 i.v. every 7 days
or Mercaptopurine	50 mg/m^2 by mouth daily or every 48 hours
Maintenance	
Reduce any of the above drug combinations to a dose and frequency which maintain white blood cell counts within the normal range	
Try alternate week therapy first, that is, a week of chemotherapy, a week without treatment, a week of chemotherapy, and so on	

Figure 8.31: Chemotherapy protocols for the treatment of acute leukaemia.

The prognosis for ALL is slightly better than for AML in both the dog and cat. Survival times of 1–3 months in dogs and 1–7 months in cats have been reported for ALL (Couto, 1992) although other authors claim better success (MacEwen *et al.*, 1977; Matus *et al.*, 1983; Gorman and White, 1987). Survival times for AML rarely exceed 2–3 months for both dogs and cats (Couto, 1985; Grindem *et al.*, 1985b).

CHRONIC LEUKAEMIAS

Epidemiology

Chronic leukaemia is less common than acute leukaemia especially in the cat where chronic lymphocytic leukaemia (CLL) is a rare disease and CML is even rarer. Most cases of CLL in the cat are FeLV negative (MacEwen, 1996). In the dog, CLL is more common than CML and most cases of CLL are derived from T lymphocytes (Vernau and Moore, 1999). CLL occurs in middle-aged to old dogs (mean 9.4 years) whereas CML occurs at any age. The male to female ratio for dogs with CLL is 2:1, but no breed predispositions have been reported.

Clinical features

Chronic leukaemia is a slowly progressive disease characterized by mild clinical signs. About 50% of cases of CLL may be asymptomatic and only detected on haematological examination. Most cases of CML and the remainder of cases of CLL present with clinical signs such as lethargy, anorexia, vomiting, pyrexia, polyuria, polydipsia and weight loss. Clinical examination may reveal pallor, mild lymphadenopathy (more common in CLL), splenomegaly, hepatomegaly or skin infiltration. Monoclonal gammopathy is associated with 25% of cases of CLL (although 10% may have reduced immunoglobulin concentrations), and hyperviscosity syndrome may therefore be present. Infection and pyrexia secondary to reduced humoral and cellular immunity are common.

A change from the proliferation of mature cells to blast cells (a blast cell crisis) often occurs as a terminal event with CML (but not CLL), months to years after diagnosis, and at this point the clinical signs become much more severe.

Diagnostic investigations

Haematology

Haematology usually shows a noticeable lymphocytosis in CLL (from 5 to more than 100 x 10^9/l) and leucocytosis with a left shift in CML. Circulating lymphocytes in patients with CLL are often normal in appearance, although slightly less mature forms can sometimes be seen. Mild anaemia and thrombocytopenia are usually present in patients with CLL and CML.

Biochemistry

Biochemistry often shows hyperproteinaemia, and serum electrophoresis may show a monoclonal gammopathy (usually owing to increased IgM concentration). Hypercalcaemia may be present.

Bone marrow

Bone marrow analysis shows a hypercellular marrow with a predominance of mature forms of the lymphoid or myeloid series (Figures 8.32 and 8.33).

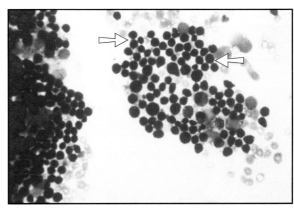

Figure 8.32: *Photomicrograph of bone marrow from dog with chronic lymphocytic leukaemia. The bone marrow is dominated by small mature lymphocytes (arrowed).*

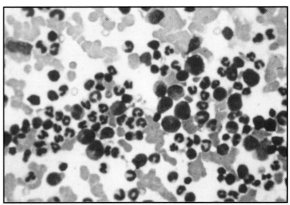

Figure 8.33: *Photomicrograph of bone marrow from dog with chronic myeloid leukaemia. The bone marrow contains increased numbers of bands and neutrophils. It can be difficult to distinguish chronic myeloid leukaemia from granulocytic hyperplasia as the appearance of the bone marrow is similar. (Picture courtesy of John Dunn.)*

Specific diagnosis

The specific diagnosis of chronic leukaemia is based on bone marrow findings and the nature of the accompanying leucocytosis. A noticeable lymphocytosis (greater than 20 x 10^9/l) is almost pathognomonic for CLL, although on occasion this may need to be differentiated from lymphoma of a lymphocytic cell type. The diagnosis of CML is often more difficult than that of CLL because of a lack of specific clinical and laboratory abnormalities characteristic of the disease.

It is often difficult to distinguish CML from leukaemoid reactions and preleukaemic syndromes on clinical findings, and careful examination of bone marrow may be necessary to reach a correct diagnosis. In patients with splenomegaly, histological examination of the spleen may be helpful.

Management

Supportive treatment

Paraneoplastic complications such as hypercalcaemia and hypergammaglobulinaemia may need to be addressed in patients with chronic leukaemia.

Specific treatment

For asymptomatic cases of CLL, there may be no need for treatment, although frequent monitoring and haematological screens are advised. For symptomatic cases of CLL and for all cases of CML, chemotherapy is the treatment of choice (Figure 8.34). In CLL, the alkylating agent chlorambucil is used in combination with prednisolone. More potent alkylating agents such as cyclophosphamide may be used in refractory cases of CLL, where they may also be combined with vincristine. CML is usually treated with either the alkylating agent busulphan or hydroxyurea, usually in combination with prednisolone.

In either CLL or CML, the aim of treatment is to restore the peripheral blood counts to within the normal range, and response to treatment is monitored by haematological findings. Once remission is achieved, maintenance therapy is continued at reduced doses and frequencies of the appropriate drugs in order to keep the white blood cell counts within the normal range.

Prognosis

The prognosis for chronic leukaemia is much more favourable than for acute leukaemia. Mean and median survival times for CLL in the dog may exceed one year (Leifer and Matus, 1985, 1986) but are usually shorter for CML, which has a greater risk of blast cell crisis.

OTHER LEUKAEMIAS

Eosinophilic and basophilic leukaemia

Eosinophilic and basophilic leukaemias are rarely reported in the dog and are usually considered as variants of CML. The diagnosis of eosinophilic leukaemia can only be made after careful exclusion of other causes of eosinophilia, and there is some doubt as to whether the condition truly exists in dogs and cats. Basophilic leukaemia must be distinguished from mast cell leukaemia because cell types

Chronic lymphocytic leukaemia	
Induction	
Chlorambucil	2–5 mg/m^2 by mouth daily for 7–14 days, then 2 mg/m^2 every 48 hours or 20 mg/m^2 by mouth as a single dose every 14 days
± Prednisolone	40 mg/m^2 by mouth daily for 7 days, then 20 mg/m^2 every 48 hours
Additional agent (for increased response)	
Vincristine	0.5 mg/m^2 i.v. every 7 days
Alternative protocol (for increased response)	
Vincristine	0.5 mg/m^2 i.v. every 7 days
and Cyclophosphamide	50 mg/m^2 by mouth every 48 hours
and Prednisolone	40 mg/m^2 by mouth daily for 7 days, then 20 mg/m^2 every 48 hours
Chronic myeloid leukaemia	
Induction	
Hydroxyurea	50 mg/kg by mouth daily for 1–2 weeks then every 48 hours **or** 80 mg/kg by mouth every 3 days until remission achieved **or** 1 g/m^2 by mouth daily until remission achieved
or Busulphan	2–6 mg/m^2 by mouth daily until remission achieved
Maintenance	
Reduce any of the above combinations of drugs to a dose and frequency which maintain white blood cell counts within the normal range	
Try alternate week therapy first, that is, a week of chemotherapy, a week without treatment, a week of chemotherapy, and so on	
After a few months try one week of treatment in three, then one week in four	

Figure 8.34: *Chemotherapy protocols for the treatment of chronic leukaemia.*

can be easily confused. Treatment of both eosinophilic and basophilic leukaemia is with corticosteroids and/or hydroxyurea.

Leukaemia of platelets and platelet precursors

Megakaryocytic leukaemia is another form of acute leukaemia rarely reported in the dog and cat, and is characterized by atypical megakaryocytes (dwarf megakaryocytes) and megakaryoblasts in the bone marrow. The corresponding chronic leukaemia, primary or essential thrombocythaemia, is even more rare and is diagnosed on the basis of persistently high platelet counts and megakaryocyte hyperplasia of the bone marrow.

Erythroid leukaemias

Erythremic myelosis is a myeloproliferative disorder, which is relatively common in cats but rare in dogs. Excessive proliferation of early erythroid precursors and nucleated erythrocytes is seen in the bone marrow, with severe anaemia, increased numbers of nucleated circulating red blood cells, moderate to severe anisocytosis and increased mean corpuscular volume. The equivalent chronic leukaemia, primary erythrocytosis (polycythaemia vera), is rare in both cats and dogs and is characterized by a persistently increased PCV, with low or normal erythropoietin activity (see Chapter 4). Erythroleukaemia is an acute leukaemia that can arise by blast transformation of erythremic myelosis. Primitive erythroid precursors predominate but myeloblasts are often present in low numbers. Erythroleukaemia occurs relatively commonly in cats but rarely in dogs.

MYELODYSPLASTIC SYNDROMES (PRELEUKAEMIA)

Some animals may present with the same vague clinical signs as seen with leukaemia, similar physical findings and haematological abnormalities such as cytopenias or abnormal circulating cells, but examination of the bone marrow fails to confirm the presence of neoplasia. The marrow is normocellular or hypercellular, with maturation arrest of the granulocytic series, erythroid abnormalities and abnormal dwarf megakaryocytes. The clinical signs and bone marrow changes may wax and wane without ever progressing. A proportion of cases, however, will develop overt myeloid leukaemia, hence the term 'preleukaemia.' Treatment of such conditions with chemotherapy is controversial because not all will progress to full leukaemia, but regular monitoring and supportive therapy with fluids and antibiotics are needed. Differentiating agents (cytosine arabinoside), haematopoietic growth factors or anabolic steroids may also be considered.

REFERENCES AND FURTHER READING

Carter RF, Kruth SA, Valli VEO and Dube ID (1990) Long-term culture of canine marrow: cytogenetic evaluation of purging of lymphoma and leukaemia. *Experimental Haematology* **18**, 995–1001

Castaigne S, Daniel MT, Tilly H, Herait P and Degos L (1983) Does treatment with Ara-C in low doses cause differentiation of leukaemic cells? *Blood* **62**, 85–86

Couto CG (1985) Clinicopathologic aspects of acute leukemias in the dog. *Journal of the American Veterinary Medical Association* **186**, 681–685

Couto CG (1992) Leukemias. In: *Essentials of Small Animal Internal Medicine*, ed. RW Nelson and CG Couto, pp. 871–878. Mosby Year Book, St Louis

Dobson JM and Gorman NT (1993) *Cancer Chemotherapy in Small Animal Practice*, ed. CJ Price, PGC Bedford and JB Sutton. Blackwell Scientific, Oxford

Facklam NR and Kociba GJ (1985) Cytochemical characterization of leukemic cells from 20 dogs. *Veterinary Pathology* **22**, 363–369

Facklam NR and Kociba GJ (1986) Cytochemical characterization of feline leukemic cells. *Veterinary Pathology* **23**, 155–161

Gardner SA (1991) Current concepts of feline immunodeficiency virus infection. *Veterinary Medicine* **86**, 300–307

Goh K, Smith RA and Proper JS (1981) Chromosomal aberrations in leukemic cats. *Cornell Veterinarian* **71**, 43–46

Gorman NT (1991) Chemotherapy. In: *Manual of Small Animal Oncology*, ed. RAS White, pp. 127–159. BSAVA Publications, Cheltenham

Gorman NT and White RAS (1987) Clinical management of canine lymphoproliferative diseases. *Veterinary Annual* **27**, 227–242

Grindem CB and Buoen LC (1989) Cytogenetic analysis in nine leukaemic cats. *Journal of Comparative Pathology* **101**, 21–30

Grindem CB, Perman V and Stevens JB (1985a) Morphological classification and clinical and pathological characteristics of spontaneous leukemia in 10 cats. *Journal of the American Animal Hospital Association* **21**, 227–236

Grindem CB, Stevens JB and Perman V (1985b) Morphological classification and clinical and pathological characteristics of spontaneous leukemia in 17 dogs. *Journal of the American Animal Hospital Association* **21**, 219–226

Grindem CB, Stevens JB and Perman V (1986) Cytochemical reactions in cells from leukemic dogs. *Veterinary Pathology* **23**, 103–109

Gulino SE (1992) Chromosome abnormalities and oncogenesis in cat leukaemias. *Cancer Genetics and Cytogenetics* **64**, 149–157

Hahn KA and Richardson RC (1995) *Cancer Chemotherapy. A Veterinary handbook*, ed. KA Hahn and RC Richardson. Williams and Wilkins, Baltimore

Henry CJ, Buss MS and Lothrop CD (1998) Veterinary uses of recombinant human granulocyte colony-stimulating factor. Part I. Oncology. *Compendium of Continuing Education for the Practising Veterinarian* **20**, 728–734

Hutson CA, Rideout BA and Pederson NC (1991) Neoplasia associated with feline immunodeficiency virus infection in cats of southern California. *Journal of the American Veterinary Medical Association* **199**, 1357–1362

Jain NC Madewell BR, Weller RE and Geissler MC (1981) Clinical-pathological findings and cytochemical characterization of myelomonocytic leukaemia in 5 dogs. *Journal of Comparative Pathology* **91**, 17–31

Leifer CE and Matus RE (1985) Lymphoid leukaemia in the dog. *Veterinary Clinics of North America: Small Animal Practice* **15(4)**, 723–739

Leifer CE and Matus RE (1986) Chronic lymphocytic leukaemia in the dog: 22 cases (1974–1984). *Journal of the American Veterinary Medical Association* **189**, 214–217

MacEwen EG (1996) Feline lymphoma and leukemias. In: *Small Animal Clinical Oncology, 2nd edn*, ed. SJ Withrow and EG MacEwen, pp. 479–495. WB Saunders, Philadelphia

MacEwen EG and Helfand SC (1993) Recent advances in the biologic therapy of cancer. *Compendium of Continuing Education for the Practising Veterinarian* **15**, 909–922

MacEwen EG, Patnaik AK and Wilkins RJ (1977) Diagnosis and treatment of canine hematopoietic neoplasms. *Veterinary Clinics of North America* **7(1)**, 105–118

Matus RE, Leifer CE and MacEwen EG (1983) Acute lymphoblastic leukaemia in the dog: a review of 30 cases. *Journal of the American Veterinary Medical Association* **183**, 859–862

Morris JS, Dunn JK and Dobson JM (1993) Canine lymphoid leukaemia and lymphoma with bone marrow involvement: a review of 24 cases. *Journal of Small Animal Practice* **34**, 72–79

Nash RA, Schnening F, Appelbaum F, Hammond WP, Boone T, Morris CF, Slichter SJ and Storb R (1991) Molecular cloning and in vivo evaluation of canine granulocyte-macrophage colony factors. *Blood* **78**, 930–937

Nolte M, Werner M, Nolte I and Georgii A (1993) Different cytogenetic findings in two clinically similar leukaemic dogs. *Journal of Comparative Pathology* **108**, 337–342

Obradovich JE, Ogilvie GK, Powers BE and Boone T (1991) Evaluation of recombinant canine granulocyte colony-stimulating factor as an inducer of granulopoiesis. *Journal of Veterinary Internal Medicine* **5**, 75–79

Obradovich JE, Ogilvie GK, Stadler-Morris S, Schmidt BR, Cooper MF and Boone TC (1993) Effect of recombinant canine granulocyte colony-stimulating factor on peripheral blood neutrophil counts in normal cats. *Journal of Veterinary Internal Medicine* **7**, 65–67

Ogilvie GK (1993a) Haematopoietic growth factors: tools for a revolution in veterinary oncology and hematology. *Compendium of Continuing Education for the Practising Veterinarian* **15**, 851-854

Ogilvie GK (1993b) Recent advances in cancer, chemotherapy and medical management of the geriatric cat. *Veterinary International* **5**, 3–12

Ogilvie GK, Obradovich JE, Cooper MF, Walters LM, Salman MD and Boone TC (1992) Use of recombinant canine granulocyte colony-stimulating factor to decrease myelosuppression associated with the administration of mitoxantrone in the dog. *Journal of Veterinary Internal Medicine* **6**, 44–47

Rosol TJ, Nagode LA, Couto CG, Hammer AS, Chew DJ, Peterson JL, Ayl RD, Steinmeyer CL and Capen CC (1992) Parathyroid hormone (PTH)-related protein, PTH, and 1, 25-dihydroxyvitamin D in dogs with cancer-associated hypercalcaemia. *Endocrinology* **131**, 1157–1164

Safran N, Perk K and Eyal O (1992) Isolation and preliminary characterisation of a novel retrovirus from a leukaemic dog. *Research in Veterinary Science* **52**, 250–255

Sykes GP, King JM and Cooper BC (1985) Retrovirus-like particles associated with myeloproliferative disease in the dog. *Journal of Comparative Pathology* **95**, 559–564

Vernau W and Moore PF (1999) An immunophenotypic study of canine leukemias and preliminary assessment of clonality by polymerase chain reaction. *Veterinary Immunology and Immunopathology* **69**, 145–164

(iv) Feline Retrovirus Infections

Andrew Sparkes and Kostas Papasouliotis

INTRODUCTION

Three exogenous contagious retroviruses are transmitted between cats (Figure 8.35): feline syncytium-forming virus (FeSFV), feline leukaemia virus (FeLV) and feline immunodeficiency virus (FIV). Of these viruses, FeSFV is generally considered to be non-pathogenic, whereas FeLV and FIV are important and common causes of disease. Infection with either FeLV or FIV can have a profound effect on haematological variables, some of which may be diagnostically helpful in alerting the clinician to the possibility of these viruses as an underlying cause of disease. Although there are many similarities in the diseases produced by these two viruses, there are also important differences in many aspects of their epidemiology, pathogenesis, diagnosis and control, and these aspects will therefore be briefly considered separately for each virus.

FELINE LEUKAEMIA VIRUS (FeLV)

Epidemiology of FeLV

Cats persistently infected with FeLV excrete large quantities of labile virus in their saliva and nasal secretions. Transmission of infection is mainly horizontal and occurs primarily during prolonged direct social interaction between infected and susceptible cats where there is opportunity for exchange of saliva (e.g. mutual grooming, sharing of food/food bowls). Vertical transmission is also possible, but persistent FeLV infection usually results in infertility, abortion or resorption of fetuses in a pregnant queen.

The outcome after exposure to FeLV depends on many factors, including the dose of virus, the viral strain and host resistance (related to the age of the cat, its immunocompetence and probably also its geno-type). In colonies of cats where FeLV is endemic, typically 30% will be persistently infected (persistently viraemic), 40% will have had self-limiting infections and be immune and 30% will have had insufficient exposure to establish infection. Of those cats with self-limiting infections, a proportion will experience transient viraemia before the immune response limits the infection, and a proportion will be latently infected (have proviral FeLV DNA integrated into certain host cells) for a period of time. Clinically and epidemiologically it is the persistently viraemic cats that are most important, although a small proportion of latently or previously infected cats may also develop FeLV-related disease.

Worldwide it is estimated that 1–3% of the general cat population is persistently infected with FeLV. However, the prevalence of infection varies according to the population of cats studied (their lifestyle and potential for exposure to FeLV), and there is also evidence of geographical and regional variations in the prevalence of FeLV. FeLV infection is most common in cats up to 5 years of age, with a declining prevalence thereafter (Hosie *et al.*, 1989).

Pathogenesis of FeLV infection

If a cat infected with FeLV fails to eliminate the infection within the first 4–6 weeks, haemolymphatic infection is established, which almost invariably results in persistent viraemia. FeLV replicates most effectively in rapidly dividing cells, having a particular tropism for the haemopoietic stem cells in the bone marrow, the intestinal crypt epithelial cells and the germinal centres of lymphoid follicles. Infection of bone marrow stem cells generally leads to large quantities of virus being produced, which overwhelms the host's immune response, leading to persistent viraemia. Within the bone marrow, those

Family	Subfamily	Virus
Retroviridae	Spumavirinae	Feline syncytium-forming virus
	Oncornavirinae	Feline leukaemia virus
	Lentivirinae	Feline immunodeficiency virus

Figure 8.35: Feline retroviruses.

cells of the myelomonocyte lineage develop an increasing virus burden as they mature, whereas in the erythrocyte precursors there is a greater viral burden in the early undifferentiated cells. The persistent viraemia of bone marrow origin is partly cell associated, with circulation of infected neutrophils, lymphocytes, monocytes and platelets, in addition to free virus being present in plasma.

Infection with FeLV can result in either cytoproliferative (neoplastic) diseases, such as lymphoma, sarcoma and myeloproliferative disorders, and/or cytosuppressive (degenerative) diseases such as immunodeficiency, anaemia and myelosuppressive disorders. The outcome of infection in any individual is partly determined by the subgroups or strains of FeLV infecting that cat.

Individual cells are infected with FeLV when the major viral envelope glycoprotein (gp70) binds to specific cellular receptors, resulting in release of the viral RNA genome into the cell cytoplasm. Under the influence of the viral reverse transcriptase and the host cell's DNA polymerase, a double-stranded DNA copy (provirus) of the single-stranded RNA viral genome is produced. The provirus is integrated into the host cell genome during cellular division and can then lead to productive infection (cellular synthesis of viral proteins, which are assembled into viral particles that bud from the cell surface). The pathogenesis of FeLV-related disease at a cellular level is not fully understood, but whereas infected cells are often able to function normally, in other cases the accumulation of certain viral proteins (e.g. p15E, gp70) within the cytoplasm may disrupt cellular function. In addition, the insertion of the proviral DNA into the host cell genome can disrupt or activate certain cellular proto-oncogenes leading to insertional mutagenesis and neoplastic transformation of the cell. Another adverse effect seen with some FeLV strains is failure to integrate the proviral DNA into the genome, leading to an accumulation of cytoplasmic viral DNA that can again disrupt cellular function and cause cytotoxicity.

According to the antigenic structure of the gp70 envelope glycoprotein, FeLV isolates are divided into three major subgroups: A, B and C. Subgroup A is the major naturally acquired transmissible form of FeLV, whereas subgroups B and C generally arise de novo in infected cats as a result of mutation of the proviral DNA and/or recombination of this DNA with endogenous FeLV-related DNA sequences present in the cat's genome. FeLV A is invariably found in all FeLV-infected cats, whereas subgroup B is found in around 50% of infected cats and subgroup C in just 1–2% of infected cats. Mixed infections with subgroups A and B are generally considered more pathogenic than infection with FeLV A alone, and infections with subgroup C lead to the rapid development of erythroid aplasia, thymic atrophy and lymphoid depletion.

Rarely, FeLV DNA may recombine with certain cellular proto-oncogenes to form the acutely transforming feline sarcoma virus (FeSV). These viruses are defective, requiring FeLV to sustain their replication, but they result in rapid neoplastic transformation of cells, with the induction of multiple malignant sarcomas.

Diseases associated with FeLV infection

Uncommonly, but particularly if infected at a young age, cats may develop FeLV-related disease and die within a few weeks of the onset of viraemia. More usually, however, FeLV-related disease occurs after a prolonged period (months to years) of asymptomatic viraemia. FeLV is a common cause of chronic disease in cats, the prevalence of viraemia in sick cats typically being 10–20% (Hosie *et al.*, 1989). Furthermore, FeLV-related disease commonly results in death of the infected cat; about 50% of infected cats die within 6 months of the diagnosis being made, and more than 80% die within 3.5 years.

Although FeLV is an oncogenic virus, the development of neoplasia accounts for only around 10–25% of FeLV-related deaths. Solid lymphomas are the most common tumours caused by FeLV infection, with thymic, alimentary, multicentric and atypical (miscellaneous) forms also being described. Most FeLV-related lymphomas are T-cell malignancies and most are subleukaemic, although a proportion will be accompanied by lymphocytic leukaemia. In addition to lymphomas, FeLV infection may result in the development of a variety of leukaemias (predominantly of erythroid or myelomonocytic origin) or myeloproliferative disorders.

Cytosuppressive (degenerative) diseases account for 75% or more of FeLV-related deaths, and of the different syndromes recognized, FeLV-associated immunosuppression is the most important, probably accounting for around 50% of all FeLV-related diseases. The pathogenesis of the immunosuppression includes defective neutrophil function, dysfunction and depletion of T lymphocytes, immune complex formation and complement depletion. The resulting immunosuppression leaves the infected cat susceptible to a wide variety of secondary and opportunistic infections.

Other manifestations of FeLV infection include anaemia (present in up to 30–50% of FeLV-infected cats), myelosuppression, enteropathy, reproductive failure, neurological disorders, fading kittens (thymic atrophy) and immune complex-related diseases (polyarthritis, glomerulonephropathies).

Specific haematological changes associated with FeLV infection

Primary infection

Most FeLV strains will cause a lymphopenia during the first 2 months after infection, with a variable effect on lymphocyte subsets. Conversely, lymphocytosis is sometimes seen, but in most cases these leucocyte changes resolve, and these variables remain normal or near normal throughout the prolonged asymptomatic period. Occasionally, with infection by more virulent FeLV strains, a persistent decrease in lymphocyte numbers (including CD4$^+$ and CD8$^+$ T cells) is seen, which contributes to the early development of immuno-suppression in these cats.

Anaemia

The development of anaemia is a common consequence of FeLV infection and may account for up to 25% of FeLV-related deaths. FeLV infection is recognized as the single most common cause of anaemia in the cat. As the haematopoietic stem cells are a major target for FeLV replication, the anaemia can be a manifestation of FeLV-induced myelodysplasia or erythroid aplasia. In other situations, the anaemia is haemolytic in origin.

Between 10% and 20% of FeLV-related anaemias are regenerative. These anaemias are characterized by anisocytosis, polychromasia, reticulocytosis, macrocytosis and the appearance of nucleated red blood cells, which can be associated with extramedullary (splenic and hepatic) erythropoiesis. Most commonly, these anaemias are either immune-mediated or due to concurrent infection with *Haemobartonella felis* (see Chapter 5). Because of the established relationship between FeLV infection and haemobartonellosis (Bobade *et al.*, 1988), evaluation of fresh (not ethyl-enediamine tetra-acetic acid-preserved) blood smears for *H. felis* is advisable in all cases of FeLV-associated anaemia. The prognosis for anaemic FeLV-infected cats is poor. Some cats may show temporary resolution of the anaemia – either spontaneously or in response to appropriate therapy – but recurrence of anaemia is common and many will eventually progress to develop lymphoma, myeloproliferative disease, leukaemia or erythroid aplasia.

Most FeLV-induced anaemias are non-regenerative and may be associated with myeloproliferative disorders, myelofibrosis and osteosclerosis, dyserythropoiesis or erythroid aplasia (which can sometimes be a part of a pancytopenia). Myeloproliferative diseases will sometimes lead to the appearance of leukaemic cells in blood smears, but more commonly the specific diagnosis of these cases requires examination of bone marrow aspirates. Some cases of dyserythropoietic anaemia exhibit high numbers of circulating nucleated red blood cells without concomitant reticulocytosis and others show a noticeable megaloblastic anaemia, which is unrelated to vitamin B12 deficiency (Figure 8.36). Although generally classified as non-regenerative, some of these anaemias may in fact show evidence of partial (but inadequate) red cell regeneration.

In the cat, 70% or more of non-regenerative anaemias are due to FeLV infection, and red cell

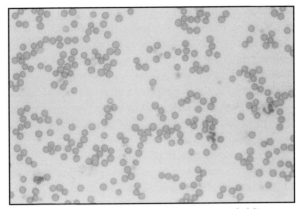

Figure 8.36: *Megaloblastic anaemia in a cat with feline leukaemia virus.*

aplasia is the most common cause, although in practice it may not be easy to distinguish red cell aplasia from certain myeloproliferative diseases and dyserythropoiesis, and these may occur concurrently in an infected cat.

Red cell aplasia is characterized by normocytic normochromic anaemia or sometimes macrocytic normochromic anaemia with reticulocytopenia of both aggregate and punctate forms. Bone marrow aspirates show a noticeable increase in the myeloid:erythroid ratio due to depletion of erythroid precursors. There is a strong association between the development of red cell aplasia and infection with FeLV subgroup C, and in experimental infections the appearance of subgroup C in plasma immediately precedes the development of progressive anaemia. It seems that FeLV C infects early erythroid precursors (burst-forming units – erythroid, and colony-forming units – erythroid) in the bone marrow, causing both depletion of these cells and also a decreased responsiveness to normal growth factors, thus the anaemia progresses despite markedly increased serum erythropoietin concentrations. There is evidence that much of the red cell aplasia attributed to infection with FeLV C is mediated by the cytotoxic and cytosuppressive effects of the gp70 envelope glyco-protein of this subgroup. Coinfection with *H. felis* may also contribute to these non-regenerative anaemias.

Lymphopenia and neutropenia

Although infection with FeLV can induce immuno-suppression through functional disturbances of both lymphocytes and neutrophils, many cats will also have depletion of these cell lines. Up to 70% of infected cats will have lymphopenia and up to 35% may have absolute leucopenia. The lymphopenia seems to involve both B and T cells.

In addition to lymphopenia, neutropenia has also been reported frequently in FeLV-infected cats, and FeLV infection should be regarded as an important differential diagnosis for any neutropenic cat. Cyclic fluctuations in the numbers of neutrophils (cyclic neutropenia), lymphocytes and other circulating cells (cyclic haematopoiesis) have been reported in some FeLV-infected cats (Swenson *et al.*, 1987). Neutropenia is an important finding as it frequently leads to secondary infections that may overwhelm the cat. Although neutropenia and/or leucopenia may be a manifestation of the cytopathic effect of FeLV infection, they may also reflect underlying myeloproliferative diseases or preleukaemic syndromes.

FeLV myeloblastopenia
FeLV-associated myeloblastopenia is clinically indistinguishable from feline panleucopenia virus infection and is reported to occur relatively frequently in FeLV-infected cats. The syndrome is characterized by profound anaemia (frequently aplastic) in combination with severe leucopenia (i.e. pancytopenia), which is accompanied by dysentery, vomiting, anorexia and depression. Affected cats invariably die. The combination of signs in these cats presumably reflects the replication of FeLV in target cells of the intestinal epithelium and bone marrow, although the picture may be complicated by secondary bacterial infection.

'Normal' leucocyte responses
Although many, if not all, FeLV-viraemic cats are immunosuppressed to some degree, this does not necessarily prevent them mounting a response to secondary or opportunistic infections. Many infected cats will therefore exhibit neutrophilic leucocytosis, perhaps with a left shift as an appropriate response to concurrent bacterial (or viral) infections.

Platelet abnormalities
Both megakaryocytes and platelets harbour FeLV. Macrothrombocytes with impaired function and decreased longevity are common in infected cats, and although this could potentially lead to bleeding disorders, such disorders have rarely been described in FeLV-infected cats. In a recent study, FeLV infection was identified in 27% (11 of 41) of thrombocytopenic cats, two of which had bleeding disorders (Jordan *et al.*, 1993).

FeLV-induced leukaemias
Leukaemias are characterized by neoplastic cells present in the peripheral circulation, and FeLV is the agent responsible for most (70-90%) feline leukaemias. Lymphoblastic (Figure 8.37) or lymphocytic leukaemia may occur alone or in combination with solid lymphomas, and other FeLV-associated leukaemias include acute and chronic myelogenous leukaemia and more rarely, monocytic, myelomonocytic, erythrocytic, megakaryocytic, eosinophilic and undifferentiated leukaemias.

Diagnosis of FeLV infection
The diagnosis of FeLV infection is usually straightforward. The clinician will be alerted to the possibility

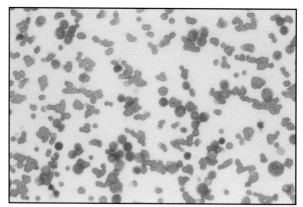

Figure 8.37: *Lymphoblastic leukaemia in a cat with feline leukaemia virus.*

of underlying FeLV as a cause of disease by the clinical history (e.g. recurrent episodes of disease suggesting immunosuppression), clinical findings and clinico-pathological changes. As most cases of FeLV-related disease occur in persistently viraemic cats, detection of infection is readily achieved by assaying blood samples for the presence of p27 – one of the core proteins of FeLV, which is almost invariably present in the plasma of persistently infected cats. Figure 8.38 lists the tests currently available in the United Kingdom for detection of this antigen and some of these are shown in Figure 8.39. Newer kits designed for 'in-house' diagnostic testing, such as the ELISA 'Snap' test (Idexx) and 'Witness' immunogold migration test (Mérial) virtually eliminate the possibility of operator error and are thus highly reliable. As with any test, on rare occasions false positives and false negatives can occur. If there is any reason to doubt the validity of a positive test result, repeating the test at a reference laboratory by using the technique of virus isolation is recommended as this is currently considered the 'gold standard' by which other tests are measured. Although false negative test results are considered extremely uncommon, if FeLV is still considered a strong possibility despite a negative 'in-house' test result, confirmation may again be sought through virus isolation. It should be remembered however, that not all cats with FeLV-related disease will be persistently viraemic, and it is estimated that 2–6% of cats that recover from FeLV infections (i.e. do not develop persistent viraemia) will go on to develop FeLV-related disease.

Treatment of FeLV-infected cats
The decision on whether to treat an FeLV-infected cat must be made on an individual basis but will be influenced by the clinical condition of the cat, the short- and long-term prognosis, the risk the infected individual poses to other cats, and the owner's wishes. Symptomatic and supportive therapy is most often provided for concurrent, secondary or opportunistic infections (e.g. *H. felis*), and it is important that these infections are correctly identified to allow specific therapy.

Detection of antigenaemia
Plate ELISA   Petchek FeLV (Idexx)
Membrane ELISA   Snap FeLV/FIV Combo (Idexx)
Rapid immunogold migration   Witness FeLV (Mérial)   SpeedCat Duo (Vetlab Supplies)
Immunofluorescence   Some commercial laboratories (e.g. VetLab   Services)
Detection of antigen in saliva
Not recommended for routine testing due to   decreased reliability
Detection of virus
Virus isolation   Feline Diagnostic Service (University of Bristol)   Feline Virus Unit (University of Glasgow)
Polymerase chain reaction (PCR) to detect   proviral DNA   Some commercial laboratories (e.g. Axiom   Laboratories)

Figure 8.38: Some diagnostic tests for feline leukaemia virus (FeLV) in the United Kingdom.
ELISA, enzyme-linked immunosorbent assay; FIV, feline immunodeficiency virus.

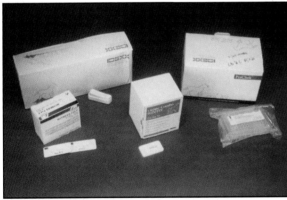

Figure 8.39: Various commercially available test kits for the diagnosis of feline leukaemia virus and feline immunodeficiency virus infections.

A wide variety of anti-viral drugs and/or those that modify biological responses have been used in an attempt to reverse the viraemia in FeLV-infected cats (reviewed by Rojko and Hardy, 1994). Although some of these agents have apparently been of benefit in individual cases, overall the response is poor, and currently no specific agent or combination of agents can be recommended.

The use of corticosteroids may have some rationale in cases of immune-mediated haemolytic anaemia, and corticosteroids may also have a beneficial effect in cases of cyclic neutropenia (perhaps through release of the bone marrow pool of neutrophils). However, it is important that covering antibiotics are used at the same time because of the risk of severe immunosuppression.

FeLV-associated lymphoma and lymphoid leukaemia may respond to appropriate chemotherapy but the 'risks versus benefits' need to be carefully assessed before commencing such therapy in a viraemic cat.

Control of FeLV

Traditionally, FeLV has been controlled in colonies of cats by the 'test and removal' policy, which has been shown to work well (Jarrett, 1994). More recently, the introduction of FeLV vaccination has meant that the general cat population can also be afforded some protection against this disease. Although vaccination is a valuable tool to help prevent infection in cats that could potentially encounter the virus, it is important to appreciate that none of the FeLV vaccines available have been shown to provide 100% protection against infection. Vaccination may clearly be desirable in cats that are considered to be 'at risk' of acquiring FeLV (e.g. cats that are allowed free access outdoors), but because vaccine efficacy is known to be less than 100%, it is important that a vaccinated cat is not deliberately exposed to the virus. Furthermore, a current vaccination certificate should not be taken in lieu of a negative FeLV blood test when screening cats before admission to a cattery. The use of vaccines does not interfere with the routine diagnostic tests for FeLV.

FELINE IMMUNODEFICIENCY VIRUS (FIV)

Epidemiology of FIV

As with FeLV infection, the source of FIV is a cat persistently infected with this virus. Like FeLV, FIV is a labile virus, which is secreted in the saliva of infected cats. In contrast to FeLV, however, the normal mucosal barrier provides a relatively strong defence against penetration by FIV, thus direct inoculation of the virus by biting is the major route of transmission. The risk of transmission by social contact is much lower than with FeLV, and although vertical transmission and transmission via milk has been shown with FIV, this is probably not epidemiologically important.

The fact that biting is the major route of transmission explains why FIV infection is much more common in male cats, free-roaming cats and non-pedigree cats. The age distribution of FIV infection also differs from FeLV, infection being uncommon in young cats (less than one year old), but the prevalence increases with age to reach a peak in the 6–10-year-old age group (Hosie *et al.*, 1989). Importantly, once a cat has been infected with FIV it will remain infected permanently. The normal immune response is unable to eliminate the virus from the body.

FIV is endemic in cat populations throughout the world. Typically, in the general cat population the prevalence of FIV in the United Kingdom and North America is 1–6% (Hopper *et al*., 1994), but the overall prevalence of infection depends on many factors, including the lifestyle of the cats studied and their population density.

Pathogenesis of FIV infection

After infection, FIV has been shown to have a tropism for both CD4$^+$ and CD8$^+$ T lymphocytes as well as macrophages and astrocytes, with cellular infection and integration of proviral DNA occurring in a similar way to FeLV infection. Noticeable viraemia is present during the first 2–4 weeks after infection, but coincidental with the development of an antibody response, the viraemia declines to low levels for many months to years until the terminal stages of disease.

After initial exposure to the virus, most FIV-infected cats exhibit a prolonged asymptomatic period, typically lasting 2–5 years, but during this time there is progressive impairment of the immune system. Although replication of the virus occurs at only a low level during most stages of infection, FIV can nevertheless be recovered from many sources, including circulating lymphocytes, lymph nodes, spleen, bone marrow, saliva, brain and cerebrospinal fluid. A depletion of CD4$^+$ T lymphocytes and an inverted CD4$^+$/CD8$^+$ T-cell ratio are characteristic early findings in FIV-infected cats, and these changes continue to progress with time (Novotney *et al*., 1990; Barlough *et al*., 1991). As early as 6 months after infection, impaired T-cell responses can be detected, and eventually the immunodeficiency caused by FIV leads to the development of clinical signs, often related to recurrent secondary or opportunistic infections.

It is clear that there are many different strains of FIV, and this is one factor that may determine the clinical effect of infection, the rapidity with which lymphocyte subset changes occur and duration of the asymptomatic period. Other factors may also be important to the development of disease, such as the age of the cat at the time of infection, exposure dose, route of infection and potential exposure to other pathogens.

Diseases associated with FIV infection

Infection with FIV is a significant cause of disease in cats, and it has been shown that the prevalence of infection among cats showing clinical signs compatible with an immunodeficiency syndrome (i.e. cats with chronic or recurrent disease) is typically 15–20% (Hopper *et al*., 1994).

Based on the staging system used to classify humans infected with human immunodeficiency virus (HIV), a five-point clinical staging of FIV-infected cats has been proposed, although the validity of this needs to be established. Experimentally, a distinct acute phase is seen around 4 weeks after infection, characterized by pyrexia of several days to weeks duration, neutropenia and generalized lymphadenopathy (lasting up to 9 months). The neutropenia may lead to the development of secondary infections, but fatalities in this stage are rare.

After acute infection, cats enter an asymptomatic stage which, as already noted, is of variable duration but generally lasts several years. Although asymptomatic, the cat has a progressively impaired immune system, which ultimately leads on to symptomatic FIV infection.

Many cats are presented for treatment or investigation during the feline equivalent of the HIV-associated persistent generalized lymphadenopathy (PGL) or AIDS-related complex (ARC) stages of the disease. The signs that develop have frequently been likened to the non-neoplastic (immunosuppressive) findings that occur in association with FeLV infection. The most common presenting signs are persistent or recurrent diseases of the oral cavity, respiratory tract and gastrointestinal tract. Non-specific signs such as lethargy, malaise, weight loss, lymphadenopathy and pyrexia are also common. Oral cavity diseases are encountered particularly frequently and include chronic gingivitis and stomatitis and periodontitis of varying severity. Some cats develop neurological signs or neoplasia as a consequence of their FIV infection, and as the disease progresses it is common to find multiple clinical signs in an infected individual.

In the terminal stages of FIV, an AIDS-like syndrome may be identified, but its classification lacks the clarity of that in HIV infection. Features consistent with this stage of the disease would include profound (greater than 20%) weight loss, multiple opportunistic infections (e.g. cryptococcosis, toxoplasmosis, poxvirus and mycobacteriosis), anaemia and leucopenia.

Specific haematological changes associated with FIV infection

Primary infection

Neutropenia with or without concomitant leucopenia is a common feature of the primary stage of FIV infection. Although many cats may pass through this stage with little or no overt clinical signs, a small proportion may develop significant disease, including secondary infections due to the neutropenia. As with FeLV, testing for FIV is advisable in any cat that presents with neutropenia.

Haematological changes are commonly seen in association with the later stages of FIV infection and these are comparable to the changes encountered in HIV-infected humans.

Anaemia

Anaemia is frequently found in the later (symptomatic) stages of FIV infection, and studies of naturally occurring disease suggest a prevalence of anaemia of between

15% and 40% in these infected cats. As with FeLV infection, FIV-induced immunosuppression will predispose cats to secondary *H. felis* infection, and it is important to consider this organism as a potential underlying cause of, or contributory factor to, anaemia. Both regenerative and non-regenerative anaemias are encountered in FIV-infected cats and, with the latter, bone marrow aspirates are indicated to rule out myeloproliferative disorders or myelodysplasia. Thrombocytopenia is occasionally seen in FIV-infected cats.

Lymphopenia and neutropenia
Lymphopenia has been reported in 30–55% of FIV-infected cats, and neutropenia in 5–35%. Both of these may contribute to a leucopenia that has been reported in 5–30% of infected cats. Along with FeLV, FIV should be considered a primary cause of neutropenia in the cat, although the pathogenesis of this and other cytopenias in FIV is poorly understood. A reversible neutropenia has been reported in six of seven FIV-infected cats that were treated with griseofulvin, and this bears similarity to the observation of antibiotic-associated neutropenias in HIV-infected humans, although again the precise pathogenesis of these changes is unclear.

The lymphopenia in FIV infection is frequently profound, and although the stress of concurrent disease may be partly responsible for this change, the selective depletion of CD4+ T cells will also contribute to this finding. From studies of FIV-infected cats, and by analogy with HIV infection, other factors likely to be involved in the pathogenesis of the various cytopenias include FIV infection of bone marrow stem cells and accessory cells, viraemia and/or viral proteins inhibiting haematopoiesis, an imbalance of bone marrow T cells, an alteration in T-cell cytokine profiles, which affect haematopoiesis and triggering of immune-mediated mechanisms.

'Normal' leucocyte responses
As with FeLV-induced immunosuppression, depending on the stage of disease, many FIV-infected cats that have concurrent or secondary infections will still elicit an overtly appropriate haematological response. Thus studies have shown leucocytosis, neutrophilia and a left shift as common findings in FIV-infected individuals, often in association with an obvious purulent or inflammatory disease process.

Haematological changes in terminal disease
Although it can be difficult to accurately clinically stage an FIV-infected cat, there is evidence that those cats with more advanced disease and those that are entering the terminal stages of disease are much more likely to have severe and multiple cytopenias present on haematological examination (Sparkes *et al.*, 1993). Results of routine haematology may therefore have some prognostic value for the individual, although it is important to interpret these findings in light of the clinical picture.

Lymphoproliferative and myeloproliferative disorders
There is clear evidence that FIV infection predisposes cats to the development of lymphoproliferative and myeloproliferative disorders, although it is not yet certain whether FIV is directly oncogenic or acts as a facilitator through disruption of the normal immune surveillance that would eliminate neoplastic cells. Although much less common than FeLV as a cause of these disorders, a similar range of haematological changes can occur.

Diagnosis of FIV infection
Unlike the diagnosis of FeLV, there is too little FIV-derived antigen present in plasma to be detected using currently available technologies. As FIV infections are persistent, routine diagnosis can be based on detection of circulating antibodies to the virus, which is generally reliable. Figure 8.40 lists the tests currently available in the United Kingdom, and some of these are shown in Figure 8.39.

Serology (detection of FIV antibodies)
Plate ELISA Petchek FIV (Idexx)
Membrane ELISA Snap FeLV/FIV (Idexx)
Rapid immunogold migration Witness FIV (Mérial) SpeedCat Duo (Vetlab Supplies)
Immunofluorescence Feline Virus Unit (University of Glasgow)
Western immunoblotting Limited to research institutes
Detection of virus
Virus isolation Limited to research institutes
Polymerase chain reaction (PCR) to identify proviral DNA Currently mainly limited to research institutes Some commercial laboratories, e.g. Axiom Laboratories

Figure 8.40: *Diagnostic tests for feline immunodeficiency virus (FIV) in the United Kingdom.*
ELISA, enzyme-linked immunosorbent assay.

As with FeLV diagnosis, several 'in-house' diagnostic kits are available for the rapid detection of FIV antibodies, and the newer 'Snap' (Idexx) and 'Witness' (Mérial) kits have done much to minimize the danger of technical error when performing these tests. Even when technical error is eliminated, false positive and false negative results are more of a concern with FIV than FeLV testing. In a cat showing clinical signs compatible with FIV infection, and perhaps with clinicopathological changes consistent with FIV, a positive result from a correctly performed test is highly likely to be reliable. However, an as yet undetermined proportion of FIV-infected cats (possibly as high as 10-15%) are seronegative on conventional testing. The reasons for this are unclear, but may include individual variation in the response to FIV infection. A terminal decline in antibody concentrations is seen in HIV infection, but there is little evidence that this is an important factor in FIV-infected cats that are sero-negative. There is currently no easy solution to the concern of cats suspected of having FIV infection that test seronegative. One approach is to repeat the sero-logical test at 2-6 monthly intervals and, as many of the rapid immunodiagnostic kits rely on detection of antibodies to a single viral protein, the use of a different test methodology looking for antibodies to alternative or multiple antigens (e.g. western blotting or immuno-fluorescence) may have some merit in these cases.

Detection of integrated proviral DNA by the polymerase chain reaction (PCR) is now available as a commercial diagnostic assay for FIV infection. This is potentially an extremely sensitive test and may be particularly useful in cases of suspected FIV infections that are seronegative by conventional tests. However, PCR is a relatively expensive test and requires strin-gent quality control to ensure reliability of test results, thus making it unsuitable for routine diagnostic use at this time. Additionally, to date there have been no published studies critically assessing the reliability of PCR for diagnosis of clinical FIV infection.

Treatment of FIV infection

As with FeLV, treatment of FIV-infected cats is largely symptomatic and supportive, although again efforts should be made to identify specific secondary or oppor-tunistic infections that can be appropriately treated. Specific treatment for haematological abnormalities is not feasible, but consideration of concurrent drug therapy and the possibility of drug-associated side effects should be considered when faced with an FIV-infected cat that is neutropenic. The reverse transcriptase inhibitor zidovudine (AZT) at a dose of 5 mg/kg twice daily has shown some efficacy in the clinical management of FIV-infected cats, although its myelosuppressive activ-ity, and in particular the induction of anaemia, may preclude its long-term continual use.

Control of FIV

As no vaccine is available for FIV, control of this disease relies on detection of infected cats and then ensuring they are managed in such a way that they are unlikely to transmit infection. This may involve the neutering of entire cats, and confining cats to prevent them wandering. Specific aspects of the control of FIV have been outlined by Hopper et al. (1994).

REFERENCES AND FURTHER READING

Barlough JE, Ackley CD, George JW, Levy N, Acevedo R, Moore PF, Rideout BA, Cooper MD and Pedersen NC (1991) Acquired immune dysfunction in cats with experimentally induced feline immunodeficiency virus infection: comparison of short-term and long-term infections. *Journal of Acquired Immune Deficiency Syndromes* **4**, 219-227

Bobade PA, Nash AS and Rogerson P (1988) Feline haemobartonellosis: clinical, haematological and pathological studies in natural infections and the relationship to infection with feline leukaemia virus. *Veterinary Record* **122**, 32-36

Hoover EA and Mullins JI (1991) Feline leukaemia virus infection and diseases. *Journal of the American Veterinary Medical Association* **199**, 1287-1297

Hopper CD, Sparkes AH and Harbour DA (1994) Feline immunodeficiency virus. In: *Feline Medicine and Therapeutics, 2nd edn*, ed. EA Chandler, CJ Gaskell and RM Gaskell, pp. 488-505. Blackwell Scientific, Oxford

Hosie MJ, Robertson C and Jarrett O (1989) Prevalence of feline leukaemia virus and antibodies to feline immunodeficiency virus in cats in the United Kingdom. *Veterinary Record* **128**, 293-297

Jarrett O (1994) Feline leukaemia virus. In: *Feline Medicine and Therapeutics, 2nd edn*, ed. EA Chandler, CJ Gaskell and RM Gaskell, pp.473-487. Blackwell Scientific, Oxford

Jordan HL, Grindem CB and Brietschwerdt EB (1993) Thrombocytopenia in cats: a retrospective study of 41 cases. *Journal of Veterinary Internal Medicine* **7**, 261-265

Macy DW (1994) Feline immunodeficiency virus. In: *The cat, diseases and clinical management, 2nd edn*, ed. RG Sherding, pp. 433-448. Churchill Livingstone, New York

Novotney C, English RV, Housman J, Davidson MG, Naisse MP, Jeng C-R, Davis WC and Tompkins MB (1990) Lymphocyte population changes in cats naturally infected with feline immunodeficiency virus. *AIDS* **4**, 1213-1218

Pedersen NC and Barlough JE (1991) Clinical overview of feline immunodeficiency virus. *Journal of the American Veterinary Medical Association* **199**, 1298-1305

Rojko JL and Hardy WD (1994) Feline leukaemia virus and other retroviruses. In: *The cat, diseases and clinical management, 2nd edn*, ed. RG Sherding, pp. 263-432. Churchill Livingstone, New York

Shelton GH, Linenberger ML and Abkowitz JL (1991) Haematologic abnormalities in cats seropositive for feline immunodeficiency virus. *Journal of the American Veterinary Medical Association* **199**, 1353-1357

Sparkes AH, Hopper CD, Millard WG, Gruffydd-Jones TJ and Harbour DA (1993) Feline immunodeficiency virus infection – clinicopathological findings in 90 naturally occurring cases. *Journal of Veterinary Internal Medicine* **7**, 85-90

Swenson CL, Kociba GJ, O'Keefe DA, Crisp MS, Jacobs RM and Rojko JL (1987) Cyclic haematopoiesis associated with feline leukaemia virus infection in two cats. *Journal of the American Veterinary Medical Association* **191**, 93-96

PART TWO

Haemostasis

Overview of Haemostasis

Mary F. McConnell

INTRODUCTION

Blood is essential for the transport of oxygen and nutrients to the tissues and the return of carbon dioxide and waste products from the tissues. Haemostasis is the maintenance of vascular integrity and blood fluidity that is necessary for the normal function of blood. When a blood vessel is injured, blood loss must be minimized by the rapid formation of a clot at the site of injury. This is achieved by the formation of a platelet plug over the injury site (primary haemostasis) and the stabilization of this plug by a mesh of fibrin formed in the coagulation cascade (secondary haemostasis). It is equally important that the clot dissolves once the blood vessel is repaired, re-establishing normal blood flow. There is a constant delicate balance between clot formation and clot dissolution (fibrinolysis), which may be disturbed in either direction in a range of pathological conditions.

PRIMARY HAEMOSTASIS

Primary haemostasis is the interaction between platelets and damaged vascular endothelium to form a platelet plug at the site of injury (Hawiger, 1990). In capillaries and venules, this initial platelet plug combined with vasoconstriction may provide adequate haemostasis. In vessels where flow and pressure are greater, it is essential to stabilize this plug with an overlying mesh of insoluble fibrin formed by the process of secondary haemostasis.

Components required for primary haemostasis

Endothelium
The vascular system is lined by endothelial cells, which sit on a basement membrane that separates the endothelial cells from the subendothelial tissues. The subendothelial tissues contain a variety of components including collagen, fibroblasts, elastic fibres and smooth muscle. Platelets do not adhere to intact healthy endothelium. Ligands such as collagen and von Willebrand factor, which are involved in platelet adhesion to endothelium,

are sequestered within the subendothelium. Intact endothelial cells secrete antithrombotic substances such as prostacyclin, which is a vasodilator and platelet inhibitor. Platelets are also repelled by the negatively charged surface of the intact endothelial cell barrier.

von Willebrand factor
von Willebrand factor (vWf) is a large protein synthesized by endothelial cells, which has two major functions (Ruggeri and Ware, 1992). It is necessary for platelet adhesion at sites of vascular damage, and it functions as a carrier molecule for factor VIII in the circulation. It consists of multiple subunits, with both smaller and larger multiple-subunit forms being synthesized. The larger molecules are the most effective at binding to platelets and are preferentially stored within the endothelial cells until released in response to a variety of stimuli, including thrombin and fibrin. Some vWf is also constantly released into the plasma and the subendothelial tissues. A small amount of vWf is synthesized by megakaryocytes and stored within platelet granules.

Platelets
Mammalian platelets are small anucleate cells 2–4 μm in diameter derived from megakaryocytes in the bone marrow. They have a plasma membrane that contains numerous types of receptors, a cytoskeleton and contractile proteins that allow them to change shape and various types of granules, some of which can release their contents when platelets are activated. The dense granules contain cations, nucleotides and amines, whereas the α-granules contain numerous proteins, including fibrinogen, vWf and factors that promote vascular repair.

Mechanism and control of primary haemostasis
When a blood vessel is damaged, the endothelial cell barrier is broken and the subendothelial tissue is exposed (Figure 9.1). This results in a localized decrease in the factors that normally prevent platelet adhesion, as well as exposure of the platelets to subendothelial substances such as collagen, which promote platelet adhesion. Simultaneously, there is localized vasocon-

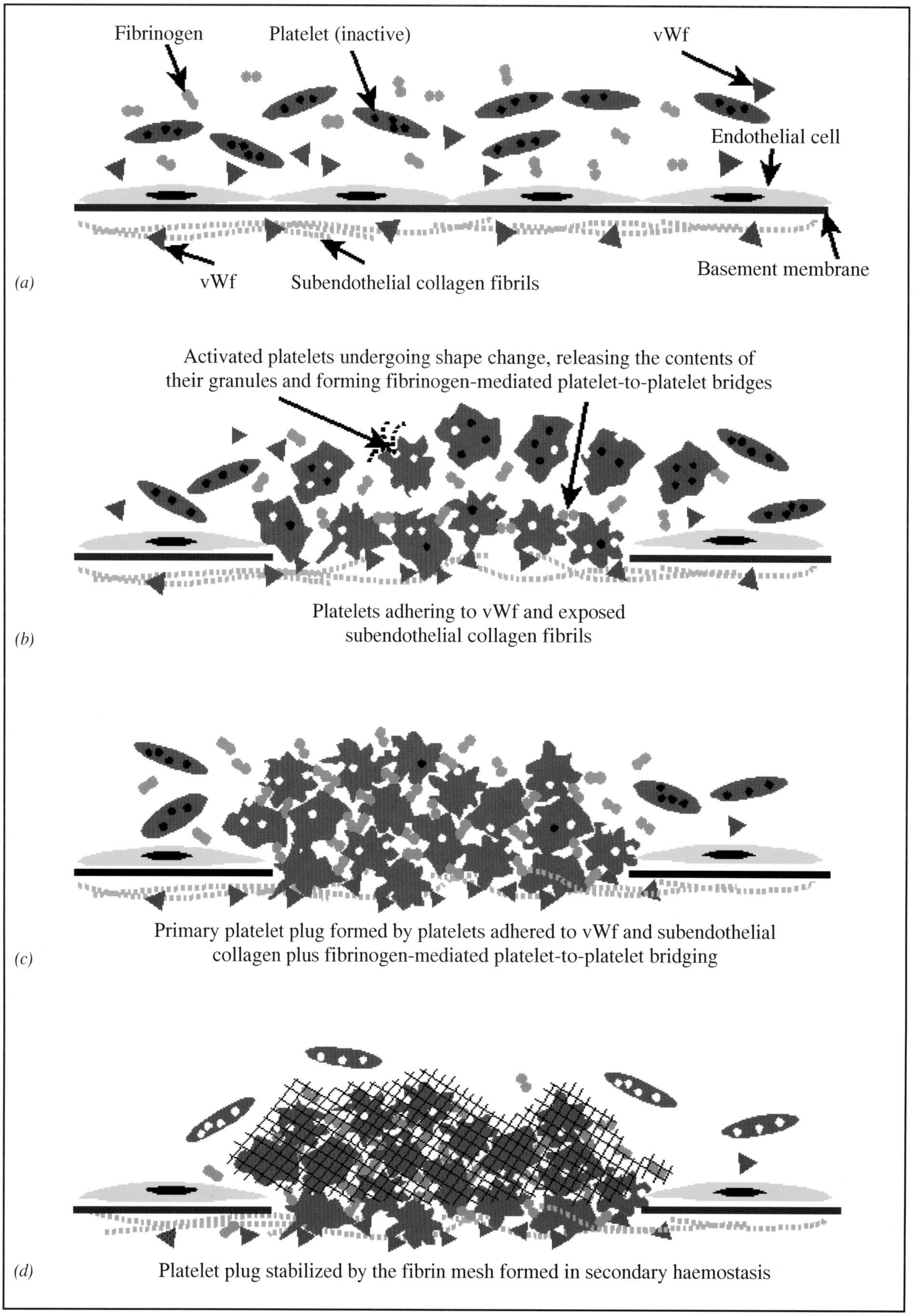

(a) Fibrinogen Platelet (inactive) vWf
Endothelial cell
vWf Subendothelial collagen fibrils Basement membrane

(b) Activated platelets undergoing shape change, releasing the contents of their granules and forming fibrinogen-mediated platelet-to-platelet bridges

Platelets adhering to vWf and exposed subendothelial collagen fibrils

(c) Primary platelet plug formed by platelets adhered to vWf and subendothelial collagen plus fibrinogen-mediated platelet-to-platelet bridging

(d) Platelet plug stabilized by the fibrin mesh formed in secondary haemostasis

Figure 9.1: *(a) Intact endothelium and components of primary haemostasis. (b) Initial response of platelets to vascular damage and exposure to subendothelial collagen fibres and von Willebrand factor (vWf). (c) Recruitment of platelets to the growing platelet plug in response to agonists released from the platelet granules and the generation of thrombin in secondary haemostasis. (d) Stabilization of the platelet plug by the fibrin mesh formed in secondary haemostasis.*

striction, which reduces the rate of blood flow. Platelets adhere to the subendothelial collagen via a specific plasma membrane receptor, and the binding of collagen to this receptor signals a message to the platelets that results in a series of events called platelet activation. Activated platelets change shape from smooth and discoid to round with numerous projecting pseudopods, which greatly increase platelet surface area. Activation exposes fibrinogen receptors on the platelet membrane and allows fibrinogen-mediated platelet-to-platelet aggregation. The contents of the dense and α-granules are released locally and help to recruit further platelets to the site of injury, where they bind to the platelets already bound to the subendothelium. The exposure of the subendothelial tissues also results in a conformational change in vWf that allows platelets to recognize and bind vWf, resulting in further adherence of platelets to the subendothelium as well as promoting further platelet activation. The primary haemostatic platelet plug over the site of vessel injury is formed by the combination of platelets adhered to the subendothelium and platelets aggregated to each other.

SECONDARY HAEMOSTASIS

Secondary haemostasis is the process of blood coagulation (Mann, 1999). Central to coagulation is the generation of thrombin, which converts soluble fibrinogen to insoluble fibrin. The fibrin is then crosslinked and forms a mesh, which stabilizes the platelet plug formed in primary haemostasis. Thrombin formation is the product of a cascade of enzymatic reactions initiated by tissue trauma and release of tissue factor. In this cascade, each coagulation factor is converted to its active form, which is then able to catalyse the next step in the cascade.

Traditionally, the coagulation cascade has been divided into the extrinsic, intrinsic and common pathways, with the intrinsic system initiated by contact activation and the extrinsic system initiated by the interaction of tissue factor and activated factor (F) VII. These two paths converge into the common pathway at the point where F X is activated. The lines between the extrinsic and intrinsic pathways have blurred as knowledge has increased, but the terms are used widely and are useful in the interpretation of in vitro coagulation tests in which the reactions may differ slightly from the coagulation cascade in vivo because of the conditions under which the assays are run. It is now known that the extrinsic tissue factor pathway is the primary pathway in the initiation of the blood coagulation cascade in vivo and that intrinsic activation is more important in sustaining the process.

Components required for secondary haemostasis

Negatively charged phospholipid surface
Activated platelets provide the negatively charged phospholipid surface that is essential for anchoring the two major enzyme-cofactor complexes (tenase and prothrombinase) formed during coagulation (Zwaal and Schroit, 1997). In resting platelets, the negatively charged membrane phospholipids are located on the inner leaflet of the lipid bilayer of the plasma membrane. When platelets are activated in primary haemostasis, these negatively charged phospholipids translocate to the outer surface of the platelet membrane where they are exposed to the circulating coagulation factors. The anchoring of the tenase and prothrombinase complexes to the platelets in the platelet plug also serves to localize the coagulation cascade and thrombin generation to the site of injury.

Ionized calcium (Ca^{++})
Ionized calcium (Ca^{++}) is essential for the formation and function of the tenase and prothrombinase complexes.

Tissue factor
Tissue factor is a glycoprotein that is part of the plasma membrane of a variety of cells, including subendothelial fibroblasts. Tissue factor is not normally present in the circulation or expressed on cell surfaces, but when subendothelial cells are damaged or activated, tissue factor is expressed and exposed to the circulating coagulation factors.

Contact activation factors
Traditionally, the contact activation factors (F XII, prekallikrein and high molecular weight kininogen) were thought to initiate the intrinsic branch of the coagulation pathway, but although the contact factors are important in in vitro clotting tests their significance in in vivo coagulation is doubtful, as deficiencies in these three contact factors are not associated with clinical bleeding disorders. They are included here because of their role in in vitro tests of coagulation. In the activated partial thromboplastin time (APTT), a surface activator is used to activate these contact factors, resulting in sequential activation of factors XI, IX, X and II (prothrombin) and fibrinogen.

These three plasma proteins may bind to negatively charged surfaces or molecular complexes where they interact to initiate a range of responses (Kaplan et al., 1997). Central to contact activation is the conversion of F XII to its active form, F XIIa. F XII is synthesized in the liver and circulates in the blood until it binds to an initiating surface and autoactivates to F XIIa. The initiating surface seems to be a negatively charged surface, most likely subendothelial basement membrane exposed during vascular injury. F XIIa is able to initiate the intrinsic coagulation pathway by converting F XI to F XIa. F XIIa also converts prekallikrein to kallikrein, which then converts high molecular weight kininogen to the inflammatory mediator bradykinin. In vivo the contact factors are more important in the initiation of inflammation and fibrinolysis than in coagulation.

F XI

F XI is synthesized by the liver and may be considered one of the contact factors. Unlike the other contact factors (F XII, prekallikrein and high molecular weight kininogen), its deficiency leads to a bleeding disorder. Although F XI can be activated by F XIIa, it is activated much more efficiently by thrombin in a positive feedback system and is more important in sustaining than initiating the coagulation cascade.

The vitamin K-dependent coagulation factors

The vitamin K-dependent clotting factors (factors II (prothrombin), VII, IX and X) are enzymes synthesized by the liver as inactive precursors (proenzymes), which are activated in the process of coagulation. They are often referred to as serine proteases because they belong to a group of enzymes that has a reactive serine at the active site. During synthesis, they undergo a vitamin K-dependent modification in which γ-carboxyglutamate is added to the protein. The γ-carboxyglutamate is negatively charged and able to bind strongly to Ca^{++}, resulting in the formation of Ca^{++}-coagulation factor complexes that bind to the negatively charged phospholipid surface of activated platelets. F VII is different to the other clotting factors in that it is poorly inhibited by the major natural anticoagulant, antithrombin III (ATIII) and 1-2% of the total F VII circulates as F VIIa (Morrisey et al., 1993). This F VIIa is available to initiate coagulation in response to endothelial damage and release of tissue factor

Cofactors F VIII and F V

Factors V and VIII are synthesized by the liver and function as non-enzymatic protein cofactors in coagulation. Once activated by thrombin or F Xa, they greatly increase the reaction rates of the tenase (F VIIIa) and prothrombinase (F Va) complexes.

Fibrinogen

Fibrinogen is a large plasma protein synthesized by the liver. It consists of two identical halves, each of which has three polypeptide chains (Aα, Bβ and γ) wound around each other to form a linear molecule. The amino ends of the Aα and Bβ chains are called fibrinopeptides A and B respectively. These fibrinopeptides are highly negatively charged and this keeps the fibrinogen molecules apart, preventing spontaneous aggregation within the circulation. Thrombin produced in the coagulation cascade cleaves the negatively charged fibrinopeptides A and B from the fibrinogen molecule to form fibrin monomers, which then spontaneously aggregate to form fibrin.

F XIII

F XIII is synthesized by the liver as an inactive precursor, which is activated by thrombin to F XIIIa at the site of clot formation. F XIIIa catalyses the formation of stable crosslinks between fibrin monomers.

Mechanism of secondary haemostasis

Secondary haemostasis is initiated by the same circumstances that initiate primary haemostasis (Figure 9.2). Tissue trauma results in exposure of the subendothelial tissues, with the primary initiating factor in secondary haemostasis being the exposure of tissue factor to the proteins of the blood coagulation system. Tissue factor initially combines with the small amount of pre-existing circulating F VIIa to form F VIIa-tissue factor complex that directly activates F X. The process is amplified as more F VII is activated by F Xa and by autoactivation, allowing the formation of more F VIIa-tissue factor complex. The function of tissue factor is to act as a regulatory protein, which greatly increases (greater than 10^7 times) the rate at which F VIIa autoactivates and activates factors IX and X. Although the F VIIa-tissue factor complex activates both factors IX and X, this does not mean that the activation of F X via F IXa and the tenase enzyme complex is redundant. Once a small amount of F Xa has been generated by direct activation of F X by the F VIIa-tissue factor complex, the F Xa molecule cooperates with the F VIIa-tissue factor complex resulting in preferred formation of F Xa via F IXa and the tenase complex.

The tenase complex consists of F VIIIa interacting with Ca^{++} and F IXa on the negatively charged surface provided by activated platelets. This anchors and localizes the tenase complex to the site of damage and allows tenase to activate F X to F Xa. F VIII is activated by F Xa and by thrombin in a positive feedback loop.

The prothrombinase complex is formed by F Xa with Ca^{++} and activated F V. This is bound on the negatively charged platelet membrane in a similar fashion to the tenase complex. F V is activated by thrombin and F Xa and is then able to bind and localize prothrombin (F II) to the site, as well as greatly increase the rate at which F Xa converts prothrombin to thrombin (F IIa). The generation of thrombin is central to normal haemostasis, and even minute amounts of thrombin result in massive amplification of the coagulation cascade via the thrombin-mediated feedback activation of factors V, VIII and XI. Thrombin is a potent platelet agonist and is important in the continued formation of the platelet plug in primary haemostasis. Thrombin rapidly converts fibrinogen into fibrin monomers and activates F XIII, which then crosslinks the fibrin monomers such that both end-to-end and side-to-side crosslinks are formed. All of the events of secondary haemostasis take place on the surface of the primary platelet plug, and the crosslinked fibrin mesh results in a firm fibrin plug that is much stronger than the primary platelet plug and resistant to proteolytic degradation by the fibrinolytic enzyme, plasmin.

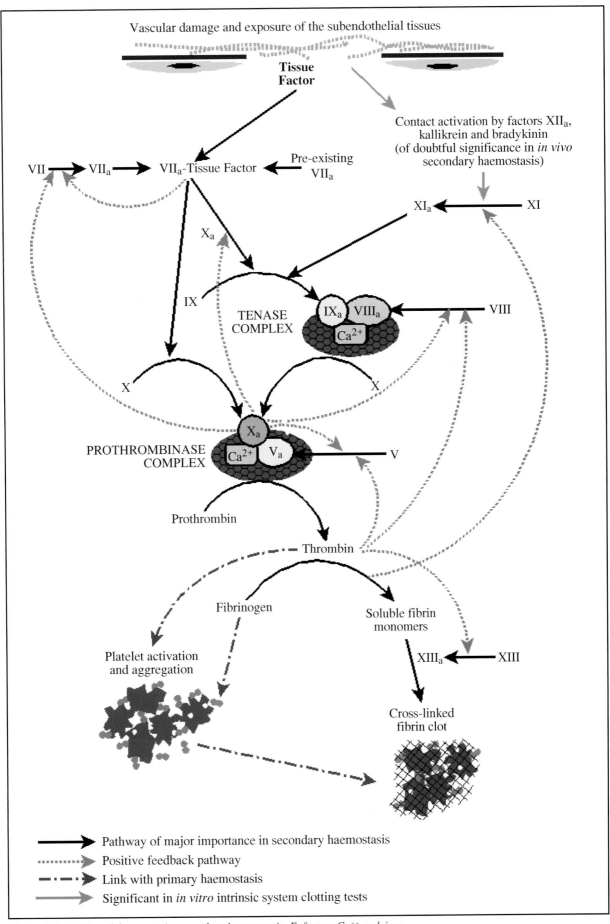

Figure 9.2: *Outline of the events in secondary haemostasis. F, factor; Ca⁺⁺, calcium.*

INHIBITORS OF COAGULATION

Blood clotting is terminated by two types of reactions. Constitutive inhibition is the constant baseline inhibition of coagulation that controls inappropriate activation of the clotting cascade. The second group of reactions are the termination reactions initiated by the clotting process. In addition to the biochemical control of coagulation, active clotting factors are rapidly diluted as the blood flows away from the site of injury, helping to limit the reaction to the local area.

Antithrombin III (ATIII)

Antithrombin III (ATIII) is the most important constitutive inhibitor of coagulation. This glycoprotein is a potent inhibitor of thrombin and factors IXa, Xa and XIa but is a poor inhibitor of F VIIa. The anticoagulant activity of circulating ATIII is greatly enhanced by binding to the heparan sulphate polymers that are located on cell surfaces. In normal haemostasis, the ATIII bound to endothelial cell heparan sulphate participates in controlling the coagulation process at the periphery of the site of vascular injury.

Tissue factor pathway inhibitor

Tissue factor pathway inhibitor (TFPI, extrinsic pathway inhibitor) is bound to endothelial cell surfaces and is also released in small amounts from activated platelets. It inhibits both the F VIIa-tissue factor complex and F Xa by forming a Ca^{++}-stabilized complex between tissue factor, F VIIa and F Xa.

Proteins C and S

Proteins C and S are vitamin K-dependent anticoagulant plasma proteins that circulate in the plasma as inactive precursors. Endothelial cells have surface receptors called thrombomodulin, which bind thrombin. When thrombin generated in the coagulation cascade binds to thrombomodulin on the surrounding intact endothelial cells, the bound thrombin loses its procoagulant activity. Instead, it becomes a potent activator of the anticoagulant protein C. The complex of activated protein C with protein S as a cofactor, Ca^{++} and a negatively charged phospholipid surface is a potent inactivator of factors Va and VIIIa, therefore inhibiting the tenase and prothrombinase complexes. Activation of protein C by thrombin–thrombomodulin is proportional to the amount of thrombin present and the extent of the coagulation response. The activated protein C–protein S complex also initiates fibrinolysis.

FIBRINOLYSIS

The final stage in haemostasis is the repair of the vascular damage and lysis of the fibrin clot to re-establish vascular patency and normal blood flow (Narayanan, 1998) (Figure 9.3). Fibrinolysis is mediated by the proteolytic enzyme, plasmin. This is synthesized by the liver and circulates an as inactive precursor, plasminogen. Once plasminogen is activated to plasmin, it degrades crosslinked fibrin within a clot to release crosslinked fibrin degradation products, including the crosslinked fragment D-dimer.

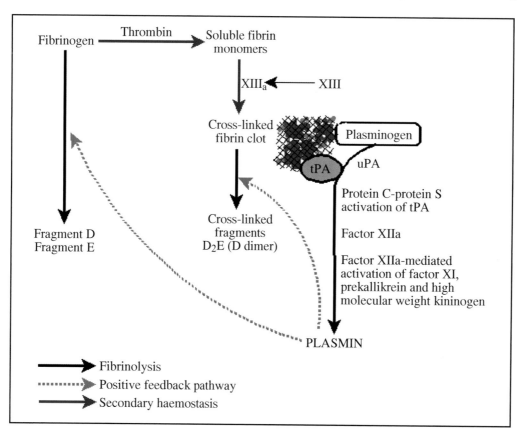

Figure 9.3: *Outline of the events in fibrinolysis. F, factor; tPA, tissue-type plasminogen activator; uPA, urokinase-type plasminogen activator.*

The most potent activators of plasminogen are tissue-type plasminogen activator (tPA) and urokinase-type plasminogen activator (uPA). Vascular endothelial cells synthesize and release tPA in response to a wide range of stimuli, including bradykinin from contact activation and catecholamines. Released tPA initially binds fibrin, which localizes the tPA to the site of thrombus formation. Only then is tPA able to bind plasminogen and activate it to plasmin. The half-life of tPA is short (about 5 minutes), and tPA is rapidly removed by the liver. The uPA is secreted primarily by the kidneys as an inactive precursor. It is activated by the contact factors kallikrein, high molecular weight kininogen and F XII as well as by plasmin, and seems to function primarily within urine and tissues. F XIIa also activates plasminogen, either directly or via activation of F XI and prekallikrein. The kallikrein then activates high molecular weight kininogen, which also converts plasminogen to plasmin.

Fibrinolysis is controlled by specific inhibitors present in the plasma that inactivate plasmin and the plasminogen activators. Plasmin is inhibited by α_2 antiplasmin and α_2 macroglobulin. Plasminogen-activator inhibitor I (PAI-1), secreted by endothelial cells, hepatocytes and platelets, is the most important inhibitor of tPA and uPA. Almost all circulating tPA is bound to PAI-1, and only the tPA captured by fibrin is able to activate plasminogen.

CONCLUSION

Haemostasis is a delicate balance between formation of a primary platelet plug at the site of vascular injury, stabilization of the platelet plug by the formation of a fibrin mesh, repair of the injury and re-establishment of normal vascular patency by fibrinolysis. There are numerous points at which both primary and secondary haemostasis are amplified to generate a rapid response. The process is localized to the site of injury, and control mechanisms ensure that the process does not extend beyond this area.

REFERENCES

Hawiger J (1990) Platelet-vessel wall interactions. Platelet adhesion and aggregation. *Atherosclerosis Reviews* **21**, 165–186

Kaplan AP, Joseph K, Shibayama Y, Reddigan S, Ghebrehiwet B and Silverberg M (1997) The intrinsic coagulation/kinin-forming cascade: assembly in plasma and cell surfaces in inflammation. *Advances in Immunology* **66**, 225–272

Mann KG (1999) Blood coagulation. *Alcoholism: Clinical and Experimental Research* **23**, 1111–1113

Morrisey JH, Macik BG, Neuenschwander PF and Comp PC (1993) Quantitation of activation factor VII levels in plasma using a tissue factor mutant selectively deficient in promoting factor VII activation. *Blood* **81**, 734–744

Narayanan S (1998) Current concepts of coagulation and fibrinolysis. *Advances in Clinical Chemistry* **33**, 133–168

Ruggeri ZM and Ware J (1992) The structure and function of von Willebrand factor. *Thrombosis and Haemostasis* **67**, 594–599

Zwaal RFA and Schroit AJ (1997) Pathophysiologic implications of membrane phospholipid asymmetry in blood cells. *Blood* **89**, 1121–1132

Haemostatic Diagnostic Techniques

Mary F. McConnell

INTRODUCTION

Adequate haemostasis depends on:

- Normal structure and function of the blood vascular system
- Adequate platelet numbers and normal platelet function
- An adequate coagulation system
- Stability of the resultant clot.

The first and last of these are rarely recognized as significant causes of haemorrhage in veterinary medicine. However, haemorrhage secondary to either quantitative and qualitative platelet defects, or defects in the coagulation system, are relatively common problems. Although the importance of a detailed history and a thorough clinical examination cannot be overemphasized, laboratory screening tests are necessary to establish the presence or absence of most haemostatic disorders. Screening tests are used to evaluate the overall activity of the haemostatic mechanism, whereas identifying problems with coagulation factors such as factor VIII deficiency (haemophilia A) requires the use of specific tests. Laboratory screening tests are invaluable in the investigation of suspected haemostatic disorders, but their limitations must be understood. Whereas some screening tests can be performed in the practice laboratory, many must be sent to a specialist veterinary diagnostic laboratory. Simple screening tests may not be sensitive enough to identify mild haemostatic disorders and, conversely, deficiency of some clotting factors (e.g. prekallikrein, factor XII) may produce abnormal screening test results although the animal is clinically normal. However, screening tests performed on samples that have been appropriately collected and processed will provide much useful information if interpreted in conjunction with the history and results of the clinical examination.

SUBMISSION OF SAMPLES TO THE LABORATORY

The correct collection, storage and processing of blood samples for haemostatic testing is critical if meaningful results are to be obtained. A clean venepuncture is essential to minimize the introduction of tissue factor into the sample as this may result in misleading results due to activation of clotting factors and/or platelets. Excessive turbulence during collection and handling, or prolonged exposure to extreme temperatures, will cause haemolysis and may affect the results, although this effect may not be clinically relevant (Moreno and Ginel, 1999). In general, samples that are clotted, collected in the incorrect anticoagulant or filled to less than 90% of the correct capacity of the collection tube are unsuitable for haemostatic screening tests. The exact requirements may differ between laboratories, and it is advisable to discuss these with the relevant laboratory beforehand. This chapter discusses the specific requirements for sample collection for each test.

TESTS OF PRIMARY HAEMOSTASIS

In primary haemostasis, interactions between the vascular endothelium and platelets result in the formation of a primary haemostatic plug, which provides a temporary seal over the injured site in the blood vessel. Platelets adhere to subendothelial collagen at the site of vascular injury via von Willebrand factor (vWf). This process activates platelets, resulting in the release of platelet granule contents, aggregation of platelets and the provision of a procoagulant surface on the platelets for the activation of coagulation factors. Vascular defects, von Willebrand's disease (vWD) and either quantitative or qualitative platelet defects result in defective primary haemostasis.

In-practice tests of primary haemostasis

Buccal mucosal bleeding time

The bleeding time is the time it takes for bleeding from a standardized superficial incision to cease. In animals, the buccal mucosal bleeding time (BMBT) is the most reliable method for measuring bleeding time. This is a useful presurgical screening test for ruling out defective primary haemostasis in an animal with no current clinical evidence of bleeding. If the animal has either thrombocytopenia or clinical evidence of defective primary haemostasis such as petechiation, caution must be exercised as it can be difficult to stop the bleeding in this location. Some experience with the technique in healthy animals is essential if meaningful and reproducible bleeding times are to be obtained. A technique for measuring the cuticle bleeding time has been described (Giles *et al.*, 1982). This is sensitive to both coagulation defects as well as primary haemostatic defects, but anaesthesia is recommended and the end point may be more difficult to determine than with the BMBT.

Method: The BMBT test is done with the animal held in lateral recumbency, with minimal physical restraint or light sedation. The upper lip is folded back and held in place by a gauze bandage; this must be tied tightly enough to impede the venous return from the lip and cause congestion (Figure 10.1). An incision is made in a non-vascular area of the mucosa with a spring-loaded cutting device (e.g. Simplate II, Organon Teknika, Cambridge, UK; Surgicutt, Ortho Diagnostic Systems, High Wycombe, UK). The edge of filter, or blotting, paper is used to absorb the blood (the paper must be held away from the edges of the incision so as not to disturb the developing clot). The time from making the incision to the cessation of bleeding is recorded.

Interpretation: The bleeding time ranges from 1.7 to 4.2 minutes for healthy dogs (Jergens *et al.*, 1987) and from 1.0 to 2.4 minutes for healthy cats (Parker *et al.*, 1988). These values may differ slightly depending on technique, and each clinician should test the method on healthy animals before using the BMBT on animals with suspected bleeding disorders. Prolonged bleeding times are seen with vWD, thrombocytopenia and qualitative platelet defects.

Estimation of platelet number and platelet morphology

Platelet numbers can be semiquantitatively estimated on examination of stained blood smears. Normal platelets appear as small (2–4 μm diameter, quarter to half the diameter of an erythrocyte) anucleate round to oval cells that stain faintly basophilic. Small reddish granules may be visible in the centre, especially in platelets from cats, which are usually larger and more visible than those from dogs.

Method: A blood smear from a sample collected in ethylenediamine tetra-acetic acid (EDTA) is stained with a Romanowsky stain such as Wright, Giemsa, Diff-Quik® or RapiDiff® and scanned under low power to determine the presence of any platelet clumps. If present, these are usually found in the feathered edge and along the sides of the smear and will result in falsely decreased platelet counts. The presence of platelet clumps does not necessarily mean that the platelet count is adequate (Grindem *et al.*, 1991). Between the feathered edge and the base of the smear is the monolayer area where the cells are evenly distributed. This area is examined and the number of platelets in several oil immersion fields counted.

Interpretation: Each platelet in an oil immersion lens field (1000 x total magnification) represents approximately 15 x 10^9 platelets/l.

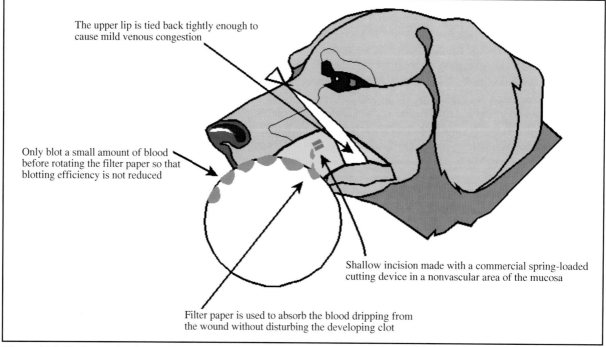

The upper lip is tied back tightly enough to cause mild venous congestion

Only blot a small amount of blood before rotating the filter paper so that blotting efficiency is not reduced

Shallow incision made with a commercial spring-loaded cutting device in a nonvascular area of the mucosa

Filter paper is used to absorb the blood dripping from the wound without disturbing the developing clot

Figure 10.1: Technique for the measurement of buccal mucosal bleeding time in the dog.

- *Normal:* 11–25 platelets/oil immersion field is equivalent to an approximate platelet count of ≥165 x 10⁹/l
- *Mild thrombocytopenia:* 6–10 platelets/oil immersion field is equivalent to an approximate platelet count of 90–150 x 10⁹/l. This number of platelets provides adequate haemostasis
- *Moderate thrombocytopenia:* 4–5 platelets/oil immersion field is equivalent to an approximate platelet count of 50–90 x 10⁹/l. This number of platelets provides adequate haemostasis, although bleeding can be expected with platelet counts of ≤50 x 10⁹/l
- *Severe thrombocytopenia:* ≤ 3 platelets/oil immersion field is equal to an approximate platelet count of <50 x 10⁹/l. Platelet counts of ≤10 x 10⁹/l are considered to be dangerously low.

Large platelets (shift platelets or megathrombocytes) may be seen in any condition in which there is excessive platelet destruction and a regenerative platelet response. Shift platelets may also be seen in infiltrative diseases of the bone marrow. Small platelets (microthrombocytosis) may be seen in iron deficiency anaemia.

Manual platelet count

Manual platelet counts are simple to perform but have an inherent coefficient of variation of 20–25%, even when performed by experienced personnel. Platelet counts performed with electronic cell counters validated for samples from dogs are more precise but are only available in specialized veterinary laboratories.

Method: A blood sample is collected in EDTA (sodium citrate can be used, but heparin causes platelet clumping). A platelet counting diluent system containing ammonium oxalate (Unopette Microcollection System for WBC/Platelet Determination, Becton-Dickinson, Oxford, UK) is filled according to the manufacturer's instructions; this dilutes the blood and lyses the erythrocytes. After complete haemolysis (about 10 minutes), a cleaned Neubauer haemocytometer is loaded by capillary action, taking care not to overfill the counting chamber. The haemocytometer is placed in a moisture chamber (a small container with a lid, such as a petri dish, and a layer of wet filter paper) for 5 to 10 minutes while the platelets settle. The platelets in the 25 small squares within the large central square are then counted on each side of the haemocytometer by using the high dry lens and a lowered condenser (Figure 10.2). The average of these two counts is the platelet count (x 10⁹/litre). All platelet counts must be confirmed by examining a stained blood smear.

Interpretation: Healthy dogs have platelet counts of 200–700 x 10⁹/l and healthy cats 300–800 x 10⁹/l.

Clot retraction

Clot retraction is a crude test of platelet function that can be done on non-thrombocytopenic samples

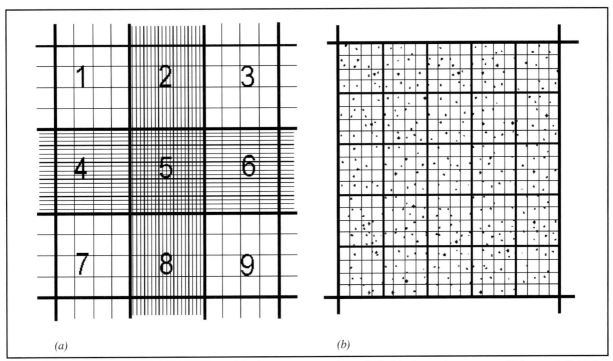

(a)   *(b)*

Figure 10.2: *Counting platelets. (a) Each side of the haemocytometer is marked with nine major squares which are subdivided into smaller squares. (b) Platelets are counted only in the central major square (5) which is subdivided into 25 minor squares, each of which is further subdivided into 16 squares. Platelets are visible as very small refractile bodies when viewed with the microscope condenser lowered. Leucocytes are larger than platelets and are readily distinguished from platelets.*

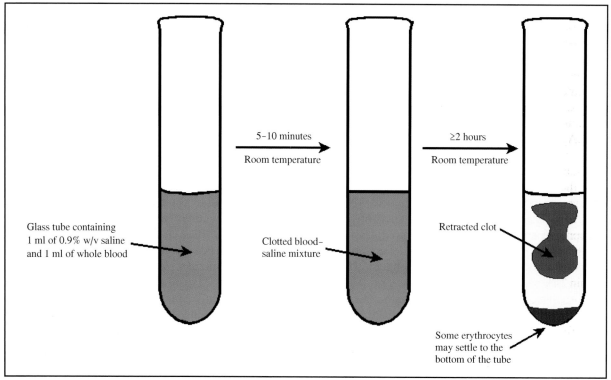

Figure 10.3: Clot retraction. Blood is added to a glass tube containing an equal volume of normal saline, and the mixture is allowed to clot. The tube is examined hourly, and the separation of the retracted clot from the serum is evaluated. Clot retraction should be complete in 2 hours, but may take longer in the saline–blood mixture.

(Figure 10.3). A blood sample collected without anticoagulant from a normal animal will clot in the tube within minutes. The contractile proteins in platelets then contract, squeezing the serum out of the clot, resulting in separation of the clot from the serum. There are several variants of this test.

Method: A sample of whole blood is placed into a glass tube and allowed to clot at room temperature. Alternatively, the blood may be added to a tube containing an equal volume of normal saline (0.9% w/v), and the saline–blood mixture is allowed to clot. Clotting should occur within 5 minutes but may take a little longer when a saline–blood mixture is used. The tube is examined hourly for evidence of separation of the clot from the serum. This saline–blood method is more sensitive than whole blood and is easier to evaluate because of the relatively smaller volume of the clot.

Interpretation: Clot retraction usually occurs within 2 hours, but may take longer in a saline–blood mixture. The clot should reduce to about 50% of its original volume, and the expected volume of serum should be at least 90% of the plasma volume that would be in the sample. Failure of clot retraction to occur indicates a severe platelet function disorder. Even though this test is subjective and not very sensitive, with experience it is useful.

Laboratory tests of primary haemostasis

Automated platelet count
Automated platelet counts are more accurate and precise than manual counts because many thousands of cells are evaluated in each sample. Platelets from cats tend to clump, which often causes inaccurate platelet counts because they are excluded. Unusually large platelets may also be excluded from a count. This is more common in cats than dogs, although it does occur as a breed variant in Cavalier King Charles Spaniels.

Platelet function tests
Platelet function testing is indicated when there is clinical evidence suggestive of defective primary haemostasis and/or a prolonged BMBT, but thrombocytopenia and vWD have been ruled out. It is essential to obtain an accurate history of all drugs the animal has received in the past 10 days to rule out their effects, especially aspirin and non-steroidal anti-inflammatory agents, which inhibit platelet function. Platelet aggregation tests must be completed within 4 hours of collection and require specialized and expensive equipment. For these reasons, specific testing of platelet function is usually only available at veterinary teaching hospitals associated with universities. The ability of the platelets to stick together (aggregate) and release the contents of their granules is tested in a platelet aggregometer by adding reagents that induce these responses in healthy platelets.

vWf antigen

The concentration of vWf antigen (vWf:Ag) in plasma may be determined by either electroimmunoassay or enzyme-linked immunosorbent assay. Blood should be collected in trisodium citrate and, if possible, the plasma separated immediately. It has been shown that vWf:Ag in plasma stored at either 4°C or 22°C is stable for up to 48 hours (Johnstone *et al.*, 1991). In whole blood, vWf:Ag is stable for 48 hours at 22°C but decreases significantly within 24 hours if stored at 4°C. It is advisable to discuss sample and shipping requirements with the laboratory before collecting the sample. vWf concentrations in dogs are increased by strenuous exercise, age, azotaemia, liver disease, parturition and the vasopressin analogue, 1-desamino-8-D-arginine vasopressin (DDAVP). Blood for vWf:Ag assays should be collected from animals at rest but should not be collected within 2 weeks of any systemic stress or illness or from females during oestrus or pregnancy.

vWf function assays

The assays measure the functional ability of vWf in plasma to agglutinate platelets by forming a bridge between adjacent platelets. Washed or formalin-fixed platelets suspended in the plasma to be tested are exposed to an agglutinating agent such as botrocetin, which alters the surface charge of the platelets allowing vWf to attach. The resulting agglutination can be measured by visual assessment, but determining the end point is difficult and the assay is best done in a platelet aggregometer. This test is largely restricted to teaching hospitals associated with universities.

TESTS OF SECONDARY HAEMOSTASIS

In secondary haemostasis the primary haemostatic plug is stabilized by the formation of cross-linked fibrin. Primary and secondary haemostasis must occur simultaneously for effective haemostasis to take place. The conversion of soluble fibrinogen to insoluble fibrin by thrombin is the final step in a cascade of enzymatic reactions in which the inactive coagulation factors are converted to active forms. This cascade is initiated by release of tissue factor from damaged cells, which combines with factor VII to form activated factor VII (the extrinsic pathway) which initiates the activation of factor X (the common pathway). The extrinsic system may serve to initiate the coagulation response, whereas the intrinsic system is responsible for sustained generation of fibrin. Although the intrinsic pathway of coagulation is triggered by activation of factor XII by exposure to subendothelial collagen and kallikrein, sustained generation of fibrin in vivo seems to depend primarily on proteolytic activation at several steps of the cascade by thrombin generated in the initial activation of the extrinsic system. Factors V and VIII, calcium and platelets as a source of negatively charged phospholipid surface are all essential cofactors in the coagulation process in vivo.

In-practice tests of secondary haemostasis

Activated clotting time

The activated clotting time (ACT) is a simple and useful screening test that measures the time it takes for fresh whole blood to clot in the presence of a substance that initiates the contact activation of coagulation. It is a measure of the intrinsic and common coagulation pathways. It is important to avoid contaminating the blood sample with tissue factor at the time of collection as this will activate the extrinsic pathway. The combination of ACT and estimated platelet count from a blood smear is the most accurate means of diagnosing disseminated intravascular coagulation (DIC) at the point of care (Bateman *et al.*, 1999).

Method: An ACT tube containing diatomaceous earth (Becton-Dickinson, Oxford, UK) is prewarmed to 37°C and venepuncture performed. To minimize contamination from tissue factor, 0.25 to 0.5 ml of blood is drawn up into the syringe and discarded, and then 2 ml of blood is drawn up and added to the ACT tube. Alternatively, if collecting directly into a vacutainer tube, the first 0.25 to 0.5 ml can be collected into one tube, which is discarded, and then the ACT tube is attached and filled. The timer is started as soon as the blood enters the ACT tube. The sample is gently mixed by inversion then placed in a 37°C heating block or water bath (60 seconds for dogs and 45 seconds for cats). It is then tilted at 10 second intervals until the first clot is observed; this may precede coagulation of the entire sample.

Interpretation: The ACT ranges from 60 to 110 seconds in normal dogs and from 50 to 75 seconds in normal cats. Prolongation of the ACT indicates a severe abnormality of the intrinsic and/or common pathways. The ACT will also be prolonged in severe thrombocytopenia ($<10 \times 10^9$ platelets/l) and hypofibrinogenaemia.

Whole blood clotting time

Whole blood cotting time (WBCT) is a less sensitive version of ACT but can be performed with the minimum of equipment. Reference ranges using a standardized procedure should be established by each practice.

Method: To minimize contamination with tissue factor, 0.25 to 0.5 ml of blood is drawn into the syringe and discarded, and then about 4 ml of blood is drawn and 1 ml is added to each of two glass tubes and a timer started. The tubes are tipped gently to 90 degrees every 30 seconds until the blood has coagulated and the average time is used.

Interpretation: The WBCT varies a little depending on the size of tubes used (the same size tubes should always be used) and the temperature, but normal dog and cat blood will clot within 6 to 7 minutes. Similar to the ACT, the WBCT will be prolonged in severe thrombocytopenia and hypofibrinogenaemia.

Laboratory tests of secondary haemostasis

These coagulation tests measure the time taken for citrated platelet-poor plasma to clot when coagulation is initiated by the addition of calcium and activating agents. Laboratories use either fibrometers, which detect when fibrin strands form and span the gap between two electrodes, or photo-optical coagulometers, which detect a change in the intensity of filtered light when clot formation occurs. Fibrin formation can also be detected by visual observation, but this technique requires considerable practice to obtain consistent results. These tests form the basis of the specialized clot-based coagulation assays used to detect specific factor deficiencies. A test kit for measuring prothrombin time (PT) designed for the human market has been evaluated in one study and found to be suitable for use with samples from dogs and cats (Monce *et al.*, 1995).

Sample requirements for clotting tests

Blood is collected into a plastic syringe, then the needle is removed and the sample added to a commercial sodium citrate tube and mixed gently by inversion. It is essential that the tube is filled exactly to the mark on the tube as an incorrect ratio of blood to sodium citrate causes misleading results. Results of these tests using blood collected from indwelling jugular catheters are not significantly different from those using blood collected by venepuncture. The plasma should be separated from the sample and frozen if the test is not to be run immediately. It has been shown, however, that blood samples from dogs collected into sodium citrate and stored at 20°C are adequate for up to 48 hours after collection, but storage of blood at 4°C results in a significant decrease in coagulant activity within 24 hours (Mansell and Parry, 1989). It is advisable to discuss sample and shipping requirements with the laboratory before collecting the sample.

Prothrombin time

The PT (one-stage PT, OSPT) identifies coagulation abnormalities of the extrinsic and common pathways. Clotting is initiated by adding calcium and tissue thromboplastin (preferably synthetic or derived from rabbit brain), which provides tissue factor and substitutes for the negatively charged phospholipid surface provided by platelets in vivo. Although there is little variation in product sensitivity or specificity between manufacturers, each laboratory must establish their own reference ranges for each species using their own

instrumentation and reagents. The use of a diluted sample may improve the sensitivity of the PT as a screening test in dogs (Mischke and Nolte, 1997).

Interpretation: The PT is sensitive to defects in the extrinsic pathway (factor VII) and/or factors in the common pathway (fibrinogen, II, V and X). Prolongation of the PT relative to the laboratory's reference range indicates a significant deficiency in clotting factor as factors must be decreased to less than 30% of normal to cause prolongation of PT. The PT is prolonged in acquired vitamin K deficiency, liver disease, specific factor deficiencies and DIC. Factor VII deficiency causes prolongation of the PT with no change in other clotting tests. Factor VII has a relatively short half-life, and the PT may therefore be the only clotting test to be prolonged in the early stages of acquired vitamin K deficiency.

Activated partial thromboplastin time

The activated partial thromboplastin time (APTT) identifies coagulation abnormalities of the intrinsic and common pathways. Clotting is initiated by adding phospholipid (which substitutes for the negatively charged phospholipid surface provided by platelets in vivo), a surface activator such as ellagic acid, silica or kaolin and excess calcium. The reagents used in the APTT vary greatly in composition and therefore in sensitivity and specificity. It is essential that each laboratory establish their own reference ranges for each species by using their own instrumentation and reagents. Dilution of the plasma does not increase the sensitivity of this test when using electro-optical detection of fibrin formation (Johnstone, 1984).

Interpretation: The APTT is sensitive to deficiencies of the intrinsic pathway factors (high-molecular weight kininogen, prekallekrein, XII, XI, IX and VIII) and the common pathway factors (fibrinogen, II, V and X). Prolongation of the APTT relative to the laboratory's reference range indicates a significant deficiency, as factors must be decreased to less than 30% of normal to cause a prolongation in the APTT. The APTT cannot be used to detect haemophiliac carriers with 40-60% or higher levels of normal factor VIII or IX activity. Clinical bleeding may occur without prolongation of the APTT or PT in mild cases of acquired vitamin K deficiency. Although factor VIII activity in animals with vWD is sometimes decreased, it is usually sufficient to give an APTT within the reference range.

TESTS OF FIBRINOLYSIS

The end product of coagulation is the formation of insoluble fibrin. The next step in the process is the repair of the damaged blood vessel, lysis of the clot and restoration of blood flow. This is achieved through dissolution of the clot by the fibrinolytic system. Both fibrinogen and fibrin are digested by the enzyme plasmin, which is derived from an inactive precursor (plasminogen) and activated by several different molecules, of which the most important is tissue plasminogen activator (tPA). If plasmin is produced on fibrin surfaces, fibrin is digested (fibrinolysis), and when plasmin is produced in the circulation, fibrinogen is digested (fibrinogenolysis). Fibrinolysis and fibrinogenolysis release fibrin(ogen) degradation products (FDPs). The FDPs have anticoagulant effects whereas plasmin also inhibits activated factors V and VIII. Except for conditions such as DIC, it is unusual for fibrinogenolysis to occur in vivo.

In-practice tests of fibrinolysis

FDPs (fibrin degradation products, fibrin split products)

Test kits that use latex particles coated with antibodies to fibrinogen fragments are rapid, accurate, sensitive and valid for use in animal species. Blood samples must be collected in the special tubes supplied with the test kit. These tubes contain thrombin to initiate clotting and remove fibrinogen, as well as protease inhibitors to prevent further fibrinolysis so that the assay only measures FDPs from the circulation.

Method: Test kits for detection of FDPs (e.g. ThromboWellco Test, Wellcome Diagnostics, Dartford, Kent, UK) provide clear instructions and all the materials necessary to perform the test. A positive test result is visualized as agglutination of the latex beads.

Interpretation: Healthy dogs have FDP concentrations of less than 10 µg/ml. Increased FDP concentrations (greater than 40 µg/ml) indicate that there is increased fibrinolysis. DIC is the most common condition in cats and dogs in which the FDP test result is positive, but concentrations of FDPs may also be increased in other disorders of fibrinolysis. DIC is a pathophysiological process that underlies many disorders ranging from sepsis to malignancy, characterized by simultaneous activation of the coagulation and fibrinolytic systems with degradation of fibrin, coagulation factors and fibrinogen by plasmin. Other conditions in which concentrations of FDPs may be increased include coagulopathy secondary to vitamin K antagonist poisoning, hepatic disease and thrombotic conditions.

Laboratory tests of fibrinolysis

Thrombin clot time

Thrombin clot time (TCT) is a useful screening test that measures the time taken for citrated plasma to clot when exogenous thrombin and calcium are added to plasma. This test only assesses the ability of exogenous thrombin to convert the fibrinogen in the plasma sample to fibrin and bypasses all other steps in the coagulation pathway. Each laboratory establishes its own protocol, but usually sufficient thrombin is added to give a TCT of 8 to 10 seconds in healthy animals.

Interpretation: The TCT is prolonged if there is either hypofibrinogenaemia (less than 1.0 g/l) or dysfibrinogenaemia, or if there is inhibition of thrombin by substances in the sample such as heparin, FDPs or abnormal serum proteins.

Fibrinogen

The simple heat precipitation method used to measure increased concentrations of fibrinogen is not sensitive enough for the accurate measurement of decreased fibrinogen concentrations, but fibrinogen assays based on clotting times are not commonly used in veterinary laboratories. When high concentrations of thrombin are added to diluted citrated plasma, the rate of clot formation is proportional to the fibrinogen concentration.

Interpretation: The fibrinogen concentration ranges from 1.5 to 3.0 g/l in normal dogs and cats. Hypofibrinogenaemia occurs primarily because of increased consumption in DIC, but decreased production of fibrinogen may occur in advanced liver disease.

Antithrombin III

Antithrombin III is a circulating natural anticoagulant, which is the main physiological inhibitor of thrombin. Heparin functions by enhancing the inhibition of thrombin by ATIII. The concentration of ATIII decreases in hypercoagulative disorders such as DIC in small animals. Common assays for ATIII activity are based on the use of a synthetic substrate attached to a chemical group that is colourless until released by proteolysis by ATIII. A chromogenic ATIII assay has been validated for samples from dogs (Mandell *et al.*, 1991). Assessment of ATIII activity is useful in animals suspected of having a hypercoagulable state.

Interpretation: In DIC, ATIII concentrations decrease in comparison to that of normal pooled citrated plasma from dogs. In one study, 85% of dogs (35 of 41) with confirmed DIC had decreased ATIII concentrations (Feldman *et al.*, 1981). ATIII also decreases in hepatic disease owing to decreased synthesis. ATIII is similar in size to albumin and is lost in protein-losing nephropathies and protein-losing enteropathies.

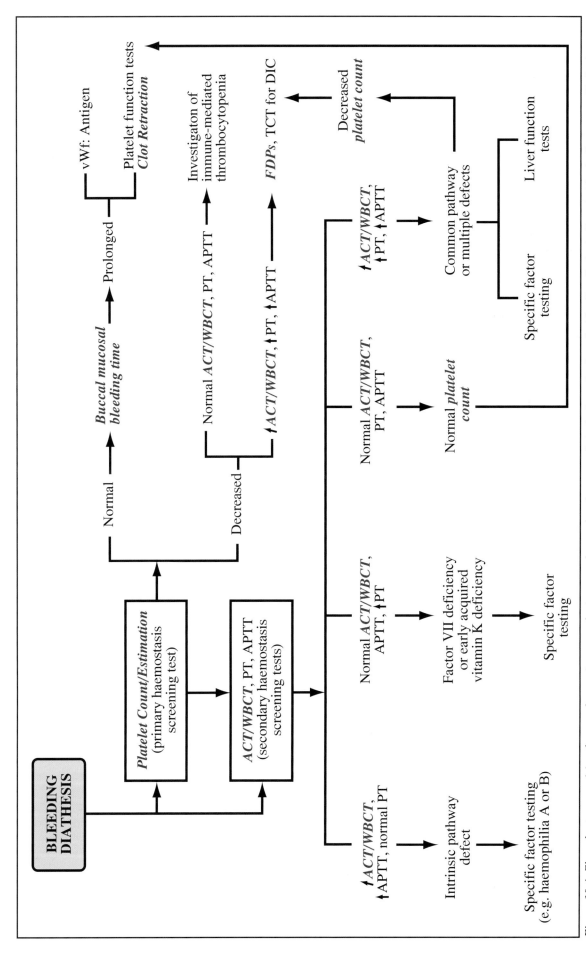

Figure 10.4: *Flow chart summarizing the use of screening tests of primary and secondary haemostasis in the investigation of a bleeding diathesis. Tests in blue italics can readily be done in veterinary practice. vWf, von Willebrand factor; ACT, activated clotting time; WBCT, whole blood clotting time; PT, prothrombin time; APTT, activated partial thromboplastin time; FDPs, fibrinogen degradation products; TCT, thrombin clot time; DIC, disseminated intravascular coagulation.*

REFERENCES AND FURTHER READING

Bateman SW, Mathews KA, Abrams-Ogg ACG, Lumsdem JH, Johnstone IB and Hillers TK (1999) Evaluation of point-of-care tests for diagnosis of disseminated intravascular coagulation in dogs admitted to an intensive care unit. *Journal of the American Veterinary Medical Association* **215**, 805-810

Feldman BF, Madewell BR and O'Neill S (1981) Disseminated intravascular coagulation: antithrombin, plasminogen, and coagulation abnormalities in 41 dogs. *Journal of the American Veterinary Medical Association* **179**, 151-154

Giles AR, Tinlin S and Greenwood R (1982) A canine model of hemophilic (factor VIII:C deficiency) bleeding. *Blood* **60**, 727-730

Grindem CB, Breitschwerdt EB, Corbett WT and Jans HE (1991) Epidemiologic survey of thrombocytopenia in dogs: a report on 987 cases. *Veterinary Clinical Pathology* **20**, 38-43

Hacker SG (1995) Approach to the diagnosis of bleeding disorders. *Compendium of Continuing Veterinary Education* **17**, 331-349

Jergens AE, Turrentine MA, Kraus KH and Johnson GS (1987) Buccal mucosal bleeding time of healthy dogs and of dogs in various pathological states, including thrombocytopenia, uremia and von Willebrand's disease. *American Journal of Veterinary Research* **48**, 1337-1342

Johnstone IB (1984) The activated partial thromboplastin time of diluted plasma: variability due to method of fibrin detection. *Canadian Journal of Comparative Medicine* **48**, 198-201

Johnstone IB, Keen J, Halbert A and Crane S (1991) Stability of factor VIII and von Willebrand factor in canine blood samples during storage. *Canadian Veterinary Journal* **32**, 173-175

Littlewood JD (1992) Differential diagnosis of haemorrhagic disorders in dogs. *In Practice* **14**, 172-180

Mandell CP, O'Neill SL and Feldman BF (1991) Antithrombin III concentrations associated with L-asparaginase administration. *Veterinary Clinical Pathology* **21**, 68-70

Mansell PD and Parry BW (1989) Stability of canine factor VIII: coagulant activity *in vitro*. *Canadian Journal of Veterinary Research* **53**, 264-267

Mischke R and Nolte I (1997) Optimization of prothrombin time measurements in canine plasma. *American Journal of Veterinary Research* **58**, 236-241

Monce KA, Atkins CE and Loughman CM (1995) Evaluation of a commercially available prothrombin time assay kit for use in dogs and cats. *Journal of the American Veterinary Medical Association* **207**, 581-584

Moreno P and Ginel PJ (1999) Effects of haemolysis, lipaemia and bilirubinaemia on prothrombin time, activated partial thromboplastin time and thrombin time in plasma samples from healthy dogs. *Research in Veterinary Science* **67**, 273-276

Parker MT, Collier LL, Kier AB and Johnson GS (1988) Oral mucosal bleeding times of normal cats and cats with Chediak-Higashi syndrome or Hageman trait (factor XII deficiency). *Veterinary Clinical Pathology* **17**, 9-12

Disorders of Platelet Number

David C. Lewis

INTRODUCTION

Platelets are small (2-4 µm) anucleate fragments of cytoplasm that are progeny of bone marrow pluripotential stem cells of the megakaryocyte lineage. Platelet production from megakaryocytes is termed thrombopoiesis. Megakaryocytes are easily recognizable in bone marrow aspirates because of their large size (20-160 µm), lobulated nuclei and abundant pale staining cytoplasm (Jain, 1993) (Figure 11.1). A variety of cytokines play important roles in thrombopoiesis, including interleukin-3 (IL-3) and interleukin-6 (IL-6), granulocyte–macrophage colony-stimulating factor and thrombopoietin (Jain, 1993). The average circulating life span of canine platelets is about 5 days (Slichter *et al.*, 1987) and of feline platelets is about 30 hours (Jacobs *et al.*, 1986). Senescent platelets are removed by fixed tissue macrophages, predominantly in the spleen and liver (Jain, 1993).

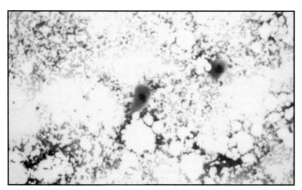

Figure 11.1: Bone marrow aspirate (10 X objective) with two mature megakaryocytes, recognizable because of their large size and lobulated nuclei. Normal cellular bone marrow aspirates from dogs contain 1–3 megakaryocytes per low power (10 x objective) field.

Platelets have important roles in thrombosis, inflammation and tissue repair; but they are best recognized for their role in haemostasis and in maintaining the structural integrity of the endothelium. In the presence of thrombocytopenia, blood leaks through structurally intact blood vessels, giving rise to spontaneous petechiae, purpura and mucosal bleeding (Figure 11.2). After blood vessel damage, local vasoconstriction resulting from nervous reflexes and local muscle spasm occurs

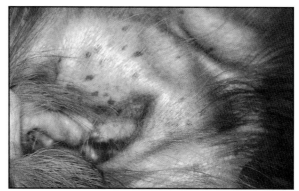

Figure 11.2: Cutaneous petechiae on the concave surface of the pinna of a dog with thrombocytopenia caused by heat stroke-induced disseminated intravascular coagulation.

and is maintained for minutes to hours by release of vasoactive substances from platelets and surrounding tissues. During this time, platelets form an occlusive plug, which stops haemorrhage. Platelets initially adhere to adhesive tissue proteins exposed as a result of vessel damage, via von Willebrand factor (Figure 11.3). After adhesion, platelets contact collagen and other activator proteins, change shape, become stimulated, adhere to one another and release biochemical substances (e.g. serotonin, adenosine diphosphate, thromboxane A_2) that maintain vasoconstriction, amplify platelet activation and recruit additional platelets to the growing haemostatic plug (Figure 11.4). This process is termed platelet aggregation. In addition to forming the initial occlusive plug to effect rapid cessation of haemorrhage (Figure 11.5), platelets play a critical procoagulant role by secreting coagulation proteins (fibrinogen, factor V) and Ca^{++} and providing a phospholipid surface (platelet factor 3) upon which coagulation reactions are accelerated. The intrinsic and extrinsic coagulation cascades lead to formation of fibrin, which stabilizes the initial platelet plug (Figure 11.6). Adhesion and aggregation of platelets is usually sufficient to stop initial haemorrhage from damaged vessels, but stabilization of the platelet plug by fibrin is required for permanent haemostasis. Fibrin stabilization of the platelet plug is not, however, required for effective cessation of haemorrhage from very small vessel wall defects. Clot retraction and tissue repair are additional functions of platelets (Jain, 1993; Hackner, 1995).

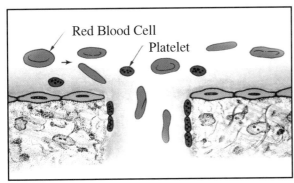

Figure 11.3: Subsequent to blood vessel damage, platelets adhere to subendothelial proteins via von Willebrand factor, become activated and change shape.

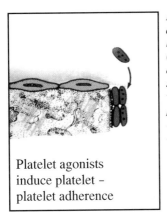

Platelet agonists induce platelet – platelet adherence

Figure 11.4: After being activated, platelets release biochemical substances (such as thromboxane A₂, adenosine diphosphate and serotonin) that amplify vasoconstriction and platelet activation and recruit additional platelets to the haemostatic plug.

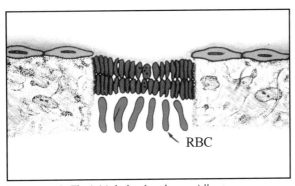

RBC

Figure 11.5: The initial platelet plug rapidly stops haemorrhage. RBC = red blood cell.

Fibrin formation proceeds and platelets contract, forming a stable haemostatic plug

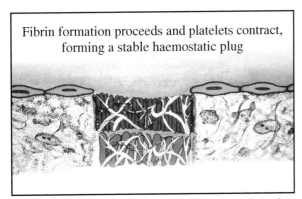

Figure 11.6: Although adhesion and aggregation of platelets are usually sufficient to stop initial haemorrhage from damaged vessels, stabilization of the platelet plug by fibrin is usually required, except for small vessel defects, for complete haemostasis.

THROMBOCYTOPENIA

Thrombocytopenia is the most common acquired haemostatic disorder in dogs, with a reported prevalence rate in canine admissions to one hospital of about 5% (Grindem *et al.*, 1991). For dogs, a reference range of platelet count of 200 to 500 x 10⁹/l, as historically reported in the literature, is used by many laboratories. However, some more recently established reference ranges use approximately 150 x 10⁹/l as the lower limit of normal (Sullivan *et al.*, 1995). Hence dogs with mild thrombocytopenia as reported by some laboratories may be normal. Greyhounds, Cavalier King Charles Spaniels and Shiba Inus have been reported to have lower platelet counts than other breeds of dog (Eksell *et al.*, 1994; Sullivan *et al.*, 1994; Smedile *et al.*, 1997; Gookin *et al.*, 1998).

Thrombocytopenia is much less common in cats than in dogs, with a reported prevalence in cats examined at one veterinary hospital of about 1% (Jordan *et al.*, 1993). In cats, a reference range of platelet count of approximately 250 to 800 x 10⁹/l is reported (Jain, 1993). Automated haematology analysers frequently result in artefactual thrombocytopenia in cats owing to the similar size of feline platelets and red cells and the tendency of feline platelets to clump (Hackner, 1995) (Figure 11.7). Platelet counts derived from a haemocytometer are more reliable than automated platelet counts in cats, although they will also be influenced by platelet clumping. Clumping can also occasionally cause problems with canine platelet counts.

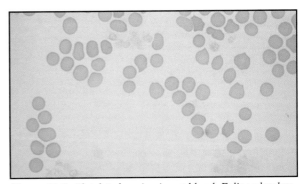

Figure 11.7: Platelet clumping in cat blood. Feline platelets have a greater tendency to clump than canine platelets. Additionally, the similar size of feline platelets and red cells results in automated platelet counts being unreliable in cats.

Causes of thrombocytopenia

The major pathophysiological causes of thrombocytopenia are:

- Decreased platelet production (due to bone marrow disease)
- Accelerated platelet destruction or utilization
- Platelet sequestration.

Decreased platelet production (bone marrow disease)

Thrombocytopenia due to bone marrow disease (Figure 11.8) is characterized invariably by pancytopenia,

Drug-induced
Cytotoxic drugs: cyclophosphamide, azathioprine, doxorubicin
Antibiotics: chloramphenicol, sulphonamide/ trimethoprim
Oestrogen
Phenylbutazone
Phenobarbitone
Albendazole
Thiazide diuretics
Phenytoin
Griseofulvin (especially in cats infected with feline immunodeficiency virus)
Propylthiouracil, methimazole
Ribavarin (cats)

Neoplasia (myelophthisis)
Originating in bone marrow: myeloproliferative or lymphoproliferative disease
Metastatic neoplasia

Infection
Canine parvovirus, distemper
Feline infectious enteritis
Feline leukaemia virus
Feline immunodeficiency virus
Sepsis, endotoxaemia
Ehrlichiosis
Systemic mycoses: histoplasmosis, blastomycosis, coccidioidomycosis, cryptococcosis
Cytauxoonosis
?Canine retroviral infection

Other
Myelofibrosis: secondary to neoplasia, sepsis or bone marrow necrosis
Haemophagocytic syndrome

Figure 11.8: Causes of decreased platelet production (bone marrow disease).

bicytopenia (thrombocytopenia in association with non-regenerative anaemia or neutropenia) or presence of abnormal blood cells or abnormal cell morphology, as detected by evaluation of a peripheral blood smear (Jain, 1993). A diagnostic guideline is to consider that the absence of these changes in a patient with thrombocytopenia is suggestive that the thrombocytopenia is due to accelerated platelet destruction or utilization. Oestrogen toxicity is an important exception to this guideline. In early oestrogen toxicity from exogenous oestrogens (mismating injections, treatment of prostatic hyperplasia or perianal gland adenomas) or endogenous oestrogens (Sertoli cell tumour), thrombocytopenia may be the only haematological abnormality found and is often accompanied by neutrophilic leucocytosis (Sherding *et al.*, 1981; Weiss and Klausner, 1990; Jain, 1993). Depending on the severity of the insult, this may be followed, after 2-4 weeks, by non-regenerative anaemia and neutropenia. This early blood picture can easily

be confused with accelerated platelet destruction from a variety of causes, in which thrombocytopenia may be the only abnormality, or may be accompanied by neutrophilia. A review of the patient's history (mismating injections and history of castration) and thorough physical examination (testicular palpation) is the best way to distinguish between these possibilities. A bone marrow aspirate can be used to confirm the diagnosis of oestrogen toxicity (few or no megakaryocytes) if necessary (Jain, 1993). Identification of the source of oestrogen would also be confirmatory. Cats are much more resistant to the toxic effects of oestrogens than are dogs.

Accelerated platelet destruction or utilization

Thrombocytopenia due to accelerated platelet destruction or utilization (Figure 11.9) can be considered by dividing the aetiologies into immune and non-immune categories. Haemorrhage does not cause thrombocytopenia in humans, and thrombocytopenia in people

Immune-mediated platelet destruction
Primary immune-mediated thrombocytopenia (also called idiopathic thrombocytopenic purpura; ITP)
Systemic lupus erythematosus (SLE)
Feline leukaemia virus, feline immunodeficiency virus
Dirofilariasis
Ehrlichiosis (*Ehrlichia canis*)
Neoplasia: particularly lymphoproliferative disease but also a variety of solid tumours
Drug-induced: especially potentiated sulphonamides but also a variety of other drugs
Rheumatoid arthritis
?*Babesia canis*
?Neonatal alloimmune thrombocytopenia
?Propylthiouracil, methimazole
?Viral infections (distemper) or modified live virus vaccines

Non-immune platelet utilization
Disseminated intravascular coagulation
Vasculitis: SLE, septicaemia, immune complex disease, *E. canis*, *E. platys*, granulocytic ehrlichiosis, *Rickettsia rickettsii*, feline infectious peritonitis, polyarteritis nodosa, canine adenovirus-1, canine herpesvirus
Haemorrhage due to anticoagulant rodenticide toxicity
Haemolytic uraemic syndrome (also called cutaneous and renal vasculopathy of Greyhounds)
Hepatozoon canis
Tularaemia
Leishmaniasis
Snake envenomation
Septicaemia
?Viral infection

Figure 11.9: Causes of accelerated platelet destruction or utilization.

subsequent to haemorrhage occurs only after transfusion with multiple units of platelet-poor blood products. Transient mild to moderate thrombocytopenia has, however, been reported in dogs subsequent to haemorrhage due to congenital and acquired bleeding disorders, and profound thrombocytopenia is occasionally observed in dogs subsequent to haemorrhage from anticoagulant rodenticide toxicity (Lewis *et al.*, 1995a). The mechanism for the thrombocytopenia in these cases is unknown. Practitioners should be aware of this possibility, because the presence of thrombocytopenia and prolonged coagulation times is often thought to be diagnostic of disseminated intravascular coagulation (DIC).

Platelet sequestration
About one third of circulating platelets are sequestered in the spleen at any one time (Jain, 1993). More platelets are sequestered as splenic size increases, and splenomegaly may cause thrombocytopenia owing to platelet sequestration (Figure 11.10). Thrombocytopenia due to splenomegaly in dogs is not well documented but is usually mild (not less than 100 x 10^9/l) and of no clinical importance. The presence of more severe thrombocytopenia in a patient with splenomegaly should stimulate a search for another mechanism for the observed thrombocytopenia. Not every case of splenomegaly will have an associated thrombocytopenia. The degree of decrease in platelet numbers in dogs with splenomegaly depends on the original platelet count and the magnitude and cause of the splenomegaly. Thrombocytopenia may be more likely

in cases of symmetrical splenomegaly, due to congestion (portal hypertension, splenic torsion) or hyperplasia (chronic infectious disease), than in asymmetrical splenomegaly due to haematomas, nodular hyperplasia or non-haematopoietic neoplasia. Thrombocytopenia is common, however, in dogs with splenic haemangiosarcoma (Grindem *et al.*, 1994). Platelet pooling may be absent in splenomegaly that is due to diffuse cellular infiltration (haematopoietic neoplasia), because of destruction of the vascular compartment by neoplastic cells.

Other causes of platelet sequestration include sepsis and hypothermia. Platelet sequestration within pulmonary vasculature may contribute to thrombocytopenia in patients with sepsis. Platelet sequestration within hepatic vasculature is reported to cause thrombocytopenia in dogs with hypothermia (Reagan and Rebar, 1995).

Clinical presentation of dogs and cats with thrombocytopenia
Clinical presentation of thrombocytopenia varies with the severity and duration of thrombocytopenia and with the underlying disease. Signs of bleeding in patients with thrombocytopenia are variable. Bleeding due to thrombocytopenia is not found unless platelet counts are less than 50 x 10^9/l, and usually less than 30 x 10^9/l. The degree of haemorrhage for any given platelet count is unpredictable; it is not unusual for dogs and cats to have platelet counts of less than 10 x 10^9/l and to have no evidence of haemorrhage (Jordan *et al.*, 1993; Hackner, 1995).

History
Historical complaints in patients with thrombocytopenia can be non-specific (e.g. anorexia and lethargy), may relate to the underlying disease causing the thrombocytopenia (e.g. fever, coughing, lymphadenopathy) or may be due to thrombocytopenia. Clients may report epistaxis, haematochezia, melaena, haematuria, haematemesis or cutaneous haemorrhages. Blindness or neurological signs may be reported owing to haemorrhage into these organs. A history of exposure to anticoagulant rodenticides or drugs (such as oestrogen, phenobarbital, phenylbutazone, potentiated sulphonamides, cytotoxic drugs, griseofulvin or methimazole) should be sought. Preventative healthcare history, including heartworm prevention and recent vaccinations, may yield helpful information. A history of travel may also provide important diagnostic clues, because infectious causes of thrombocytopenia can have variable geographical prevalence.

Physical examination findings
Mucosal and cutaneous petechiae, purpura and ecchymoses are characteristic of a disorder of primary haemostasis (Hackner, 1995). Petechiae are pinpoint extravasations of blood from intact blood vessels

Neoplasia
Myeloproliferative and lymphoproliferative disease, haemangiosarcoma, haemangioma, mast cell tumour, metastatic neoplasia
Congestion
Splenic torsion (primary or associated with gastric dilation–volvulus), portal hypertension (hepatic cirrhosis, portosystemic vascular anomaly)
Haematoma
Lymphoid/macrophage hyperplasia
Systemic lupus erythematosus, immune-mediated haemolytic anaemia, chronic bacterial, fungal or rickettsial infections
Splenitis
Hypothermia
Sequestration in multiple vessels
Sepsis
Sequestration in pulmonary and/or hepatic vasculature

Figure 11.10: Causes of platelet sequestration.

(Figure 11.11). Purpura are confluent petechiae, up to about 1 cm in diameter. Ecchymoses are small haemorrhagic spots, larger than petechiae, often associated with trauma (Figure 11.12). The terms purpura and ecchymoses can be used interchangeably. Although thrombocytopenia is the most common cause of such clinical signs, altered platelet function (thrombocytopathia) and vascular disorders (vasculitis, hypertension) may cause similar bleeding manifestations (Figure 11.13). Petechiae are commonly

seen in dogs with thrombocytopenia but are rare in cats with thrombocytopenia (Jordan *et al.*, 1993). Disorders of secondary haemostasis, such as haemophilia A or anticoagulant rodenticide toxicity, do not cause petechiae, purpura or ecchymoses but rather larger areas of haemorrhage, such as haematomas, body cavity haemorrhages (haemothorax, haemoperitoneum) and haemarthroses. Bleeding from mucosal surfaces, such as epistaxis, oral cavity haemorrhage, haematemesis, haematuria, haematochezia or melaena, although not specific, are also commonly seen in patients with thrombocytopenia (Figure 11.14). Bleeding from mucosal surfaces can be due to a disorder of primary or secondary haemostasis (Figure 11.15). Mucosal surface bleeding can also be due to localized disease, for example, nasal tumours causing epistaxis or gastric ulcers causing melaena (Figure 11.16). Bleeding at multiple sites would enable the presence of a haemostatic disorder to be confirmed (Hackner, 1995).

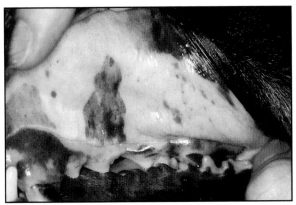

Figure 11.11: Oral mucosal petechiae (pinpoint extravasations of blood from intact blood vessels) in a dog with primary immune-mediated thrombocytopenia. Reproduced from Feldman, Zinkl and Jain (2000) Schalm's Veterinary Hematology, 5th edition, *with permission of Lippincott, Williams and Wilkins.*

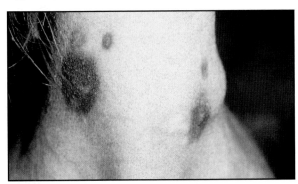

Figure 11.12: Cutaneous purpura and ecchymoses in a dog with immune-mediated thrombocytopenia. Purpura are confluent petechiae, up to about 1 cm diameter. Ecchymoses are small haemorrhagic spots, larger than petechiae, often associated with trauma. The terms purpura and ecchymoses can be used interchangeably.

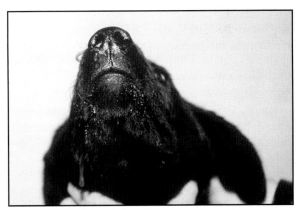

Figure 11.14: Epistaxis in a dog with anticoagulant rodenticide toxicity. Epistaxis can be due to local disease, a primary haemostatic disorder such as thrombocytopenia or a secondary haemostatic disorder such as haemophilia A.

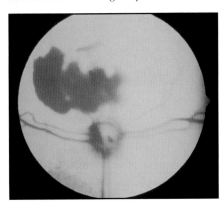

Figure 11.13: Retinal haemorrhage in a cat with systemic hypertension.

Disorders of primary haemostasis (platelet or vascular abnormalities)
Petechiae and ecchymoses common
Haematomas rare
Bleeding from mucous membranes
Bleeding disproportionate to degree of trauma
Bleeding from multiple sites

Disorders of secondary haemostasis (coagulation factor abnormalities; except von Willebrand factor)
Petechiae and ecchymoses rare
Haematomas common
Bleeding from mucous membranes
Bleeding into muscles, joints and body cavities
Bleeding disproportionate to degree of trauma
Bleeding from multiple sites
Rebleeding common

Figure 11.15: Diagnostic clues from bleeding manifestations.

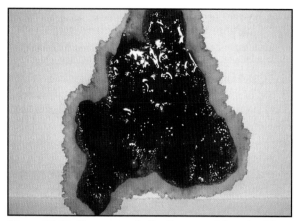

Figure 11.16: Haematemesis ('coffee grounds' vomitus) in a patient with thrombocytopenia. Mucosal surface bleeding, such as haematemesis, can be due to primary haemostatic disorders, secondary haemostatic disorders or local disease.

Other physical examination findings associated with specific causes of thrombocytopenia may include lymphadenopathy, hepatosplenomegaly and fever.

Laboratory evaluation of patients with thrombocytopenia

Peripheral blood smear evaluation

Substantial information in patients with thrombocytopenia can be gleaned from evaluation of a peripheral blood smear. This is a rapid and reliable method to assess adequacy of platelet numbers and to assess the presence of platelet clumping. Each platelet in the peripheral blood smear is equivalent to about 15×10^9 platelets per litre, and less than three to four platelets per oil immersion field (without platelet clumping at the feather edge or along the sides of the blood smear) indicates significant thrombocytopenia (Jain, 1993). Platelet clumping is a common cause of spurious thrombocytopenia, especially in cats. Platelet clumping can be minimized by careful venepuncture and prompt (within 6 hours) analysis. Ethylenediamine tetra-acetic acid (EDTA) is the preferred anticoagulant for platelet enumeration (Jain, 1993), although EDTA-induced platelet clumping causing spurious thrombocytopenia has been observed in dogs. In the presence of platelet clumping, neither manual nor automated platelet counts will be accurate (Figure 11.17). In the presence of platelet clumping, the likelihood of thrombocytopenia needs to be subjectively assessed on the basis of the platelet count or estimate and the degree of clumping. Large densely stained platelets on a blood smear (megathrombocytes) suggest active thrombopoiesis in response to accelerated platelet destruction or utilization (Sullivan *et al.*, 1995) (Figure 11.18). Infectious organisms, such as *Ehrlichia canis* morulae in leucocytes, *E. platys* morulae in platelets or cytoplasmic distemper inclusion bodies in leucocytes or red cells, may rarely be seen on

evaluation of peripheral blood smears (Figure 11.19). The subjective impression of leucopenia or presence of abnormal cells, such as 'blast cells,' on evaluation of a peripheral blood smear is suggestive of bone marrow disease. The presence of many fragmented red cells (schistocytes or schizocytes) would support DIC, haemangiosarcoma or heartworm disease as likely causes for thrombocytopenia.

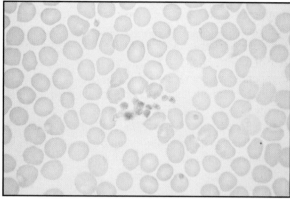

Figure 11.17: Platelet clumping, evident in this blood smear from canine blood anticoagulated with heparin, invalidates a platelet estimate or count. Ethylenediamine tetra-acetic acid is the preferred anticoagulant for platelet enumeration.

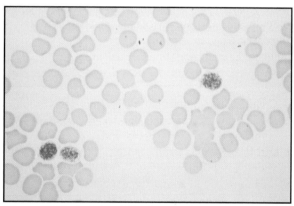

Figure 11.18: Peripheral blood smear from a dog with thrombocytopenia showing large platelets (megathrombocytes). Megathrombocytes are indicative of accelerated platelet production (thrombopoiesis) in response to accelerated platelet destruction or utilization.

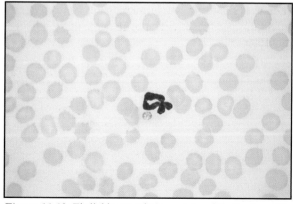

Figure 11.19: Ehrlichia morula in a neutrophil of a dog with thrombocytopenia.

Platelet count

Despite the value of evaluation of peripheral blood smears, a platelet count is still important to quantify thrombocytopenia precisely. Spurious thrombocytopenia owing to platelet clumping (see Peripheral blood smear evaluation) can be minimized by careful venepuncture and prompt (within 6 hours) analysis. Spurious thrombocytopenia can also occur in platelet counts from automated haematology analysers owing to exclusion of small or large platelets because of inappropriate machine settings or calibration. In addition, automated cell counters often do not provide accurate platelet counts in cats because of the similar size of feline platelets and red cells. Spurious thrombocytopenia has been reported in Cavalier King Charles Spaniels owing to the presence of many large platelets (Brown et al., 1994). For these reasons thrombocytopenia should be verified by examination of a peripheral blood smear to assess platelet numbers and to check for platelet clumping, especially in patients without clinical signs of bleeding.

Complete blood count

Thrombocytopenia due to bone marrow disease is typically characterized by leucopenia and non-regenerative anaemia accompanying the thrombocytopenia (pancytopenia). Decreases in two cells lines (so called bicytopenia; thrombocytopenia and neutropenia or thrombocytopenia and non-regenerative anaemia) or abnormalities in peripheral blood cell morphology is also suggestive of bone marrow disease. An important exception to these guidelines is in the early stages (first 2-3 weeks) of oestrogen toxicity, in which thrombocytopenia due to decreased platelet production is often accompanied by leucocytosis and a normal haematocrit. In dogs with oestrogen toxicity, pancytopenia may or may not develop after 3-4 weeks, depending on the magnitude of the toxic insult (Weiss and Klausner, 1990; Jain, 1993). Neutrophilia with or without a left shift is often seen in animals with thrombocytopenia due to accelerated platelet destruction or utilization, and a stress haemogram may be evident in some cases. Leucopenia in affected cats is suggestive of a viral aetiology for thrombocytopenia (feline leukaemia virus (FeLV), feline immunodeficiency virus (FIV), feline infectious peritonitis (FIP), panleucopenia) (Jordan et al., 1993).

Anaemia in dogs and cats with thrombocytopenia could be due to bone marrow disease, haemorrhage as a result of thrombocytopenia, immune-mediated haemolytic anaemia (IMHA) accompanying immune-mediated thrombocytopenia (IMT) or microangiopathic haemolytic anaemia accompanying DIC, heartworm disease or haemangiosarcoma. Anaemia due to haemorrhage or IMHA may be regenerative or non-regenerative depending on the time course of events and the presence of immunological targeting of red cell precursors.

Mean platelet volume

Mean platelet volume (MPV) is measured by automated haematology analysers and may be reported together with the results of complete blood counts (CBCs). MPV in dogs is reported to range between 7.5 fl and 10 fl (Waner et al., 1989; Northern and Tvedten, 1992; Sullivan et al,. 1995) and in cats between 12.1 fl and 15.1 fl (Boyce et al., 1986; Jain, 1993). An increased MPV (macrothrombocytosis) suggests active thrombopoiesis in response to thrombocytopenia due to accelerated platelet destruction or utilization (Sullivan et al., 1995). Macrothrombocytosis associated with decreased automated platelet counts (but not manual counts) has been reported in Cavalier King Charles Spaniels (Brown et al., 1994). Thrombocytopenia in cats with FeLV infection may also be associated with an increased MPV (Boyce et al., 1986). A low MPV (microthrombocytosis), due to platelet fragmentation or preferential destruction of larger more heavily antibody-sensitized platelets, may be found in some dogs in the early stages of IMT (Northern and Tvedten, 1992).

Bone marrow evaluation (aspiration and biopsy)

Bone marrow evaluation is not routinely necessary in patients with thrombocytopenia. Indications for bone marrow evaluation include pancytopenia or abnormal peripheral blood cell morphology. Bicytopenia (two cell lines decreased; thrombocytopenia with non-regenerative anaemia or neutropenia) may or may not be indicative of bone marrow disease. Bone marrow evaluation can be used to determine whether thrombocytopenia is due to impaired platelet production (decreased numbers of megakaryocytes in bone marrow) or accelerated platelet destruction or utilization (increased numbers of megakaryocytes in bone marrow) (Jain, 1993). Normal bone marrow contains around three megakaryocytes per low power (10 x objective) field (Joshi and Jain, 1976). Large numbers of megakaryocytes in bone marrow indicate that platelet production is adequate, and therefore thrombocytopenia is due to accelerated platelet destruction or utilization (Jain, 1993) (Figure 11.20). The presence of decreased numbers of megakaryocytes in bone marrow must be interpreted in light of the quality and cellularity of the bone marrow aspirate. This may need to be confirmed by repeating the aspirate (Figure 11.21) or by procuring a bone marrow core biopsy. Evidence of phagocytosis of platelets by bone marrow macrophages would be supportive of IMT or haemophagocytic syndrome, which has been associated with infectious and neoplastic diseases in dogs and cats (Walton et al., 1996). Major haemorrhage is unusual subsequent to bone marrow aspiration or core biopsy, even in dogs with profound thrombocytopenia, and can be readily controlled with local pressure. Hence, thrombocytopenia is not a contraindication to bone marrow aspiration or core biopsy.

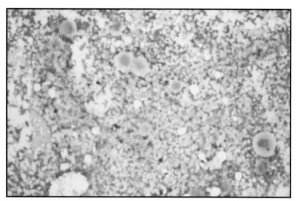

Figure 11.20: Bone marrow aspirate from a dog with thrombocytopenia showing hypercellular bone marrow and increased numbers of megakaryocytes, indicating that thrombocytopenia is due to accelerated peripheral platelet destruction or utilization. Normal canine bone marrow contains 1–3 megakaryocytes per low power (10 x objective) field.

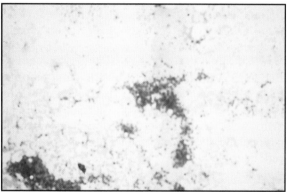

Figure 11.21: Bone marrow aspirate from a dog with thrombocytopenia showing decreased numbers of megakaryocytes. This could be indicative of thrombocytopenia due to impaired platelet production or could be due to a non-representative sample of bone marrow. This bone marrow sample was diluted with peripheral blood and may not be representative of bone marrow as a whole.

Coagulation profile

Although not routinely necessary, tests of coagulation may be indicated to investigate the possibility of thrombocytopenia related to DIC or anticoagulant rodenticide toxicity. A prolonged activated clotting time (ACT), which can readily be done in-house, in a dog or cat with thrombocytopenia is suggestive of DIC or anticoagulant rodenticide toxicity. Severe thrombocytopenia itself (<10 x 10^9/l), however, will cause slight prolongation of the ACT. In addition to the platelet count, a more complete coagulation profile can include prothrombin time (PT), activated partial thromboplastin time (APTT), thrombin clotting time, measurement of fibrin or fibrinogen degradation products (FDPs) and evaluation of a blood smear for schistocytes (fragmented red cells). Fibrinogen concentrations may be included in a CBC (heat precipitation method) or can be more accurately determined by a modified thrombin clotting time. Measurement of antithrombin III concentrations may be offered by some laboratories and can be a useful adjunct in investigating possible DIC (Feldman *et al.*, 1981; Bateman *et al.*, 1999).

Mucosal bleeding time or cuticle bleeding time will be prolonged in the presence of major thrombocytopenia and will not add more information. The bleeding time tests are more useful for investigating platelet function defects and von Willebrand's disease.

Detection of antiplatelet antibodies

A variety of tests have been used to detect serum antibodies (usually IgG) with the capability of binding to platelets (platelet bindable IgG) and more recently to detect IgG bound to the dog's own megakaryocytes or platelets (platelet-bound IgG). No such tests have yet been developed for use in cats. It is important to recognize that none of these tests are specific for primary IMT and do not enable dogs with primary IMT (no underlying cause) to be differentiated from dogs with secondary IMT (Lewis *et al.*, 1995c). The PF3 test is based on the principle that normal canine platelets will be damaged by platelet-bindable IgG in the plasma sample being evaluated and will release PF3, causing an acceleration of the APTT (Jain and Kono, 1970). Unfortunately, the PF3 test has poor sensitivity and specificity for IMT and is of little diagnostic use in evaluating patients with thrombocytopenia (Jain and Kono, 1970; Williams and Maggio-Price, 1984). The direct megakaryocyte immunofluorescence test detects IgG bound to bone marrow megakaryocytes from affected dogs (Joshi and Jain, 1976). The sensitivity of the direct megakaryocyte immunofluorescence test in dogs with IMT is variable; sensitivities of 30% to 80% are reported (Joshi and Jain, 1976). A major disadvantage is that a bone marrow aspirate, which is not routinely needed in patients with thrombocytopenia, is needed to perform the test.

Flow cytometry tests for detection of serum platelet-bindable IgG and platelet-bound IgG have been developed for use in dogs and are presently available to practitioners in the United States to assist in evaluating patients with thrombocytopenia (Lewis *et al.*, 1995b). Detection of platelet-bound IgG is the most sensitive test for IMT (sensitivity around 90%) and can be performed in dogs with even profound thrombocytopenia (5 to 10 x 10^9/l), but still does not enable primary causes of IMT to be differentiated from secondary causes. Detection of platelet-bindable IgG in serum is much less sensitive than detection of IgG already bound to a dog's platelets, but may be helpful in those cases in which sufficient numbers of patient platelets are unable to be isolated for testing (Lewis *et al.*, 1995c).

Serology

Cats: FeLV and FIV testing are indicated in cats with confirmed thrombocytopenia. A syndrome of lethargy, anorexia, weight loss, lymphadenopathy, polyarthritis, anaemia, thrombocytopenia and hyperglobulinaemia has been reported in cats in North America. These cats have had positive titres to ehrlichial organisms and respond to doxycycline therapy (Bouloy *et al.,* 1994; Peavey *et al.,* 1997). Pyogranulomatous vasculitis in cats with FIP can result in thrombocytopenia due to accelerated platelet consumption, however the utility of FIP titres in reaching a diagnosis of FIP is controversial.

Dogs: Depending on geographical location and travel history, physical examination findings and initial laboratory data, testing for *Ehrlichia canis*, *E. platys*, *E. equi*, *Rickettsia rickettsii*, leptospirosis and *Dirofilaria immitis* may be indicated in dogs with thrombocytopenia. An antinuclear antibody titre is indicated in dogs with physical examination findings and screening laboratory testing supportive of systemic lupus erythematosus (SLE).

Other tests

Biochemical profile: A biochemical profile is indicated to look for evidence of systemic disease. Examples include evidence of kidney and liver disease in dogs with leptospirosis or rickettsial infections, hypercalcaemia in dogs with lymphoma, hypoalbuminaemia, hypercholesterolaemia and/or azotaemia in dogs with glomerulonephritis, which may be associated with SLE.

Urinalysis: Proteinuria may be indicative of immune complex disease such as SLE, dirofilariasis, ehrlichiosis, lymphoma, chronic bacterial infections (e.g. endocarditis, discospondylitis, prostatitis) or systemic fungal infections.

Radiology: Radiography and ultrasonography may be indicated to investigate the possibility of splenomegaly, neoplasia or infectious disease.

Diagnostic approach to the patient with a disorder of primary haemostasis

In patients that present with signs consistent with a primary haemostatic disorder (petechiae, purpura, ecchymoses or mucosal haemorrhages), the following diagnostic approach is suggested:

1. Evaluate a peripheral blood smear for platelet numbers, platelet clumping and platelet size
2. Confirm the magnitude of thrombocytopenia by performing a platelet count (a manual platelet count can be used to recheck electronic counts, especially in cats)
3. For an initial data base include a careful review of the patient's history, including exposure to drugs or toxins (oestrogens, phenylbutazone, phenobarbital, other drugs, anticoagulant rodenticides); heartworm status and travel history; CBC and platelet count; biochemical profile and urinalysis

4. Further diagnostics:
   i. Bone marrow aspirate if indicated by CBC, history (drug exposure) or physical examination findings (e.g. testicular abnormality suggesting the possibility of a Sertoli cell tumour). If there is evidence of impaired platelet production (decreased numbers of megakaryocytes) without evident aetiology from bone marrow aspirates, then a bone marrow core biopsy and serology for *E. canis* (dogs) and FeLV and FIV (cats) is indicated
   ii. If there is no evidence of impaired platelet production from initial CBC, then a coagulation profile to test for DIC, tests for platelet-bound or serum platelet-bindable IgG and serology for *E. canis*, *E. platys*, *E. equi*, *R. rickettsii*, leptospirosis and *D. immitis* in dogs and FIV, FeLV, *E. risticii* and *E. equi* in cats may be indicated
   iii. Response to treatment (e.g. glucocorticoids, tetracyclines) can be used as a diagnostic test and while awaiting the results of other diagnostic tests.

Treatment of thrombocytopenia

In addition to specific therapy, which is dictated by the cause of thrombocytopenia, supportive care to minimize haemorrhage and its consequences is important. Supportive care includes cage rest and prevention of trauma, minimization of injections, use of the oral or intravenous route in preference to the subcutaneous or intramuscular routes for drug administration and transfusion therapy for provision of platelets and/or red blood cells.

Platelet transfusions

Platelet transfusions are rarely necessary in dogs and cats with thrombocytopenia (Williams and Maggio-Price, 1984). Platelet transfusions are indicated for patients with profound thrombocytopenia that develop neurological signs and are suspected to have central nervous system (CNS) haemorrhage, and before surgery in patients with platelet counts of less than $50 \times 10^9/l$. Patients with severe bleeding manifestations due to profound thrombocytopenia are also candidates for platelet transfusions.

Fresh whole blood or platelet components (platelet-rich plasma, platelet concentrate) can be used as sources of platelets for transfusion. Administration of a single unit of fresh whole blood, platelet-rich plasma or platelet concentrate has the potential to increase the platelet count of a 20 kg dog by as much as 30 to $40 \times 10^9/l$.

In patients with thrombocytopenia due to accelerated platelet destruction or utilization (e.g. IMT, DIC), platelets have dramatically reduced circulating life spans (minutes to hours) and transfused platelets are destroyed rapidly (Carr *et al.*, 1986). In these cases, multiple units of platelet-rich plasma or platelet concentrate (prepared from fresh whole blood by centrifugation) are required to maintain platelet counts greater than 10 x 10⁹/l and to stop ongoing haemorrhage. This is impractical and cost prohibitive in most situations. The administration of a single unit of fresh whole blood, platelet-rich plasma or platelet concentrate to these patients is ineffective.

Red cell transfusions
Red cell transfusions are indicated in patients with thrombocytopenia in which anaemia is severe.

Commonest causes of thrombocytopenia

Thrombocytopenia in dogs
Thrombocytopenia is about five times more common in dogs than it is in cats (Grindem *et al.*, 1991). The commonest causes of thrombocytopenia in dogs in North America (Cockburn and Troy, 1986; Grindem *et al.*, 1991, 1994) are reported to be:

- IMT (either primary or secondary)
- Infectious diseases, including rickettsial diseases (*E. canis* and Rocky Mountain spotted fever), heartworm disease and systemic mycoses (cryptococcosis, coccidioidomycosis, blastomycosis, histoplasmosis)
- Neoplasia (especially lymphoma and haemangiosarcoma).

Thrombocytopenia in cats
Thrombocytopenia in cats is uncommon (Jordan *et al.*, 1993). The commonest reported causes of confirmed thrombocytopenia in cats (Shelton *et al.*, 1990; Hart and Nolte, 1994; Peterson *et al.*, 1995) include:

- Infectious diseases, including FeLV, FIV, FIP, *Toxoplasma gondii* and *Haemobartonella felis*
- Neoplasia, especially lymphoproliferative and myeloproliferative diseases
- Thromboembolism related to cardiac disease.

DIC has been identified as the pathophysiological cause for thrombocytopenia in about 10% of cases of feline thrombocytopenia (Jordan *et al.*, 1993). The aetiology for thrombocytopenia in cats is frequently undetermined, for example, 20% of cases in one study were idiopathic (Jordan *et al.*, 1993).

Specific causes of thrombocytopenia

Primary immune-mediated thrombocytopenia
Primary IMT is discussed fully in Chapter 14(i).

Secondary immune-mediated thrombocytopenia
Secondary IMT has been described in dogs with SLE, neoplasia and certain infectious diseases, and subsequent to drug administration (Mackin, 1995b; Lewis

and Meyers, 1996). In cats, IMT may occur secondary to FeLV or FIV infection (Shelton *et al.*, 1990).

Although any drug can potentially provoke secondary IMT, potentiated sulphonamides, the gold salt auranofin and cephalosporins have been documented to cause IMT in dogs. Drug-induced IMT usually develops after weeks to months of treatment, resolves within 2 weeks of cessation of the drug and does not recur in the absence of the drug. IMT is a common feature of SLE. Other clinical and laboratory manifestations of SLE, such as polyarthritis, dermatitis, mucocutaneous ulceration, peripheral neuropathy, polymyositis, glomerulonephritis, IMHA, neutropenia and antinuclear antibodies usually enable SLE to be distinguished from primary IMT. IMT is well documented in dogs with lymphoproliferative and non-haematopoietic neoplasia. Immune-mediated platelet destruction may contribute to thrombocytopenia in dogs infected with *E. canis*, *Babesia canis*, *D. immitis* and distemper virus (Lewis *et al.*, 1995; Mackin, 1995b; Waner *et al.*, 1995).

Neoplasia
Thrombocytopenia is frequently associated with neoplasia in dogs, particularly lymphoproliferative neoplasia and haemangiosarcoma (Grindem *et al.*, 1994). Mechanisms for thrombocytopenia associated with neoplasia are multiple and include disseminated or local platelet consumption, splenic sequestration, myelophthisis, bone marrow suppression by chemotherapy, radiation therapy or tumour elaborated oestrogens and immune-mediated platelet destruction. IMT is well documented in dogs with lymphoproliferative and non-haematopoietic neoplasms (Helfand *et al.*, 1985) and may precede the discovery of neoplasia, leading to an erroneous diagnosis of primary IMT.

Disseminated intravascular coagulation
Thrombocytopenia is a common finding in dogs and cats with DIC (Feldman *et al.*, 1981; Grindem *et al.*, 1991; Jordan *et al.*, 1993; Bateman *et al.*, 1999). DIC in dogs is most frequently associated with septicaemia, disseminated malignancy, massive trauma, heat stroke and vasculitis (e.g. leptospirosis, Rocky Mountain spotted fever, immune-mediated vasculitis). In cats, liver disease, FIP, malignancy and thromboembolism related to cardiac disease are the most commonly reported causes of DIC (Jordan *et al.*, 1993; Peterson *et al.*, 1995). Assessment of a coagulation profile, including PT, APTT, FDPs, fibrinogen concentration and antithrombin III concentrations, and evaluation of a blood smear for schistocytes will enable most cases of DIC to be diagnosed.

Infectious disease
Viral, bacterial, protozoal, fungal and parasitic diseases may cause thrombocytopenia in dogs and cats. In North America, infectious diseases are reported to

account for 20% to 60% of dogs with thrombocytopenia. *E. canis*, Rocky Mountain spotted fever, leptospirosis and dirofilariasis are frequently diagnosed infectious causes of thrombocytopenia in dogs in North America (Breitschwerdt, 1988; Grindem *et al.*, 1991). Thrombocytopenia is a common haematological abnormality associated with bacteraemia in humans but is less commonly reported in bacteraemic dogs. Mild thrombocytopenia is a frequent occurrence subsequent to modified-live distemper vaccination and is less commonly observed in naturally occurring cases of distemper. Immune-mediated platelet destruction may contribute to thrombocytopenia in dogs infected with *E. canis, B. canis, D. immitis* and distemper virus (Lewis *et al.*, 1995c; Mackin, 1995b; Waner *et al.*, 1995).

Haemolytic uraemic syndrome
Haemolytic uraemic syndrome (HUS), a disorder of platelet hyperaggregability with intravascular platelet thrombi and widespread tissue ischaemia, has been reported in dogs, especially greyhounds. Clinical and laboratory findings in HUS, including neurological signs, renal failure, microangiopathic haemolytic anaemia (schistocytosis), thrombocytopenia and fever, make it distinguishable from primary IMT (Holloway and Senior, 1993; Hertzke *et al.*, 1995).

Breed-related thrombocytopenia
Greyhounds, Cavalier King Charles Spaniels and Shiba Inus can have platelet counts that are lower than in other breeds of dog (Eksell *et al.*, 1994; Sullivan *et al.*, 1994; Smedile *et al.*, 1997; Gookin *et al.*, 1998).

THROMBOCYTOSIS

Thrombocytosis, defined as a platelet count above the reference range, is a much less common abnormality than thrombocytopenia. Thrombocytosis, other than primary thrombocytosis, is usually of no clinical significance. The causes of thrombocytosis are summarized in Figure 11.22.

Mechanisms and causes of thrombocytosis

Thrombocytosis due to splenic contraction
The spleen normally contains about 30% of the circulating platelet pool, which is recognized by the body as being a constituent of total platelet numbers (Jain, 1993). Any cause of splenic contraction, for example, excitement, exercise or acute blood loss, will result in a transient increase in platelet numbers in the circulating blood, which may or may not cause mild thrombocytosis.

Post-splenectomy thrombocytosis
Splenectomy will result in a more permanent increase in platelet numbers, which may or may not cause mild thrombocytosis (Jain, 1993).

Thrombocytosis due to splenic contraction (physiological)
Excitement
Exercise
Acute blood loss
Trauma
Rebound thrombocytosis
Response to prior thrombocytopenia
Post-splenectomy thrombocytosis
Reactive thrombocytosis
Inflammatory conditions
Infection
Neoplasia: haematopoietic and solid tumours
Chronic blood loss
Hyperadrenocorticism or administration of glucocorticoids
Primary thrombocytosis
Platelet leukaemias
Essential thrombocythaemia
Megakaryoblastic leukaemia
Polycythaemia vera, other myeloproliferative and lymphoproliferative diseases
Myelodysplasia and myelofibrosis

Figure 11.22: *Causes of thrombocytosis.*

Rebound thrombocytosis
Subsequent to resolution of thrombocytopenia from any cause, rebound thrombocytosis may occur owing to the residual effect of increased concentrations of thrombopoietin and other cytokines stimulating thrombopoiesis.

Reactive thrombocytosis
Although thrombopoietin provides the major physiological stimulus, thrombopoiesis can also be stimulated by a variety of cytokines, such as IL-3 and IL-6, granulocyte–macrophage colony-stimulating factor and erythropoietin. Reactive thrombocytosis may occur due to non-specific stimulation of thrombopoiesis associated with increased concentrations of these cytokines in a variety of inflammatory conditions, infections, solid tumours, chronic blood loss and hyperadrenocorticism (Jain, 1993; Reagan and Rebar, 1995).

Primary thrombocytosis
Platelet leukaemia or essential thrombocythaemia (a myeloproliferative disease affecting mature platelet precursors) and megakaryoblastic leukaemia (which affects a more immature cell of the platelet lineage) are rare diseases but cause profound thrombocytosis (platelet counts often greater than 1000 x 10⁹/l). Megakaryoblastic leukaemia can also cause thrombocytopenia. Essential thrombocythaemia is characterized by large numbers of circulating platelets (including

bizarre forms), increased numbers of megakaryocytes in bone marrow and no identifiable cause for reactive thrombocytosis (Hopper *et al.*, 1989). Circulating megakaryoblasts and bizarre platelet forms, which may infiltrate other tissues, are typically seen in megakaryoblastic leukaemia (Canfield *et al.*, 1993). In cats, platelet or megakaryoblastic leukaemias may be due to FeLV infection. Platelets, red cells and white cells originate from common bone marrow precursor cells (pluripotential and multipotential bone marrow stem cells) and thrombocytosis may occur in association with polycythaemia vera, lymphoproliferative or myeloproliferative disease or myelodysplasia if an early stem cell is affected.

Clinical presentation

The clinical presentation of animals with thrombocytosis varies primarily with the underlying disease. Physiological and reactive thrombocytosis is usually transient and without clinical consequence. Although both thrombotic and haemorrhagic tendencies may occur in patients with primary thrombocytosis, bleeding is more commonly seen. Splenomegaly is common in animals with primary thrombocytosis (Jain, 1993).

Thrombosis may occur owing to the increase in platelet numbers, in addition to enhanced platelet function. Clinical signs depend on the thrombosed organ. Pulmonary thrombosis frequently causes tachypnoea and dyspnoea. Pulmonary thrombosis can also cause right-sided congestive heart failure secondary to pulmonary hypertension, with ascites, jugular distension and peripheral oedema; and haemoptysis may also be seen. Mesenteric thrombosis can result in abdominal pain, vomiting and diarrhoea. Portal vein thrombosis may lead to ascites. CNS thrombosis leads to sudden onset of neurological signs, such as seizures, altered mental state and paresis, which depends on the location of the thrombus in the CNS.

Bleeding in patients with primary thrombocytosis is due to defective platelet function. Haemorrhagic signs reflect a disorder of primary haemostasis and may include bleeding from mucosal surfaces, mucosal and cutaneous petechiae, purpura and ecchymoses (Jain, 1993).

REFERENCES AND FURTHER READING

Bateman SW, Mathews KA, Abrams-Ogg ACG, Lumsden JH, Johnstone IB, Hillers TK and Foster RA (1999) Diagnosis of disseminated intravascular coagulation in dogs admitted to an intensive care unit. *Journal of the American Veterinary Medical Association* **215**, 798-804

Bouloy RP, Lappin MR, Holland CH, Thrall MA, Baker D and O'Neil S (1994) Clinical ehrlichiosis in a cat. *Journal of the American Veterinary Medical Association* **204**, 1475-1478

Boyce JT, Kociba GJ, Jacobs RM and Weiser MG (1986) Feline leukemia virus-induced thrombocytopenia and macrothrombocytosis in cats. *Veterinary Pathology* **23**, 16-20

Breitschwerdt EB (1988) Infectious thrombocytopenia in dogs. *Compendium of Continuing Education for the Practising Veterinarian* **10**, 1177-1190

Brown SJ, Simpson KW, Baker S, Spagnoletti MA and Elwood CM (1994) Macrothrombocytosis in Cavalier King Charles Spaniels. *Veterinary Record* **135**, 281-283

Canfield PJ, Church DB and Russ IG (1993) Myeloproliferative disorders involving the megakaryocytic line. *Journal of Small Animal Practice* **34**, 296-301

Carr JM, Kruskall MS, Kaye JA and Robinson SH (1986) Efficacy of platelet transfusions in immune thrombocytopenia. *American Journal of Medicine* **80**, 1051-1054

Cockburn C and Troy GC (1986) A retrospective study of 62 cases of thrombocytopenia in the dog. *Southwest Veterinarian* **37**, 133-141

Eksell P, Haggstrom J, Kvart C and Karlsson A (1994) Thrombocytopenia in the Cavalier King Charles Spaniel. *Journal of Small Animal Practice* **35**, 153-155

Feldman BF, Madewell BR and O'Neill S (1981) Disseminated intravascular coagulation: antithrombin, plasminogen, and coagulation abnormalities in 41 dogs. *Journal of the American Veterinary Medical Association* **179**, 151-154

Gookin JL, Bunch SE, Rush LJ and Grindem CB (1998) Evaluation of microcytosis in 18 Shibas. *Journal of the American Veterinary Medical Association* **212**, 1258-1259

Grindem CB, Breitschwerdt EB, Corbett WT and Jans HE (1991) Epidemiologic survey of thrombocytopenia in dogs: a report on 987 cases. *Veterinary Clinical Pathology* **20**, 38-43

Grindem CB, Breitschwerdt EB, Corbett WT, Page RL and Jans HE (1994) Thrombocytopenia associated with neoplasia in dogs. *Journal of Veterinary Internal Medicine* **8**, 400-405

Hackner SG (1995) Approach to the diagnosis of bleeding disorders. *Compendium of Continuing Education for the Practising Veterinarian* **17**, 331-349

Hart SW and Nolte I (1994) Hemostatic disorders in feline immunodeficiency virus-seropositive cats. *Journal of Veterinary Internal Medicine* **8**, 355-362

Helfand SC, Couto CG and Madewell BR (1985) Immune-mediated thrombocytopenia associated with solid tumors in dogs. *Journal of the American Animal Hospital Association* **21**, 787-794

Hertzke DM, Cowan LA, Schoning P and Fenwick BW (1995) Glomerular ultrastructural lesions of idiopathic cutaneous and renal glomerular vasculopathy of greyhounds. *Veterinary Pathology* **32**, 451-459

Holloway SA and Senior DF (1993) Hemolytic-uremic syndrome in dogs. *Journal of Veterinary Internal Medicine* **7**, 220-227

Honeckman AL, Knapp DW and Reagan WJ (1996) Diagnosis of canine immune-mediated hematologic disease. *Compendium on Continuing Education for the Practising Veterinarian* **18**, 113-125

Hopper PE, Mandell CP, Turrel JM, Jain NC, Tablin F and Zinkl JG (1989) Probable essential thrombocythemia in a dog. *Journal of Veterinary Internal Medicine* **3**, 79-85

Jacobs RM, Boyce JT, and Kociba GJ (1986) Flow cytometric and radioisotopic determinations of platelet survival time in normal cats and feline leukemia virus-infected cats. *Cytometry* **7**, 64-69

Jain NC (1993) *Essentials of Veterinary Hematology*. Lea and Febiger, Philadelphia

Jain NC and Kono CS (1970) The platelet factor-3 test for detection of canine antiplatelet antibody. *Veterinary Clinical Pathology* **9**, 10-14

Jordan HL, Grindem CB and Breitschwerdt EB (1993) Thrombocytopenia in cats: a retrospective study of 41 cases. *Journal of Veterinary Internal Medicine* **7**, 261-265

Joshi BC and Jain NC (1976) Detection of antiplatelet antibody in serum and on megakaryocytes of dogs with autoimmune thrombocytopenia. *American Journal of Veterinary Research* **37**, 681-685

Lewis DC and Meyers KM (1996) Canine idiopathic thrombocytopenic purpura. *Journal of Veterinary Internal Medicine* **10**, 207-218

Lewis DC, Bruyette DS and Kellerman DL (1995a) Thrombocytopenia subsequent to anticoagulant rodenticide-induced hemorrhage in dogs. (Abstract.) *Journal of Veterinary Internal Medicine* **9**, 188

Lewis DC, McVey DS, Shuman WS and Muller WB (1995b) Development and characterization of a flow cytometric assay for detection of platelet-bound immunoglobulin G in dogs. *American Journal of Veterinary Research* **56**, 1555-1558

Lewis DC, Meyers, KM, Callan MB, Bücheler J and Giger U (1995c) Detection of platelet-bound and serum platelet-bindable antibodies for diagnosis of idiopathic thrombocytopenic purpura in dogs. *Journal of the American Veterinary Medical Association* **206**, 47-52

Mackin A (1995a) Canine immune-mediated thrombocytopenia. Part I. *Compendium of Continuing Education for the Practising Veterinarian* **17**, 353-364

Mackin A (1995b) Canine immune-mediated thrombocytopenia. Part II. *Compendium of Continuing Education for the Practising Veterinarian* **17**, 515-535

Northern J and Tvedten NW (1992) Diagnosis of microthrombocytosis and immune-mediated thrombocytopenia in dogs with thrombocytopenia: 68 cases (1987-1989). *Journal of the American Veterinary Medical Association* **200**, 368-372

Peavey GM, Holland CJ, Dutta SK, Smith G, Moore A, Rich LJ, Lappin MR and Richter K (1997) Suspected ehrlichial infection in five cats from a household. *Journal of the American Veterinary Medical Association* **210**, 231-234

Peterson JL, Couto CG and Wellman ML (1995) Hemostatic disorders in cats: a retrospective study and review of the literature. *Journal of Veterinary Internal Medicine* **9**, 298-303

Reagan WJ and Rebar AH (1995) Platelet disorders. In: *Textbook of Veterinary Internal Medicine, 4th edn*, ed. SJ Ettinger and EC Feldman, pp. 1964-1976. WB Saunders, Philadelphia

Shelton GH, Linenberger ML, Grant CK and Abkowitz JL (1990) Hematologic manifestations of feline immunodeficiency virus infection. *Blood* **76**, 1104-1109

Sherding RG, Wilson GP and Kociba GJ (1981) Bone marrow hypoplasia in eight dogs with Sertoli cell tumor. *Journal of the American Veterinary Medical Association* **178**, 497-501

Slichter SJ, Deeg HJ and Kennedy MS (1987) Prevention of platelet alloimmunization in dogs with systemic cyclosporine and by UV-irradiation or cyclosporine-loading of donor platelets. *Blood* **69**, 414-418

Smedile LE, Houston DM, Taylor SM, Post K and Searcy GP (1997) Idiopathic asymptomatic thrombocytopenia in Cavalier King Charles Spaniels: 11 cases (1983-1993). *Journal of the American Animal Hospital Association* **33**, 411-415

Sullivan PS, Evans HL and McDonald TP (1994) Platelet concentration and hemoglobin function in Greyhounds. *Journal of the American Veterinary Medical Association* **205**, 838-841

Sullivan PS, Manning KL and McDonald TP (1995) Association of mean platelet volume and bone marrow megakaryocytopoieses in thrombocytopenic dogs: 60 cases (1984-1993). *Journal of the American Veterinary Medical Association* **206**, 332-334

Walton RM, Modiano JF, Thrall MA and Wheeler SL (1996) Bone marrow cytological findings in 4 dogs and a cat with hemophagocytic syndrome. *Journal of Veterinary Internal Medicine* **10**, 7-14

Waner T, Harrus S, Weiss DJ, Bark H and Keysary A (1995) Demonstration of serum antiplatelet antibodies in experimental acute canine ehrlichiosis. *Veterinary Immunology and Immunopathology* **48**, 177-182

Waner T, Yuval D and Nyska A (1989) Electronic measurement of canine mean platelet volume. *Veterinary Clinical Pathology* **18**, 84-86

Weiss DJ and Klausner JS (1990) Drug-associated aplastic anemia in dogs: eight cases (1984-1988). *Journal of the American Veterinary Medical Association* **196**, 472-475

Williams DA and Maggio-Price L (1984) Canine idiopathic thrombocytopenic purpura: clinical observations and long-term follow up in 54 cases. *Journal of the American Veterinary Medical Association* **185**, 660-663

Disorders of Platelet Function

Tracy Stokol

INTRODUCTION

The most commonly encountered platelet disorders in veterinary practice are quantitative abnormalities, particularly thrombocytopenia. Defects in platelet function, i.e. thrombopathias (thrombocytopathies), are much less common and difficult to diagnose as they require specialized tests, most of which are not readily available to the general practitioner. Abnormalities in platelet function have, however, been documented in domestic animals and result in abnormal bleeding in affected individuals. Thrombopathias should always be suspected if an animal is bleeding excessively but has a normal platelet count and coagulation profile. Knowledge of normal platelet physiology and function is helpful in understanding the different forms of disturbed platelet function.

PLATELET STRUCTURE

Platelets are small anucleate cells produced by megakaryocytes in the bone marrow and pulmonary vasculature. While circulating they have a characteristic discoid shape. Despite its small size, the platelet is a complex cell, composed of an outer membrane enclosing a cytoplasm rich in organelles and membranous structures (Figure 12.1). The platelet can be divided into several compartments or zones, each having a distinctive role in platelet function. These compartments are the outer membrane, the sol–gel zone, the organelle zone and the membrane systems.

The outer membrane

The outer membrane is a biphospholipid membrane, throughout which cholesterol is uniformly dispersed. Phospholipids within the membrane are distributed asymmetrically; this asymmetry is maintained by specific proteins in the membrane. In the resting platelet, the outer layer is rich in phosphatidylcholine and sphingomyelin, whereas the inner layer is rich in phosphatidylserine and phosphatidylethonalamine. This asymmetry is essential for proper platelet function, as alterations in the distribution of the phospholipids (specifically, the preferential movement

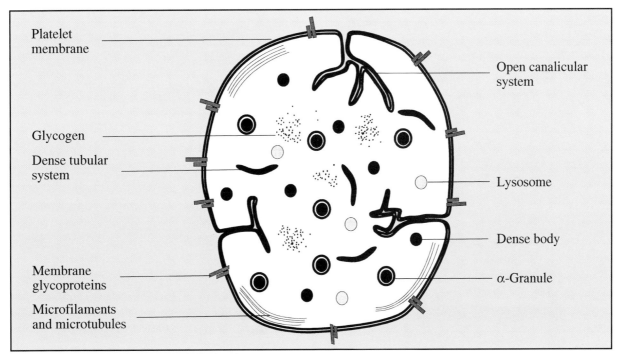

Figure 12.1: *Schematic illustration of platelet ultrastructure.*

of phosphatidylserine to the outer layer of the membrane) that occur on platelet activation converts the platelet into a procoagulant molecule. Numerous glycoproteins (GP) are embedded within the lipid membrane. These act as receptor molecules, allowing the platelet to interact with other cells and the subendothelial matrix. The glycoproteins are labelled consecutively with roman numerals and belong to several different gene families, including integrins, leucine-rich glycoproteins, selectins, the immunoglobulin superfamily and quadraspanins. Figure 12.2 lists the glycoprotein families with known roles in platelet function.

The different outer membrane components have specific roles in platelet function. The translocation of phosphatidylserine to the outer membrane provides a binding surface for activated coagulation factors (especially those associated with the activation of factor X and prothrombin) and promotes their catalytic activity (Figure 12.3). This is essential for propagation of the coagulation cascade. The exposure of phosphatidylserine is also termed 'platelet procoagulant activity,' and used to be called platelet factor 3 (PF3). Arachidonic acid is produced by the action of phospholipase A_2 on membrane phospholipids (particularly phosphatidylcholine). Arachidonic acid is the initial substrate in a series of reactions that result in eicosanoid (prostaglandin) synthesis (Figure 12.4). The most important platelet eicosanoid is thromboxane A_2, a potent mediator of platelet aggregation and recruitment. The surface glycoproteins, especially the complexes of GPIb-IX and GPIIb-IIIa, act as receptors for both soluble (e.g. fibrinogen) and insoluble (e.g. collagen) ligands and are essential for platelet aggregation and platelet adhesion to the vascular subendothelium. A qualitative or quantitative defect in these receptors results in abnormal platelet function.

Platelet glycoprotein	Ligand	Role in platelet function
Integrins		
GPIIb-IIIa ($\alpha_{IIb}\beta_3$)	Fibrinogen, von Willebrand factor (vWf), fibronectin, vitronectin	Aggregation and spreading
Vitronectin receptor ($\alpha_v\beta_3$)	Vitronectin, fibrinogen, fibronectin, thrombospondin	Adhesion (low shear)
GPIa-IIa ($\alpha_2\beta_1$)	Collagen	Adhesion (low shear)
GPIc-IIa ($\alpha_5\beta_1$)	Fibronectin	Adhesion (low shear)
GPIc-IIa region ($\alpha_6\beta_1$)	Laminin	Adhesion (low shear)
Leucine-rich glycoproteins		
GPIb-IX	vWf	Adhesion (high shear) and shape change
GPV	Forms a complex with GPIb-IX	Binding site for α-thrombin Interacts with vWf
Selectins		
P-selectin (α-granule)	Lectins	Leucocyte–platelet interactions

Figure 12.2: *Glycoprotein receptors on the platelet membrane and their role in platelet function.*

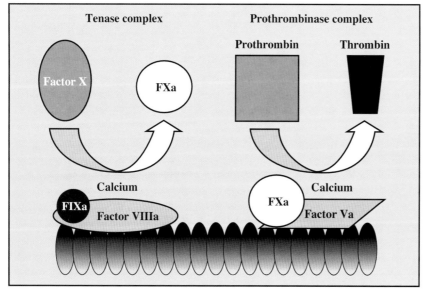

Figure 12.3: *Schematic illustration of assembly of the tenase and prothrombinase complexes on the platelet surface. During platelet activation, phosphatidylserine is enriched in the outer leaflet of the platelet membrane. The tenase complex consists of the platelet membrane-associated assembly of activated factor IX (FIXa), activated factor VIII (factor VIIIa), phosphatidylserine and ionized calcium (calcium) and is responsible for the activation of factor X. Similarly, the prothrombinase complex consists of a composite of activated factor X (FXa), activated factor V (factor Va), phosphatidylserine and ionized calcium and is responsible for the activation of prothrombin to thrombin.*

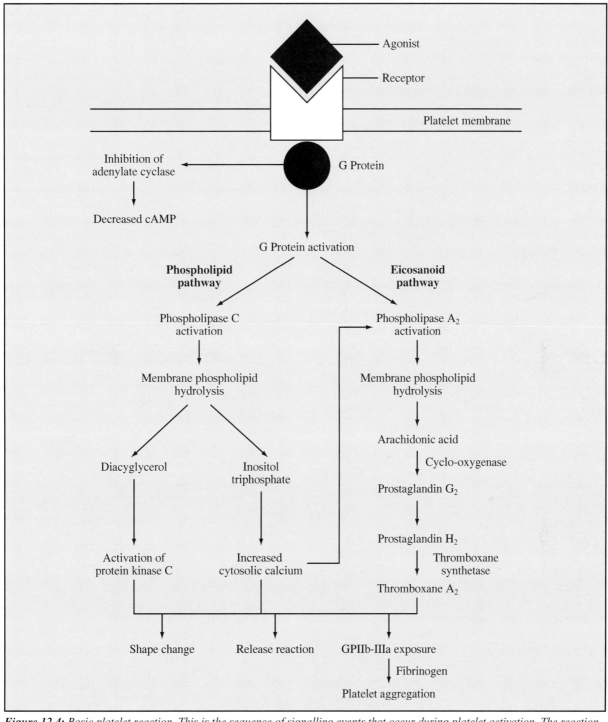

Figure 12.4: *Basic platelet reaction. This is the sequence of signalling events that occur during platelet activation. The reaction is initiated when an agonist binds to its specific receptor on the platelet membrane. Through messengers called G proteins this binding activates the enzymes phospholipase C (phospholipid pathway) and phospholipase A₂ (arachidonate or eicosanoid pathway) and causes a rapid influx of extracellular calcium. In the phospholipid pathway, phospholipase C hydrolyses phosphatidylinositol 4,5-biphosphate in the platelet membrane to diacylglycerol and inositol 1,4,5-phosphate. Diacylglycerol activates protein kinase C, which, through secondary messengers, leads to platelet aggregation, shape change and secretion. Inositol triphosphate increases cytosolic calcium concentrations by promoting calcium release from the dense tubular system. The increased intracellular calcium has several effects, including shape change, granule secretion and activation of GPIIb-IIIa. In the eicosanoid pathway, phospholipase A₂ catalyses the release of arachidonic acid from phospholipids (especially phosphatidylcholine) in the platelet membrane, leading to the synthesis of prostaglandin endoperoxides and thromboxane A₂. Thromboxane A₂ plays a critical role in platelet recruitment and granule secretion. Although these two pathways of platelet activation are illustrated as relatively distinct from one another, they do interact with, and amplify, each other. The inositol triphosphate-mediated increase in intracellular calcium concentration also activates phospholipase A₂. A lipase converts diacylglycerol into arachidonic acid. Both arachidonic acid and thromboxane A₂ can also activate phospholipase C. A separate effect of agonist-receptor binding is the inhibition of adenylate cyclase, thus decreasing cyclic adenosine monophosphate (cAMP) concentrations and promoting calcium release from the dense tubular system.*

The sol–gel zone

The sol-gel zone contains microfilaments and microtubules, which form the platelet cytoskeleton and are responsible for maintenance of the normal discoid shape. These fibres provide the means by which the platelet can undergo a change in shape and exteriorize the contents of the granules by the so-called 'release reaction'. This zone also contains glycogen, the principle energy source for the platelet.

The organelle zone

The organelle zone contains two platelet-specific granules, the α-granules and δ-granules (dense bodies), as well as common organelles such as mitochondria, peroxisomes and lysosomes. Figure 12.5 lists the contents of the platelet-specific granules. The α-granule proteins are secreted during the release reaction and participate in both platelet aggregation (von Willebrand factor (vWf) and fibrinogen) and fibrin formation (fibrinogen, factor XI and factor V). The dense bodies are the storage site for the non-metabolic pool of adenosine triphosphate (ATP), adenosine diphosphate (ADP), serotonin and calcium. Two thirds of the platelet's adenine nucleotides are in this storage pool, with an ATP:ADP ratio of 2:3. The metabolic pool has an ATP:ADP ratio of 8:1. Deficiency within the storage pool, resulting from reduced or absent dense bodies, is characterized by an increased ATP:ADP ratio in the storage pool approaching that of the metabolic pool.

Membrane systems

The platelet contains two important membrane systems: the open surface-connected canalicular system and the dense tubular system (see Figure 12.1). The open canalicular system, produced by invaginations of the platelet membrane, maintains direct contact with the plasma and is the likely site of endocytosis of plasma proteins into the platelet. The contents of both α-granules and dense bodies are exocytosed into the open canalicular system during the release reaction. The dense tubular system (composed of residual smooth endoplasmic reticulum) actively sequesters calcium by means of a calcium pump, the activity of which is enhanced by cyclic adenosine monophosphate (cAMP). The concentration of cyclic AMP is regulated by two enzymes: adenylate cyclase, which increases cAMP concentrations, and phosphodiesterase, which destroys cAMP. Calcium release from the dense tubular system is essential for platelet activation, the release reaction and aggregation. Therefore, agents that stimulate adenylate cyclase, such as prostacyclin, increase cAMP concentrations, which promotes calcium sequestration in the dense tubular system and inhibits aggregation and release. The dense tubular system also contains a platelet-specific peroxidase and enzymes involved in prostaglandin synthesis.

α-Granules
Adhesive proteins – promote platelet aggregation and adhesion to subendothelium and leucocytes von Willebrand factor*, fibronectin* Fibrinogen† Thrombospondin, vitronectin, P-selectin
Growth modulators – stimulate the growth and proliferation of smooth muscle cells and fibroblasts and the deposition of extracellular matrix material (roles in inflammation, wound repair and atherosclerosis) Platelet-derived growth factor, transforming growth factor β Platelet factor 4, connective tissue activating peptide III, thrombospondin C1 – inhibitor, high molecular weight kininogen
Coagulation factors – participate in fibrin formation and fibrinolysis Fibrinogen Factor V*, factor XI* High molecular weight kininogen Plasminogen activator inhibitor I, Protein S

δ-Granules (dense bodies)
Adenosine triphosphate
Guanine triphosphate
Adenosine diphosphate
Guanine diphosphate
Calcium
Serotonin
Pyrophosphate

Figure 12.5: *Contents of platelet-specific granules. *Substances produced by megakaryocytes. †Along with albumin and immunoglobulin G, fibrinogen is endocytosed by platelets and packaged into α-granules.*

PLATELET FUNCTION

Haemostasis (see Chapter 9) can be separated into two different processes: primary and secondary haemostasis. Platelets act mostly in primary haemostasis where they plug sites of vascular injury by adhering to, and aggregating around, breaches in vessel walls. This role is, however, a vastly simplified one. Platelets also participate actively in the coagulation cascade by the release of stored coagulation factors and by the exposure of phosphatidylserine. The latter promotes the coagulation cascade by providing a scaffold on which coagulation can proceed and by optimising the activity of coagulation factors. It is becoming increasingly clear that platelets contribute significantly to pathological vascular events including inflammation, thrombosis, atherosclerosis and cancer metastasis. Defects in platelet function are, however, recognized clinically by the abnormal bleeding symptoms that result from failure of platelets to form an adequate platelet plug in primary haemostasis. Therefore, only the role of platelets in haemostasis will be discussed here.

Platelet function in haemostasis can be separated into several steps: adhesion, aggregation, the release reaction and platelet procoagulant activity (Figure 12.6). Although these processes are discussed separately, these events occur simultaneously in the vasculature, and this distinction is an artificial one.

Adhesion

Under normal circumstances, the endothelium prevents platelet interaction with the vessel wall by acting as a physical barrier and secreting platelet inhibitors, prostacyclin and nitric oxide. Vessel injury disrupts the endothelium and exposes the thrombogenic subendothelium to circulating cells. Immediately, platelets adhere to the vessel wall

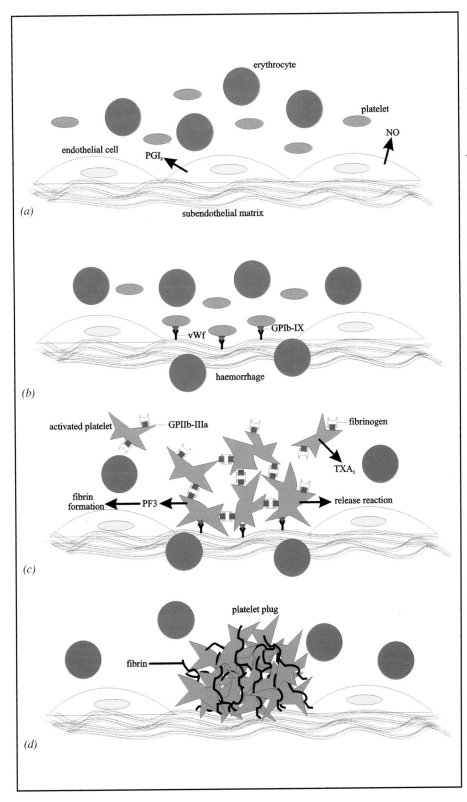

Figure 12.6: *Schematic illustration of primary haemostasis. (a) The intact endothelium prevents platelet adherence by acting as a physical barrier and releasing inhibitors of platelet function, including prostacyclin (PGI$_2$) and nitric oxide (NO). These substances inhibit platelet function by increasing platelet concentrations of cyclic adenosine monophosphate and cyclic guanosine monophosphate, respectively. (b) When the endothelium is disrupted, platelets adhere to the exposed subendothelium. Under conditions of high shear, platelets adhere through an interaction between GPIb-IX and von Willebrand factor (vWf). (c) Under conditions of low shear, platelets adhere, through integrin receptors, to collagen, laminin and fibronectin in the subendothelial matrix. Adhesion activates platelets through the basic platelet reaction, resulting in shape change, the release reaction and thromboxane A$_2$ (TXA$_2$) generation. This culminates in platelet recruitment, further platelet activation and aggregation. Platelet aggregation occurs when fibrinogen binds to its receptor, GPIIb-IIIa, on the platelet membrane. Consequently, the primary platelet plug is produced by a fused mass of platelets. Platelet procoagulant activity (PF3) becomes available (through translocation of phosphatidylserine to the outer leaflet of the platelet membrane) on platelet activation and promotes secondary haemostasis, resulting in the formation of fibrin. (d) Fibrin solidifies the primary platelet plug, forming a stable thrombus.*

through the interaction of glycoprotein receptors in the unstimulated platelet membrane with ligands in the vascular subendothelial matrix. The type of receptors and ligands differ depending on the site of vessel damage and, more specifically, on the shear rate of blood flow in that area. Studies performed in vitro indicate that under conditions of low shear, as found in the venous circulation or areas of blood stasis, platelets adhere to collagen, laminin and fibronectin through integrin receptors. Under conditions of high shear, as found in the arterioles and microcirculation, adhesion is accomplished by vWf and GPIb-IX (Figure 12.2). Humans with abnormalities in either vWf (von Willebrand's disease) or GPIb-IX (Bernard–Soulier syndrome) exhibit defective platelet adhesion under conditions of high shear, illustrating the importance of this interaction and providing a physiological basis for the haemorrhage observed in these two conditions. von Willebrand's disease has been diagnosed in several breeds of dogs, however an animal model of Bernard–Soulier syndrome has not been identified. The interaction of vWf with GPIb-IX triggers platelet activation and subsequent aggregation through a complex series of intracellular signal transduction events termed the basic platelet reaction (Figure 12.4). This reaction involves two separate but interacting pathways, one involving phospholipid hydrolysis (phospholipase C pathway) and the other, arachidonic acid metabolism (arachidonate or eicosanoid pathway). An important consequence of triggering both pathways is the activation (by conformational change) of the fibrinogen receptor, GPIIb-IIIa, which culminates in platelet aggregation.

Aggregation

Under physiological conditions, platelet aggregation occurs after platelets have attached and spread along the subendothelium or have interacted with certain agonists, such as thrombin or ADP. These interactions initiate the basic platelet reaction, resulting in activation of GPIIb-IIIa. Platelet aggregation is mediated by the binding of soluble plasma proteins, particularly fibrinogen, to GPIIb-IIIa (in the presence of divalent cations) on the same or adjacent platelets, thus effectively crosslinking the platelets. Plasma and platelet vWf (released from α-granules) may contribute to this aggregation in healthy humans. Aggregation is potentiated by other mediators, including thrombin, ADP (released from dense bodies, damaged endothelial cells or erythrocytes), serotonin, platelet activating factor and thromboxane A_2. Therefore, unlike adhesion, aggregation is an active process, requiring both platelet metabolism and stimulation by one or more specific agonists.

Platelet aggregation can be measured in vitro by platelet aggregometers. In these devices, aggregation is initiated when one or more agonists bind to specific receptors in the platelet membrane. Figure 12.7 lists the various types of platelet agonists. Strong agonists, like collagen and thrombin, induce aggregation through both the phospholipase C (hydrolysis of phospholipid) and eicosanoid pathways (generation of thromboxane A_2). They can trigger granule secretion even when aggregation is inhibited. Weak agonists, like ADP, activate the eicosanoid pathway and rely on thromboxane A_2 for aggregation. They cannot cause phospholipid hydrolysis and require aggregation for secretion to occur. The aggregation initiated by these weak agonists is inhibited by drugs that interfere with eicosanoid synthesis, such as aspirin.

Agonist	Aggregation inhibited by aspirin
Weak agonists	
Adenosine diphosphate	Yes
Epinephrine (adrenaline)	Yes
Platelet-activating factor	Partial
Arachidonic acid	Yes
Vasopressin (antidiuretic hormone)	Partial
Thromboxane A_2	No
Strong agonists	
Collagen	At low concentrations of agonist
Thrombin	At low concentrations of agonist
Calcium ionophores	No

Figure 12.7: Platelet agonists.

Release reaction

The release reaction involves the secretion of the α-granule and dense body constituents into the open canalicular system. The released constituents can then participate in platelet aggregation and fibrin formation. The release reaction can be measured by detecting the amount of ^{14}C-serotonin or ATP released during aggregation.

Procoagulant activity

The generation of platelet procoagulant activity requires an influx of calcium and is associated with the redistribution of phosphatidylserine to the outer platelet membrane leaflet and the shedding of membrane vesicles from the platelet surface. The translocation of phosphatidylserine provides a binding site for activated coagulation factors and is essential for the generation of activated factor X and thrombin. Platelets also secrete enzymes and cofactors during the release reaction, all of which participate in thrombin generation. Similarly, factor XIII is released from the platelet cytoplasm and crosslinks fibrin.

DIAGNOSIS OF THROMBOPATHIAS

Thrombopathias should be suspected in an animal with excessive haemorrhage typical of primary haemostatic disorders (Figure 12.8) and a normal platelet count and coagulation profile. In many thrombopathias, spontaneous bleeding is uncommon, haemorrhage typically being induced by trauma or surgery.

Petechiae and purpura

Mild to moderate bleeding from mucosal surfaces
    Gastrointestinal
    Genitourinary
    Nasal
    Gingival

History of easy bruising and haematoma
    formation

Excessive bleeding after trauma, surgery and
    venepuncture

Figure 12.8: Clinical findings in thrombopathias.

The minimal data base in patients with excessive haemorrhage includes a complete history (including sex, age and breed of dog, family history, details of previous bouts of haemorrhage, possible access to anticoagulant rodenticides or drugs), a thorough physical examination (noting the type and distribution of haemorrhage and the presence of underlying disease), a platelet count, a blood smear examination for platelet morphology and a coagulation profile (i.e. activated partial thromboplastin time, prothrombin time and fibrinogen concentration). If all these tests are within reference limits, the animal should be evaluated for a thrombopathia (Figure 12.9). Unfortunately, many of the tests for thrombopathias are only performed at referral institutions and are not readily available to the general practitioner. Some of these tests will be mentioned briefly here (see also Chapter 10).

Buccal mucosal bleeding time*
Clot retraction*
von Willebrand factor testing
Glass bead retention test
Platelet aggregation
Platelet release (^{14}C-serotonin and ATP)
Platelet procoagulant activity
Platelet function analysers
Platelet ATP:ADP ratio
Platelet glycoproteins (gel filtration, immunoblot,
    flow cytometry)

Figure 12.9: Tests for diagnosis of thrombopathias.
*Can be performed in private practice.

Buccal mucosal bleeding time

The buccal mucosal bleeding time (BMBT) is a relatively simple in vivo test of primary haemostasis. The BMBT is the length of time needed for haemorrhage to cease from a small standardized cut in the buccal mucosa made with a special disposable device (Simplate II, Organon Teknika, Jessup, MD, USA or Surgicutt™, International Technidyne Corporation, Edison, NJ, USA). The technique has been well described in the veterinary literature (Parker *et al.*, 1988; Stokol and Parry, 1993).

von Willebrand factor
Evaluation of von Willebrand factor (vWf) is discussed in Chapter 14.

Clot retraction
Clot retraction is a crude and subjective test of platelet number and function. Abnormal retraction may be due to hypofibrinogenaemia, thrombocytopenia and thrombopathia.

Glass bead retention
In the glass bead retention test, platelet numbers are determined before and after a standard volume of venous blood is passed at a standard rate through a plastic column packed with glass beads. Retention is dependent on vWf, ADP release from haemolysed erythrocytes, normal platelet function and coagulation. Platelet retention is decreased in thrombopathias and vWD (Brassard and Meyers, 1991). This test is, however, difficult to standardize and is not recommended as there are more specific tests for the diagnosis of these disorders.

Platelet aggregation
Platelet aggregation is induced in vitro in response to agonists. This process occurs in a machine known as a 'platelet aggregometer,' of which there are two types: optical and impedance. The optical aggregometer is sensitive to changes in light transmission, whereas the impedance method is sensitive to changes in electrical resistance across two electrodes produced by platelet aggregates. Special optical aggregometers, lumiaggregometers, measure ATP release simultaneously with aggregation. The impedance method, which also measures whole blood platelet aggregation, is thought to be a more accurate indicator of the physiological processes occurring in vivo than the optical method, which uses platelet-rich plasma.

Platelet release and ATP:ADP ratio
The release reaction can be assessed by determination of total platelet ATP and ADP content and by the release of ATP or ^{14}C-serotonin from dense bodies during aggregation. In storage pool defects, dense bodies and their associated nucleotides are reduced or absent; therefore the ATP:ADP ratio of the storage pool increases.

Analysers of platelet function
New instruments have been developed that assess platelet function by simulation of in vivo vessel injury. Anticoagulated blood is passed through an aperture cut in a collagen-coated membrane impregnated with ADP

or adrenaline. These instruments measure the time taken (closure time) for platelets to adhere to the membrane, activate and produce a platelet plug, thus closing the aperture. In human patients this process depends on vWf and normal platelet function. Preliminary testing in dogs has shown that, with the ADP channel, the closure time is abnormally long in dogs with vWD, Glanzmann's thrombasthenia and Basset Hound thrombopathia (MB Brooks, personal communication).

Platelet procoagulant activity

In the past, procoagulant activity of platelets was measured by the PF3 test, an obsolete assay that was used primarily for detection of antiplatelet antibodies. Currently, procoagulant activity of platelets can be determined in human patients using a prothrombinase assay or flow cytometry. These procedures have not been evaluated in companion animals.

Platelet glycoproteins

Platelet glycoproteins can be separated by gel filtration and labelled. With advances in immunological techniques, the presence or absence of these glycoproteins,

as well as their state of activation, can be assessed with monoclonal antibodies in procedures such as flow cytometry and immunoblotting (Welles *et al.*, 1994; Boudreaux *et al.*, 1996).

DEFECTS IN PLATELET FUNCTION

Thrombopathias can be inherited or acquired. Acquired disorders are far more common, especially those induced by drug treatment or disease. Thrombopathias typically are associated with haemorrhage and a decrease in platelet function. However, there are many disorders (such as diabetes mellitus, immune-mediated haemolytic anaemia, pancreatitis, nephrotic syndrome and hyperadrenocorticism) that are associated with thrombosis. Although thrombosis is usually due to endothelial injury, deficient or abnormal coagulation inhibitors and abnormalities of fibrinolysis, there is no doubt that platelet hyperaggregability is a contributing factor in thrombus formation. Thrombotic disorders will not be discussed further because hyperfunctional platelets have been implicated in thrombosis in only a few animal diseases (Figure 12.10).

Disease	Proposed mechanism of platelet dysfunction
Decreased platelet function	

Neoplasia
    Acute megakaryoblastic leukaemia
    Essential thrombocythaemia
    Polycythaemia vera
	
	Defective adhesion and aggregation
	Defective adhesion and aggregation
	Defective adhesion and aggregation

Dysproteinaemias (lymphoma, multiple myeloma)	Paraprotein (IgG, IgM, IgA) coats platelets causing defective adhesion, aggregation and procoagulant activity

Infectious agents
    Ehrlichia canis
 	
    Ehrlichia platys
	
	Decreased adhesion, procoagulant activity, ?antibody-mediated dysfunction
	Decreased aggregation (secondary to platelet activation with subsequent exhaustion)

Hepatic disease	Decreased aggregation attributed to a variety of causes
Renal disease	Decreased adhesion
Pancreatitis	Decreased aggregation (secondary to platelet exhaustion after initial hyperresponsiveness and DIC)
Disseminated intravascular coagulation (DIC)	Fibrinogen degradation products coat platelets interfering with function
Immune-mediated thrombocytopenia	Decreased aggregation
Increased platelet function	
Nephrotic syndrome	Enhanced arachidonic acid availability
Neoplasia	?
Feline hypertrophic cardiomyopathy	?

Infectious agents
    Rickettsia rickettsi
    Dirofilaria immitis
	
	?Due to larger more functional platelets
	?Parasite liberates biogenic amines, which interact with platelet surface

Feline infectious peritonitis virus	Unknown: ?Direct viral interaction with platelets, and DIC

Figure 12.10: Animal diseases associated with acquired thrombopathias.

Disorder	Defect
Glanzmann's thrombasthenia	Decreased GPIIb-IIIa expression due to defects in GPIIb gene
Basset Hound thrombopathia	Increased cyclic adenosine monophosphate (?abnormal phosphodiesterase), ?variant of Glanzmann's thrombasthenia
Spitz dog thrombopathia	?Variant of Glanzmann's thrombasthenia
Storage pool deficiency (American Cocker Spaniel)	?Defective adenosine diphosphate transport in dense body
von Willebrand's disease	Deficiency or abnormality in von Willebrand factor
Chediak–Higashi syndrome (cats)	Storage pool deficiency (absent dense bodies), phospholipase C signalling defect
Canine cyclic haematopoiesis (grey Collies)	Defective uptake and storage of serotonin, and signal transduction defect

Figure 12.11: *Inherited thrombopathias in animals.*

Thrombopathias are more readily recognized in dogs than in cats. In general, cats do not often exhibit excessive haemorrhage, which may be attributed to their small size and lifestyle. Inherited disorders should be suspected in a young animal, especially if family members display similar bleeding tendencies and there is no history of drug treatment. Thrombopathias can affect any component of platelet function from adhesion to aggregation. Defects can involve quantitative or qualitative abnormalities in membrane proteins needed for platelet adhesion and interplatelet interactions, aberrant cAMP metabolism, impaired synthesis of proaggregatory prostaglandin metabolites, decreased or absent granule pools, and low concentrations or abnormal function of essential cofactors such as vWf and fibrinogen.

Inherited thrombopathias
Many inherited thrombopathias have been characterized in human medicine, however only a few have been diagnosed in companion animals (Figure 12.11). Some of these will be discussed in detail.

von Willebrand's disease
Although vWD does not affect platelets directly, vWf is essential for platelet adhesion to the subendothelium and, to a lesser extent, platelet aggregation. The clinical signs in this disorder are therefore similar to thrombopathias (see Chapter 14).

Glanzmann's thrombasthenia
Glanzmann's thrombasthenia has been diagnosed in Otterhounds and a Great Pyrenees (Boudreaux *et al.*, 1996). The defect seems to be autosomal recessive, and affected dogs have excessive mucosal haemorrhage (Figure 12.12). Haemostatic testing shows a normal to mildly decreased platelet count, normal to increased mean platelet volume and prolonged BMBT. Characteristic features include decreased platelet retention, absent platelet aggregation to collagen, ADP, platelet activating factor and thrombin, and decreased granule secretion. Change in shape does occur. Clot

retraction is abnormal, which helps differentiate this disorder from Basset Hound thrombopathia. Flow cytometric studies have shown a noticeable reduction in GPIIb-IIIa on the platelet surface in both Otterhounds and Great Pyrenees. In the Otterhound, there is a single nucleotide change in exon 12 of the GPIIb gene, which disrupts a calcium-binding domain and forms an unstable GPIIb-IIIa complex, preventing its expression on the platelet surface (Boudreaux and Catalfmo, 1999). An mRNA splicing defect in exon 13 of the GPIIb gene has been identified in the Great Pyrenees. This defect also disrupts a calcium-binding domain and results in a truncated protein, which destabilizes the GPIIb-IIIa complex (Lipscomb *et al.*, 1999).

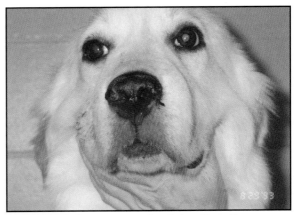

Figure 12.12: *Spontaneous epistaxis in a Great Pyrenees with Glanzmann's thrombasthenia. (Photograph courtesy of Dr M. Boudreaux, Auburn University.)*

Basset Hound thrombopathia
Basset Hound thrombopathia is unique to this breed and does not have a human counterpart. Clinical signs in affected dogs consist of petechiae, aural haematomas and prolonged haemorrhage with shedding of deciduous teeth. These signs are generally observed at oestrus and after trauma or surgery. An autosomal recessive condition, Basset Hound thrombopathia is characterized by decreased platelet retention and absent platelet aggregation in response to all agonists,

except thrombin, to which there is a delayed onset and reduced rate of aggregation. Platelet ^{14}C-serotonin release is decreased in response to collagen, but normal to ADP and thrombin. Change in shape does occur and clot retraction is normal. The precise aetiology of the defect is unknown, although abnormal calcium metabolism or a variant of Glanzmann's thrombasthenia are possible causes. Platelets from affected dogs have increased basal cAMP concentrations, which have been attributed to impaired phosphodiesterase activity. Increased cAMP inhibits intracellular calcium release, agonist-receptor binding and agonist-induced phospholipid hydrolysis (Boudreaux *et al.*, 1986).

Spitz dog thrombopathia
Thrombopathia has been described by Boudreaux *et al.* (1994) in young Spitz dogs with chronic intermittent mucosal bleeding. The disorder closely resembles Basset Hound thrombopathia, except that platelet secretion in response to ADP is absent in the Spitz.

Storage pool deficiency in American Cocker Spaniels
American Cocker Spaniel dogs with storage pool deficiency have moderate to severe haemorrhage after trauma, venepuncture or surgery. They have normal platelet counts, a prolonged BMBT, decreased platelet aggregation and ^{14}C-serotonin release in response to collagen, and an increased platelet ATP:ADP ratio. Dense bodies are visible on electron microscopy. The disorder has been attributed to a selective defect in ADP transport in dense granules. Haemorrhage is often severe enough to require fresh platelet transfusions (Callan *et al.*, 1995).

Acquired thrombopathias
Acquired thrombopathias should be suspected in animals with specific diseases known to be associated with platelet dysfunction (see Figure 12.10) and in animals that have been treated with certain drugs (Figure 12.13). The risk of bleeding is unpredictable and typically less severe and consistent than in animals with inherited disorders. Although abnormal platelet function occurs in these diseases, there may be other causes for the excessive haemorrhage seen in these conditions (thrombocytopenia, for example). However, it should be recognized that platelets are potentially not functioning normally in these situations, and drugs that may exacerbate platelet dysfunction should therefore be avoided.

Drugs
An enormous variety of drugs can interfere with platelet function (George and Shattil, 1991). The most commonly used of these is aspirin, which in some situations is prescribed precisely for its antiplatelet effects, such as in the prevention of thromboembolism in feline cardiomyopathy and canine heartworm disease. Aspirin inhibits platelet function by irreversibly acetylating platelet cyclo-oxygenase, thus preventing

Inhibitors of prostaglandin synthesis

Cyclo-oxygenase inhibitors
    Aspirin
    Non-steroidal anti-inflammatory drugs
      (phenylbutazone, indomethacin, ibuprofen)
Thromboxane synthetase inhibitors (diazoxiben)

Drugs that increase concentrations of cyclic adenosine monophosphate (cAMP) or cyclic guanosine monophosphate (cGMP)

Adenylate cyclase or guanylate cyclase activators
    Prostaglandin I_2, E_1 and D_2 (cAMP)
    Nitric oxide, nitroglycerin, nitroprusside
      (cGMP)
Phosphodiesterase inhibitors
    Dipyridamole
    Methylxanthines (caffeine, theophylline,
      aminophylline)

Calcium antagonists

Diltiazem, nifepidine, verapamil
Barbiturates (?interfere with agonist-receptor
  binding and prevent increase in cytosolic
  calcium concentration)

Membrane-active drugs (interfere with platelet receptors)

Antibiotics (penicillin, ampicillin, ticarcillin,
  gentamicin, sulphonamides, cephalothrin,
  cefmetazole, moxalactam)
Antihistamines (phenothiazines)
Plasma expanders (dextran, hetastarch,
  pentastarch)
Propanolol, isoproterenol
Anaesthetic agents (procaine, lignocaine,
  halothane, glycerol guiacolate)

Unknown
Heparin Ticlopidine (?interfere with fibrinogen-receptor   exposure) Oestrogens, chondroitin sulphate, carbenicillin

Figure 12.13: Drugs that can interfere with platelet function. Most of these have been reported in humans and not in animals.

generation of thromboxane A_2, which is needed for secretion and aggregation. Other non-steroidal anti-inflammatory agents (e.g. phenylbutazone) reversibly inhibit cyclo-oxygenase activity. Aspirin is unique, however, as its effect lasts for the life span of the platelet (7–10 days in the dog). Therefore when using aspirin, platelet function is inhibited for at least 7 days after drug treatment ceases. Aspirin should be avoided as an analgesic in dogs with inherited haemostatic disorders such as vWD and haemophilia A.

Disseminated intravascular coagulation
Disseminated intravascular coagulation (DIC) is caused by the systemic activation of thrombin resulting in

widespread coagulation, with resultant microcirculatory thromboembolism and multiorgan failure. DIC is not a primary disorder; it is initiated by an underlying disease process, typically septicaemia, pancreatitis, heat stroke, surgery, viral infections, neoplasia, transfusion reactions or tissue necrosis. DIC is initiated by increased tissue factor expression by monocytes and endothelial cells, mediated by cytokines or endothelial cell injury. Some tumours (e.g. mucinous adenocarcinoma) and snake venoms can initiate DIC by directly activating coagulation factors such as factor X. As a result, there is widespread activation of coagulation, with fibrin deposition and thrombus formation. Consequently, there is consumption of platelets, fibrinogen and coagulation factors with secondary fibrinolysis and generation of fibrin (fibrinogen) degradation products (FDPs). Erythrocytes shear as they traverse damaged blood vessels, producing a microangiopathic haemolytic anaemia. Clinical signs may be related to tissue hypoxia, infarction or haemorrhage. Typically, haemorrhage is attributed to depletion of platelets and coagulation factors and abnormal fibrin polymerization, but there is often concurrent platelet dysfunction. Platelet dysfunction is mediated by FDPs (especially fragments D and E), which have a high affinity for platelet membranes and compete with fibrinogen for platelet receptors, thus impairing aggregation.

Immune-mediated thrombocytopenia

Some dogs with immune-mediated thrombocytopenia (IMT) have abnormal platelet aggregation, which is mediated by IgG antibodies (Kristensen *et al.*, 1994). In chronic IMT in humans, most antibodies are directed against GPIIb-IIIa and GPIb-IX (McMillan *et al.*, 1987), and studies in dogs by Lewis and Meyers (1996) indicate that, in some dogs with IMT, there is an autoantibody against GPIIb-IIIa. As this glycoprotein has an essential role in platelet aggregation, it is not surprising that dogs with IMT have concurrent platelet dysfunction. For unknown reasons, in IMT the clinical signs of haemorrhage do not always correlate with the platelet count. It may be that the clinical signs of IMT depend on the extent of platelet dysfunction as well as the severity of the thrombocytopenia. Further studies need to be performed in this area.

Renal disease

Mucosal bleeding, reduced platelet retention and a prolonged BMBT are features of natural and experimental uraemia in dogs. These abnormalities correlate with the extent of azotaemia. Platelet aggregation is either normal or mildly decreased, implicating defective adhesion as the main haemostatic abnormality (Brassard *et al.*, 1994). The amount and multimeric composition of vWf are normal, indicating that the adhesion defects are not due to vWf abnormalities (Brassard and Meyers, 1994).

Hepatic disease

Hepatic disease is often associated with prolonged haemorrhage, attributable to a combination of reduced synthesis of coagulation factors, DIC and platelet dysfunction. Dogs with various types of hepatic disease have defective platelet aggregation in whole blood, and display excessive haemorrhage related to platelet dysfunction (Willis *et al.*, 1989). This dysfunction is thought to be due to circulating FDPs, increased bile acids, altered platelet phospholipids, enhanced nitric oxide production (from hyperammonaemia) and increased proportions of older less active platelets (Bowen *et al.*, 1988; Willis *et al.*, 1989).

MANAGEMENT

Assessment of the risk of bleeding in thrombopathias is difficult, as none of the platelet function tests accurately predicts the likelihood of haemorrhage. The BMBT is considered by some to be the best indicator of 'in vivo' haemostatic competence in patients with thrombopathias. The BMBT can be used as a screening test in animals considered at risk of bleeding owing to platelet dysfunction (e.g. dogs being treated with aspirin) before invasive surgery. Those patients with a prolonged BMBT are considered to be more likely to bleed during surgery than those with a BMBT within reference intervals. However, there have been no studies to determine if a prolonged BMBT is associated with increased surgical haemorrhage in animals. In a patient with clinical signs referable to platelet dysfunction, suitable precautions should be taken before invasive surgical procedures. These include treatment of the underlying disease in acquired thrombopathias, cessation of drug treatment, attention to strict surgical haemostasis and platelet transfusions. Ideally, platelet-rich plasma or platelet concentrates should be infused, however fresh whole blood is the only form of transfusion therapy readily available to the general practitioner. This should be used judiciously, and ideally all animals should be typed or crossmatched to minimize transfusion reactions. Infusion therapy in inherited thrombopathias is only palliative, and if haemorrhage is severe, euthanasia may be warranted.

REFERENCES AND FURTHER READING

Colman RW, Hirsh J, Marder VJ and Salzman EW (1994) *Hemostasis and thrombosis: Basic principles and clinical practice, 3rd edn.* JB Lippincott, Philadelphia

Boudreaux MK, Dodds WJ, Slauson DO and Catalfmo JL (1986) Evidence for the regulatory control of canine platelet phosphodiesterase. *Biochemical and Biophysical Research Communications* **140**, 589-594

Boudreaux MK, Crager C, Dillon AR, Stanz K and Toivio-Kinnucan M (1994) Identification of an intrinsic platelet function defect in Spitz Dogs. *Journal of Veterinary Internal Medicine* **8**, 93-98

Boudreaux MK, Kvam K, Dillon AR, Bourne C, Scott M, Schwartz KA and Toivio-Kinnucan M (1996) Type I Glanzmann's thrombasthenia in a Great Pyrenees dog. *Veterinary Pathology* **33**, 503–511

Boudreaux MK and Catalfmo JL (1999) Evaluation of the genes encoding for GP complex IIB-IIIA in Otterhounds with thrombasthenic thrombopathia (abstract). *Veterinary Pathology* **36**, 483

Bowen DJ, Clemmons RM, Meyer DJ and Dorsey-Lee MR (1988) Platelet functional changes secondary to hepatocholestasis and elevation of serum bile acids. *Thrombosis Research* **52**, 649–654

Brassard JA and Meyers KM (1991) Evaluation of the buccal bleeding time and platelet glass bead retention as assays of hemostasis in the dog: the effects of acetylsalicylic acid, warfarin and von Willebrand Factor deficiency. *Thrombosis Haemostasis* **65**, 191–195

Brassard JA and Meyers KM (1994) von Willebrand factor is not altered in azotemic dogs with prolonged bleeding time. *Journal of Laboratory and Clinical Medicine* **124**, 55–62

Brassard JA, Meyers KM, Person M and Dhein CR (1994) Experimentally induced renal failure in the dog as an animal model for uremic bleeding. *Journal of Laboratory and Clinical Medicine* **124**, 48–54

Callan MB, Bennett JS, Phillips DK, Haskins ME, Hayden JE, Anderson JG and Giger U (1995) Inherited platelet δ-storage pool disease in dogs causing severe bleeding: an animal model for a specific ADP deficiency. *Thrombosis and Haemostasis* **74**, 949–953

De Gopegui RR and Feldman BF (2000) Platelets and von Willebrand's Disease. In: *Textbook of Veterinary Internal Medicine*, 5th edn, ed. SJ Ettinger and EC Feldman, pp. 1817–1828. WB Saunders, Philadelphia

George JN and Shattil SJ (1991) The clinical importance of acquired abnormalities of platelet function. *New England Journal of Medicine* **321**, 27–36

Kristensen AT, Weiss DJ and Klausner JS (1994) Platelet dysfunction associated with immune-mediated thrombocytopenia in dogs. *Journal of Veterinary Internal Medicine* **8**, 323–327

Lewis DC and Meyers KM (1996) Studies of platelet-bound and serum platelet-bindable immunoglobulins in dogs with idiopathic thrombocytopenic purpura. *Experimental Haematology* **24**, 696–701

Lipscomb D, Boudreaux M and Bourne C (1999) Comparison of the αIIb nucleotide sequence from platelet cDNA of thrombasthenic and normal dogs (abstract). *Veterinary Pathology* **36**, 482

McMillan R, Tani P, Millard F, Berchtold P, Renshaw L and Woods VL (1987) Platelet-associated and plasma anti-glycoprotein autoantibodies in chronic ITP. *Blood* **70**, 1040–1045

Parker MT, Collier LL, Kier AB and Johnson GS (1988) Oral mucosa bleeding times of normal cats and cats with Chediak-Higashi syndrome or Hageman trait (factor 12 deficiency). *Veterinary Clinical Pathology* **17**, 9–12

Roth GJ (1992) Platelets and blood vessels: the adhesion event. *Immunology Today* **13**, 100–105

Stokol T and Parry BW (1993) Canine von Willebrand Disease: a review. *Australian Veterinary Practitioner* **23**, 94–103

The British Society for Haematology Haemostasis and Thrombosis Task Force (1988) Guidelines on platelet function testing. *Journal of Clinical Pathology* **41**, 1322–1330

Welles EG, Bourne C, Tyler JW and Boudreaux MK (1994) Detection of activated feline platelets in platelet-rich plasma by use of fluorescein-labeled antibodies and flow cytometry. *Veterinary Pathology* **31**, 553–560

Willis SE, Jackson ML, Meric SM and Rousseaux CG (1989) Whole blood platelet aggregation in dogs with liver disease. *American Journal of Veterinary Research* **50**, 1893–1897

Disorders of Secondary Haemostasis

Janet D. Littlewood

INTRODUCTION

Secondary haemostasis is the process by which soluble fibrinogen is converted into insoluble fibrin. This process occurs on the phospholipid surface of activated platelets at the site of vascular injury and stabilizes the primary haemostatic platelet plug in a meshwork of fibrin strands. The conversion of fibrinogen to fibrin is achieved by the proteolytic action of thrombin, which is formed from prothrombin by the sequential activation of proteases in conjunction with essential cofactors, which together are known as coagulation, or clotting, factors. The term 'coagulation cascade' is used to describe this sequential activation, with thrombin itself further activating inactive factors and thus amplifying the process (Figure 13.1). The coagulation cascade can be conveniently considered to consist of an extrinsic pathway, an intrinsic pathway and a final common pathway, although in vivo the intrinsic and extrinsic pathways are not separate but interactive. However, as the in vitro tests described earlier (see Chapter 10) measure distinct components of the clotting process, this concept of two pathways is helpful in the classification and investigation of clotting disorders.

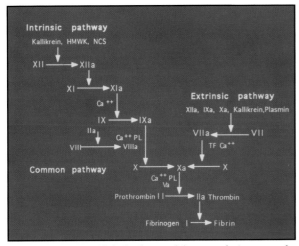

Figure 13.1: *A simplified scheme of the coagulation cascade. HMWK, high molecular weight kininogen; NCS, negatively charged surface; Ca⁺⁺, calcium; PL, phospholipid; TF, tissue factor.*

The extrinsic pathway comprises the activation of factor VII (F VII), principally by tissue factor (TF), a lipoprotein that is derived from various cell and tissue types. Activated F VII and TF with calcium ions (Ca⁺⁺) comprise the 'tissue factor' complex, which activates factor X (F X). The intrinsic pathway is triggered by negatively charged surfaces, the subendothelium in vivo, glass or added activators (e.g. kaolin) in vitro, followed by sequential protease activation, culminating in the production of the 'tenase' complex, which consists of activated factor IX (F IXa), activated cofactor VIII (F VIIIa), phospholipid and Ca⁺⁺. The activation of prothrombin by F Xa, F Va, phospholipid and Ca⁺⁺ and the subsequent conversion of fibrinogen to fibrin is known as the common pathway.

Inherited disorders of coagulation are usually deficiencies of single clotting factors due to genetic mutations, although multiple factor defects may occur. Acquired disorders of coagulation are generally multiple factor deficiencies and may occur in conjunction with platelet disorders in the consumptive coagulopathies.

CLINICAL FINDINGS IN COAGULOPATHIES

The manifestation of abnormal bleeding in coagulation defects is generally similar, irrespective of the specific factor defects, but distinct from the clinical signs resulting from platelet abnormalities (Figure 13.2). Animals with coagulopathies often bleed at a single site rather than showing widespread haemorrhage. Deep bleeds into soft tissues, joints and body cavities are seen, as opposed to mucosal or surface bleeding. Soft tissue swelling may indicate the presence of haematomata, with lameness and joint swelling being features of haemarthroses. Haemothorax and haemomediastinum result in dyspnoea and dullness on chest percussion, and occasionally severe respiratory compromise may result from submucosal haemorrhage affecting the trachea and retropharyngeal region. Abdominal pain and malaise are the cardinal signs of intraperitoneal or visceral haemorrhage.

Haematomata common
Often single site of haemorrhage
Bleeds into body cavities
Mucosal or surface bleeds rare
Delayed bleeding or rebleeding
Venepuncture often uncomplicated

Figure 13.2: *Typical clinical features of coagulopathies.*

The history of the patient may be helpful in discriminating between inherited and acquired disorders (Figure 13.3). Both inherited and acquired disorders of coagulation may be exacerbated by concurrent illness. Other historical features of importance include recent drug therapy and potential exposure to toxins; these have been reviewed by Littlewood (1989, 1992) and Couto (1999).

Inherited coagulation defects	Acquired coagulation defects
Onset at young age	Onset at any age
History of previous bleeding episodes	Often no previous problems, uneventful operations
Relatives may show bleeding abnormality	Usually no affected relatives

Figure 13.3: *Differentiation of inherited and acquired coagulopathies.*

Further investigations

Primary haemostatic function is normal in uncomplicated coagulation defects, and the buccal mucosal bleeding time in patients is usually within the normal range (less than 5 minutes). During bleeding episodes, however, it is not uncommon for the platelet count to decrease due to consumption at the site of vessel injury, and in cases of disseminated intravascular coagulation (DIC), defects of primary and secondary haemostasis coexist.

Laboratory investigation should include the screening assays of coagulation: prothrombin time (PT), activated partial thromboplastin time (APTT) and thrombin clotting time (TCT). Further details of these and other tests of haemostasis are covered in Chapter 10. Further elucidation of the exact nature of

the coagulation defect can be achieved by the performance of APTT correction assays, whereby normal plasma, aluminium hydroxide-adsorbed plasma and normal serum are added to the patient's plasma and APTT assays performed (Figure 13.4). Assays of specific factors are required to quantify the exact nature of the defect.

MANAGEMENT OF COAGULOPATHIES

Ideally, patients with defects of coagulation factors should be treated by replacement of the missing clotting factors. In practice, treatment usually entails giving fresh plasma or thawed fresh frozen plasma taken from donor dogs or cats. Although there are several animal blood banking facilities in North America, there is no commercial source of blood products in the United Kingdom. However, several referral institutions and practices maintain donor animals.

Whole blood transfusions limit the amount of clotting factors that can be given and carry the accompanying risk of reactions of red cell incompatibility either after first or, significantly, subsequent transfusions (see Chapters 15 and 16). As a guide, the aim is to increase the concentration of clotting factors in the circulation to at least 25% of normal to achieve haemostasis. This can be accomplished by infusion of 10–15 ml/kg of normal plasma, although significant blood loss may increase the requirement for plasma replacement. Infusions should be repeated twice daily until haemorrhage is controlled and resolving. Broad-spectrum antibiosis is indicated as extravasated blood provides an ideal medium for bacterial growth.

Where specific contributory factors or underlying diseases are identified, then these must be addressed and treated appropriately. In the case of some of the inherited coagulopathies, the use of inhibitors of fibrinolysis to stabilize fibrin clots at the site of vessel injury has been found to be of great benefit (AR Giles, personal communication; JD Littlewood, unpublished observations). The author has used tranexamic acid (Cyclokapron, Kabi) at a dose rate of 15–20 mg/kg orally 2–4 times daily. This drug is used to control

	APTT clotting times			
Test plasma + normal plasma	Corrected	Corrected	Corrected	Uncorrected
Test plasma + adsorbed plasma	Corrected	Corrected	Uncorrected	Uncorrected
Test plasma + normal serum	Corrected	Uncorrected	Corrected	Uncorrected
Possible factor deficiency	XI, XII, PK, HMWK	I, II, V, VIII	II, VII, IX, X	Circulating inhibitor

Figure 13.4: *Correction assays for activated partial thromboplastin time (APTT). PK, prekallikrein; HMWK, high molecular weight kininogen.*

external haemorrhage (e.g. dental, prostatic) in human haemophilic patients and, owing to the risk of thromboembolic complications, would not be used in the management of internal bleeds. This risk, however, seems to be minimal in veterinary patients, probably owing to their enhanced fibrinolytic system compared with that of humans. It should be noted that this product is not licensed for veterinary use.

INHERITED COAGULOPATHIES

The major features of the most common inherited coagulopathies of the dog and cat are summarized in Figure 13.5.

Haemophilia A
Haemophilia A, also known as 'classic' haemophilia, is due to a deficiency in clotting factor VIII (F VIII) and is the commonest of the inherited coagulopathies. This condition is covered in detail in Chapter 14.

Haemophilia B
Haemophilia B is also known as Christmas disease. The condition is due to a deficiency in clotting factor IX (F IX). Like F VIII deficiency, this is a sex-linked condition, with affected animals being male and the offspring of carrier females. The size of the gene on the X chromosome is considerably smaller than the gene for F VIII, and the frequency of occurrence of gene mutations in populations is proportionately less. Haemophilia B is therefore less common than haemophilia A.

F IX acts at the same point in the coagulation cascade as F VIII (see Figure 13.1), the activated forms of both proteins contributing to the 'tenase' complex, which activates F X. The clinical manifestations of F VIII and F IX deficiency are identical. The inheritance pattern is similarly identical. All the daughters of an affected male will be obligate carriers of the disease, but his sons will be normal. There is a 50% probability of the offspring of a carrier female inheriting the defective chromosome, and on average half of her sons will be affected and half of her daughters will be carriers of the disease.

Factor deficiency	Breeds affected	Inheritance	Prothrombin time	Activated partial thromboplastin time	Thrombin clotting time
I	Various dogs	Autosomal dominant and recessive	Prolonged	Prolonged	Prolonged
VII	Beagles Alaskan Malamute Crossbreed	Autosomal dominant	Prolonged	Normal	Normal
VIII	Many pure- and crossbred dogs Various cat breeds	Sex-linked recessive	Normal	Prolonged	Normal
IX	Several breeds and crossbred dogs British Shorthair, Siamese and DSH-cross cats	Sex-linked recessive	Normal	Prolonged	Normal
X	American Cocker Spaniel Jack Russell Terrier DSH cat	?Autosomal recessive	Prolonged	Prolonged	Normal
XI	Pyrenean Mountain Dog Kerry Blue Terrier	Autosomal dominant; only homozygotes bleed	Normal	Prolonged	Normal
XII	Various cat breeds	Autosomal dominant; no bleeding tendency	Normal	Prolonged	Normal
Vitamin K-dependent	Devon Rex cat	?Autosomal recessive	Prolonged	Prolonged	Normal

Figure 13.5: Summary of features of common inherited coagulopathies.

Because F IX deficiency is a defect of the intrinsic pathway, the APTT is prolonged but the PT and TCT are normal. The APTT is not corrected by addition of adsorbed plasma, and an assay of specific factors shows F IX deficiency, which may be severe (less than 1% of pooled normal plasma) or moderate (2–10% of pooled normal plasma). Mild forms of the disease have not been reported in dogs or cats.

Haemophilia B has been reported in 11 breeds of dog in the United States (Verlander *et al.*, 1984) and more recently the disease has also been described in a family of German Shepherd Dogs (Feldman *et al.*, 1995). In the United Kingdom a moderately severe form of the disease was identified in a spaniel-cross dog (Littlewood *et al.*, 1986). The dam of this dog was confirmed as a carrier, with only half of the normal plasma activity of F IX, and a male sibling that had died at a few weeks of age was assumed to have been affected also. The dog was successfully maintained as a family pet and had only occasional bleeding episodes as a result of trauma and subsequent to dental extractions. These episodes were managed by plasma transfusion, and the dog survived to old age.

At a molecular level the defect has been shown as a post-transcriptional defect (High *et al.*, 1987), a point mutation (Evans *et al.*, 1989) and, in other cases, deletion mutations (Mauser *et al.*, 1996; Brooks *et al.*, 1997; Gu *et al.*, 1999), one of which was associated with the production of inhibitors against transfused canine F IX. Dogs with haemophilia B have been used in studies of gene replacement therapy (reviewed by Dodds and Womack, 1997), with a recent report of long-term F IX expression (more than 17 months) after adeno-associated viral vector gene transfer in dogs with haemophilia B (Herzog *et al.*, 1999).

Haemophilia B has been reported in British shorthaired cats (Dodds, 1984) and Siamese cats (W J Dodds, personal communication). A combined defect of F IX and F XII was described in a litter of Siamese-cross domestic shorthaired kittens (Dillon and Boudreaux, 1988).

Factor X deficiency

Factor X (Stuart-Power factor) deficiency has been reported in a family of American Cocker Spaniels (Dodds, 1973) and in a Jack Russell Terrier (Cook *et al.*, 1993). The condition has been identified in a domestic shorthaired cat that presented with seizures, bleeding associated with jugular venepuncture and a history of prolonged bleeding after declawing (Gookin *et al.*, 1997). Although not confirmed by imaging techniques, the neurological abnormalities were assumed to have been the result of intracranial haemorrhage, which is reported in some human infants with F X deficiency.

As F X is a common pathway defect, both PT and APTT are prolonged but the TCT is normal. The Russell's viper venom test (RVVT), a direct activator of F X, is prolonged, and the diagnosis is confirmed by specific F X assay.

The pattern of inheritance in humans is autosomal recessive, with either gender being affected with the disease. The severity of bleeding episodes in dogs with F X deficiency is variable, and severely affected animals tend to die young, although moderately affected dogs may survive to adulthood.

Factor XI deficiency

Factor XI (plasma thromboplastin antecedent) deficiency presents as a severe and often lethal bleeding disorder. The condition has been reported in Springer Spaniels and Pyrenean Mountain Dogs (Dodds and Kull, 1971; Dodds, 1977) and in Kerry Blue Terriers (Knowler *et al.*, 1994). The inheritance pattern is autosomal, with F XI activity in homozygotes of less than 10%, and of the order of 25–50% in heterozygotes, the latter being asymptomatic. An acquired form of the condition has been reported in a cat (Feldman *et al.*, 1983). The APTT is prolonged as this is a defect of the intrinsic pathway, but the PT and TCT are normal. The diagnosis is confirmed by specific F XI assay.

Factor VII deficiency

Deficiency of F VII is well recognized in certain families of laboratory Beagles and has also been described in the Alaskan Malamute (Spurling, 1980) and a crossbred dog (Macpherson *et al.*, 1999). The bleeding tendency is usually mild. The pattern of inheritance is autosomal dominant, but heterozygotes are asymptomatic. The extrinsic pathway-screening test, the PT, is prolonged in cases of F VII deficiency, but the APTT and TCT are normal.

Hypofibrinogenaemia (F I) deficiency

Deficiencies of fibrinogen are reported occasionally and have been identified in several dogs by the coagulation laboratory at the Animal Health Trust, Newmarket, UK (unpublished observations). One such case was a 1-year-old male Cocker Spaniel that presented with a history of recurrent episodes of joint stiffness and epistaxis. The dog was referred for investigation of respiratory distress. Tachypnoea and pallor were evident on clinical examination, together with scleral and retinal haemorrhages. Radiographs revealed alveolar densities due to pulmonary haemorrhage (Figure 13.6). The fibrinogen concentration in this dog was 0.4 g/l (normal range 2–4 g/l). The dog subsequently had seizures, and lesions consistent with infarcts due to cerebrovascular accidents were identified on magnetic resonance imaging (MRI) scans.

The PT, APTT and TCT assays were all prolonged and plasma fibrinogen concentration was low. The acute episode of haemorrhage was managed by plasma transfusion, and low doses of tranexamic acid (an inhibitor of fibrinolysis) on a prophylactic basis were successful in minimizing the occurrence of bleeding episodes.

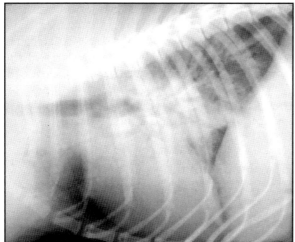

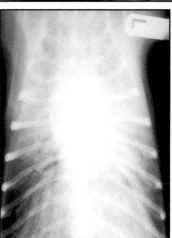

Figure 13.6: Factor I deficiency (hypofibrinogenaemia): lateral and dorsoventral chest radiographs showing an alveolar pattern with air bronchograms due to intrapulmonary haemorrhage.

Vitamin K-dependent coagulopathy
A multifactorial vitamin K-dependent coagulopathy has been described in the Devon Rex cat. Although a complex coagulopathy has been recognized in the breed for some time (Evans, 1985), the true nature of the condition was elucidated by Maddison *et al.* (1990) in related Devon Rex cats in Australia. The condition has also been confirmed in a Devon Rex cat (Figure 13.7) in the United Kingdom (Littlewood *et al.*, 1995).

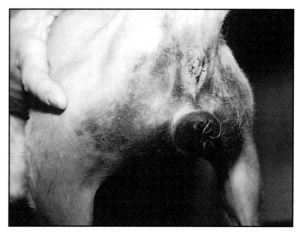

Figure 13.7: Vitamin K-dependent coagulopathy of Devon Rex cats: perineal bruising and scrotal haematoma in an affected male cat after surgery. (Photograph courtesy of Steve Shaw.)

Both autosomal recessive and autosomal dominant patterns of inheritance of hypofibrinogenaemia have been documented, but the recessive condition may be a variant of congenital afibrinogenaemia and the dominant disease may actually be heterozygous afibrinogenaemia (Fogh and Fogh, 1988).

Factor XII deficiency
Factor XII (Hageman factor) deficiency has been reported in cats on several occasions (Kier *et al.*, 1980; Peterson *et al.*, 1995), and a combined deficiency of F VIII and F XII was encountered in a family of cats (Littlewood and Evans, 1990) in addition to the combined F IX and F XII deficiencies described above (Dillon and Boudreaux, 1988). Although a deficiency of F XII results in dramatic prolongation of the APTT, it is not associated with a symptomatic bleeding tendency and is, in effect, a laboratory abnormality. The importance of this was shown in the family of haemophilic cats where the presence of F XII deficiency complicated the identification of kittens affected with haemophilia A (Littlewood and Evans, 1990). The pattern of inheritance is autosomal, with homozygotes having a severe deficiency of F XII activity and heterozygotes having about 50% of normal plasma F XII activity.

Clinical signs of this coagulopathy include prolonged haemorrhage after surgery and trauma, although the risk of bleeding in an individual cat seems to be variable. Cats of both genders are affected. Two-to three-fold prolongation of the PT and APTT occurs, with reduced activity of all the vitamin K-dependent clotting factors. Factors II, IX and X are reduced to less than 20% of pooled normal plasma in the cat, and F VII to less than 50% of normal. Subsequent biochemical investigations have shown a defect in hepatic vitamin K metabolism in affected animals. An autosomal recessive pattern of inheritance is proposed.

Giving vitamin K1 (phytomenadione, Konakion, Roche; not licensed for veterinary use) orally at a dose rate of 5 mg daily successfully corrects the abnormalities in clotting factors and controls the bleeding tendency, and can be given long term.

The prevalence of the condition in the breed is not known, although the PT assay would provide a simple screening test to identify affected animals. These cats could then be removed from breeding programmes, but treated prophylactically with vitamin K1 to prevent the risk of haemorrhage.

Other inherited coagulopathies
Other rare inherited disorders of clotting factors are occasionally reported (Fogh and Fogh, 1988; Peterson *et al.*, 1995; Brooks, 1999).

ACQUIRED COAGULOPATHIES

Vitamin K-dependent coagulopathies

Vitamin K antagonism
The commonest acquired disorder of coagulation is due to the depletion of vitamin K-dependent clotting factors resulting from the ingestion of coumarin rodenticides, which are vitamin K antagonists (see Chapter 14).

Vitamin K deficiency
Vitamin K is a fat-soluble vitamin and deficiencies resulting in a coagulopathy are reported in cats secondary to maldigestion and malabsorption conditions such as exocrine pancreatic deficiency (Perry *et al.*, 1991), severe infiltrative enteritis (Edwards and Russell, 1987) and bile duct obstruction (Pederson and Holzworth, 1987).

Hepatic disease
The liver is the site of synthesis of many of the plasma clotting factors, as well as inhibitors of coagulation, and is the site of conversion of the vitamin K-dependent factors into their active forms. Widespread damage to the liver parenchyma may thus result in deficiencies of many clotting factors. In addition, the liver is responsible for the removal and inactivation of any activated clotting factors that may escape from the site of vascular injury into the circulation. Both qualitative and quantitative alterations in platelets may occur in liver disease. Clinically significant haemostatic abnormalities tend to be associated with acute insults to the liver, although it is considered prudent to check clotting variables before embarking on surgical intervention in patients with chronic hepatic disease (Bradylak, 1988). Defects of coagulation factors have been described in dogs with cirrhosis, similar to those occurring in human hepatic cirrhosis (Mischke *et al.*, 1998).

Clinical signs of liver disease such as hepatomegaly and anterior abdominal discomfort accompany the haemorrhagic tendency. Since multiple clotting factors are depleted, prolongation of both the PT and APTT is seen. If activated clotting factors are not cleared from the circulation, intravascular coagulation and a consumptive coagulopathy may result (see Chapter 14: Disseminated intravascular coagulation). The presence of liver damage and liver dysfunction is confirmed by increased concentrations of liver enzymes (alanine aminotransferase, gamma glutamyl transferase, alkaline phosphatase) and bile acids. Jaundice (hyperbilirubinaemia) may be evident.

Treatment is primarily supportive, and the prognosis depends on the nature and reversibility of the hepatic disease.

Disseminated intravascular coagulation
The diagnostically and therapeutically challenging condition of disseminated intravascular coagulation is characterized by widespread intravascular coagulation and ongoing fibrinolysis. This results in the consumption of both platelets and clotting factors, together with the activation of fibrinolysis, depletion of natural inhibitors of coagulation such as antithrombin III (ATIII) and release of substances that interfere with fibrin polymerization. Affected animals thus present with a bleeding tendency due to defects in primary, secondary and tertiary haemostasis. The condition, predisposing factors, diagnosis and management are covered fully in Chapter 14.

Circulating inhibitors of clotting factors

Heparin
Canine mast cells contain significant amounts of heparin, the physiological inhibitor of coagulation. Some animals with mast cell tumours may release heparin into the circulation resulting in a haemorrhagic tendency.

Heparin, in conjunction with ATIII, primarily inhibits activated F X but also other plasma proteases. Prolongation of both PT and APTT is seen, and addition of normal plasma to patient plasma fails to correct the clotting times. The bleeding tendency can be managed by plasma transfusion, but the prognosis relates to that of the underlying malignancy.

Antibodies to clotting factors

Lupus anticoagulant
A lupus-type anticoagulant, which in humans is due to the presence of circulating autoantibodies directed against phospholipids, has been reported in one dog with thromboembolic disease (Stone *et al.*, 1994). Although coagulation tests show a defect in the intrinsic pathway, with prolongation of the APTT, patients are at risk of thrombotic disease rather than abnormal bleeding. The dog described with this condition had pulmonary thromboembolism and immune-mediated haemolytic anaemia.

Factor VIII inhibitors
Acquired inhibitors to F VIII are present in 6% of human patients with haemophilia A in the United Kingdom, with 12% of severely affected haemophiliacs having inhibitors (Rizza, 1984). Similar spontaneous inhibitor (antibody) formation has been documented in haemophilic dogs transfused with dog F VIII (Giles *et al.*, 1984; Pijnappels *et al.*, 1986). In addition, antibodies to heterologous F VIII, which cross react with canine F VIII, have been described in haemophilic dogs that have received human and/or pig F VIII concentrates (Littlewood and Barrowcliffe, 1987; Littlewood, 1988).

Autoantibodies to F VIII may develop in human patients, resulting in acquired haemophilia A. A circulating inhibitor to F VIII, presumed to be an antibody, has been identified in the plasma from a dog with a haemorrhagic diathesis at the Animal Health Trust, Newmarket, United Kingdom (unpublished observations).

Factor XI inhibitor

An acquired coagulopathy has been described in a cat due to the development of inhibitors against F XI (Feldman *et al.*, 1983).

REFERENCES

Bradylak SF (1988) Coagulation disorders and liver disease. *Veterinary Clinics of North America: Small Animal Practice* **18**, 87-93

Brooks M (1999) Hereditary bleeding disorders in dogs and cats. *Veterinary Medicine* **94**, 555-564

Brooks MB, Gu W and Ray K (1997) Complete deletion of factor IX gene and inhibition of factor IX activity in a Labrador Retriever with hemophilia B. *Journal of the American Veterinary Medical Association* **211**, 1418-1421

Cook AK, Werner LL, O'Neill SL, Brooks M and Feldman BF (1993) Factor X deficiency in a Jack Russell terrier. *Veterinary Clinical Pathology* **22**, 68-71

Couto CG (1999) Clinical approach to the bleeding dog or cat. *Veterinary Medicine* **94**, 450-459

Dillon AR and Boudreaux MK (1988) Combined factors IX and XII deficiencies in a family of cats. *Journal of the American Veterinary Medical Association* **193**, 833-834

Dodds WJ (1973) Canine factor X (Stuart-Power factor) deficiency. *Journal of Laboratory and Clinical Medicine* **82**, 560-566

Dodds WJ (1977) Inherited hemorrhagic defects. In: *Current Veterinary Therapy VI*, ed. RW Kirk, pp. 438-445. WB Saunders, Philadelphia

Dodds WJ (1984) Hemophilia in cats. *Cat World (USA)* November, p. EE13

Dodds WJ and Kull JE (1971) Canine factor XI (plasma thromboplastin antecedent) deficiency. *Journal of Laboratory and Clinical Medicine* **78**, 746-752

Dodds WJ and Womack JE (1997) Molecular genetics, gene transfer and therapy. *Advances in Veterinary Medicine* **No 40**

Edwards DF and Russell RG (1987) Probable vitamin K-deficient bleeding in two cats with malabsorption syndrome secondary to lymphocytic-plasmacytic enteritis. *Journal of Veterinary Internal Medicine* **1**, 97-101

Evans JP, Brinkhaus KM, Brayer GD, Reisner HM and High KA (1989) Canine hemophilia B resulting from a point mutation with unusual consequences. *Proceedings of the National Academy of Sciences of the USA* **86**, 10095-10099

Evans RJ (1985) *Feline Medicine*, ed. EA Chandler and CJ Gaskell. Blackwell, Oxford

Feldman BF, Soares CJ, Kitchell BE, *et al.* (1983) Hemorrhage in a cat caused by inhibition of factor XI (plasma thromboplastin antecedent). *Journal of the American Veterinary Medical Association* **182**, 589-591

Feldman DG, Brooks MB and Dodds WJ (1995) Hemophilia B (factor IX) deficiency in a family of German shepherd dogs. *Journal of the American Veterinary Medical Association* **206**, 1901-1905

Fogh JM and Fogh IT (1988) Inherited coagulation disorders. *Veterinary Clinics of North America: Small Animal Practice* **18**, 231-244

Giles AR, Tinlin S, Hoogendoorn H, Greenwood P and Greenwood R (1984) Development of factor VIII:C antibodies in dogs with hemophilia A (factor VIII:C deficiency). *Blood* **63**, 451-456

Gookin JL, Brooks MB, Catalfamo JL, Bunch SE and Muñana KR (1997) Factor X deficiency in a cat. *Journal of the American Veterinary Medical Association* **211**, 576-579

Gu W, Brooks M, Catalfamo J, Ray J and Ray K (1999) Two distinct mutations cause severe hemophilia B in two unrelated canine pedigrees. *Thrombosis and Haemostasis* **82**, 1270-1275

Herzog RW, Yang EY, Couto LB, Hagstrom JN, Elwell D, Fields PA, Burton M, Bellinger DA, Read MS, Brinkhous KM, Podsakoff GM, Nichols TC, Kurtzman GJ and High KA (1999) Long-term correction of canine hemophilia B by gene transfer of blood coagulation factor IX mediated by adeno-associated viral vector. *National Medicine* **5**, 56-63

High KA, Evans JP, Ware JL, Stafford DW and Roberts HR (1987) Hemophilia in canines is due to a post-transcriptional defect. *Thrombosis and Haemostasis* **58**, 337, 1218 [Abstract]

Kier AB, Bresnaham JF, White FJ and Wagner JE (1980) The inheritance pattern of factor XII deficiency in domestic cats. *Canadian Journal of Comparative Medicine* **44**, 309-314

Knowler C, Giger U, Dodds WJ and Brooks M (1994) Factor XI deficiency in Kerry blue terriers. *Journal of the American Veterinary Medical Association* **205**, 1557-1561

Littlewood JD (1988) Factor VIII - phospholipid mixtures and factor VIII inhibitors: studies in haemophilic dogs. PhD thesis, University of Cambridge

Littlewood JD (1989) Inherited bleeding disorders of dogs and cats. *Journal of Small Animal Practice* **30**, 140-143

Littlewood JD (1992) Differential diagnosis of haemorrhagic disorders in dogs. *In Practice* **14**, 172-180

Littlewood JD and Barrowcliffe TW (1987) The development and characterisation of antibodies to human factor VIII in haemophilic dogs. *Thrombosis and Haemostasis* **57**, 314-321

Littlewood JD and Evans RJ (1990) A combined deficiency of factor VIII and contact activation defect in a family of cats. *British Veterinary Journal* **146**, 30-35

Littlewood JD, Matic SE and Smith N (1986) Factor IX deficiency (haemophilia B, Christmas disease) in a cross-bred dog. *Veterinary Record* **118**, 400-401

Littlewood JD, Shaw SC and Coombes LM (1995) Vitamin K-dependent coagulopathy in a British Devon Rex cat. *Journal of Small Animal Practice* **36**, 115-118

Macpherson R, Scherer J, Ross ML and Gentry PA (1999) Factor VII deficiency in a mixed breed dog. *Canadian Veterinary Journal* **40**, 503-505

Maddison JE, Watson ADJ, Eade IG and Exner T (1990) Vitamin K-dependent multifactor coagulopathy in Devon Rex cats. *Journal of the American Veterinary Medical Association* **197**, 1495-1497

Mauser AE, Whitlark J, Whitmey KM and Lothrop CD (1996) A deletion mutation causes hemophilia B in Lhaso Apso dogs. *Blood* **88**, 3451-3455

Mischke R, Pohle D, Schoon HA, Fehr M and Nolte I (1998) Changes in blood coagulation in dogs with hepatic cirrhosis. *Deutsche Tierarztliche Wochenschrift* **105**, 43-47

Pederson NC and Holzworth J (1987) *Diseases of the Cat*, ed. NC Pederson and J Holzworth, pp. 146-181. WB Saunders, Philadelphia

Perry LA, Williams DA, Pidgeon GL *et al.* (1991) Exocrine pancreatic insufficiency with associated coagulopathy in a cat. *Journal of the American Animal Hospital Association* **27**, 109-114

Peterson JL, Couto CG and Wellman ML (1995) Hemostatic disorders in cats: a retrospective study and review of the literature. *Journal of Veterinary Internal Medicine* **9**, 298-303

Pijnappels MIM, Briet E, van der Zweet GTh, Huisden R, van Tilburg NH and Eulderink F (1986) Evaluation of the cuticle bleeding time in canine haemophilia A. *Thrombosis and Haemostasis* **55**, 70-73

Rizza CR (1984) The management of haemophiliacs who have antibodies to factor VIII. *Scandinavian Journal of Haematology* **33 (Suppl 40)**, 187-193

Spurling NW (1980) Hereditary disorders of haemostasis in dogs: a critical review of the literature. *Veterinary Bulletin* **50**, 151-173

Stone MS, Johnstone IB, Brooks M, Bollinger TK and Cotter SM (1994) Lupus-type "anticoagulant" in a dog with hemolysis and thrombosis. *Journal of Veterinary Internal Medicine* **8**, 57-61

Verlander JW, Gorman NT and Dodds WJ (1984) Factor IX deficiency (hemophilia B) in a litter of Labrador retrievers. *Journal of the American Veterinary Medical Association* **185**, 83-84

Disorders of Haemostasis:
Selected Topics

(i) Immune-Mediated Thrombocytopenia

David C. Lewis

INTRODUCTION

Immune-mediated thrombocytopenia (IMT) is a disease in which antibodies bound to the surface of platelets result in premature platelet destruction by macrophages (Mackin 1995a; Lewis and Meyers, 1996a). IMT may occur alone or in association with systemic lupus erythematosus (SLE); rheumatoid arthritis; neoplasia; viral, bacterial, rickettsial or parasitic infections; or drug administration (Helfand *et al.*, 1985; Axthelm and Krakowka, 1987; Chong, 1991; Kristensen *et al.*, 1994; Lewis *et al.*, 1995b). In cats, IMT can occur in association with feline leukaemia virus (FeLV) or feline immunodeficiency virus (FIV) infection (Shelton *et al.*, 1990). IMT in the absence of other identifiable disease is referred to as primary IMT or idiopathic thrombocytopenic purpura (also called ITP). Primary IMT is an autoimmune disease and the term autoimmune thrombocytopenia (AITP) is also used to describe this disease (Lewis and Meyers, 1996b). Primary IMT may occur alone or in conjunction with immune-mediated haemolytic anaemia (IMHA; Evans' syndrome).

Primary IMT is common in dogs and the prevalence may approach as high as 1% of hospitalized patients (Cockburn and Troy, 1986; Jans *et al.*, 1990; Grindem *et al.*, 1991). Primary IMT has been reported in cats, but is rare (Jordan *et al.*, 1993).

PATHOGENESIS

Platelet destruction in dogs with IMT is mediated by antibodies (primarily IgG) bound to the platelet surface (Figure 14.1) (Lewis *et al.*, 1995d); in primary IMT these antibodies are thought to be directed against normal host antigens on the surface of the platelet (antiplatelet autoantibodies) (Lewis and Meyers, 1996b). The pathogenesis of most secondary causes of IMT is unknown. It is not known why the humoral immune system targets host platelet antigens in dogs with primary IMT, but genetic predisposition, gender and environmental factors (including infectious agents, pollutants and stress) may all play a part.

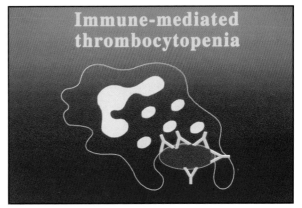

Figure 14.1: Pathogenesis of immune-mediated thrombocytopenia. Antibodies (primarily IgG) bound to the surface of platelets result in accelerated platelet destruction by macrophages in the spleen and liver. Reproduced from Feldman, Zinkl and Jain (2000) Schalm's Veterinary Hematology, 5th edition, *with permission of Lippincott, Williams and Wilkins.*

Genetic predisposition to primary IMT in dogs is suggested by a high prevalence of the disease in Cocker Spaniels, miniature and toy Poodles and Old English Sheepdogs, and reports of primary IMT in families of Cocker Spaniels, Hungarian Vizslas, Scottish Terriers and longhaired Dachshunds (Dodds, 1983; Grindem *et al.*, 1991; Day and Penhale, 1992; Lewis *et al.*, 1995d).

Gender (female) predilection to many autoimmune diseases is recognized, and primary IMT occurs in females around twice as frequently as in males (Wilkins *et al.*, 1973; Williams and Maggio-Price, 1984; Jackson and Kruth, 1985; Lewis *et al.*, 1995d). Cause and effect associations between environmental factors and primary IMT in dogs have not been defined.

IMT is primarily a disorder of accelerated platelet destruction. Average platelet life span in dogs is about 5 days; in primary IMT platelet life span is reduced to hours or minutes (Shulman and Jordan, 1987). Platelet production (thrombopoiesis) is usually appropriately accelerated (as much as five times normal) although, in some cases, thrombopoiesis may be impaired (Joshi and Jain, 1977; Ballem *et al.*, 1987). After Fc receptor interaction, platelets are destroyed by macrophages in the spleen and liver (Figure 14.2). In addition to being

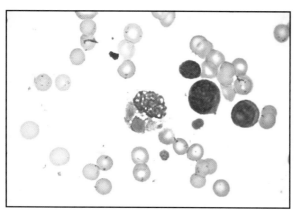

Figure 14.2: Splenic aspirate from a dog with primary immune-mediated thrombocytopenia and immune-mediated haemolytic anaemia, showing a macrophage phagocytosing two platelets and a red cell. The other nucleated cells present are red cell precursors. Reproduced from Feldman, Zinkl and Jain (2000) Schalm's Veterinary Hematology, 5th edition, with permission of Lippincott, Williams and Wilkins.

a major site of platelet destruction in primary IMT, the spleen is an important source of antiplatelet autoantibodies (McMillan *et al.*, 1974).

Platelet function in primary IMT is usually enhanced (Harker and Slichter, 1972), owing to accelerated thrombopoiesis producing a larger and more haemostatically competent platelet population, although platelet function may be impaired in some cases (Kristensen *et al.*, 1994).

CLINICAL FEATURES

Signalment

Primary IMT can occur in dogs of all ages (the reported age range is 8 months to 15 years), but is most common in middle-aged dogs (Wilkins *et al.*, 1973; Williams and Maggio-Price, 1984; Lewis *et al.*, 1995d). Females, spayed or intact, are affected twice as frequently as males (Wilkins *et al.*, 1973; Williams and Maggio-Price, 1984; Jackson and Kruth, 1985; Lewis *et al.*, 1995d). A high prevalence of primary IMT is reported in Cocker Spaniels; German Shepherd Dogs; miniature, toy, and standard Poodles; and Old English Sheepdogs, although any breed of dog, including crossbreeds, can be affected (Dodds, 1983; Grindem *et al.*, 1991; Day and Penhale, 1992; Lewis *et al.*, 1995d). Primary IMT has been reported in cats, but is rare (Jordan *et al.*, 1993).

History

The most frequently reported complaints with IMT are anorexia, lethargy, weakness, epistaxis, haematochezia and mucosal haemorrhage (Jackson and Kruth, 1985). Episodes of primary IMT have been preceded by stressors such as kennelling, extremes of environmental temperature, hormonal changes (oestrus, pseudo-

cyesis, parturition) and surgery (Dodds, 1983; Jackson and Kruth, 1985). A seasonal distribution has not been reported.

Physical examination

Frequent findings in IMT are mucosal and cutaneous petechiae, purpura, ecchymoses, hyphaema, retinal haemorrhages, melaena, haematemesis, epistaxis and pallor of the mucous membranes (Wilkins *et al.*, 1973; Williams and Maggio-Price, 1984; Feldman *et al.*, 1985; Jackson and Kruth, 1985) (Figures 14.3 to 14.6). Central nervous system or intraocular haemorrhage can lead to neurological signs or blindness, respectively. The degree of haemorrhage for any given platelet count is unpredictable. Dogs with primary IMT may have a platelet count of less than 10 x 10⁹/l without evidence of haemorrhage. Fever, splenomegaly, hepatomegaly and lymphadenopathy are uncommon in dogs with primary IMT (Wilkins *et al.*, 1973; Williams and Maggio-Price, 1984; Feldman *et al.*, 1985; Jackson and Kruth, 1985).

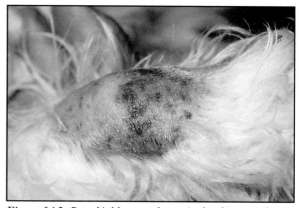

Figure 14.3: Petechial haemorrhages in the skin over the carpus of a West Highland White Terrier with primary immune-mediated thrombocytopenia.

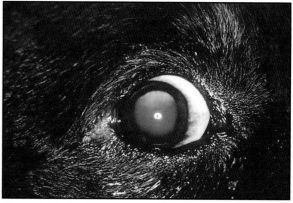

Figure 14.4: Hyphaema in a Rottweiler with primary immune-mediated thrombocytopenia. Blindness can be the presenting complaint in dogs with intraocular haemorrhage due to thrombocytopenia. Reproduced from Feldman, Zinkl and Jain (2000) Schalm's Veterinary Hematology, 5th edition, with permission of Lippincott, Williams and Wilkins.

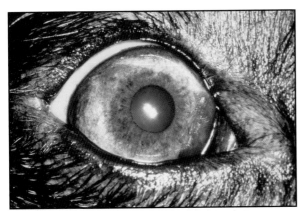

Figure 14.5: *Iris petechiae in a dog with primary immune-mediated thrombocytopenia. Reproduced from Feldman, Zinkl and Jain (2000)* Schalm's Veterinary Hematology, *5th* edition, *with permission of Lippincott, Williams and Wilkins.*

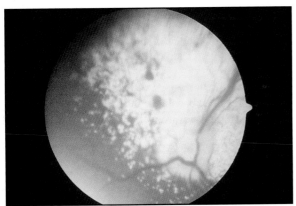

Figure 14.6: *Retinal petechiae in a dog with primary immune-mediated thrombocytopenia.*

DIAGNOSIS

Complete blood count and platelet count

Dogs with primary IMT usually have marked thrombocytopenia ($<30 \times 10^9/l$) on presentation (Wilkins *et al.*, 1973; Williams and Maggio-Price, 1984; Grindem *et al.*, 1991; Northern and Tvedten, 1992). Examination of a peripheral blood smear is a reliable way to assess the presence of thrombocytopenia, although a platelet count is necessary to quantify its severity (Jain, 1993). Megathrombocytes (large densely stained platelets suggestive of active thrombopoiesis) and microthrombocytes may be seen on peripheral blood smears from dogs with IMT (Sullivan *et al.*, 1995).

Total and differential leucocyte counts are variable in dogs with ITP. Neutrophilia with a left shift may be present owing to non-specific bone marrow response to thrombocytopenia or anaemia or owing to chemotactic activity of platelet-activating factor or leukotrienes (Joshi and Jain, 1976; Williams and Maggio-Price, 1984). A stress leucogram may be evident (Wilkins *et al.*, 1973; Joshi and Jain, 1976). Anaemia, due to haemorrhage or concurrent IMHA, may be present and may be regenerative or non-

regenerative depending on the time course of red cell loss and the presence of immunological targeting of red cell precursors. Immune-mediated haemolytic anaemia is reported in about 20% of dogs with primary IMT (Wilkins *et al.*, 1973; Williams and Maggio-Price, 1984; Jackson and Kruth, 1985).

A variety of criteria have been used to confirm a diagnosis of primary IMT in dogs, including:

- Severity of thrombocytopenia
- Presence of microthrombocytosis
- Normal to increased numbers of megakaryocytes in bone marrow
- Detection of antiplatelet autoantibodies
- Increased platelet counts subsequent to administration of immunosuppressive doses of glucocorticoids
- Exclusion of other causes of thrombocytopenia.

Severity of thrombocytopenia

Although thrombocytopenia in dogs with primary IMT is typically severe, thrombocytopenia associated with other diseases (e.g. disseminated intravascular coagulation, rickettsial infection) can also be marked (Waddle and Littman, 1988; Harvey, 1990). The degree of thrombocytopenia cannot alone be considered a dependable diagnostic indicator of primary IMT.

Microthrombocytosis

Microthrombocytosis, the presence of a predominant population of small platelets, is reported to be a specific indicator of primary IMT in dogs (specificity 95%) but is detected in less than 50% of cases (Northern and Tvedten, 1992).

Microthrombocytosis may result from preferential destruction of larger more heavily IgG-sensitized platelets by macrophages or complement, or platelet fragmentation after immune injury. Although microthrombocytosis may increase diagnostic suspicion for IMT in dogs, it is unlikely to be helpful in differentiating primary from secondary causes of IMT.

Bone marrow evaluation

The value of bone marrow evaluation in dogs with primary IMT is equivocal. Bone marrow disease is unlikely in the absence of leucopenia, non-regenerative anaemia or abnormal blood cell morphology, and bone marrow evaluation is therefore not routinely indicated in dogs with thrombocytopenia (Jones and Boyko, 1985; Jain, 1993). The presence of normal to increased numbers of bone marrow megakaryocytes may suggest that thrombocytopenia is due to accelerated platelet destruction or utilization, but this finding is not specific for primary IMT (Jain, 1993) (Figure 14.7). Furthermore, some dogs with primary IMT may have decreased numbers of bone marrow megakaryocytes owing to failure of bone marrow samples to provide a representative sample of bone

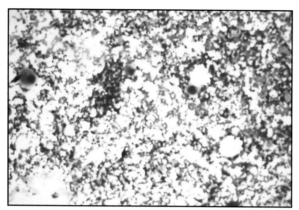

Figure 14.7: *Bone marrow aspirate from a dog with primary IMT. Bone marrow is hypercellular with increased numbers of megakaryocytes, an appropriate thrombopoietic response to accelerated peripheral platelet destruction or utilization.*

marrow or owing to immunological targeting of megakaryocytes (Joshi and Jain, 1976; Williams and Maggio-Price, 1984). One study reported that dogs with primary IMT and decreased numbers of bone marrow megakaryocytes had a poorer prognosis (Williams and Maggio-Price, 1984). Thrombocytopenia is not a contraindication for bone marrow aspiration or core biopsy, as severe haemorrhage is unusual and can be readily controlled with local pressure.

Measurement of mean platelet volume (MPV) can also be used to gauge the adequacy of platelet production. Increased MPV is a sensitive and specific indicator of the adequacy of bone marrow response in dogs with thrombocytopenia (Sullivan *et al.*, 1995).

Detection of antiplatelet autoantibodies

A variety of tests have been used to detect serum antiplatelet antibodies in dogs with thrombocytopenia. These antibodies are usually of the IgG class and may be referred to as 'platelet-bindable IgG.' Tests for the detection of IgG bound to the dog's own megakaryocytes or platelets ('platelet-bound IgG') have also been reported. It is important to realize that none of these tests enable dogs with primary IMT to be distinguished from dogs with secondary IMT.

Platelet factor 3 test

The platelet factor 3 (PF3) test is based on the principle that normal canine platelets will be damaged by platelet-bindable IgG in the plasma sample being tested and release PF3, causing acceleration of the partial thromboplastin time (Jain and Kono, 1970). Unfortunately, the PF3 test has variable sensitivity (from 28% to 80%) in dogs with primary IMT, lacks specificity and is of little diagnostic use in evaluating patients with thrombocytopenia (Jain and Kono, 1970; Wilkins *et al.*, 1973; Joshi and Jain, 1976; Williams and Maggio-Price, 1984).

Megakaryocyte direct immunofluorescence test

The megakaryoctye direct immunofluorescence test detects IgG bound to megakaryocytes and has variable sensitivity (from 30% to 80%) in dogs with primary IMT (Joshi and Jain, 1976; Jackson and Kruth, 1985; Kristensen *et al.*, 1994). A major disadvantage is that a bone marrow aspirate is required and this is otherwise not routinely necessary in patients with thrombocytopenia.

Detection of platelet-bound IgG

Detection of increased concentrations of platelet-bound IgG is extremely sensitive (about 90%) for primary IMT (Lewis *et al.*, 1995d) (Figure 14.8). Because of the high sensitivity of tests for platelet-bound IgG, a diagnosis of primary IMT is unlikely if the test result is negative. A positive test result for platelet-bound IgG in dogs with thrombocytopenia implicates an immune pathogenesis for thrombocytopenia but is not specific for primary IMT. Positive test results for platelet-bound IgG have been reported in dogs with thrombocytopenia associated with SLE, *Ehrlichia canis* infection, dirofilariasis, sulphadiazine/trimethoprim administration and cancer (lymphoproliferative disease and haemangiosarcoma) (Lewis *et al.*, 1995c,d).

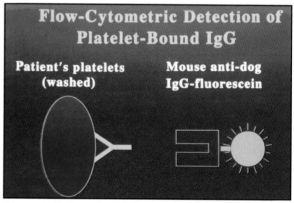

Figure 14.8: *Detection of platelet-bound IgG by flow cytometry. Platelets from affected dogs are washed, incubated with fluorescein-conjugated anti-dog IgG, washed again, and analysed for fluorescence by flow cytometry.*

Detection of platelet-bindable IgG in serum

Tests for platelet-bindable IgG are less sensitive (approximate sensitivity 60%) than tests for platelet-bound IgG, probably because most platelet-bindable IgG is already bound to platelets and little remains free in the circulation. However, these tests may be helpful in those cases in which sufficient numbers of platelets cannot be isolated for testing. A positive test result for platelet-bindable IgG is not specific for primary IMT (Kristensen *et al.*, 1994; Lewis *et al.*, 1995c).

Flow cytometry assays for detecting platelet-bound IgG and platelet-bindable IgG in serum are presently available to practitioners in the United States to assist in evaluating dogs with thrombocytopenia (Lewis *et al.*, 1995c).

Response to glucocorticoid therapy

Most (about 70%) of dogs with ITP will have platelet counts greater than 100 x 10^9/l within 7 days of initiating immunosuppressive glucocorticoid treatment (Williams and Maggio-Price, 1984; Jackson and Kruth, 1985; Jans *et al.*, 1990). However, because the principal action of glucocorticoids is to impair macrophage phagocytosis of antibody-sensitized platelets, primary and secondary IMTs may respond similarly.

Exclusion of other causes of thrombocytopenia

Although patient signalment, history, clinical findings and laboratory tests are helpful in increasing diagnostic suspicion, none is specific for primary IMT. Ultimately a diagnosis of ITP is made by excluding other causes of thrombocytopenia, although absolute certainty of a diagnosis of ITP is unattainable. Other causes of thrombocytopenia need to be excluded to reduce diagnostic uncertainty enough to enable the clinician to make optimal and timely decisions about treatment. The degree to which other causes of thrombocytopenia must, or can, be excluded varies with each patient and each client.

Splenomegaly

Thrombocytopenia due to splenomegaly is mild (not less than 100 x 10^9/l), which enables it to be easily distinguished from primary IMT (Jain, 1993). Splenomegaly is unusual in dogs with primary IMT.

Disseminated intravascular coagulation

Thrombocytopenia is a frequent finding in dogs with disseminated intravascular coagulation (DIC) (Feldman *et al.*, 1981). The absence of overt signs of illness in dogs with thrombocytopenia makes DIC unlikely. Evaluation of a coagulation profile, including prothrombin time, partial thromboplastin time, fibrin degradation products, antithrombin III concentrations and evaluation of a peripheral blood smear for schistocytes enable most cases of DIC to be diagnosed.

Haemolytic uraemic syndrome (HUS)

Haemolytic uraemic syndrome (HUS), a disorder of platelet hyperaggregability with intravascular platelet thrombi and widespread tissue ischaemia, has been reported in dogs (Holloway and Senior, 1993; Hertzke *et al.*, 1995). Clinical and laboratory findings in HUS, including neurological signs, renal failure, microangiopathic haemolytic anaemia (schistocytosis), thrombocytopenia and fever, make it distinguishable from primary IMT.

Anticoagulant rodenticide toxicity

Moderate to severe thrombocytopenia has been described in some dogs with haemorrhage subsequent to ingestion of anticoagulant rodenticide toxins (Lewis *et al.*, 1995a). Bleeding manifestations typical of secondary haemostatic disorders and abnormal coagulation profiles enable differentiation from dogs with primary IMT.

Neoplasia

Thrombocytopenia is frequently associated with neoplasia in dogs, particularly lymphoproliferative neoplasia and haemangiosarcoma (Helfand *et al.*, 1985; Grindem *et al.*, 1994), but can occur with a variety of solid neoplasms. Mechanisms for thrombocytopenia associated with neoplasia include DIC; splenic sequestration; myelophthisis; IMT; and bone marrow suppression by chemotherapy, radiation therapy or tumour-elaborated oestrogens. IMT is well documented in dogs with lymphoproliferative and solid neoplasia and may precede the discovery of neoplasia (Helfand *et al.*, 1985).

Systemic lupus erythematosus

IMT may be a component of SLE in dogs. Other clinical and laboratory manifestations of SLE, such as polyarthritis, dermatitis, polymyositis, glomerulonephritis, neutropenia, IMHA, lupus erythematosus cells and antinuclear antibodies would enable a diagnosis of ITP to be excluded (Scott *et al.*, 1983).

Drug-associated IMT

The gold salt auranofin, cephalosporins, and trimethoprim/sulphonamide have been associated with IMT in dogs (Bloom *et al.*, 1985, 1988; Lewis *et al.*, 1995d). Any drug can potentially provoke IMT. Drug-induced IMT usually develops after weeks to months of therapy, resolves within 2 weeks of cessation of administration of the drug and does not recur; hence it should be readily distinguishable from primary IMT (Chong, 1991). Any unnecessary medications should be discontinued in dogs with IMT.

Infectious disease

In North America, infectious diseases are reported to account for 20–60% of dogs with thrombocytopenia (Cockburn and Troy, 1986; Grindem *et al.*, 1991). Ehrlichiosis, Rocky Mountain spotted fever and dirofilariasis are frequently diagnosed infectious causes of thrombocytopenia in dogs (Cockburn and Troy, 1986; Grindem *et al.*, 1991). Mild thrombocytopenia is a frequent occurrence subsequent to modified live distemper vaccination (McAnulty and Rudd, 1985). Immune-mediated platelet destruction may contribute to thrombocytopenia in dogs infected with *Ehrlichia canis, Babesia canis, Dirofilaria immitis* or distemper virus (Axthelm and Krakowka, 1987; Lewis *et al.*, 1995d; Waner *et al.*, 1995).

Spurious thrombocytopenia

Spurious thrombocytopenia is a consideration in dogs with asymptomatic thrombocytopenia. Causes of spurious thrombocytopenia include platelet clumping owing to poor sampling technique, eythelenediamine tetra-acetic acid (EDTA)-induced platelet clumping and exclusion of large or small platelets owing to inappropriate machine settings or calibration (Jain,

1993). Macrothrombocytosis in Cavalier King Charles Spaniels can result in spurious thrombocytopenia (Brown *et al.*, 1994). Abnormal platelet counts should always be verified by examination of a peripheral blood smear.

Breed-related thrombocytopenia
Greyhounds, Cavalier King Charles Spaniels and Shiba Inus may normally have lower platelet counts than dogs of other breeds (Eksell *et al.*, 1994; Sullivan *et al.*, 1994; Smedile *et al.*, 1997; Gookin *et al.*, 1998).

TREATMENT

Supportive care
Cage rest and minimization of trauma are important. Drugs and fluids should be given enterally if feasible; the intravenous route is otherwise preferred.

Transfusion therapy
Life-threatening haemorrhage is uncommon in dogs with primary IMT (Wilkins *et al.*, 1973; Williams and Maggio-Price, 1984). Hypovolaemia or anaemia should be treated by administration of crystalloid or colloid solutions, packed red cells or whole blood. Platelet transfusions in dogs with IMT are rarely necessary but are indicated in dogs with central nervous system haemorrhage (dogs with severe thrombocytopenia and sudden onset of neurological signs) to control bleeding until platelet numbers are able to be increased by other therapies (Figure 14.9). In this circumstance, transfusion of multiple units of platelets is necessary because transfused platelets are destroyed rapidly (Carr *et al.*, 1986). The inaccessibility of platelet components makes this therapy impractical for most veterinarians.

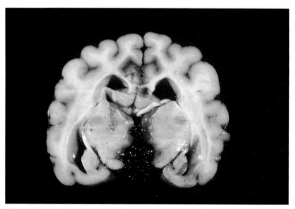

Figure 14.9: *Intracranial haemorrhage, which caused rapid onset of altered mentation and seizures in this dog with immune-mediated thrombocytopenia, may occur with severe thrombocytopenia and is frequently fatal. Reproduced from Feldman, Zinkl and Jain (2000) Schalm's Veterinary Hematology, 5th edition, with permission of Lippincott, Williams and Wilkins.*

Glucocorticoids
Glucocorticoids are the initial therapy of choice for dogs with ITP. The initial beneficial effect of glucocorticoids in dogs with IMT is primarily inhibition of macrophage destruction of antibody-sensitized platelets (Branehog and Weinfeld, 1974). Autoantibody production may also be impaired. Glucocorticoids also increase capillary resistance to haemorrhage, often reducing the severity of haemorrhage before platelet counts increase (Freund *et al.*, 1983). Glucocorticoids may also stimulate platelet production in some patients with IMT (Gernsheimer *et al.*, 1989).

Prednisolone or prednisone (2 mg/kg orally every 12 hours) is the most frequently used immunosuppressive agent for the treatment of IMT (Wilkins *et al.*, 1973; Williams and Maggio-Price, 1984; Feldman *et al.*, 1985; Jackson and Kruth, 1985; Jans *et al.*, 1990), although some clinicians favour dexamethasone (0.1–0.6 mg/kg every 24 hours) (Dodds, 1983; Williams and Maggio-Price, 1984). Most dogs with primary IMT attain a platelet count greater than 100 x 10⁹/l within 7 days of commencing glucocorticoid therapy (Williams and Maggio-Price, 1984; Jackson and Kruth, 1985; Jans *et al.*, 1990). Initial glucocorticoid therapy should ideally be continued until the platelet count normalizes, although this may not be achievable in some dogs, followed by tapering of the dose over weeks to months to find the minimal effective maintenance dose. Tapering too rapidly may cause disease exacerbation. Giving prednisone on alternate days during dose tapering may cause less hypothalamic–pituitary–adrenal axis suppression than giving dexamethasone on alternate days. Platelet counts should be monitored frequently while tapering glucocorticoid therapy, and glucocorticoid tapering should continue as long as the platelet count does not decline below the reference range. In many cases, glucocorticoids can be discontinued once the disease is in remission.

Adjunctive treatments
A variety of additional treatments, including cyclophosphamide, azathioprine, vincristine, danazol, cyclosporin, human immunoglobulin and splenectomy, have been used in conjunction with glucocorticoids to treat dogs with primary IMT. These treatments are generally reserved for dogs failing to respond to glucocorticoids, those with recurrent disease or those experiencing unacceptable glucocorticoid-induced adverse effects.

Vincristine
Vincristine given to dogs with primary IMT results in prompt (within 1 week) increases in platelet numbers (Greene *et al.*, 1982; Helfand *et al.*, 1984). One mechanism of action of vincristine is to diminish phagocytosis of platelets by macrophages by impairing macrophage microtubule assembly. To accentuate targeting of macrophages, vincristine can be incubated

with homologous platelets in vitro (vincristine-loaded platelets) or infused intravenously over 6–8 hours to achieve in vivo platelet uptake (Ahn *et al.*, 1984; Helfand *et al.*, 1984). Vincristine may also increase platelet counts by stimulating thrombopoiesis (Mackin *et al.*, 1995). Vincristine can have inhibitory effects on platelet function via disruption of platelet microtubules, however this has not been shown to be clinically important (Mackin *et al.*, 1995).

Cyclophosphamide

Although the role of cyclophosphamide as an immunosuppressive agent has been questioned, based on its inability to impair lymphocyte mitogenesis in normal dogs (Ogilvie *et al.*, 1988), it is frequently used for treating dogs with primary IMT. Cyclophosphamide is given orally or intravenously, in conjunction with glucocorticoids, at a dose of 200 mg/m² each week until an adequate response is attained. In humans with primary IMT, an adequate response may take 1 to 16 weeks (Reiner *et al.*, 1995). The efficacy of cyclophosphamide in dogs with primary IMT is not documented.

Azathioprine

Azathioprine is given (2 mg/kg orally) once daily initially and, once the desired clinical response is obtained, tapered in tandem with glucocorticoids to a maintenance dose of 0.5 to 1 mg/kg every 48 hours (Ogilvie *et al.*, 1988). An adequate response may take as long as 6 to 16 weeks in human patients (Quiquandon *et al.*, 1990). The efficacy of azathioprine in dogs with primary IMT is not documented.

Splenectomy

In humans with primary IMT, splenectomy results in a higher cure rate than any medical regimen and is performed early in the course of disease if glucocorticoids do not result in long-term remission. In dogs with primary IMT, splenectomy is reserved for those dogs that fail to respond to, or relapse after medical therapy. Rates of remission of clinical disease in dogs with primary IMT subsequent to splenectomy vary from 0% (0/4) to 80% (4/5), with a mean response rate of about 25% (Williams and Maggio-Price, 1984; Feldman *et al.*, 1985; Jackson and Kruth, 1985; Jans *et al.*, 1990).

Danazol

Danazol, a synthetic androgen with low capacity for masculinization, reduces the number of Fc receptors on macrophages and may act synergistically with glucocorticoids by displacing them from glucocorticoid-binding globulin. Documentation of danazol treatment of dogs with primary IMT is limited. Two dogs with primary IMT refractory to prednisone (1 mg/kg orally every 12 hours) had platelet counts higher than 100 x 10⁹/l within 1 to 2 weeks of starting danazol (5 mg/kg orally every 12 hours) in conjunction with prednisone (Bloom *et al.*, 1989; Roseler and Mason, 1994).

Cyclosporin

Cyclosporin inhibits T lymphocytes by inhibiting calcium-dependent transcription of interleukin-2 (IL-2). Experience with cyclosporin is limited; there is one preliminary report of cyclosporin treatment of dogs with primary IMT. Cyclosporin (15–30 mg/kg daily, to maintain trough blood concentrations of 400–600 ng/ml), in addition to other immunosuppressive therapies, was given to four dogs with ITP refractory to glucocorticoids. Three dogs achieved normal platelet counts after 3–5 weeks; one of these dogs died from systemic aspergillosis (Cook *et al.*, 1994).

Human immunoglobulin

Platelet count increases in humans with primary IMT subsequent to intravenous administration of human immunoglobulin (IVIG) are more rapid than platelet responses to oral prednisone therapy, and IVIG is frequently used as emergency therapy in humans with primary IMT (Blanchette *et al.*, 1992). Human IVIG binds to dog mononuclear cells and can modulate immune responses in dogs (Scott-Moncrieff *et al.*, 1995). One dog with IMHA and IMT had resolution of thrombocytopenia subsequent to IVIG therapy (Scott-Moncrieff *et al.*, 1995). Human IVIG is presently undergoing trials in dogs with ITP and/or IMHA.

Although the rationale for the use of vincristine, cyclophosphamide, azathioprine, danazol, cyclosporin, IVIG and splenectomy in the treatment of dogs with primary IMT may be valid, the proclaimed efficacy of these treatments is based largely on subjective clinical impressions. Until appropriately controlled clinical trials test the efficacy and place of these treatments in the management of dogs with primary IMT, clinicians should use the therapies with which they have most experience.

Goals of treatment

The goal of treatment in dogs with primary IMT is to withdraw all therapy while maintaining disease remission. This may not be attainable in all cases, and some dogs require long-term immunosuppressive therapy to maintain remission. Maintenance of a normal platelet count in the absence of therapy is the status most likely to be associated with immunological absolution. Dogs with lower platelet counts (partial remission) are more likely to be in a compensated thrombocytolytic state, maintaining platelet numbers in the face of accelerated platelet destruction.

PROGNOSIS

Most (over 70%) of dogs with primary IMT, with or without concurrent IMHA, will have platelet count increases to greater than 100 x 10⁹/l subsequent to initial therapy (glucocorticoids alone or in conjunction with vincristine, cyclophosphamide, azathioprine or fresh whole blood or platelet transfusions) (Williams and Maggio-Price, 1984; Jackson and Kruth, 1985; Jans *et al.*, 1990). Based on reported cases from referral hospitals, which may not be representative of cases seen by practitioners in the field, about 30% of dogs with ITP die or are euthanased during the initial episode of thrombocytopenia or during disease recurrence (Wilkins *et al.*, 1973; Williams and Maggio-Price, 1984; Jackson and Kruth, 1985; Jans *et al.*, 1990). About 40% of dogs have recurrent clinical signs of primary IMT. The remaining dogs are either cured, have subclinical disease or are lost to follow-up. The prognosis for dogs with primary IMT and IMHA may be considerably worse than for dogs with primary IMT only (Jackson and Kruth, 1985).

REFERENCES AND FURTHER READING

Ahn YS, Harrington WJ, Mylvaganam R, Allen LM and Pall LM (1984) Slow infusion of vinca alkaloids in the treatment of idiopathic thrombocytopenic purpura. *Annals of Internal Medicine* **100**, 192-196

Axthelm MK and Krakowka S (1987) Canine distemper virus-induced thrombocytopenia. *American Journal of Veterinary Research* **48**, 1269-1275

Ballem PJ, Segal AM, Stratton JR, Gernsheimer T, Adamson JW and Slichter SJ (1987) Mechanisms of thrombocytopenia in chronic autoimmune thrombocytopenic purpura. Evidence of both impaired platelet production and increased platelet clearance. *Journal of Clinical Investigation* **80**, 33-40

Blanchette VS, Kirby MA and Turner C (1992) Role of intravenous immunoglobulin G in autoimmune hematologic disorders. *Seminars in Hematology* **29**, 72-82

Bloom JC, Blackmer SA, Bugelski PJ, et al. (1985) Gold-induced immune thrombocytopenia in the dog. *Veterinary Pathology* **22**, 492-499

Bloom JC, Meunier LD, Thiem PA and Sellers TS (1989) Use of danazol for treatment of corticosteroid-resistant immune-mediated thrombocytopenia in a dog. *Journal of the American Veterinary Medical Association* **194**, 76-77

Bloom JC, Thiem PA, Sellers TS, Deldar A and Lewis HB (1988) Cephalosporin-induced immune cytopenia in the dog: demonstration of erythrocyte-, neutrophil-, and platelet-associated IgG following treatment with cefazedone. *American Journal of Hematology* **28**, 71-78

Branehog I and Weinfeld A (1974) Platelet survival and platelet production in idiopathic thrombocytopenic purpura (ITP) before and during treatment with corticosteroids. *Scandinavian Journal of Haematology* **12**, 69-79

Brown S, Simpson KW, Baker S, Spagnoletti MA and Elwood CM (1994) Macrothrombocytosis in Cavalier King Charles Spaniels. *Veterinary Record* **135**, 281-283

Carr JM, Kruskall MS, Kaye JA and Robinson SH (1986) Efficacy of platelet transfusions in immune thrombocytopenia. *American Journal of Medicine* **80**, 1051-1054

Chong BH (1991) Drug-induced immune thrombocytopenia. *Platelets* **2**, 173-181

Cockburn C and Troy GC (1986) A retrospective study of 62 cases of thrombocytopenia in the dog. *Southwest Veterinarian* **37**, 133-141

Cook AK, Bertoy EH, Gregory CR and Stewart AF (1994) Effect of oral cyclosporine (CS) in dogs with refractory immune-mediated anemia (IMA) or thrombocytopenia (ITP). (Abstract). *Journal of Veterinary Internal Medicine* **8**, 170

Day MJ and Penhale WJ (1992) Immune-mediated disease in the old English sheepdog. *Research in Veterinary Science* **53**, 87-92

Dodds WJ (1983) Immune-mediated diseases of the blood. *Advances in Veterinary Science and Comparative Medicine* **27**, 163-196

Eksell P, Haggstrom J, Kvart C and Karlson A (1994) Thrombocytopenia in the Cavalier King Charles Spaniel. *Journal of Small Animal Practice* **35**, 153-155

Feldman BF, Handagama P and Lubberink AA (1985) Splenectomy as adjunctive therapy for immune-mediated thrombocytopenia and hemolytic anemia in the dog. *Journal of the American Veterinary Medical Association* **187**, 617-619

Feldman BF, Madewell BR and O'Neill S (1981) Disseminated intravascular coagulation: antithrombin, plasminogen, and coagulation abnormalities in 41 dogs. *Journal of the American Veterinary Medical Association* **179**, 151-154

Freund LA, Berild D and Hainau B (1983) Haemostatic effect of prednisolone in thrombocytopenia. *Scandinavian Journal of Haematology* **31**, 485-487

Gernsheimer T, Stratton J, Ballem PJ and Slichter SJ (1989) Mechanisms of response to treatment in autoimmune thrombocytopenic purpura. *New England Journal of Medicine* **320**, 974-980

Gookin JL, Bunch SE, Rush LJ and Grindem CB (1998) Evaluation of microcytosis in 18 Shibas. *Journal of the American Veterinary Medical Association* **212**, 1258-1259

Greene CE, Scoggin J, Thomas JE and Barsanti JA (1982) Vincristine in the treatment of thrombocytopenia in five dogs. *Journal of the American Veterinary Medical Association* **180**, 140-143

Grindem CB, Breitschwerdt EB, Corbett WT and Jans HE (1991) Epidemiologic survey of thrombocytopenia in dogs: a report on 987 cases. *Veterinary Clinical Pathology* **20**, 38-43

Grindem CB, Breitschwerdt EB, Corbett WT, Page RL and Jans HE (1994) Thrombocytopenia associated with neoplasia in dogs. *Journal of Veterinary Internal Medicine* **8**, 400-405

Harker LA and Slichter SJ (1972) The bleeding time as a screening test for evaluation of platelet function. *New England Journal of Medicine* **287**, 155-159

Harvey JW (1990) Ehrlichia platys infection (infectious cyclic thrombocytopenia of dogs). In: *Infectious Diseases of the Dog and Cat*, ed. CE Greene, pp. 415-418. WB Saunders, Philadelphia

Helfand SC, Couto CG and Madewell BR (1985) Immune-mediated thrombocytopenia associated with solid tumors in dogs. *Journal of the American Animal Hospital Association* **21**, 787-794

Helfand SC, Jain NC and Paul M (1984) Vincristine-loaded platelet therapy for idiopathic thrombocytopenia in a dog. *Journal of the American Veterinary Medical Association* **185**, 224-226

Hertzke DM, Cowan LA, Schoning P and Fenwick BW (1995) Glomerular ultrastructural lesions of idiopathic cutaneous and renal glomerular vasculopathy of greyhounds. *Veterinary Pathology* **32**, 451-459

Holloway SA and Senior DF (1993) Hemolytic-uremic syndrome in dogs. *Journal of Veterinary Internal Medicine* **7**, 220-227

Jackson ML and Kruth SA (1985) Immune-mediated hemolytic anemia and thrombocytopenia in the dog: a retrospective study of 55 cases diagnosed from 1969 through 1983 at the Western College of Veterinary Medicine. *Canadian Veterinary Journal* **26**, 245-250

Jain NC (1993) *Essentials of Veterinary Hematology*. Lea and Febiger, Philadelphia

Jain NC and Kono CS (1970) The platelet factor-3 test for detection of canine antiplatelet antibody. *Veterinary Clinical Pathology* **9**, 10-14

Jans HE, Armstrong PJ and Price GS (1990) Therapy of immune-mediated thrombocytopenia. A retrospective study of 15 dogs. *Journal of Veterinary Internal Medicine* **4**, 4-7

Jones EC and Boyko WJ (1985) Diagnostic value of bone marrow examination in isolated thrombocytopenia. *American Journal of Clinical Pathology* **84**, 665-667

Jordan HL, Grindem CB and Breitschwerdt EB (1993) Thrombocytopenia in cats: a retrospective study of 41 cases. *Journal of Veterinary Internal Medicine* **7**, 261-265

Joshi BC and Jain NC (1976) Detection of antiplatelet antibody in serum and on megakaryocytes of dogs with autoimmune thrombocytopenia. *American Journal of Veterinary Research* **37**, 681-685

Joshi BC and Jain NC (1977) Experimental immunologic thrombocytopenia in dogs: a study of thrombocytopenia and megakaryocytopoiesis. *Research in Veterinary Science* **22**, 11-17

Kristensen AT, Klausner JS, Weiss DJ, Laber J and Christie DJ (1994a) Detection of antiplatelet antibody with a platelet immunofluorescence assay. *Journal of Veterinary Internal Medicine* **8**, 36-39

Kristensen AT, Weiss DJ and Klausner JS (1994b) Platelet dysfunction associated with canine immune-mediated thrombocytopenia (ITP). *Journal of Veterinary Internal Medicine* **8**, 323-327

Kristensen AT, Weiss DJ, Klausner JS, Laber J and Christie DJ (1994c) Comparison of microscopic and flow cytometric detection of platelet antibody in dogs suspected of having immune-mediated thrombocytopenia. *American Journal of Veterinary Research* **55**, 1111-1114

Lewis DC and Meyers KM (1996a) Canine idiopathic thrombocytopenic purpura. *Journal of Veterinary Internal Medicine* **10**, 207–218

Lewis DC and Meyers KM (1996b) Studies of platelet-bound and serum platelet-bindable immunoglobulins in dogs with idiopathic thrombocytopenic purpura. *Experimental Hematology* **24**, 696–701

Lewis DC, Bruyette DS and Kellerman DL (1995a) Thrombocytopenia subsequent to anticoagulant rodenticide-induced hemorrhage in dogs. (Abstract.) *Journal of Veterinary Internal Medicine* **9**, 188

Lewis DC, McVey DS and Callan MB (1995b) Flow-cytometric detection of platelet-bound and serum platelet-bindable IgG in dogs with immune-mediated thrombocytopenia. (Abstract.) *Journal of Veterinary Internal Medicine* **9**, 189

Lewis DC, McVey DS, Shuman WS and Muller WB (1995c) Development and characterization of a flow-cytometric assay for detection of platelet-bound immunoglobulin G in dogs. *American Journal of Veterinary Research* **12**, 1555–1558

Lewis DC, Meyers KM, Callan MB, Bucheler J and Giger U (1995d) Detection of platelet-bound and serum platelet-bindable antibodies in the diagnosis of canine ITP. *Journal of the American Veterinary Medical Association* **206**, 47–52

Mackin A (1995a) Canine immune-mediated thrombocytopenia. Part I. *Compendium of Continuing Education for the Practicing Veterinarian* **17**, 353–364

Mackin A (1995b) Canine immune-mediated thrombocytopenia. Part II. *Compendium of Continuing Education for the Practicing Veterinarian* **17**, 515–535

Mackin AJ, Allen DG and Johnstone IB (1995) Effects of vincristine sulfate and prednisone on platelet numbers and function in clinically normal dogs. *American Journal of Veterinary Research* **56**, 100–108

McAnulty JF and Rudd RG (1985) Thrombocytopenia associated with vaccination of a dog with a modified-live paramyxovirus vaccine. *Journal of the American Veterinary Medical Association* **186**, 1217–1219

McMillan R, Longmire RL, Yelenosky R, Donnell RL and Armstrong S (1974) Quantitation of platelet-binding IgG produced in vitro by spleens from patients with idiopathic thrombocytopenic purpura. *New England Journal of Medicine* **291**, 812–817

Northern J and Tvedten HW (1992) Diagnosis of microthrombocytosis and immune-mediated thrombocytopenia in dogs with thrombocytopenia: 68 cases (1987–1989). *Journal of the American Veterinary Medical Association* **200**, 368–372

Ogilvie GC, Felsburg PJ and Harris CW (1988) Short-term effect of cyclophosphamide and azathioprine on selected aspects of the canine blastogenic response. *Veterinary Immunology and Immunopathology* **18**, 119–127

Quiquandon I, Fenaus P, Caulier MT, Pagniez D, Huart JJ and Bauters F (1990) Re-evaluation of the role of azathioprine in the treatment of adult chronic idiopathic thrombocytopenic purpura: a report on 53 cases. *British Journal of Haematology* **74**, 223–228

Reiner A, Gernsheimer T and Slichter SJ (1995) Pulse cyclophosphamide therapy for refractory autoimmune thrombocytopenic purpura. *Blood* **2**, 351–358

Roseler BJ and Mason KV (1994) Use of danazol and corticosteroids for the treatment of immune-mediated thrombocytopaenia in a dog. *Australian Veterinary Practitioner* **24**, 126–130

Scott DW, Walton DK, Manning TO, Smith CA and Lewis RM (1983) Canine lupus erythematosus. I. Systemic lupus erythematosus. *Journal of the American Animal Hospital Association* **19**, 461–479

Scott-Moncrieff JC, Regan WJ, Glickman LT, DeNicola DB and Harrington D (1995) Treatment of nonregenerative anemia with human γ-globulin in dogs. *Journal of the American Veterinary Medical Association* **206**, 1895–1900

Shulman NR and Jordan JV (1987) Platelet kinetics. In: *Hemostasis and Thrombosis, Basic Principles and Clinical Practice*, ed. RW Colman, J Hirsh, VJ Marder and EW Salzman, pp. 452–529. JB Lippincott, Philadelphia

Smedile LE, Houston DM, Taylor SM, Post K and Searcy GP (1997) Idiopathic, asymptomatic thrombocytopenia in Cavalier King Charles Spaniels: 11 cases (1983–1993). *Journal of the American Animal Hospital Association* **33**, 411–415

Sullivan PS, Evans HL and McDonald TP (1994) Platelet concentration and hemoglobin function in greyhounds. *Journal of the American Veterinary Medical Association* **205**, 838–841

Sullivan PS, Manning K and McDonald TP (1995) Association of mean platelet volume and bone marrow megakaryocytopoiesis in thrombocytopenic dogs: 60 cases (1984–1993). *Journal of the American Veterinary Medical Association* **206**, 332–334

Waddle JR and Littman MP (1988) A retrospective study of 27 cases of naturally occurring canine ehrlichiosis. *Journal of the American Animal Hospital Association* **24**, 615–620

Waner T, Harrus S, Weiss DJ, Bark H and Keysary A (1995) Demonstration of serum antiplatelet antibodies in experimental acute canine ehrlichiosis. *Veterinary Immunology and Immunopathology* **48**, 177–182

Wilkins RJ, Hurvitz AL and Dodds WJ (1973) Immunologically mediated thrombocytopenia in the dog. *Journal of the American Veterinary Medical Association* **163**, 277–282

Williams DA and Maggio-Price L (1984) Canine idiopathic thrombocytopenic purpura: clinical observation and long-term follow-up in 54 cases. *Journal of the American Veterinary Medical Association* **185**, 660–663

(ii) von Willebrand's Disease

Tracy Stokol

INTRODUCTION

von Willebrand's disease (vWD) is caused by a deficiency of, or abnormality in, a large plasma glycoprotein called von Willebrand factor (vWf). It is the most common inherited disorder of haemostasis in dogs and has been diagnosed in one cat (French *et al.*, 1987). In the United States, vWD has been detected in over 50 breeds of dog, with a high prevalence in Dobermanns, Pembroke Welsh Corgis, Scottish Terriers and Shetland Sheepdogs (Brooks, 1992). In the United Kingdom, vWD has been diagnosed in 16 breeds of dog, particularly Dobermanns, Irish Wolfhounds and German Shepherd Dogs (Littlewood, 1991), of which several have exhibited clinical signs of bleeding. Knowledge of the pathogenesis, diagnosis and treatment of vWD is therefore essential for practitioners.

STRUCTURE AND FUNCTION OF vWF

In humans, vWf is produced by endothelial cells and megakaryocytes. These cells store vWf in specific organelles known as Weibel–Palade bodies (endothelial cells) or α-granules (megakaryocytes). These organelles release vWf in response to endothelial cell damage and various agonists, including thrombin. Maintenance of plasma concentrations of vWf is achieved by a constant basal secretion of vWf from endothelial cells. These cells also secrete vWf directly into the subendothelial matrix, where it binds to matrix components such as type VI collagen and elastin-associated microfibrils.

In plasma, vWf circulates in a non-covalently bound complex with coagulation factor VIII (FVIII). As these two proteins are found as a complex, vWf was formerly called FVIII-related antigen, but this term is misleading and now obsolete. In dogs, vWf is produced by endothelial cells, with a negligible amount detectable in platelets (in contrast to human platelets). Production of vWf by megakaryocytes has not been proven in dogs.

vWf is composed of a series of protein polymers called multimers, which consist of repeating subunits linked by disulphide bonds. Each subunit contains binding sites for platelet glycoprotein receptors (GPIb-IX and GPIIb-IIIa) and components of the subendothelial matrix (e.g. collagen). The number of subunits in each multimer varies, imparting a range of molecular weights (from 0.5 to 20 million daltons) to the multimers. The multimeric structure is important because the multimers with higher molecular weight, owing to their large size and multiple binding sites, are the most effective in haemostasis.

vWf is essential in primary haemostasis where it functions primarily as an adhesion molecule between platelets and the subendothelial matrix, between platelets and fibrin produced in the coagulation cascade and between individual platelets that are part of a platelet aggregate (Figure 14.10). The association of vWf with FVIII serves to protect FVIII from proteolytic degradation, to transport FVIII to sites of vascular injury and to promote the secretion of FVIII. Any quantitative or qualitative abnormality in vWf therefore results in an inadequate platelet plug, permitting continued haemorrhage from an injured blood vessel.

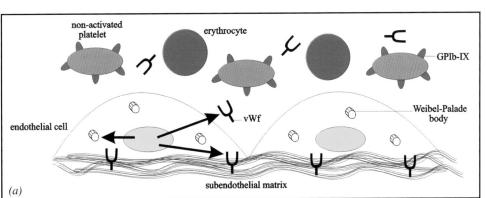

Figure 14.10: The role of von Willebrand factor (vWf) in haemostasis. (a) Endothelial cells secrete vWf into plasma, the subendothelial matrix and Weibel–Palade bodies. (continued overleaf)

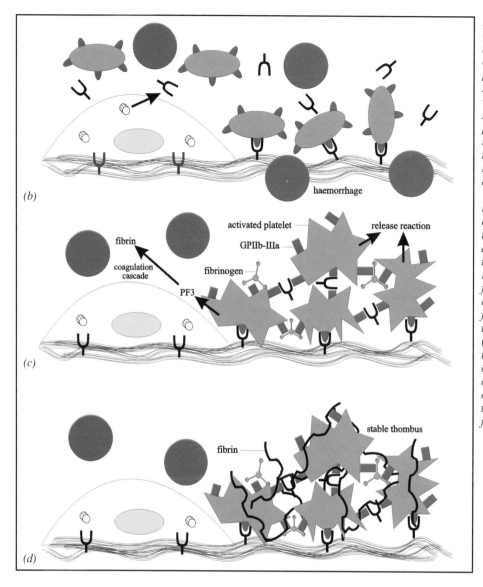

Figure 14.10 (continued):
(b) Vascular trauma disrupts the endothelium and, under conditions of high shear, plasma vWf binds to the subendothelial matrix, which, with the original subendothelial vWf, mediates platelet adhesion by interacting with GPIb-IX on the non-activated platelet membrane. Stimulated endothelial cells release Weibel–Palade vWf, which increases the local concentration of vWf at the trauma site. (c) Adhesion activates platelets, exposing the platelet receptor GPIIb-IIIa, which binds to both fibrinogen and vWf, thus crosslinking platelets, forming aggregates called the primary platelet plug. (d) The coagulation cascade is activated simultaneously, culminating in the formation of fibrin, which, with the aid of vWf, is incorporated into the growing platelet plug to form a stable thrombus.

CLINICAL SIGNS OF vWD

Clinically, vWD manifests as excessive bleeding from mucosal surfaces (haematuria, epistaxis, melaena, uterine or gingival haemorrhage; Figure 14.11) or excessive bleeding after surgery or trauma (including clipping of claws). These signs can be seen in any disorder of primary haemostasis (Figure 14.12), although for unknown reasons petechial haemorrhages (which usually typify these diseases) are rarely seen in vWD. This may be a useful clue when trying to differentiate these disorders. Other signs that have been attributed to vWD include lameness, intracranial haemorrhage and poor wound healing. The disease can be diagnosed at any age but typically is detected in young dogs, especially in countries where early neutering is practised and in breeds subjected to cosmetic surgery at a young age. vWD is inherited as an autosomal trait, so there is no sex predisposition for the disease.

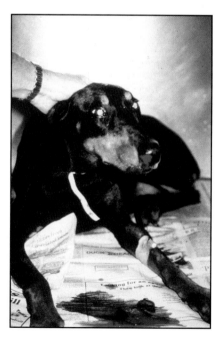

Figure 14.11:
Spontaneous epistaxis in a Dobermann Pinscher with severe von Willebrand's disease.

Quantitative platelet abnormalities
    Thrombocytopenia

Qualitative platelet abnormalities
    Inherited or acquired thrombopathias

Vessel wall defects (e.g. Ehlers–Danlos syndrome)

von Willebrand's disease

Figure 14.12: Disorders of primary haemostasis.

The clinical expression of vWD is variable and depends on several factors that decrease vWf concentrations and/or impair vWf or platelet function (Figure 14.13). The extent of vWf deficiency and the type of vWD are the most important variables governing the likelihood and severity of haemorrhage (Figure 14.14). Generally, the lower the vWf concentration the greater the likelihood of haemorrhage. An absolute deficiency of vWf (type III vWD) results in severe haemorrhage, often requiring vWf replacement therapy. Less dramatic reductions occur in type I vWD and consequently the clinical expression is milder. Studies by Johnson *et al.* (1985), Brooks *et al.* (1992) and Stokol *et al.* (1995) showed that most bleeding Dobermanns have vWf antigen (vWf:Ag) concentrations of less than 35%, or

Extent of deficiency in von Willebrand factor
Type of vWD
Concurrent disease
• Hepatic disease
• Renal disease
• Hypothyroidism
Drug treatment

Figure 14.13: Factors affecting the clinical expression of von Willebrand's disease (vWD).

35 canine units per decilitre. In Australia, this concentration is used as an arbitrary cut-off point below which dogs are regarded as being at risk of haemorrhage. A similar cut-off point of 40% is used in the United Kingdom (Littlewood *et al.*, 1987; Holmes *et al.*, 1996). These cut-off values should only be used as guidelines, as some dogs will haemorrhage despite having higher concentrations of vWf. Conversely, not all dogs 'at risk' will haemorrhage. The severest haemorrhage occurs in Dobermanns with low concentrations of vWf:Ag (<20%). These findings cannot be extrapolated to other breeds. For unknown reasons, Airedale Terriers do not show clinical signs of vWD, despite some dogs having low concentrations of vWf:Ag.

Expression of disease is most severe in type III vWD, in which there is an absolute deficiency of vWf. Dogs with type II vWD lack the higher molecular weight multimers of vWf and consequently haemorrhage severely, although their total concentrations of vWf:Ag are normal or mildly decreased.

Underlying diseases or drugs that impair platelet function (see Chapter 12) can precipitate or worsen haemorrhage in dogs with vWD. Much has been made of an association between vWD and hypothyroidism in dogs (Avgeris *et al.*, 1990; Dodds, 1991). Definitive proof that hypothyroidism produces an acquired form of vWD is, however, lacking, and recent studies do not support this contention (Johnstone *et al.*, 1993; Lumsden *et al.*, 1993; Panciera and Johnson, 1994, 1996). Anecdotally, hypothyroidism does seem to influence the frequency and severity of haemorrhage in dogs with vWD, because previously asymptomatic animals may bleed if they develop concurrent hypothyroidism. Thyroid supplementation should not be used for treatment or prophylaxis in vWD, unless dogs prove to be hypothyroid by thyroid function testing.

Type	Breed	Characteristics
Type I	Most breeds, including Dobermann Pinschers, Manchester Terriers, Pembroke Welsh Corgis, Poodles and Airedale Terriers	Quantitative reduction in von Willebrand factor (vWf) All multimers present but reduced in amount ?Autosomal recessive Clinical expression depends on breed Individual patients responsive to DDAVP (desmopressin)
Type II	German Shorthair Pointers and German Wirehair Pointers	Variable quantitative reduction in vWf Abnormal multimers: reduced proportion of large multimers ?Autosomal recessive Severe clinical expression No response to DDAVP
Type III	Scottish Terriers, Chesapeake Bay Retrievers, Shetland Sheepdogs and Dutch Kooiker dogs	Absolute deficiency of vWf in plasma and endothelial cells Total or near total lack of multimers Autosomal recessive, except Shetland Sheepdog (?2 mutations) Most severe clinical expression No response to DDAVP

Figure 14.14: Types of von Willebrand's disease in the dog.

DIAGNOSIS OF vWD

vWD can only be diagnosed by using laboratory tests for direct evaluation of vWf or by testing for mutations in the vWf gene. Routine coagulation profiles (platelet counts, activated partial thromboplastin and prothrombin times) in animals with vWD are within reference limits. Any dog (especially of a breed with a high prevalence of vWD) with a history of haemorrhage and a normal coagulation profile and platelet count should be tested for vWD. There are several diagnostic tests for vWD (Figure 14.15), including genetic tests, quantitative tests based on immunological assays and qualitative tests based on the ability of

Quantitative assays to measure the amount of von Willebrand factor antigen*
Laurell electroimmunoassay
Enzyme-linked immunosorbent assay
Qualitative assays to measure the functional activity of von Willebrand factor
Platelet adhesion
Buccal mucosal bleeding time*
Glass bead retention test
PFA-100 platelet function analyser
Platelet aggregation in response to agonists
Botrocetin
Polybrene
Further characterization of vWD
Multimeric analysis
Crossed immunoelectrophoresis
Genetic analysis*

Figure 14.15: *Diagnostic tests for von Willebrand's disease (vWD). *Generally available to veterinary surgeons in practice.*

vWf to participate in platelet aggregation in response to specific agonists in vitro. vWD is classified into different types depending on the multimeric composition of vWf, principally using the technique of multimeric analysis (which involves separation of vWf into its constituent multimers in a gel; Figure 14.16). In veterinary medicine, vWD is usually diagnosed by quantifying plasma vWf (termed vWf:Ag) in immunoassays with anti-vWf antibodies. In certain dog breeds, the mutation in the vWf gene can be detected by using new molecular techniques (Rieger *et al.*, 1998; Venta *et al.*, 2000).

Measurement of vWf:Ag

The Laurell rocket electroimmunoassay is the most widely used technique for measuring vWf:Ag (available in the United Kingdom through the Animal Health Trust, Newmarket), although enzyme-linked immunosorbent assays (ELISAs) are replacing this older assay. The results obtained by either immunoassay are used to define the patient's vWD status (Figure 14.17); however, neither assay measures the functional activity of vWf. This can only be assessed in vivo by using the buccal mucosal bleeding time (BMBT), or in vitro by platelet aggregation.

To obtain valid results for vWf:Ag, strict attention should be paid to the collection and handling of samples. vWf is an acute phase reactant protein, and values therefore increase in response to stress, excitement or disease. Incorrect collection and handling can initiate coagulation in vitro and artifactually increase or decrease vWf:Ag values. Values also change when blood samples are either refrigerated or stored at room temperature. It is therefore essential that blood is collected via clean venepuncture from a healthy unstressed dog and placed into a tube containing citrate anticoagulant (the tube must be filled to the appropriate level so that

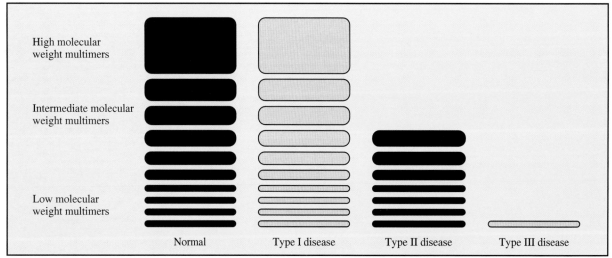

Figure 14.16: *The classification of von Willebrand's disease is based on the multimeric analysis of von Willebrand factor (vWf). A normal multimeric distribution shows a mixture of low, intermediate and high molecular weight multimers. In type I disease, there is a quantitative decrease in multimer biosynthesis, thus all multimers are present but the concentrations are decreased. Type II disease is characterized by an absence of high and intermediate molecular weight multimers. In type III disease there is a total or near total absence of vWf.*

vWf:Ag concentration	Category of von Willebrand's disease
Dobermann Pinscher	
60–150%	Normal
50–60%	Equivocal[*]
<50%	Likely carrier of vWf gene defect
<30%	Carrier 'at risk' of haemorrhage
Scottish Terrier	
60–150%	Normal
50–60%	Equivocal
<50%	Likely carrier of vWf gene defect
Undetectable[‡]	Homozygous affected

Figure 14.17: *Interpretation of results for von Willebrand factor antigen (vWf:Ag) in Dobermann Pinschers and Scottish Terriers in the United Kingdom, based on information from the Animal Health Trust, Newmarket (ranges differ in the United States (Brooks, 1992) and Australia (Stokol and Parry, 1993). *vWD status questionable, i.e. the dog could be a carrier or could be normal (genetic testing is advised in these dogs and in dogs with low normal vWf:Ag concentrations that are to be used for breeding). ‡vWf:Ag concentration below assay sensitivity.*

a blood:citrate ratio of 9:1 is achieved). The sample should be immediately centrifuged and the supernatant plasma harvested and transported, on ice, to the laboratory within 24 hours of collection. If despatch is delayed, the plasma sample should be frozen and transported on dry ice.

Buccal mucosal bleeding time

The BMBT is a useful in vivo test of primary haemostasis as a whole and is not specific for vWD. It is an insensitive test for routine diagnosis of vWD, because dogs with mild decreases in vWf:Ag concentrations may have a normal BMBT (Stokol and Parry, 1993). The BMBT will, however, be prolonged in many Dobermanns with moderate or severe decreases in vWf:Ag concentrations. Most Dobermanns with vWf:Ag concentrations of less than 20% will have prolonged BMBTs, indicating a compromised primary haemostatic system. The BMBT may be used as a presurgical assessment of the competence of primary haemostasis in Dobermanns of unknown vWD status (Figure 14.18). A prolonged BMBT warrants prophylactic treatment. Normal surgical haemostasis should not be taken for granted in a dog with a normal BMBT, as phenothiazines and anaesthetic agents may impair platelet function and precipitate surgical bleeding in a dog with a mild decrease in vWf:Ag concentrations. Therefore, the BMBT should not replace testing for vWf:Ag, and knowledge of the patient's vWf:Ag concentration (as well as a known history of haemorrhagic tendencies) is the most reliable guide to the need for prophylactic treatment before elective surgery.

Genetic testing

With the advent of molecular technology, precise defects in the gene encoding vWf have been identified in various dog breeds, including the Doberman Pinscher, Manchester Terrier, Pembroke Welsh Corgi, Poodle, Shetland Sheepdog, Dutch Kooiker and Scottish Terrier. In the dog breeds with type I vWD, there is a similar splicing defect in an intron in the vWf gene. In the Dobermann, this defect results in decreased synthesis of vWf by endothelial cells (Meinkoth and Meyers, 1995). In Scottish Terriers, a single base deletion causes a frameshift mutation with generation of a new stop codon and a severely truncated protein,

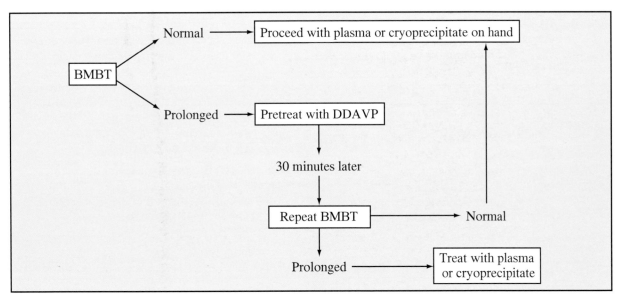

Figure 14.18: *Protocol outlining the presurgical use of buccal mucosal bleeding time (BMBT) and desmopressin (DDAVP) in Dobermanns of unknown status for von Willebrand's disease and those 'at risk' of haemorrhage due to the disease (concentrations of von Willebrand factor antigen <30 or 35%).*

resulting in severe type III vWD (Venta *et al.*, 2000). In Dutch Kooikers with type III vWD, there is a splicing defect in intron 16, which generates a premature stop codon in the vWf gene (Rieger *et al.*, 1998). Currently, tests for identification of vWf gene mutations are being offered for certain dog breeds in the United States (VetGen LLC, Ann Arbor, MI). The principal use of these tests is for the accurate identification of carriers for the selection of breeding stock, especially those dogs with 'equivocal' results for vWf:Ag concentrations. Genetic testing should not be used as the sole diagnostic test for vWD, because genetic status cannot be used to predict vWf:Ag concentrations, and there is no evidence linking genetic status to clinical signs of haemorrhage. In contrast, there is a well documented association between vWf:Ag concentrations and tendency to bleed.

TREATMENT OF vWD

Treatment for vWD is palliative, with the goal being short-term prevention or control of haemorrhage. The objective is to increase plasma vWf:Ag concentrations to a level that will either prevent or stop haemorrhage. This is usually accomplished by infusion of plasma products that contain vWf, although desmopressin, a drug that increases plasma vWf:Ag concentrations, can also be used.

Infusion therapy
Cryoprecipitate, a concentrated form of vWf and FVIII, is the treatment of choice for vWD. Cryoprecipitate provides the greatest amount of vWf in a small plasma volume, is associated with few side effects and is more efficacious in increasing plasma vWf:Ag concentrations and shortening the BMBT than any other form of infusion therapy. The preparation of cryoprecipitate is described in Chapter 15. Figure 14.19 provides guidelines for infusion therapy. Fresh frozen plasma is the best alternative to cryoprecipitate and, with the right

equipment, is easy to prepare. To prevent sensitization of the recipient to donor antigens and to minimize the risk of transfusion reactions, fresh whole blood should be avoided in vWD, especially as these dogs frequently have repeated bouts of haemorrhage and require repeated treatment. Fresh whole blood, typed or crossmatched, can be used to treat vWD, but whenever possible should be reserved for those cases with a specific need for red blood cells (e.g. severe anaemia).

Desmopressin
Desmopressin (1-deamino-8-arginine vasopressin; DDAVP) is a synthetic analogue of arginine vasopressin (antidiuretic hormone). Desmopressin increases plasma vWf:Ag and FVIII values by inducing the release of vWf from Weibel–Palade bodies in endothelial cells. This drug will only work in dogs with endothelial stores of vWf (i.e. type I vWD) and is ineffective in dogs with type III vWD, who lack vWf stores. Repeat injections produce a diminishing response owing to depletion of stores, therefore the drug has limited use in the treatment of the haemorrhagic episodes of vWD. Desmopressin is recommended as presurgical prophylaxis in Dobermanns 'at risk,' and in Dobermanns of unknown vWD status with a prolonged BMBT. It can also be used to increase vWf:Ag concentrations in donor dogs before obtaining blood for transfusion purposes. Synthetic vasopressin is available in tablet form or as an aqueous solution for injection. Intranasal preparations are also available as solutions or sprays, which are more cost effective than the aqueous solution for injection. The intranasal preparations are injected subcutaneously 30 minutes before surgery, at a dose of 1 μg/kg diluted to a 1 ml volume with sterile saline. This dose may shorten the BMBT in Dobermanns with vWD for up to 4 hours. However, response to the drug is unpredictable in dogs with vWD (some dogs may not respond at all) and DDAVP should not be relied upon to achieve surgical haemostasis. Plasma or cryoprecipitate should be available in the event of excessive surgical haemorrhage.

Product	Dose	Prophylaxis	Treatment
Cryoprecipitate	1 unit/10–15 kg bodyweight*	Give immediately before surgery. If surgery is prolonged (more than 2 hours), give additional units during surgery	Twice daily (minimum) until haemorrhage ceases
Fresh frozen plasma	6–10 ml/kg bodyweight	Give one dose immediately before surgery and a second dose if surgery is prolonged (more than 2 hours)	Twice daily (minimum) until haemorrhage ceases
Whole blood	13–22 ml/kg bodyweight	Give one dose before, and a second dose during, surgery	As needed until haemorrhage ceases

*Figure 14.19: Guidelines for infusion therapy in dogs with von Willebrand's disease. *Dosing is empirical as the amount of von Willebrand factor antigen (vWf:Ag) in each unit of cryoprecipitate varies, depending on the vWf:Ag concentration in the donor and the efficiency of the preparation technique. Pretreatment of donors with desmopressin optimizes the yield of vWf:Ag from the cryoprecipitate (Sato and Parry, 1998).*

REFERENCES AND FURTHER READING

Avgeris S, Lothrop CD and McDonald TP (1990) Plasma von Willebrand factor concentration and thyroid function in dogs. *Journal of the American Veterinary Medical Association* **196**, 921–924

Brooks M (1992) Management of canine von Willebrand's disease. *Problems in Veterinary Medicine* **4**, 636–646

Brooks M, Dodds WJ and Raymond SL (1992) Epidemiologic features of von Willebrand's disease in Doberman Pinschers, Scottish Terriers, and Shetland Sheepdogs: 260 cases (1984–1988). *Journal of the American Veterinary Medical Association* **200**, 1123–1127

De Gopegui RR and Feldman BF (1997) von Willebrand's disease. *Comparative Haematology International* **7**, 187–196

Dodds WJ (1991) Blood substitutes. *Advances in Veterinary Science and Comparative Medicine* **36**, 257–290

French TW, Fox LE, Randolph JF and Dodds WJ (1987) A bleeding disorder (von Willebrand's disease) in a Himalayan cat. *Journal of the American Veterinary Medical Association* **190**, 437–439

Holmes NG, Shaw SC, Dickens HF, Coombes LM, Ruder EJ, Littlewood JD and Binns MM (1996) von Willebrand's disease in UK Dobermanns: possible correlation of a polymorphic DNA marker with disease status. *Journal of Small Animal Practice* **37**, 307–308

Johnson GS, Schlink GT, Fallon RK and Moore CP (1985) Hemorrhage from the cosmetic otoplasty of Doberman Pinschers with von Willebrand's disease. *American Journal of Veterinary Research* **46**, 1335–1340

Johnson GS, Turrentine MA and Kraus KH (1988) Canine von Willebrand's disease. *Veterinary Clinics of North America: Small Animal Practice* **18**, 195–229

Johnstone IB, O'Grady MR, Lumsden JH and Horne RH (1993) Thyroid supplementation effect on plasma von Willebrand factor/factor VIII in Doberman Pinschers (abstract). *Journal of Veterinary Internal Medicine* **7**, 130

Littlewood JD (1991) Von Willebrand's disease in the dog. *Veterinary Annual* **31**, 163–172

Littlewood JD, Herrtage ME, Gorman NT and McGlennon MJ (1987) von Willebrand's disease in the United Kingdom. *Veterinary Record* **121**, 463–468

Lumsden JH, O'Grady MR, Johnstone IB and Horne R (1993) Prevalence of hypothyroidism and von Willebrand's disease in Doberman Pinschers and the observed relationship between thyroid, von Willebrand and cardiac status (abstract). *Journal of Veterinary Internal Medicine* **7**, 115

Meinkoth JH and Meyers KM (1995) Measurement of von Willebrand factor-specific mRNA and release and storage of von Willebrand factor from endothelial cells of dogs with type-1 von Willebrand's disease. *American Journal of Veterinary Research* **56**, 1577–1585

Meyers KM, Wardrop KJ and Meinkoth J (1992) Canine von Willebrand's disease: pathobiology, diagnosis, and short-term treatment. *Compendium of Continuing Education for the Practicing Veterinarian* **14**, 13–22

Montgomery RR and Coller BS (1994) von Willebrand disease. In: *Hemostasis and Thrombosis: Basic Principles and Clinical Practice, 3rd edn*, ed. RW Colman, J Hirsh, VJ Marder and EW Salzman, pp. 134–168. JB Lippincott, Philadelphia

Panciera DL and Johnson GS (1994) Plasma von Willebrand factor antigen concentration in dogs with hypothyroidism. *Journal of the American Veterinary Medical Association* **205**, 1550–1553

Panciera DL and Johnson GS (1996) Plasma von Willebrand factor antigen concentrations and buccal mucosal bleeding time in dogs with experimental hypothyroidism. *Journal of Veterinary Internal Medicine* **10**, 60–64

Rieger M, Schwarz HP, Turecek PL, Dorner F, Van Mourik JA and Mannhalter C (1998) Identification of mutations in the canine von Willebrand factor gene associated with type III von Willebrand disease. *Thrombosis and Haemostasis* **80**, 332–337

Sato I and Parry BW (1998) Effect of desmopressin on plasma factor VIII and von Willebrand factor concentrations in Greyhounds. *Australian Veterinary Journal* **76**, 809–812

Stokol T and Parry BW (1993) Canine von Willebrand disease: a review. *Australian Veterinary Practitioner* **23**, 94–103

Stokol T, Parry BW and Mansell PD (1995) von Willebrand's disease in Dobermann dogs in Australia. *Australian Veterinary Journal* **72**, 257–262

Venta PJ, Yuzbasiyan-Gurkan V, Brewer GJ and Schall WD (2000) Mutation causing von Willebrand's disease in Scottish Terriers. *Journal of Veterinary Internal Medicine* **14**, 10–19

(iii) Haemophilia A

Janet D. Littlewood

INTRODUCTION

Haemophilia A, or classic haemophilia, results from the deficiency or absence of factor VIII (F VIII), an essential cofactor in the activation of F X by F IXa.

FUNCTION OF FACTOR VIII

Human F VIII has a molecular weight of about 330 kD and an approximate plasma concentration of 200 ng/ml. The specific activity of canine F VIII is about four times greater than that of human F VIII (Littlewood, 1988a). The protein circulates in plasma, non-covalently bound to von Willebrand factor (vWf), which confers stability on the F VIII molecule. This association has given rise to confusion in the early literature about the separate identity and functions of these two plasma proteins. F VIII is activated by the action of thrombin, and further thrombin cleavage, together with activated protein C (enhanced by protein S) results in inactivation by proteolysis. F VIII is synthesized largely in the liver but is also produced by other cell types. F VIII activity is assessed by biological assays. The one-stage assay utilizes F VIII-deficient plasma as a substrate and compares the activity of dilutions of patient plasma with that of a standard of known F VIII activity by a modified activated partial thromboplastin time (APTT) test. Two-stage clotting methods and chromogenic assays can also be used to assess F VIII potency. International standards for animal plasmas do not exist, and patient plasma is usually compared with a pool of normal plasma collected from at least 10 healthy animals of mixed age, sex and breed. Many laboratories calibrate each new pool of plasma with the previous pool to standardize results from that laboratory, and will cross calibrate with other laboratories with recognized expertise and experience in coagulation assays.

Antigen detection assays using polyclonal and monoclonal antisera exist for human F VIII, and some of these reagents cross react with F VIII from animal sources (Rotblat *et al.*, 1983). Human patients with moderate and mild disease usually have identifiable F VIII antigen (F VIII:Ag), indicating the presence of an abnormal F VIII molecule with reduced function, whereas most of the severely affected patients have no F VIII:Ag measurable because of complete absence of F VIII synthesis.

PREVALENCE AND INHERITANCE

Haemophilia A was recognized in humans by the ancient Egyptians and is clearly documented in the Talmud. The disease is inherited in a sex-linked manner, with affected males and female carriers. It is the commonest of the severe inherited bleeding disorders, with a UK prevalence in the order of 16 per 100,000 of the male population. About 30% of patients have no family history and represent new mutations. The nature of the genetic defect has been elucidated in many human families with haemophilia. Gene deletions and various point mutations have been identified.

The prevalence in dogs and cats is not known, but haemophilia A is the commonest of the inherited coagulopathies. It has been reported in many breeds of dogs, including crossbreeds. It is likely that most of the cases identified represent new mutations, since in the severe form the condition is self-limiting, with affected males rarely surviving to adulthood and reproductive capability. In the German Shepherd Dog, however, a moderately severe form of the disease occurs, and affected males may survive to adulthood and be used at stud. This has led to dissemination of the disease in this breed across the world (Fogh *et al.*, 1984; Johnstone and Norris, 1984; Fogh, 1988; Littlewood, 1988b; Parry *et al.*, 1988). It should be noted that severe forms of the disease have also been identified in this breed, but not in the same families; all of the moderately affected animals are descendants of a single dog, Canto von der Wienerau. Screening programmes are in place in several countries and have been successful in eliminating the problem in Australia (Mansell, 1991). Cytogenetic analysis in these German Shepherd Dogs has shown that the defect is not due to a gross chromosomal abnormality or large gene deletion (Clarke and Parry, 1997), as one would expect when there is not complete absence of functional protein.

The disease is also reported in cats (Cotter *et al.*, 1978; Littlewood, 1986). Moderate haemophilia has also been recognized in a cat that survived castration. The cat, however, bled excessively after surgical removal of a lump, which proved to be a resolving haematoma on histological examination (Littlewood, 1999).

CLINICAL SIGNS

In humans, severe, moderate and mild forms of haemophilia A are recognized (Figure 14.20). Severe and moderate forms are recognized in dogs and cats, and it is likely that mild forms also occur but go unrecognized.

Severe disease

In the severe form of the disease it is often possible to identify affected puppies in a litter at birth due to persistent naval bleeding (Figure 14.21). Haematomata are common in young puppies once they begin to interact with littermates. Gingival haemorrhage is often seen when deciduous teeth are shed (Figure 14.22). Shifting and recurrent lameness are common in both moderate and severe forms, with degenerative osteoarthrosis developing as a sequel to these haemarthroses. Muscle haematomata are also common. Subcutaneous bleeds can be extensive due to the loose nature of the subcutis in the dog (Figure 14.23). Mediastinal haemorrhage (Figure 14.24), haemothorax and retroperitoneal bleeding are common causes of death in affected animals.

	Plasma factor VIII (% of normal)	Bleeding manifestation
Severe	<2	Prolonged severe bleeding after injury, spontaneous haemarthroses and muscle haemorrhages, life-threatening 'cavity' bleeds
Moderate	2–15	Severe bleeding after surgery or major injury, some bleeding after minor trauma, occasional haemarthroses and spontaneous bleeding
Mild	15–25	Bleeding only after major trauma and surgery

Figure 14.20: Classification of haemophilia (after Rizza, 1977).

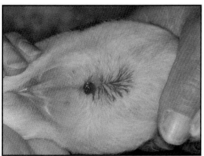

Figure 14.21: Persistent umbilical haemorrhage in a haemophilic puppy.

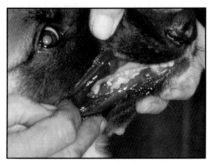

Figure 14.22: Gingival haemorrhage due to shedding of deciduous teeth.

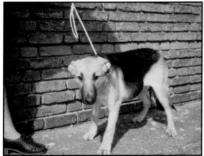

Figure 14.23: Extensive subcutaneous haematoma affecting the left thoracic and abdominal wall of a dog, hanging below the normal outline of the ventrum.

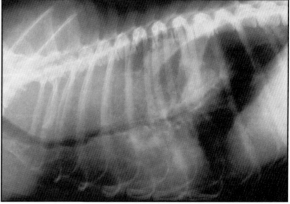

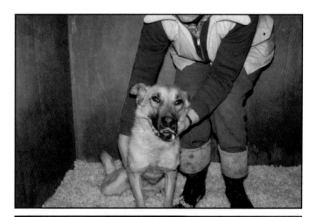

Figure 14.24: Mediastinal haemorrhage causing left-sided Horner's syndrome, dysphagia, dyspnoea and coughing in a dog. The lateral thoracic radiograph shows the anterior mediastinal haematoma, causing noticeable depression and compression of the trachea and caudal displacement of cranial lung lobes.

Moderate disease

In moderately affected animals there is often some episode of trauma that results in the bleeding tendency being recognized, although there is often a history of recurrent lameness or other suspicious signs if owners are questioned carefully. Abnormal bleeding has also been encountered during ovariohysterectomy of carrier bitches, as it is possible for carrier females to have F VIII concentrations as low as 25–30% of normal, due to random suppression of X chromosomes. This would be a manifestation of mild haemophilia in a heterozygote. Affected haemophilic female dogs that are homozygotic can be bred, when an affected male is mated with a carrier female. An acute bleeding disorder due to low F VIII-coagulant activity was described in a female dog of mixed breed as a spontaneous occurrence (Murtaugh and Dodds, 1988), but it is not known if this was a heterozygotic or homozygotic defect.

The bleeding tendency in haemophilic cats is much less severe than in dogs, probably due to the smaller size of cats and differences in behaviour between the two species (Cotter *et al.*, 1978; Littlewood, 1986).

TREATMENT

Cryoprecipitates

Management of bleeding episodes is difficult in severely affected animals, and owners often request euthanasia once the disease is diagnosed. The aim should be to increase plasma F VIII concentrations to at least 25–30% of normal to achieve haemostasis (Giles *et al.*, 1982; Pijnappels *et al.*, 1986). Transfusions of normal plasma from dogs at a rate of 15 ml/kg should achieve this, but greater volumes may be required, and over-transfusion can become a problem. Plasma cryoprecipitate contains a higher concentration of F VIII, and some centres make their own cryoprecipitate from fresh frozen plasma. A comparison between fresh frozen plasma and cryoprecipitate showed similar increases in F VIII clotting activity with both products, but the incidence of side effects (mild pruritus, pallor, weakness) was less with cryoprecipitate (Stokol and Parry, 1998). Adverse reactions usually are a feature of animals that have received multiple transfusions, and can be avoided by pretreatment with an antihistamine such as chlorpheniramine (Littlewood, 1988a). Commercial F VIII concentrates from humans and pigs are haemostatically effective in animals (Littlewood, 1988a; Lutze *et al.*, 1999), but the administration of heterologous proteins induces the formation of antibodies and the risk of anaphylaxis at subsequent infusion (Littlewood and Barrowcliffe, 1987; Littlewood, 1988a). Infusions should be given twice daily until bleeding has stopped and the haematoma is resolving. Antibiotic cover is indicated.

Tranexamic acid

Inhibitors of fibrinolysis can be useful in the management of bleeding episodes in haemophilic dogs (AR Giles, unpublished observations; Littlewood, 1988a). The author has used tranexamic acid (Cyclokapron, Kabi) at a dose rate of 15–20 mg/kg orally 2–4 times daily. This drug is used to control external haemorrhage (e.g. dental, prostatic) in human haemophilic patients and, owing to the risk of thromboembolic complications, would not be used in the management of internal bleeds. This risk, however, seems to be minimal in veterinary patients, probably owing to their enhanced fibrinolytic system compared with humans. It should be noted that this product is not licensed for veterinary use.

Gene therapy

Gene therapy has been used successfully in F VIII-deficient dogs (Connelly *et al.*, 1996). The gene for human F VIII in an adenoviral vector corrected the haemophilic phenotype as assessed by clotting times and the cuticle bleeding time. Expression of the gene product was only short term, lasting 1–2 weeks, owing to the development of an antibody response and a human F VIII-specific inhibitor.

CARRIER DETECTION

Asymptomatic heterozygotes provide a genetic reservoir for the disease. In human medicine, DNA analysis by the use of probes that detect diagnostically useful restriction fragment length polymorphisms, enables the identification of carrier females in many families with haemophilia A. However, studies using these probes in German Shepherd Dogs with moderate haemophilia showed no differences in the restriction patterns between normal and affected males for any of the probe combinations, although all probes used hybridized to the dogs' genomic DNA (Clark *et al.*, 1997). Whether the probes would be useful in other haemophilic dog families is unknown.

Carrier status

Carrier status is ascribed by taking into account pedigree evidence of haemophilic antecedents, plasma F VIII concentration and the production of affected progeny. According to these criteria a bitch can be classified as a suspected, probable or obligate heterozygote (Figure 14.25). Whereas coagulation assays will accurately distinguish between normal and affected males, the same is not true of females. This is because of the wide variability of F VIII expression in female heterozygotes due to the random suppression of X chromosomes in somatic cells. Measurement of plasma F VIII activity in females can only provide a statistical probability for the status of that animal. Although some studies have found that carrier bitches

Pedigree evidence	Factor VIII	Number of haemophilic pups born	Diagnosis
Father is haemophilic	–	–	Obligate heterozygote
–	–	2	Obligate heterozygote
Suggestive	Low	1	Obligate heterozygote
Suggestive	Low	–	Probable heterozygote
Suggestive	–	1	Probable heterozygote
–	Low	1	Probable heterozygote
Suggestive	–	–	Suspected heterozygote
–	Low	–	Suspected heterozygote
–	–	1	Suspected heterozygote

Figure 14.25: *Identification of heterozygotic carrier bitches.*

	Probability of non-carrier status
Immediate probability	50%
Plasma F VIII activity 15–60%	11%
One plasma F VIII test >60%	82%
Two plasma F VIII tests >60%	98%
One plasma F VIII test >60%, one test <60%	64%
Two plasma F VIII tests >60%, one test <60%	93%

Figure 14.26: *Factor VIII (F VIII) concentrations in daughters of obligate carriers.*

	Probability of non-carrier status
Immediate probability	50%
1 unaffected son	66%
2 unaffected sons	80%
3 unaffected sons	89%
4 unaffected sons	94%
5 unaffected sons	97%
6 unaffected sons	98%
If daughter has F VIII >60% and:	82%
1 unaffected son	90%
2 unaffected sons	95%
3 unaffected sons	97%
4 unaffected sons	98%
If daughter has F VIII 15–60% and:	11%
1 unaffected son	20%
2 unaffected sons	34%
3 unaffected sons	50%
4 unaffected sons	67%
5 unaffected sons	80%
6 unaffected sons	89%
7 unaffected sons	94%

Figure 14.27: *Identification of carrier status in daughters of carriers by production of unaffected sons. F VIII, factor F VIII.*

express only half the plasma F VIII activity of normal bitches (Fogh, 1988; Littlewood, 1988b), others have found functional assays of less use in the differentiation between normal and carrier animals (Littlewood, 1988a; Mansell and Parry, 1992). Figure 14.26 shows the inference of carrier status from F VIII assays in the daughters of obligate heterozygotes, and Figure 14.27 shows the influence on the probability figures of production of normal male offspring.

If a bitch has a high probability of non-carrier status, owners should be advised that if she is to be used for breeding then all the male pups in the first litter should be tested for APTT and/or F VIII activity. A bitch with a F VIII concentration greater than 60% who produces four normal male offspring has a 99% probability of non-carrier status. Blood testing of males before their use at stud is an effective way of identifying affected animals and preventing further dissemination of the genetic defect into subsequent generations in breeds with mild to moderate manifestations of disease.

REFERENCES

Clark P, Bowden DK and Parry BW (1997) Studies to detect carriers of haemophilia A in German shepherd dogs using diagnostic DNA polymorphisms in the human factor VIII gene. *Veterinary Journal* **153**, 71–74

Clark P and Parry BW (1997) Cytogenetic analysis of German Shepherd Dogs with haemophilia A. *Australian Veterinary Journal* **75**, 521–522

Connelly S, Mount J, Mauser A, Gardner JM, Kaleko M, McClelland A and Lothrop CD (1996) Complete short-term correction of canine hemophilia A by in vivo gene therapy. *Blood* **88**, 3846–3853

Cotter SM, Brenner RM and Dodds WJ (1978) Hemophilia A in three unrelated cats. *Journal of the American Veterinary Medical Association* **172**, 166–168

Fogh JM (1988) A study of hemophilia A in German shepherd dogs in Denmark. *Veterinary Clinics of North America: Small Animal Practice* **18**, 245–254

Fogh JM, Nygaard L, Andreson E *et al.* (1984) Hemophilia in dogs, with special reference to hemophilia A among German shepherd dogs in Denmark. I. Pathophysiology, laboratory tests and genetics. *Nordisk Veterinaermedicin* **36**, 235–240

Giles AR, Tinlin S and Greenwood R (1982) A canine model of hemophilic (factor VIII:C deficiency) bleeding. *Blood* **60**, 727–730

Johnstone IB and Norris AM (1984) A moderately severe expression of classical hemophilia in a family of German shepherd dogs. *Canadian Veterinary Journal* **25**, 191–194

Littlewood JD (1986) Haemophilia A (factor VIII deficiency) in the cat. *Journal of Small Animal Practice* **27**, 541–546

Littlewood JD (1988a) Factor VIII - phospholipid mixtures and factor VIII inhibitors: studies in haemophilic dogs. PhD thesis, University of Cambridge

Littlewood JD (1988b) Haemophilia A (factor VIII deficiency) in German shepherd dogs. *Journal of Small Animal Practice* **29,** 117-128

Littlewood JD (1999) Diseases of the blood and blood-forming organs. In*: Textbook of Small Animal Medicine,* ed. JK Dunn, pp. 765-819. Blackwell Scientific, Oxford

Littlewood JD and Barrowcliffe TW (1987) The development and characterisation of antibodies to human Factor VIII in haemophilic dogs. *Thrombosis and Haemostasis* **57,** 314-321

Lutze G, Kutschmann K, Thomae K, Lutze G and Franke D (1999) Successful treatment of canine haemophilia A with porcine factor VIII. *Praktische Tierarzt* **80,** 664-670

Mansell PD (1991) Diagnosis of haemophilia A in dogs, with particular reference to the disease in German shepherd dogs in Australia. PhD thesis, University of Melbourne

Mansell PD and Parry BW (1992) Carrier detection in human and canine hemophilia A. *Veterinary Bulletin* **62,** 999-1007

Murtaugh RJ and Dodds WJ (1988) Hemophilia A in a female dog. *Journal of the American Veterinary Medical Association* **193,** 351-352

Parry BW, Howard MA, Mansell PD and Holloway SA (1988) Haemophilia A in German shepherd dogs. *Australian Veterinary Journal* **65,** 276-279

Pijnappels MIM, Briet E, van der Zweet GTh, Huisden R, van Tilburg NH and Eulderink F (1986) Evaluation of the cuticle bleeding time in canine haemophilia A. *Thrombosis and Haemostasis* **55,** 70-73

Rizza CR (1977) Clinical management of haemophilia. *British Medical Bulletin* **33,** 225-230

Rotblat F, Goodhall AH, O'Brien DP, Rawlings E, Middleton S and Tuddenham EG (1983) Monoclonal antibodies to human procoagulant factor VIII. *Journal of Laboratory Clinical Medicine* **101,** 736-746

Stokol T and Parry BW (1998) Efficacy of fresh-frozen plasma and cryoprecipitate in dogs with von Willebrand's disease or hemophilia A. *Journal of Veterinary Internal Medicine* **12,** 84-92

(iv) Anticoagulant Rodenticides

Andrew Mackin

INTRODUCTION

Poisoning with anticoagulant rodenticides is one of the most common toxicities encountered by veterinary practitioners and is also one of the most common acquired causes of haemostatic disorders in small animal practice. Potential or actual poisonings with anticoagulant rodenticide currently account for almost 10% of the enquiries received by the Veterinary Poisons Information Service (VPIS) in London, which handles the bulk of such enquiries in the United Kingdom (A Campbell, personal communication). Anticoagulant toxicity often presents as a life-threatening emergency, with published mortality rates of between 10% and 20% despite there being a readily available and highly effective antidote, vitamin K (Green and Thomas, 1995; Robben *et al.*, 1998; Sheafor and Couto, 1999). Based on practitioner feedback, the VPIS estimates that in the United Kingdom current mortality rates from poisoning with anticoagulant are at least 5% (A Campbell, personal communication). Mortality rates are probably high for two reasons: because it can be difficult to obtain a prompt diagnosis and because treatment with vitamin K is often of inadequate dosage and duration (Mount, 1988). This chapter describes the relevant pathophysiological features of poisoning with anticoagulant rodenticide and presents a logical diagnostic and therapeutic approach for practitioners.

ROLE OF VITAMIN K IN HAEMOSTASIS

Four of the major coagulation proteins, factors II (prothrombin), VII, IX and X, depend on vitamin K for functional clotting activity (Mount *et al.*, 1986), as do several proteins with anticoagulant activity, namely proteins C and S (Green and Thomas, 1995). This group of vitamin K-dependent coagulant and anticoagulant proteins are known as the prothrombin complex. Like most other clotting factors, the proteins in the prothrombin complex are manufactured by the liver. The proteins are manufactured by hepatocytes in an inactive precursor form and to become functional must contain the amino acid glutamic acid in its carboxylated form (γ-carboxyglutamic acid). Carboxylation of glutamic acid in the proteins of the prothrombin complex requires the presence of vitamin K. In the absence of vitamin K, these proteins are only present in non-functional forms (Mount and Feldman, 1982).

Vitamin K-dependent clotting factors are important components of the clotting cascade: factor IX in the intrinsic pathway, factor VII in the extrinsic pathway and factors II and X in the common pathway of secondary haemostasis (Figure 14.28). Functional deficiency of any one of these clotting factors leads to significant impairment of secondary haemostasis, whereas deficiency of all four factors, with a combined effect on all of the major coagulation pathways, is likely to be clinically catastrophic.

In the normal animal, vitamin K (a fat-soluble vitamin) is obtained from both dietary sources and bacterial synthesis within the gut lumen, typically in a quinone form, and is absorbed in the small intestine together with ingested fatty acids (Mount and Feldman, 1982; Green and Thomas, 1995). The vitamin is then stored in various forms within hepatocytes. Only one form, the hydroquinone form of vitamin K, is involved in the carboxylation of the non-functional precursors of factors II, VII, IX and X into their active forms. As part of this carboxylation process, the active hydroquinone form of the vitamin is converted into an inactive epoxide form (Figure 14.29). Since the normal intestinal uptake of vitamin K is insufficient to meet the ongoing demand generated by activation of clotting factors, the animal must continuously enzymatically regenerate the active hydroquinone form of vitamin K from its various inactive forms to maintain adequate concentrations of the functional vitamin. The inactive epoxide form of vitamin K is converted via an epoxide reductase reaction into a quinone form, and a subsequent reductase reaction converts the various inactive quinone forms of the vitamin (those derived from both reduction of epoxides and dietary and bacterial origins) into the active hydroquinone form. A breakdown in any of the above enzymatic reactions (collectively known as the vitamin K-enzyme complex) rapidly leads to a deficiency in the functional hydroquinone form of vitamin K, which in turn leads

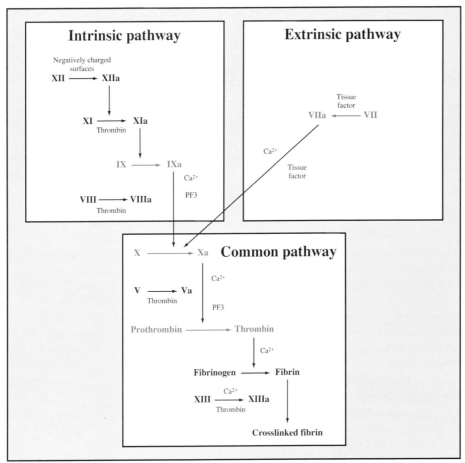

Figure 14.28: *The vitamin K-dependent clotting factors, II (prothrombin), VII, IX and X, are involved in all the major pathways of secondary haemostasis: the intrinsic pathway (IX), the extrinsic pathway (VII), and the common pathway (II and X).*

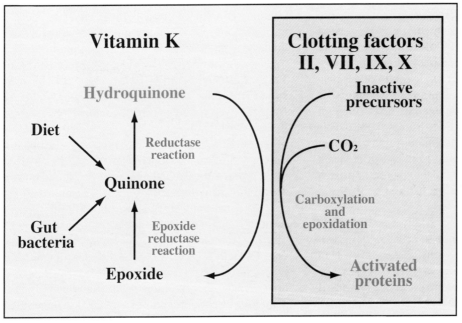

Figure 14.29: *The active hydroquinone form of vitamin K is required for the carboxylation and epoxidation process that forms functional factors II, VII, IX and X from their inactive precursor proteins. As part of this process for activation of clotting factors, the hydroquinone is converted into the inactive epoxide form of vitamin K, and the active form must then be regenerated by a complex series of enzymatic reductions. Anticoagulant rodenticides act predominantly by inhibiting the epoxide reductase reaction.*

to a deficiency in the active forms of the vitamin K-dependent clotting factors (Mount and Feldman, 1982). By contrast, if the vitamin K-enzyme complex is intact, reduced dietary intake of vitamin K is unlikely to lead to impaired haemostasis in the normal animal, since intestinal bacterial synthesis of the vitamin is sufficient to replenish body stores.

INHIBITION OF THE VITAMIN K-ENZYME COMPLEX

Anticoagulant rodenticides inhibit the enzymatic process that regenerates the active hydroquinone form of vitamin K, predominantly via inhibition of the epoxide reductase reaction (Mount and Feldman, 1982).

Severe and complete enzyme inhibition can lead to a deficiency in active vitamin K in less than 24 hours, after which the inactive precursors of vitamin K-dependent clotting factors are unable to be converted into their functional forms. Defective secondary haemostasis and susceptibility to bleeding occur as soon as pre-existing circulating amounts of these factors are consumed (Schulman *et al.*, 1986). Since the circulating half-lives of factors VII, IX, X and II in the dog are about 6, 14, 16 and 40 hours respectively, impaired secondary haemostasis can potentially occur as soon as one day after ingestion of an anticoagulant rodenticide, depending on the type and potency of the ingested toxin (Forbes *et al.*, 1973; Mount *et al.*, 1986; Schulman *et al.*, 1986).

Inhibition of the vitamin K-enzyme complex is not the only means by which vitamin K deficiency can lead to bleeding disorders. Since vitamin K is fat soluble and taken up by the small intestine concurrently with fatty acids, conditions that cause maldigestion and/or malabsorption of dietary fat can also cause vitamin K deficiency. Potential causes of poor intestinal absorption of vitamin K include severe infiltrative bowel disease, lymphangiectasia, exocrine pancreatic insufficiency and biliary obstruction (since bile acids are an essential component of micelle formation, which facilitates intestinal absorption of lipid) (Mount and Feldman, 1982; Mount, 1986; Hammer and Couto, 1991; Green and Thomas, 1995). Prolonged antibiotic therapy, particularly with second and third generation cephalosporins, has also been reported to lead to mild vitamin K deficiency secondary to reduced synthesis of the vitamin by intestinal bacteria (Mount and Feldman, 1982; Hammer and Couto, 1991; Green and Thomas, 1995). Unlike inhibition of the vitamin K-enzyme complex, decreased bacterial synthesis or impaired intestinal absorption of vitamin K is unlikely to lead to acute haemostatic defects since hepatocytes have some stores of vitamin K in its inactive forms.

ANTICOAGULANT RODENTICIDES

The original anticoagulant rodenticides, which were first commercially developed in the 1940s, are known as first generation rodenticides. First generation rodenticides are further divided into the hydroxycoumarin group, of which warfarin is the best known example, and the indandione group, which includes diphacinone. Over the years, as the rodent population developed resistance to the original rodenticides, newer forms of the hydroxycoumarins were created, which bypassed the rodents' mechanisms of resistance. These newer anticoagulants are known as second generation rodenticides and include products such as brodifacoum (Figure 14.30), difenacoum and bromadiolone (Mount and Feldman, 1982; Green and Thomas, 1995). Figure 14.31 sum-

marizes the rodenticides that belong to each of these major groups (Beasley and Buck, 1983; Mount *et al.*, 1986; Mount, 1988; Dorman, 1990). Experimental studies and extensive clinical experience have shown that anticoagulant rodenticides are highly poisonous and frequently fatal when ingested by dogs and cats at doses that can be easily attained at home (Forbes *et al.*, 1973; Schulman *et al.*, 1986; Woody *et al.*, 1992; Berry *et al.*, 1993; Lewis *et al.*, 1997). Many more poisonings have been reported in dogs than in cats, and recent data from the London VPIS show about 10 veterinary enquires regarding potential anticoagulant rodenticide toxicities in dogs for every one enquiry in cats (A Campbell, personal communication).

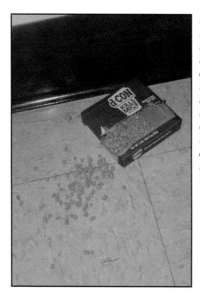

Figure 14.30: Brodifacoum rodenticide bait trays are torn open and placed in locations accessible to rodents. Almost half of the contents of this bait tray (far in excess of a lethal dose) was ingested by a young Pomeranian.

First generation hydroxycoumarins
Warfarin*
Dicoumarin*
Coumafuryl (Fumarin)
Coumatetralyl*
First generation indanediones
Diphacinone* (Diphenacin)
Chlorphacinone*
Pindone
Valone
Second generation hydroxycoumarins
Brodifacoum*
Bromadiolone*
Difenacoum*
Miscellaneous
Sulphaquinoxaline

Figure 14.31: Common anticoagulant rodenticides. *Enquiries for dog and cat exposures made to the Veterinary Poisons Information Service (London) between 1994 and 1996 (A Campbell, personal communication). The most commonly encountered rodenticides were bromadiolone and difenacoum, followed by, in descending order of frequency, coumatetralyl, chlorphacinone, warfarin, brodifacoum, diphacinone and dicoumarin.*

First generation rodenticides, particularly those in the hydroxycoumarin group, are generally less potent than second generation rodenticides. Multiple ingestions of first generation rodenticides over a period of time are usually considered necessary to cause a coagulopathy, although a single exposure to a massive dose (e.g. ingestion of the contents of a full container of toxin) may be enough to cause bleeding, especially if the toxin is an indandione. Clinical signs of toxicity are unlikely to develop until at least 4–5 days after ingestion of a first generation hydroxycoumarin (Forbes *et al.*, 1973), although bleeding may occur as little as one day after massive exposure to some members of the indandione group (Mount *et al.*, 1986). Secondary poisoning from ingestion of poisoned rodents is unlikely to occur with the less potent first generation rodenticides. Warfarin, the prototype first generation hydroxycoumarin, has a half-life of a little over 12 hours and, once exposure is discontinued, toxicity is unlikely to persist for more than a week (Mount *et al.*, 1986). By contrast, the indanediones generally have a half-life of 4–5 days, and toxicity may therefore potentially persist for over a month after ingestion of the poison (Mount *et al.*, 1986; Schulman *et al.*, 1986; Mount and Kass, 1989).

Second generation hydroxycoumarins such as brodifacoum are, in contrast to their first generation cousins, highly potent. A single dose of brodifacoum can cause bleeding within a day of ingestion, and the toxin can persist in an animal's system for up to a month (Mount *et al.*, 1986; Woody *et al.*, 1992). Secondary poisoning is feasible (Mount, 1988). Over the past 10 years the use of second generation rodenticides has grown noticeably, and reported poisonings of dogs and cats have correspondingly increased (Woody *et al.*, 1992; Berry *et al.*, 1993; Peterson and Streeter, 1996; Lewis *et al.*, 1997). Currently, most of the calls received by the London VPIS are enquiries about poisoning with second generation rodenticides (A Campbell, personal communication).

Sulphaquinoxaline, a coccidiostatic sulphonamide used in the poultry industry, caused a serious coagulopathy in several dogs that ingested treated drinking water (Neer and Savant, 1992). Like the anticoagulant rodenticides, sulphaquinoxaline is a potent inhibitor of the vitamin K epoxide reductase enzyme. The toxic effects of sulphaquinoxaline persist for less than a week after ingestion. Because of its anticoagulant properties, sulphaquinoxaline has been incorporated into several rodenticides (Mount *et al.*, 1986).

The potent anticoagulant properties of the inhibitors of the vitamin K-enzyme complex are not necessarily undesirable in some clinical circumstances. Numerous hydroxycoumarins and indanediones are used as anticoagulants in human medicine, and in veterinary medicine the carefully controlled and monitored use of warfarin in cats and dogs has been recommended for the prevention and treatment of thrombotic conditions such as aortic or pulmonary thromboembolism (Beasley and Buck, 1983).

CLINICAL SIGNS OF ANTICOAGULANT RODENTICIDE TOXICITY

The clinical signs of poisoning with anticoagulant rodenticides are typical of those associated with defective secondary haemostasis (see Chapter 13). Poisoned animals typically present with acute episodes of major haemorrhage into body cavities (Mount *et al.*, 1986). Commonly reported sites of major haemorrhage include the pleural cavity (Figure 14.32), the mediastinum, the pericardium, the abdominal cavity (Figure 14.33) and the joints (Forbes *et al.*, 1973; Schulman *et al.*, 1986; Berry *et al.*, 1993; Lewis *et al.*, 1997; Petrus and Henik, 1999). Patients are often in hypovolaemic shock secondary to acute blood loss and, if they survive the initial episode of haemorrhage, will develop a typical blood loss anaemia (Sheafor and Couto, 1999; see Chapter 3). Acute severe dyspnoea secondary to haemothorax, haemomediastinum and pulmonary parenchymal haemorrhage is common (Mount *et al.*, 1986; Berry *et al.*, 1993; Lewis *et al.*, 1997; Sheafor and Couto, 1999). The development of large subcutaneous or intramuscular haematomas is often reported, either spontaneously or secondary to such simple procedures as the collection of blood samples and intramuscular injections (Mount *et al.*, 1986; Schulman *et al.*, 1986; Woody *et al.*, 1992; Peterson and Streeter, 1996; Sheafor and Couto, 1999). Frequently, there may also be clinical signs of haemorrhage into the gastrointestinal, respiratory and genitourinary tracts, including oral bleeding, haematemesis, melaena, haemoptysis, epistaxis, haematuria and vaginal or preputial bleeding (Berry *et al.*, 1993; Padgett *et al.*, 1998; Sheafor and Couto, 1999). Cutaneous bruising and ocular haemorrhage (conjunctival and scleral bruising, hyphaema) may be observed. Clinical signs can frequently be diagnostically challenging. Patients often present either with no external signs of haemorrhage despite having either acute life-threatening dys-

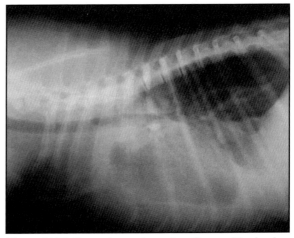

Figure 14.32: *Severe haemothorax in a German Shepherd Dog that ingested brodifacoum several days earlier.*

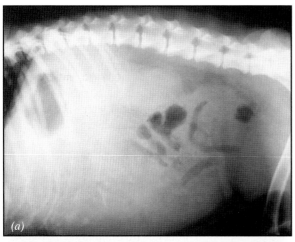

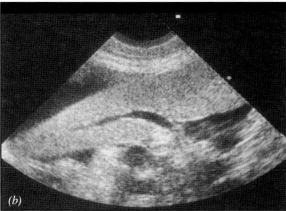

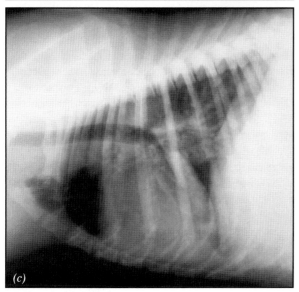

Figure 14.33: *Diagnostic images from a crossbred dog that was a housemate to the German Shepherd Dog with haemothorax shown in Figure 14.32. The crossbreed had also had access to brodifacoum and presented with acute hypovolaemic shock several days after the German Shepherd Dog was diagnosed and treated. (a) Abdominal radiographs showed noticeable abdominal fluid distension with a loss of normal radiographic detail. (b) Abdominal ultrasonography confirmed that the organs were surrounded by a large amount of free abdominal fluid, which was presumed to be blood. (c) Thoracic radiographs showed only mild pleural and pulmonary parenchymal haemorrhage. Final diagnosis was profound haemoperitoneum and mild pleural and pulmonary haemorrhage secondary to brodifacoum poisoning.*

pnoea or hypovolaemic shock, or with unexpected manifestations that reflect a hidden site of haemorrhage, such as coughing (pulmonary, mediastinal, tracheal or laryngeal haemorrhage), lameness (bleeding into joints or muscles) or neurological abnormalities (haemorrhage in the central nervous system) (Peterson and Streeter, 1996).

An understanding of the pathophysiological mechanisms underlying poisoning with anticoagulant rodenticides would suggest that primary haemostasis should be intact, and therefore that petechial (pin point) mucosal and cutaneous haemorrhages should be unexpected findings. Indeed, although several review papers have stated that rodenticide poisoning could cause petechial haemorrhages (Mount *et al.*, 1986), this type of bleeding was not reported in several clinical papers (Schulman *et al.*, 1986; Berry *et al.*, 1993; Lewis *et al.*, 1997; Sheafor and Couto, 1999). Interestingly, however, several recent clinical papers have reported that a majority of dogs who presented with poisoning with anticoagulant rodenticides had transient mild to marked thrombocytopenia of undetermined aetiology, although no patients exhibited petechial haemorrhages (Berry *et al.*, 1993; Lewis *et al.*, 1997; Sheafor and Couto, 1999).

Clinicians should always remember that, even in patients with severely impaired haemostasis secondary to rodenticide poisoning, spontaneous bleeding may not as yet have occurred (Mount *et al.*, 1986). Toxicological trials have observed that despite having noticeably prolonged clotting times, some experimental dogs displayed minimal bleeding, probably because they had been cage rested (Mount and Kass, 1989; Woody *et al.*, 1992). Even the first bleeding episode in a patient with defective secondary haemostasis can be severe, acute and potentially fatal, therefore apparently healthy animals with suspected or proved ingestion of anticoagulants should always be regarded at risk until diagnostic testing determines the status of their coagulation cascade (Mount, 1988; Hammer and Couto, 1991).

DIAGNOSIS

In those patients that have known access to anticoagulant rodenticides and that present with the clinical signs classically associated with advanced coagulopathies (e.g. haematoma formation, haemothorax, haemoperitoneum), establishing a diagnosis is usually straightforward. Poisoned animals that do not immediately succumb to hypovolaemic shock develop typical acute blood loss anaemia and hypoproteinaemia within a day of commencing bleeding. The anaemia becomes regenerative (characterized by anisocytosis, polychromasia and reticulocytosis) about 5 days later (Mount *et al.*, 1986; Berry *et al.*, 1993). Even if external haemorrhage is not evident, careful history taking and physical examination usually enables localization of sites of internal bleeding. Dyspnoea due to bleeding into the spaces and structures within the thoracic cavity is particularly common. Thoracic radiographs frequently show abnormalities such as pleural effusion due to haemothorax, an increase in mediastinal soft tissue opacity due to haemomediastinum, patchy generalized mixed alveolar/interstitial opacities caused by pulmonary parenchymal haemorrhage and narrowing of the tracheal lumen due to extratracheal and intratracheal bleeding (Berry *et al.*, 1993; Sheafor and Couto, 1999). Abdominal radiographs may show abdominal distension and loss of soft tissue detail due to haemoperitoneum (Sheafor and Couto, 1999). Additional diagnostic tests that may be needed to confirm and localize internal bleeding include abdominal, thoracic and cardiac ultrasonography and aspiration of fluid from suspected haematomas, swollen joints and the pleural, pericardial and/or abdominal spaces. Clinicians should, however, be aware that the aspiration of blood from a body cavity that fails to clot should never be considered proof of a coagulopathy. In patients with normal haemostasis with an episode of internal haemorrhage (post traumatic, for example), blood that has remained within a body cavity for a significant time will have clotted and the resultant clot will have been dissolved by the fibrinolytic system. Since most of the platelets and clotting factors within the cavity will have been consumed by this process, blood collected by paracentesis will fail to clot.

Animals that have ingested toxic amounts of anticoagulant rodenticide can often seem to be clinically normal for several days before bleeding commences. Prompt and specific diagnostic evaluation of the clotting cascade is always indicated in any dog or cat that may have ingested an anticoagulant, including the apparently healthy companions of animals that are already showing clinical signs of toxicity. Evaluation of haemostasis is similarly indicated in those animals that present with clinical signs consistent with rodenticide poisoning, even if the owners cannot readily identify a source of the toxin.

Standard screening tests of secondary haemostasis (see Chapter 10) that should be performed in all patients with possible poisoning with anticoagulant rodenticides include the activated clotting time (ACT), which can be performed simply and rapidly in house, the activated partial thromboplastin time (APTT) and the one-stage prothrombin time (OSPT). Since the vitamin K-dependent clotting factors are involved in all of the major coagulation pathways, severe rodenticide poisoning usually causes prolongation of the OSPT (which tests the extrinsic and common pathways) and the ACT and APTT (which test the intrinsic and common pathways) (Schulman *et al.*, 1986; Berry *et al.*, 1993; Lewis *et al.*, 1997). Factor VII is the vitamin K-dependent clotting factor with the shortest

circulating half-life and, since factor VII is a component of the extrinsic pathway, the OSPT may become prolonged before the ACT and APTT in early or mild cases of toxicity (Mount *et al.*, 1986; Mount and Kass, 1989; Woody *et al.*, 1992). In most patients with obvious toxicity, however, all three tests of coagulation will be noticeably prolonged.

Combined prolongation of the OSPT, ACT and APTT is not unique to poisoning with anticoagulant rodenticides. It can occur in other conditions that cause vitamin K deficiency (e.g. biliary obstruction, severe intestinal malabsorption) and in processes that lead to either a failure of production of multiple clotting factors (severe liver failure) or a generalized accelerated consumption of factors (disseminated intravascular coagulation). Far less frequently, a combined prolongation of the coagulation tests occurs due to congenital deficiencies of either a single clotting factor within the common pathway or multiple factors within both the intrinsic and extrinsic pathways, or due to the presence of a circulating inhibitor of coagulation such as heparin. Isolated prolongation of the OSPT alone is highly suggestive of early or mild poisoning with anticoagulant rodenticides, although a congenital deficiency of factor VII (a condition that is rare and often subclinical) could cause the same haemostatic abnormality. Most of the conditions that can mimic the haemostatic abnormalities caused by the anticoagulant rodenticides can be excluded by thorough history taking, physical examination and simple diagnostic tests including haematology, serum biochemistry, thoracic and abdominal radiography and, if indicated, liver function tests. A more complete haematological and haemostatic profile should enable identification of disseminated intravascular coagulation (see Chapter 14v), which often causes microangiopathic haemolytic anaemia (recognized as schistocytes on a blood smear), thrombocytopenia, hypofibrinogenaemia and increased concentrations of fibrin degradation products. Clinicians should remember, however, that rodenticides can themselves cause thrombocytopenia, due to unknown causes.

Response to treatment with vitamin K should differentiate coagulopathies due to a deficiency of functional vitamin K from other disorders of haemostasis (Forbes *et al.*, 1973; Mount *et al.*, 1986). Poisoning with anticoagulant rodenticides responds to the appropriate oral or parenteral doses of vitamin K, whereas vitamin K deficiency caused by poor intestinal absorption of the vitamin may only respond well to drugs given parenterally. Samples for evaluation of haemostasis should always be collected before commencement of treatment, and treatment can then be started before the results are obtained. An ACT, which is almost invariably prolonged in animals actively bleeding from rodenticide poisoning, can always be performed rapidly in practice and treatment commenced before laboratory evaluation of OSPT and APTT.

More specialized tests can establish a specific diagnosis of poisoning with anticoagulant rodenticide even if a source of the toxin can not be identified. In situations of vitamin K deficiency of any cause, the non-functional vitamin K-dependent clotting factors build up in hepatocytes and 'spill over' into the circulation. These non-functional factors are known as PIVKA or proteins induced by vitamin K absence, and are only detectable in the serum of patients with vitamin K deficiency. Measurement of PIVKA may be available in some specialist centres, and the assay is considered to be even more sensitive than the OSPT for detecting early poisonings (Mount, 1986). Alternatively, researchers have shown that once vitamin K is given to an animal with anticoagulant rodenticide toxicity, large amounts of the epoxide form of vitamin K are produced in the hepatocytes as the active hydroquinone form of the vitamin is used to regenerate essential functional clotting factors. The epoxide then 'spills over' into the circulation as the ongoing inhibition of the vitamin K epoxide reductase enzyme by the toxin prevents metabolism of this inactive form of vitamin K (Mount and Kass, 1989). A surge in serum concentrations of vitamin K epoxide 4 to 8 hours after the administration of vitamin K therefore specifically confirms a diagnosis of poisoning with anticoagulant rodenticide. To date, however, measurement of vitamin K epoxide has only been available as a research tool. Finally, specialist toxicology laboratories may on request assay to detect the presence of specific anticoagulants in stomach contents, unclotted blood, urine or tissues such as the liver or kidney (Beasley and Buck, 1983; Mount *et al.*, 1986; Mount, 1988; Dorman, 1990; Poppenga and Braselton, 1990; Woody *et al.*, 1992; Green and Thomas, 1995; Peterson and Streeter, 1996; Robben *et al.*, 1998).

TREATMENT

Vitamin K

Since vitamin K is a specific and highly effective antidote for inhibitors of the vitamin K-enzyme complex, administration of vitamin K is the mainstay of treatment of poisoning with anticoagulant rodenticides. Coagulation parameters return to normal within one or at most two days of the commencement of appropriate doses of vitamin K (Hammer and Couto, 1991; Woody *et al.*, 1992) and remain within normal limits provided that the vitamin is given for as long as the toxin is within the patient's system. Since the first generation hydroxycoumarins such as warfarin have a half-life of less than a day and are therefore rapidly cleared from the body, treatment for more than a week is rarely necessary. By contrast, animals poisoned with the more potent and longer-acting indanediones and second generation hydroxycoumarins may require treatment for many weeks.

Vitamin K_1 (phytonadione, phylloquinone or phytomenadione) is the formulation of choice for treating anticoagulant poisoning (Beasley and Buck, 1983; Mount *et al.*, 1986; Hammer and Couto, 1991). Vitamin K_3 (menadione or menophthone), although much cheaper than vitamin K_1 is also much less effective and should therefore never be used as a substitute for vitamin K_1 (Beasley and Buck, 1983; Mount and Feldman, 1982; Schulman *et al.*, 1986; Hammer and Couto, 1991). Treatment of severely affected patients usually commences with the parenteral (subcutaneous) administration of vitamin K_1, which is then switched to oral therapy as they recover (Mount and Feldman, 1982). Vitamin K_1 should never be given intravenously as this route can cause an anaphylactic reaction (Mount and Feldman, 1982; Schulman *et al.*, 1986). Even in life-threatening emergencies, intravenous administration of the vitamin does not significantly hasten recovery as the animal still needs time to regenerate functional clotting factors. Although intramuscular administration of vitamin K is recommended by some clinicians, it is associated with an increased risk of haematoma formation (Hammer and Couto, 1991). Although most clinicians switch to oral vitamin K_1 within a day or two of commencing treatment, subcutaneous therapy can be continued if the oral form of the vitamin is not readily available or if there are concerns regarding the efficacy of intestinal absorption of vitamin K (infiltrative bowel disease or biliary obstruction, for example) (Mount, 1988; Hammer and Couto, 1991). Oral vitamin K is best given with a fatty meal to facilitate intestinal uptake (Hammer and Couto, 1991).

The standard vitamin K_1 dosage recommended for the treatment of poisoning with first generation hydroxycoumarin rodenticides is a loading dose of 5 mg/kg s.c. (often given at multiple sites) followed 12 hours later by an ongoing maintenance regimen of 2.5 mg/kg s.c. or orally given as a twice daily divided dose for one week (Mount *et al.*, 1986; Hammer and Couto, 1991). The same dosing regimen is recommended for animals exposed to the indanediones or second generation hydroxycoumarins, but the maintenance regimen is continued for 2 to 3 weeks and an OSPT is re-evaluated 2 days after therapy is discontinued (Mount *et al.*, 1986; Hammer and Couto, 1991). Maintenance therapy is continued for two further weeks if the OSPT is still prolonged (Hammer and Couto, 1991). Monitoring of therapeutic response by measurement of an ACT, which can be cheaply performed in house, is less desirable because the test is less sensitive than the OSPT to early relapses of haemostatic dysfunction (Mount *et al.*, 1986). The ACT must therefore be performed at least 4 days after discontinuing vitamin K (Mount, 1988).

Vitamin K therapy of too inadequate a dosage or duration to treat the more potent forms of anticoagulant rodenticide effectively is a major cause of unexpected morbidities and mortalities. For this reason, some clinicians recommend that, if cost is not a major issue and owner compliance cannot be absolutely guaranteed, a 'double dose' maintenance regimen of vitamin K_1 (5 mg/kg split twice daily) should be given to those patients poisoned by the more potent rodenticides (Mount and Feldman, 1982; Robben *et al.*, 1998). One experimental study, however, has shown that although this higher dose is well tolerated in most dogs, individual animals may develop a Heinz body haemolytic anaemia (Fernandez *et al.*, 1984). Whenever owners do not wish to repeat test haemostasis to monitor response to therapy, vitamin K_1 should be given for at least 3 weeks, and the animal should then be strictly rested for a further week after treatment is discontinued (Mount *et al.*, 1986). Patients should be treated for suspected poisoning with a potent anticoagulant if the source of the toxin cannot be identified.

Transfusion

However promptly vitamin K therapy is commenced in a patient poisoned with anticoagulant rodenticide, functional clotting factors may not be generated for one or even two days (Schulman *et al.*, 1986; Hammer and Couto, 1991; Peterson and Streeter, 1996). Severely affected patients can therefore rapidly succumb to life-threatening haemorrhage despite receiving vitamin K. In these patients, functional clotting factors must be provided by transfusion to ensure survival over the first day of treatment with vitamin K. Compared with many of the other clotting factors, the vitamin K-dependent factors are relatively stable with storage. They are still viable in plasma extracted from refrigerated whole blood stored under standard conditions for at least a month (Stone and Cotter, 1992; see Chapter 15). Missing clotting factors and red blood cells may therefore be provided by either fresh or stored whole blood if patients present with hypovolaemic shock or acute blood loss anaemia, and vitamin K-dependent factors alone may be provided by any of the standard plasma products (fresh, stored, frozen or fresh frozen plasma) if the patient does not require concurrent red cells (Mount and Feldman, 1982; Schulman *et al.*, 1986; Hammer and Couto, 1991).

Other

Induction of emesis or gastric lavage to remove gastric contents may prevent toxicity in animals with recent suspected or confirmed ingestion of rodenticides (Mount *et al.*, 1986; Schulman *et al.*, 1986; Hammer and Couto, 1991). These are, however, of little use and may in fact precipitate gastrointestinal bleeding once the toxin has caused impairment of haemostasis. Haemostatic function in animals with possible exposure to toxin should be regularly monitored, either by measurement of an ACT or, preferably, an OSPT, for at least one week after suspected exposure, and vitamin K therapy commenced if defects are detected.

In patients with confirmed anticoagulant toxicity, haemorrhage can be minimized by strict cage rest and avoidance of unnecessary venepuncture, catheterization, surgery and other potentially traumatic procedures until vitamin K (with or without transfusion) corrects haemostatic defects. Patients with acute hypovolaemic shock may require intravenous isotonic crystalloids, hypertonic saline, bovine polymerized haemoglobin or whole blood, whereas dyspnoeic animals may need oxygen supplementation (Mount *et al.*, 1986; Green and Thomas, 1995). Therapeutic thoracocentesis is indicated in animals with severe dyspnoea due to haemothorax, and pericardiocentesis is indicated in patients with cardiac tamponade due to haemopericardium (Mount *et al.*, 1986; Schulman *et al.*, 1986; Hammer and Couto, 1991; Petrus and Henik, 1999). Aspiration of blood from body cavities should, however, be avoided unless absolutely necessary, because of the associated risk of traumatically precipitating further haemorrhage (Mount *et al.*, 1986; Schulman *et al.*, 1986; Green and Thomas, 1995). Aspirated blood can be used for emergency autotransfusion in animals with acute severe blood loss (Figure 14.34). It should be remembered, however, that the autotransfused blood will not provide functional vitamin K-dependent clotting factors. Autotransfusions should always be provided through an in-line filter to remove microthrombi (Green and Thomas, 1995).

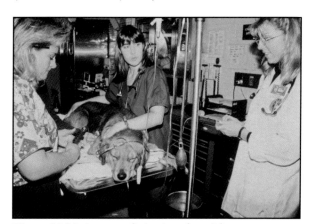

Figure 14.34: Autotransfusion in a dog with severe haemothorax secondary to poisoning with anticoagulant rodenticide. Blood is being aspirated from the thoracic cavity and collected into multiple large syringes. The contents of the syringes are then given intravenously into the same patient through an in-line filter. No anticoagulant is needed for this process.

PROGNOSIS

Provided that patients do not present in extremis or that bleeding has not occurred in a location that could cause irreversible damage (the central nervous system, for example), poisoning with anticoagulant rodenticides should be a readily treatable condition. The unacceptably high mortality rates associated with this poisoning probably reflect delays in obtaining a correct diagnosis and failure to treat the condition aggressively enough. Practitioners should therefore be aware of the typical clinical signs of defective secondary haemostasis and the diagnostic tests that are indicated in affected patients. They should also be prepared to treat acute emergencies with blood products as well as vitamin K_1 and, in animals exposed to second generation rodenticides, to provide the vitamin for extended periods.

REFERENCES

Beasley VR and Buck WB (1983) Warfarin and other anticoagulant poisonings. In: *Current Veterinary Therapy VIII: Small Animal Practice,* ed. RW Kirk, pp. 101-106. WB Saunders, Philadelphia

Berry CR, Gallaway A, Thrall DE and Carlisle C (1993) Thoracic radiographic features of anticoagulant rodenticide toxicity in fourteen dogs. *Veterinary Radiology and Ultrasound* **34**, 391-396

Dorman DC (1990) Anticoagulant, cholecalciferol and bromethalin-based rodenticides. *Veterinary Clinics of North America: Small Animal Practice* **20**, 339-352

Fernandez FR, Davies AP, Teachout DJ, Krake A, Christopher MM and Perman V (1984) Vitamin K-induced Heinz body formation in dogs. *Journal of the American Animal Hospital Association* **20**, 711-720

Forbes CD, Thomson C, Prentice CRM, McNicol GP and McEwan AD (1973) Experimental warfarin poisoning in the dog. *Journal of Comparative Pathology* **83**, 173-180

Green RA and Thomas JS (1995) Hemostatic disorders: coagulopathies and thrombosis. In: *Textbook of Veterinary Internal Medicine, 4th edn,* ed. SJ Ettinger and EC Feldman, pp. 1946-1963. WB Saunders, Philadelphia

Hammer AS and Couto CG (1991) Disorders of hemostasis and principles of transfusion therapy. In: *Small Animal Medicine,* ed. DG Allen, pp. 173-194. JB Lippincott, Philadelphia

Lewis DC, Bruyette DS, Kellerman DL and Smith SA (1997) Thrombocytopenia in dogs with anticoagulant rodenticide-induced hemorrhage: eight cases (1990-1995). *Journal of the American Animal Hospital Association* **33**, 417-422

Mount ME (1986) Proteins induced by vitamin K absence or antagonists ('PIVKA'). In: *Current Veterinary Therapy IX: Small Animal Practice,* ed. RW Kirk, pp. 513-515. WB Saunders, Philadelphia

Mount ME (1988) Diagnosis and therapy of anticoagulant rodenticide intoxication. *Veterinary Clinics of North America: Small Animal Practice* **18**, 115-130

Mount ME and Feldman BF (1982) Vitamin K and its therapeutic importance. *Journal of the American Veterinary Medical Association* **180**, 1354-1356

Mount ME and Kass PH (1989) Diagnostic importance of vitamin K_1 and its epoxide measured in serum of dogs exposed to an anticoagulant rodenticide. *American Journal of Veterinary Research* **50**, 1704-1709

Mount ME, Woody BJ and Murphy MJ (1986) The anticoagulant rodenticides. In: *Current Veterinary Therapy IX: Small Animal Practice,* ed. RW Kirk, pp. 156-165. WB Saunders, Philadelphia

Neer TM and Savant RL (1992) Hypoprothrombinemia secondary to administration of sulfaquinoxaline to dogs in a kennel setting. *Journal of the American Veterinary Medical Association* **200**, 1344-1345

Padgett SL, Stokes JE, Tucker RL and Wheaton LG (1998) Hematometra secondary to anticoagulant rodenticide toxicity. *Journal of the American Animal Hospital Association* **34**, 437-439

Peterson J and Streeter V (1996) Laryngeal obstruction secondary to brodifacoum toxicosis in a dog. *Journal of the American Veterinary Medical Association* **208**, 352-355

Petrus DJ and Henik RA (1999) Pericardial effusion and cardiac tamponade secondary to brodifacoum toxicosis in a dog. *Journal of the American Veterinary Medical Association* **215**, 647-648

Poppenga RH and Braselton WE (1990) Effective use of analytical laboratories for the diagnosis of toxicological problems in small animal practice. *Veterinary Clinics of North America: Small Animal Practice* **20**, 293-306

Robben JH, Kuijpers EAP and Mout HCA (1998) Plasma superwarfarin levels and vitamin K_1 treatment in dogs with anticoagulant rodenticide poisoning. *Veterinary Quarterly* **20**, 24-27

Schulman A, Lusk R, Lippincott CL and Ettinger SL (1986) Diphacinone-induced coagulopathy in the dog. *Journal of the American Veterinary Medical Association* **188**, 402-405

Sheafor SE and Couto GC (1999) Anticoagulant rodenticide toxicity in 21 dogs. *Journal of the American Animal Hospital Association* **35**, 38-46

Stone MS and Cotter SM (1992) Practical guidelines for transfusion therapy. In: *Current Veterinary Therapy XI: Small Animal Practice,* ed. RW Kirk and JD Bonagura, pp. 475-479. WB Saunders, Philadelphia

Woody BJ, Murphy MJ, Ray AC and Green RA (1992) Coagulopathic effects and therapy of brodifacoum toxicosis in dogs. *Journal of Veterinary Internal Medicine* **6**, 23-28

(v) Disseminated Intravascular Coagulation

Steven A. Holloway

INTRODUCTION

Disseminated intravascular coagulation (DIC) is a serious complicating event in the pathophysiology of many diseases. Reported death rates in fulminant DIC are high, and the diagnosis of DIC has often been regarded as forecasting the death of the patient. So much has the catastrophic nature of DIC been emphasized that DIC is often regarded as an individual disease, without proper consideration of the initiating illness. DIC should be regarded as a mechanism of disease secondary to other severe clinical disorders.

For many clinicians, DIC is a confusing disorder. Much of the confusion stems from the fact that many of the diseases causing DIC vary in severity and prognosis, the clinical signs are variable, there is a lack of consensus regarding the appropriate laboratory tests to confirm a diagnosis and there is varied opinion regarding appropriate treatment regimens. This chapter explains the pathogenesis of DIC and discusses the clinical signs related to the condition and its laboratory diagnosis and treatment.

DISSEMINATED INTRAVASCULAR COAGULATON

Definition
Bick (1994) defined DIC as a systemic thrombohaemorrhagic disorder found in association with well defined clinical situations and laboratory evidence of procoagulant activation, fibrinolytic activation and inhibitor consumption and biochemical evidence of end-stage organ damage.

Pathophysiology of DIC: blood clotting mechanism
The homeostatic mechanisms that control bleeding after blood vessel injury involve the complex interaction of the coagulation and anticoagulation systems. It is convenient to view the process of blood clotting as the generation of the powerful serine protease, thrombin (Figure 14.35). Thrombin cleaves the soluble plasma protein, fibrinogen, so that an insoluble meshwork of fibrin strands develops, enmeshing red cells and adherent platelets and forming a stable clot. The clotting mechanism is triggered by injury to blood vessels and involves the coordinated interaction of over 20 different proteins in the clotting cascade. The end result of this process is the generation of active thrombin and the formation of fibrin. Injury to the vessel wall causes platelet aggregation and provides a specialized surface that initiates and localizes the clotting mechanism. Although the arrest of bleeding after injury is initiated within a few seconds, it is not complete for several hours and is limited to the site of injury by the anticoagulation system. In the context of preventing DIC, the limitation of the clotting mechanism to the active site of injury is important. Once generated, thrombin has powerful proteolytic properties, accelerating the formation of activated clotting factors including thrombin from prothrombin and causing the aggregation of platelets. Once a critical amount of thrombin is formed, a cycle develops that causes more clotting to occur and amplification of the coagulation cascade. This process would ultimately lead to DIC if it were not for the presence of intravascular anticoagulants in the normal animal.

The anticoagulation system
The anticoagulation system represents the mechanism whereby the blood coagulation pathways are downregulated. Once activated, the extent and control of the clotting mechanism is limited by the relative local concentrations of activated coagulant and anticoagulant proteins. Anticoagulant proteins include antithrombin III (ATIII) and proteins C and S. ATIII is an α_2 globulin that binds and inactivates serine proteases, including thrombin (Figure 14.35). Complexes of ATIII and protease are then removed by the mononuclear phagocyte system (MPS). The antiprotease activity of ATIII is enhanced by heparin and heparin-like substances, and these are normally produced by perivascular mast cells. About 80% of the total anticoagulant effect of plasma comes from ATIII. Additional plasma proteins, including α_1 antitrypsin and α_2 macroglobulin, also remove activated serine proteases from the circulation.

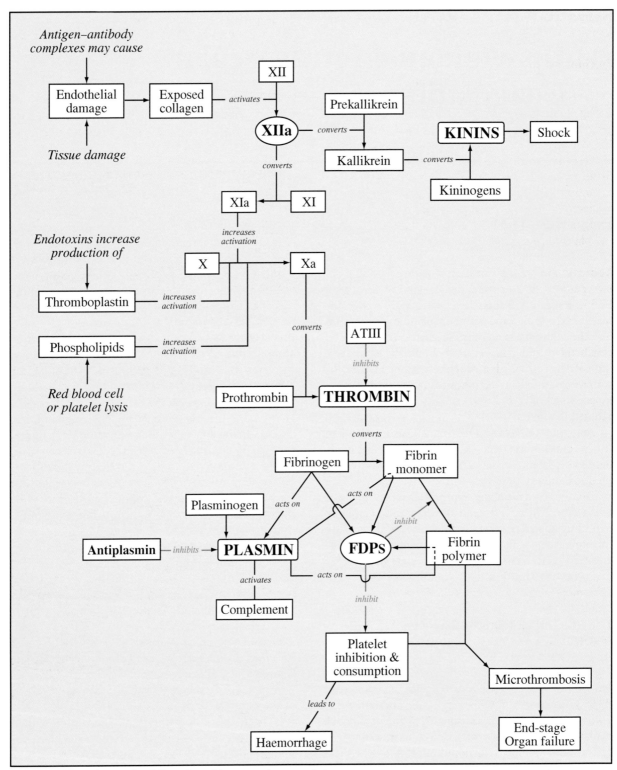

Figure 14.35: *Pathogenesis of disseminated intravascular coagulation.*
ATIII, antithrombin III; FDPs, fibrinogen degradation products; XIIa, activated factor XII.

Once thrombin is formed from prothrombin, a large amount of it is adsorbed to the newly generated fibrin strands and prevents dissemination of the clotting process. Thrombomodulin, a protein bound to the endothelium, binds thrombin. The binding of thrombomodulin with thrombin not only removes thrombin but the complex so formed activates plasma protein C, which then acts as an anticoagulant by inactivating the activated factors V and VIII. Another plasma protein, protein S, acts as a cofactor for protein C. Finally, a major limitation to the process of clotting is the removal and dilution of activated clotting factors by the microcirculatory flow of blood. The constant flow of blood past the site of activation of clotting removes activated clotting factors and facilitates the removal of inhibitor protease complexes from the circulation by the MPS.

Fibrinolysis

The final stage of the coagulation process is fibrinolysis, which is initiated by the action of thrombin during clotting, together with the release of plasminogen activators from the damaged blood vessel wall. These plasminogen activators convert plasminogen to the active form, plasmin, which then digests the fibrin clot. Plasmin protease inhibitors include α_1 antitrypsin, tissue plasmin inhibitor (TPI) and α_2 macroglobulin. These rapidly inactivate any circulating active serine proteases including thrombin and plasmin (Figure 14.35).

Activation of the coagulation system

The pathophysiology of DIC is shown in Figure 14.35. Essentially there are three processes that can initiate activation of the coagulation system: endothelial injury exposing subendothelial collagen, which then activates factor XII (Hageman factor) and subsequently activates the intrinsic clotting system; release of tissue thromboplastin from damaged tissue, which activates the extrinsic clotting system; and mechanisms involving the direct release of procoagulants into the circulation causing activation of the clotting cascade. This includes substances such as snake venoms and phospholipids from damaged red cells.

DIC occurs when the clotting mechanism becomes activated widely throughout the circulation. This widespread activation of the coagulation system consumes the essential protease inhibitors, allowing thrombin and plasmin to circulate systemically. Circulating thrombin may then generate fibrin monomers from fibrinogen and these are polymerized to form fibrin in the circulation. The deposition of fibrin in the microcirculation in turn entraps platelets and leads to vascular thrombosis, ischaemia and end-stage organ failure.

The systemic circulation of plasmin causes cleavage of fibrin into fibrinogen degradation products (FDPs). Circulating FDPs may then interfere with fibrin monomer polymerization. FDPs may also bind to platelet membranes and induce a platelet function defect that further contributes to haemorrhage (Bick, 1994). Additionally, circulating plasmin activates the complement cascade, causing red cell and platelet lysis and the release of additional procoagulant substances. Furthermore, activation of the complement system increases vascular permeability, contributing to hypotension and shock and further activation of factor XII. Activated factor XII contributes to the generation of circulating kinins (including bradykinin) and subsequently increased vascular permeability, hypotension and shock. Shock promotes microcirculatory or venous stasis, which further promotes microthrombosis by allowing the accumulation of activated clotting proteins and preventing the removal of activated clotting factors by the MPS (Slappendel, 1988; Bick, 1994).

Aetiology

DIC occurs in association with a wide variety of clinical entities. Figure 14.36 summarizes those disorders most commonly associated with DIC in small animals.

Neoplasia
Thyroid carcinoma
Mammary carcinoma
Haemangiosarcoma (see Figure 14.37)
Lymphoma
Myeloproliferative diseases
Inflammatory
Pancreatitis
Chronic active hepatitis
Haemorrhagic gastroenteritis
Severe burns
Infectious
Bacterial sepsis
Aflatoxicosis
Canine infectious hepatitis (canine adenovirus 1 infection)
Leptospirosis
Canine parvovirus infection
Feline infectious peritonitis
Canine babesiosis (*Babesia canis*)
Canine ehrlichiosis (*Ehrlichia canis*)
Rocky Mountain spotted fever (*Rickettsia* spp.)
Canine angiostrongylosis
Canine heartworm disease
Immune mediated
Immune-mediated haemolytic anaemia
Glomerulonephritis
Systemic lupus erythematosus
Other
Heat stroke
Tumour lysis syndrome
Venomous snake bite
Shock
Cardiac failure
Severe trauma

Figure 14.36: *Common clinical disorders associated with disseminated intravascular coagulation in small animals.*

Clinical signs

DIC occurs with a variety of diseases, and depending on the interplay of the processes of coagulation and fibrinolysis, clinical signs are related to haemorrhage or thrombosis (Green, 1981; Greene, 1983; Bick, 1994). Depending on the extent, severity and speed of onset of the initiating disease, DIC may have variable clinical signs ranging from an acute fulminant process to a chronic low grade process. Severe fulminant DIC is characterized by generalized bleeding from body orifices, mucosal petechiae or ecchymoses and haematuria. Additionally, organ failure frequently occurs after obstruction of the microcirculation by fibrin thrombi. In particular, acute oliguric renal failure, dyspnoea, bloody vomitus, diarrhoea and coma are frequent clinical signs in DIC. It is important for the clinician to realize that haemorrhage occurs as a late event in the pathogenesis of DIC. Severe DIC may manifest as organ failure before serious haemorrhage develops. For example, a patient with heat stroke may develop oliguric renal failure and respiratory distress resulting from microthrombosis in these organs before the onset of haemorrhage. Laboratory tests may confirm the presence of DIC before the onset of haemorrhage.

In contrast, chronic DIC may be associated with minimal clinical signs, or signs related to microcirculatory thrombosis may occur and an increasing bleeding tendency may be seen. As would be expected, chronic DIC is often noted in diseases characterized by a protracted course of tissue or endothelial damage, such as malignant metastatic or autoimmune disease (Figure 14.37). In these cases abnormal coagulation may be detected, but clinical signs may be mild or inapparent because of a compensatory increase in the production of platelets and clotting factors. In such instances low grade consumption of platelets and clotting factors may occur, predisposing to potentially disastrous bleeding complications after surgery. Similarly, after the treatment of large volume tumours with chemotherapeutic agents, the destruction of large amounts of tumour and release of procoagulants may contribute to the progression from chronic DIC to acute fulminant DIC.

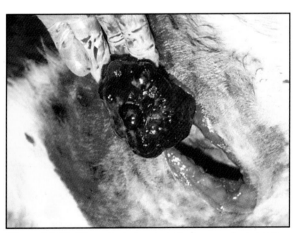

Figure 14.37: Disseminated metastatic haemangiosarcoma in the thorax of a dog with disseminated intravascular coagulation (DIC). Many animals with disseminated malignancies have laboratory evidence of subacute or chronic DIC, which may or may not be clinically manifested.

Diagnosis

A presumptive diagnosis of DIC should be considered when:

- Clinical signs of a bleeding disorder are apparent
- Clinical signs relating to multiple organ failure develop after an initial problem predisposing to DIC, for example, gastric dilation–volvulus, heat stroke, sepsis, pancreatitis, chemotherapy for neoplasia
- An initial problem predisposing to DIC exists and laboratory evidence of coagulation abnormalities are present, for example, thrombocytopenia or prolonged coagulation tests. A useful in-house screening test for detecting abnormalities in the intrinsic and common clotting pathway factors is the activated clotting time (ACT) (Figure 14.38).

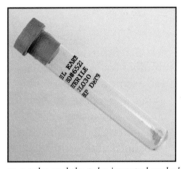

Figure 14.38:
Activated clotting test (ACT). Measurement of clotting by the ACT provides a useful in-house screening test for the presumptive diagnosis of disseminated intravascular coagulation (DIC). Whole blood is added to a tube and the tube inverted and placed in a water bath at 37°C. Every 15 seconds the tube is inverted and inspected for the presence of a clot. The time taken to clot is the ACT. Prolongation of the ACT (>120 seconds in dogs and >90 seconds in cats) should alert the clinician to the possibility of DIC.

The definitive diagnosis of DIC should include at least three of the following:

- Moderate to severe thrombocytopenia (<100,000 x 10^9 platelets/l)
- Prolongation of the activated partial thromboplastin time (APTT) and prothrombin time (PT) to greater than 25% of control pooled normal plasma
- Reduction of ATIII by 60% or less
- Increase in FDPs to greater than 1:10 dilution (Figure 14.39)
- Detection of increased concentrations of fibrin monomers.

Other supportive evidence may include:

- Hypofibrinogenaemia
- The presence of fragmented red blood cells, such as schistocytes, in blood smears (Figure 14.40)
- The presence histologically of fibrin microthrombi, particularly involving the capillary and venous circulations.

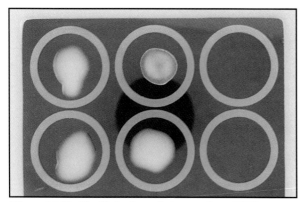

Figure 14.39: *The fibrin degradation products (FDPs or FSPs) test is a semiquantitative slide agglutination test that uses rabbit anti-human FDP antiserum. The test can be used in dogs because rabbit antiserum cross reacts with canine FDPs, but the test gives variable results in cats. The results are scored (– 4 to +4) by comparing the extent of agglutination in the patient's blood with positive control standards. The presence of increased concentrations of FDPs suggests the possibility of DIC but should be performed in conjunction with the measurement of coagulation times and a platelet count for a definitive diagnosis of DIC.*

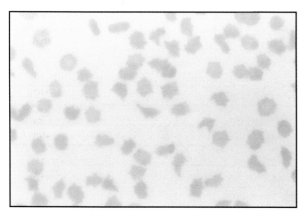

Figure 14.40: *Schistocytes in the blood smear of a dog with disseminated intravascular coagulation. Fragmentation of red cell membranes by fibrin strands in the microcirculation occurs frequently in DIC.*

The above criteria have been adapted from Feldman *et al.* (1981), Green (1981), Greene (1983) and Bick (1994).

Increases in concentrations of circulating fibrin monomers or FDPs should not by themselves be considered diagnostic of DIC. Increased concentrations of FDPs or fibrin monomers occur in a variety of other clinical situations in human medicine including pulmonary thromboembolism, haemolytic uraemic syndrome (HUS) and myocardial infarction. Similar increases in concentrations of FDPs has been seen in canine pulmonary thromboembolism and in renal disease resembling HUS in the dog (Holloway *et al.*, 1993).

Localized intravascular coagulation with platelet and fibrin thrombus formation, thrombocytopenia and coagulation factor deficiencies has been recognized in humans with giant cavernous haemangiomas, haemangiosarcomas or disseminated vascular malignancies (Kasabach–Merrit syndrome) (Bick, 1992). Similar localized consumptive coagulopathies have been documented in the dog and such animals may develop a clinical pathology profile consistent with a diagnosis of DIC (Rishniw and Lewis, 1994). It is important to realize that some dogs with skin tumours or vascular tumours of internal organs may develop a severe localized consumptive coagulopathy. In such cases the differentiation of a localized consumptive coagulopathy from DIC must be based on clinical examination and diagnostic imaging techniques.

It is important for the clinician to maintain a high index of clinical suspicion that DIC may develop secondarily in many severe medical illnesses. In many cases a presumptive diagnosis of DIC is often required for effective treatment of DIC to be instituted. This may precede all laboratory criteria being fulfilled that would allow a definitive diagnosis of DIC. On the basis of these aforementioned criteria, DIC may be divided into several categories (Figure 14.41).

Clinical signs	Laboratory findings
Acute fulminant DIC	
Unexplained haemorrhage from three unrelated body sites Severe bleeding and end-stage organ failure	Noticeably prolonged ACT, PT and PTT Increased concentration of FDPs or fibrin monomers Noticeably decreased ATIII concentration Severe thrombocytopenia Schistocytes present on blood smears
Acute DIC without evidence of haemorrhage	
Clinical signs related to end-stage organ failure apparent, including oliguria, dyspnoea, jaundice	Noticeably prolonged ACT, PT and PTT Increased concentration of FDPs or fibrin monomers Noticeably decreased ATIII concentration Severe thrombocytopenia Schistocytes present on blood smears

Figure 14.41: *Clinical staging of disseminated intravascular coagulation (DIC).* **(continued overleaf)**
ACT, activated clotting time; PT, prothrombin time; PTT, partial thromboplastin time; ATIII, antithrombin III.
Adapted from Bick (1994), Feldman et al. *(1981) and Greene (1983).*

Clinical signs	Laboratory findings
Subacute DIC	
No clinical signs of severe haemorrhage or overt end-stage organ failure but petechial haemorrhages may be evident on mucous membranes May be an increased tendency towards haemorrhage after venepuncture or trauma	Moderate to severe thrombocytopenia usually present Coagulation times (ACT, PT, PTT) may be normal, shortened or mildly prolonged FDPs or fibrin monomers may be present ATIII concentration may be normal or decreased Serial evaluation of coagulation profiles is strongly recommended
Chronic DIC	
Minimal clinical signs	Coagulation times (ACT, PT, PTT) may be normal, mildly prolonged or shortened Concentration of FDPs may be mildly increased Platelet count may be normal or increased

Figure 14.41 continued: Clinical staging of disseminated intravascular coagulation (DIC).
ACT, activated clotting time; PT, prothrombin time; PTT, partial thromboplastin time; ATIII, antithrombin III.
Adapted from Bick (1994), Feldman et al. *(1981) and Greene (1983).*

Treatment

Aggressive and prompt treatment is always required in the management of DIC. The most important principle is to remove or inhibit the initiating disease process. Removal of procoagulant stimuli significantly reduces the intravascular clotting process and improves the chances of controlling life-threatening thrombosis or haemorrhage. Factors such as hypovolaemia, hypoxaemia, endotoxaemia and acidaemia contribute to the development of DIC, and these should be treated appropriately (Figure 14.42).

Principle of treatment	Action
Aetiology specific	
	Diagnose initiating disease and establish prognosis
Improvement of microcirculatory flow	
Volume expansion	Intravenous fluid replacement as required
	Correct anaemia and hypoalbuminaemia with whole blood or plasma transfusion
	Colloidal volume expansion using Pentastarch (20 ml/kg/day)
Cardiac support	Dobutamine (5–10 µg/kg/min i.v. infusion)
	Monitor electrocardiogram for arrhythmia
Renal support (if oliguric)	Dopamine (2–5 µg/kg/min i.v. infusion) and furosemide 2–5 mg /kg i.v. Monitor fluid therapy, central venous pressure and urine output
Treatment of metabolic acidosis	Sodium bicarbonate as required
Treatment of hypoxia	Supplemental oxygen
Treatment of coagulopathy	
Fulminant and acute DIC	Whole blood or fresh frozen plasma transfusions (may need to repeat fresh frozen plasma several times to restore ATIII concentration) Heparin 50–100 IU/kg in first bag (incubate 30 minutes before transfusion) Heparin 250–500 IU/kg tid s.c. Heparin 250–500 IU/kg tid s.c. Monitor ATIII, PT, PTT if possible
Subacute DIC	Heparin 75–150 IU/kg tid s.c.
Chronic DIC	Heparin 25–150 IU/kg tid s.c.

Figure 14.42: Treatment of disseminated intravascular coagulation (DIC).
ATIII, antithrombin III; PT, prothrombin time; PTT, partial thromboplastin time.

The second principle of treating DIC is to limit the intravascular clotting process. Again, failure to remove or lessen the initiating disease will almost always be associated with the eventual failure of factor replacement or anticoagulant therapy to alleviate DIC. A logical approach to the treatment of DIC is to individualize treatment options after assessment of the severity of clinical signs and laboratory abnormalities in the patient (Figure 14.42). Foremost, the primary disease must be diagnosed and treated promptly. If treatment for the initiating disease is likely to be protracted or if the intravascular clotting process cannot be stopped by treatment of the primary disease, then the intravascular clotting process must be blunted. The clinician should bear in mind that thrombosis, and not haemorrhage, is more often the process that has a major effect on mortality in DIC. Thromboses develop in small vessels and usually manifest as progressive end-stage organ failure. In this context the use of heparin to reduce the process of intravascular coagulation is logical. Subcutaneous heparin is given to most patients with DIC, the dosage based on an assessment of the severity of the condition (Figures 14.41 and 14.42). The use of subcutaneous low dose heparin provides the advantage of ease of administration and avoids the potential complications associated with rapid increases and decreases in blood heparin concentrations associated with intravenous heparin therapy. Furthermore, clinical data from humans with DIC suggest that low dose subcutaneous heparin is more effective than larger doses of intravenous heparin (Bick, 1994).

Much of the controversy surrounding the treatment of DIC concerns the use of factor replacement and heparin anticoagulant therapy. To summarize the controversy, heparin may make bleeding worse and factor replacement may potentiate organ thrombosis and the generation of FDPs. The author believes that if fulminant DIC is present, the patient should be given factor replacement in the form of a whole blood or plasma transfusion. The use of heparin alone is likely to be minimally effective when ATIII concentrations are severely reduced. The development of haemorrhage in DIC suggests exhaustive consumption of platelets, clotting factors and the natural anticoagulants, particularly ATIII. In this situation transfusion of fresh frozen plasma or fresh blood is required to replace clotting factors and ATIII. Heparin may then be given to prevent the consumption of the administered coagulation factors and potentiate the effect of infused ATIII. Whole blood has the advantage of providing platelets, although the platelet count is unlikely to be increased by more than 10 to 30 x 10^9/l for each 500 ml of blood transfused in an average sized dog.

A potential problem associated with the use of whole blood or plasma for factor replacement is the rapid degradation of coagulation factors, particularly fibrinogen, by plasmin. The subsequent generation of FDPs may further exacerbate haemorrhage, and the formation of fibrin thrombi further compromises the microvascular circulation. In humans with DIC the administration of ATIII concentrates has proved an effective method of restoring ATIII concentrations in patients with fulminant DIC, without adding components that may potentially worsen the condition. Unfortunately, ATIII concentrates for animals are not currently available to veterinarians. Although no studies have been performed, the use of cryosupernatant may be superior in fulminant DIC at restoring ATIII without providing fibrinogen. If the patient continues to haemorrhage, repeated plasma or possibly cryosupernatant infusions should be given. Usually if therapy is successful haemorrhage will stop. Continued haemorrhage, despite therapy for the underlying disease and rational therapy for DIC, is likely to be associated with a poor prognosis and reflects failure to control the underlying disease process.

REFERENCES AND FURTHER READING

Aronsohn M (1985) Cardiac hemangiosarcoma in the dog: a review of 38 cases. *Journal of the American Veterinary Medical Association* **187**, 922–926
Bick RL (1992) Coagulation abnormalities in malignancy: a review. *Seminars in Thrombosis and Hemostasis* **18**, 353–372
Bick RL (1994) Disseminated intravascular coagulation. Objective criteria for diagnosis and management. *Medical Clinics of North America* **78**, 511–543
Brooks MB, Matus RE, Leifer CE and Patnaik AK (1987) Use of splenectomy in the management of lymphoma in dogs: 16 cases (1976-1985). *Journal of the American Veterinary Medical Association* **191**, 1008–1010
Burrows CF (1977) Canine hemorrhagic gastroenteritis. *Journal of the American Animal Hospital Association* **13**, 451–458
Feldman BF, Madewell BR and O'Neill S (1981) Disseminated intravascular coagulation: antithrombin, plasminogen, and coagulation abnormalities in 41 dogs. *Journal of the American Veterinary Medical Association* **179**, 151–154
Green RA (1981) Hemostasis and disorders of coagulation. *Veterinary Clinics of North America: Small Animal Practice* **11**, 289–319
Greene CE (1975) Disseminated intravascular coagulation in the dog: a review. *Journal of the American Animal Hospital Association* **11**, 674–687
Greene CE (1983) Management of DIC and thrombosis. In: *Current Veterinary Therapy VIII*, ed. RW Kirk, pp. 401–405. WB Saunders, Philadelphia
Greene CE, Barsanti JA and Jones BD (1977) Disseminated intravascular coagulation complicating aflatoxicosis in dogs. *Cornell Veterinarian* **67**, 29–49
Hammer AS, Couto CG, Swardson C and Getzy D (1991) Hemostatic abnormalities in dogs with hemangiosarcoma. *Journal of Veterinary Internal Medicine* **5**, 11–14
Hargis AM and Feldman BF (1991) Evaluation of hemostatic defects secondary to vascular tumors in dogs: 11 cases (1983-1988). *Journal of the American Veterinary Medical Association* **198**, 891–894
Holloway SA (1992) Heatstroke in dogs. *Compendium of Continuing Education* **14**, 1598–1604
Holloway SA, Senior DF, Roth L and Tisher CC (1993) Hemolytic uremic syndrome in dogs. *Journal of Veterinary Internal Medicine* **7**, 220–227
Kangstrom LE (1989) Snake bite (*Vipera berus*) in dogs and cats. *Svensk Veterinartidning* **41**, 8–9
Millis DL, Hauptman JG and Fulton RJ (1993) Abnormal hemostatic profiles and gastric necrosis in canine gastric dilatation-volvulus. *Veterinary Surgery* **22**, 93–97

Moore DJ and Williams MC (1979) Disseminated intravascular coagulation: a complication of *Babesia canis* infection in the dog. *Journal of the South African Veterinary Association* **50,** 265-275

Rishniw M and Lewis DC (1994) Localized consumptive coagulopathy associated with cutaneous hemangiosarcoma in a dog. *Journal of the American Animal Hospital Association* **30,** 261-264

Slappendel RJ (1988) Disseminated intravascular coagulation. *Veterinary Clinics of North America: Small Animal Practice* **18,** 169-184

Susaneck SJ, Allen TA, Hoopes J, Withrow SJ and Macy DW (1983) Inflammatory mammary carcinoma in the dog. *Journal of the American Animal Hospital Association* **19,** 971-976

Weller RE, Theilen GH and Madewell BR (1982) Chemotherapeutic responses in dogs with lymphosarcoma and hypercalcemia. *Journal of the American Veterinary Medical Association* **181,** 891-893

Zenoble RD and Gabbert NH (1977) A possible case of disseminated intravascular coagulation and splenic hemangiosarcoma. *Canine Practice* **4,** 52-55

PART THREE

Transfusion Medicine

Practical Blood Transfusion

Anthony Abrams-Ogg

INTRODUCTION

Transfusion is defined as intravenous therapy with whole blood or blood products. Whole blood refers to blood that has not been separated into various products. Historically, transfusion therapy has relied on the use of whole blood, and such use remains the most practical means of giving a transfusion in many veterinary clinics.

Blood products include blood components and blood derivatives. Blood components are blood products prepared either by centrifugation or, less commonly, by apheresis. The most frequently used components are packed red blood cells (RBCs) and plasma. In many clinical situations a patient in need of a transfusion requires only a specific component of blood. The use of blood components allows several patients to benefit from one blood donation and reduces the risks of transfusion reactions to unnecessary components. During the past decade there has been increasing interest in veterinary transfusion medicine, spurred on by advances in veterinary oncology and critical care, such that blood components are routinely prepared by certain institutions and commercial enterprises in some countries.

Both whole blood and blood components may be used shortly after collection ('fresh' products) or after storage ('stored' or 'banked' products). Before World War II, blood banking was not extensively practised in human medicine. Donors were called in as needed and blood collected and immediately transfused. This remains the most common practice in veterinary medicine, although, as with blood component preparation, an interest in blood banking has flourished in the recent past. Blood banking allows immediate access to whole blood and blood components. Blood collection and component preparation can be labour intensive and time consuming. It may not be feasible or optimal to obtain and process blood on demand. For clinics that only occasionally need to perform a transfusion, blood banking is probably neither cost nor time effective as a certain percentage of stored components will have to be discarded because of limited shelf life. However, for emergency clinics and clinics with a large caseload requiring transfusion therapy, blood banking is essential.

Blood derivatives are blood protein products prepared by using biochemical methods (e.g. ethanol extraction) to process large pools of donor plasma. Blood derivatives, which include albumin solutions, intravenous immunoglobulins and specific factor concentrates, have had relatively limited use in veterinary medicine compared with blood components, and most products used have been of human origin.

Transfusion may be more broadly defined to include therapy with blood substitutes, which are produced by using biotechnological methods. Blood substitutes include artificial colloids, oxygen transporters, platelet substitutes and human coagulation proteins produced by recombinant DNA technology. The first two have been used in veterinary medicine.

This chapter reviews the practical aspects of transfusion therapy in the dog and cat. It is organized in a temporal fashion, beginning with the blood donor and blood donation followed by blood processing and banking, transfusion and transfusion reactions. Lastly, autotransfusion is discussed. Many of the recommendations are based on current human blood banking and transfusion standards. It may not be possible for some veterinary clinics to meet these standards, especially in emergency situations. As with all therapy, the risks associated with a transfusion must be weighed against the potential benefits. Meeting less than ideal standards increases risks, but in the author's opinion a potentially life-saving transfusion should not be withheld because ideal transfusion practices cannot be followed.

THE BLOOD DONOR

Source
Blood donors may be obtained from several sources. Each clinic must decide on the optimal source for its needs, and local regulations regarding animal use should be reviewed. In the United Kingdom, practitioners are advised to ensure that their source of donors is compatible with Home Office guidelines.

Clinic owned
The simplest approach for ensuring access to blood donors is to keep such animals in the clinic. The

number of animals depends on anticipated needs. For most general practices one to two dogs and cats will suffice. Some ethical concerns have been expressed about donor animal lifestyles, but these are easily addressed. The donors at the Ontario Veterinary College (OVC), for example, are animals that were destined for euthanasia. The animals are used as donors for 2 years and then adopted into the community. The dogs are exercised regularly outside, and the cats are free to roam in an environmentally enriched room. In determining the costs of this approach, the cost of food, use of space in the clinic and staff time should be taken into account.

Donor programme

An alternative to clinic-owned animals is the use of pets owned by the clinic's staff. An extension of this approach is a donor programme, where client-owned animals donate blood in exchange for benefits such as free annual examinations, vaccinations and pet food. Pet owners can be 'on-call' if fresh blood is required, and/or their animals can donate blood regularly if the clinic practises blood banking. Such programmes can be excellent practice builders, although a slight risk is present for an adverse consequence of donation. The risk is more so with cats, which need to be sedated or anaesthetized for donation. Given the ease of keeping donor cats in the clinic, using clinic-owned cats may be preferable to using client-owned cats. It must be made clear to owners to what extent costs of dealing with unrelated medical problems will be subsidized, if at all. The cost of such a programme, including lost revenue, must be calculated against the costs of keeping donors in the hospital.

Animal control facilities

An animal shelter or pound may allow blood donation from stray or surrendered animals awaiting adoption. There are two principal disadvantages with the use of such donors. Firstly, because of unknown history, time constraints and expense, there is usually inadequate screening for infectious and metabolic diseases. Secondly, there are ethical and public relations concerns.

Terminal donors

These are animals that are being euthanased, either at animal control or research facilities or at clinics for behaviour problems or medical disorders that do not affect the quality of donated blood. The same concerns exist as for non-terminal donations from pound-source animals. The main advantage of terminal donors is that large volumes of blood (up to 50% estimated blood volume) can be collected.

Commercial blood bank

Commercial small animal blood banks exist in some countries, which supply selected blood products.

The canine donor

The ideal canine blood donor is a friendly, clinically normal, nulliparous, large breed dog with normal body weight, and has easily accessible veins and a universal donor blood type (see Canine blood groups). Greyhounds are often used for these reasons and because of availability when retired from the track. (The life span of Greyhound RBCs is shorter than that of other breeds (Novinger *et al.*, 1996). It is not known if the survival of Greyhound RBCs after transfusion is lower than in other breeds. If it is, it is unlikely that this has any detrimental effect on the immediate benefits of a transfusion.) Donors should be young to middle aged; dogs up to 8 years of age are used at the OVC.

A donor should weigh 28 kg or more so that a standard blood donation can be given without excessive volume depletion (see Blood donation). Smaller dogs can donate when a smaller transfusion volume is being considered (e.g. paediatric transfusion). A high donor packed cell volume (PCV) is desirable when RBC transfusion is planned, whereas a lower PCV is desirable when plasma and platelet products are being made. Greyhounds normally have high PCVs and low to low–normal platelet counts.

Temperament

Blood can be collected from an uncooperative dog by using sedation or general anaesthesia, but regular blood donors should be sufficiently tractable to permit donation with either manual restraint or light sedation, especially if they are client-owned. Many dogs habituate to the procedure, and sedation can be discontinued.

Clinical evaluation

Donors are considered to be clinically normal on the basis of standard history and physical examination findings. These should be reviewed before each donation and the donation cancelled if there is any suspicion of a relevant disorder. Typical reasons for cancelling a donation include bite wounds or acute vomiting and diarrhoea. Similarly, blood should be discarded from a dog that develops a fever or other signs of potentially infectious disorders within a week of blood donation. In a client-owned donor programme, owners are advised to report such events. Annual laboratory evaluation consisting of a complete blood count, serum biochemistry profile, urinalysis and faecal examination for parasites is often recommended, but the value of such screening is not known. Certainly the donor's PCV and total solids protein should be measured before each donation.

Pregnancy: Pregnant bitches should not be used as donors, as donation poses an undesirable stress on the donor and fetuses. Furthermore, bitches that have had previous pregnancies should not be used. The concern is that there is a risk that a DEA (dog erythrocyte antigen) 1.1 negative bitch (see Canine blood groups) bred to a DEA 1.1 positive dog may develop anti-DEA 1.1 antibodies. This increases the risk of a minor incompatibility reaction.

Vaccination status: Blood donors should be current on vaccinations, but these should not be given within 10–14 days of a planned donation because of the potential for modified live vaccines to alter platelet number and function.

Infections and parasites: Donors should be free of parasites and infectious diseases, especially those that are blood borne. Depending on risk of infection based upon geographical location and other factors, dogs may be tested for infection with *Brucella canis, Borrelia burgdorferi, Ehrlichia* spp., *Rickettsia rickettsii, Bartonella vinsonii, Babesia* spp., *Trypanosoma cruzi, Leishmania* spp. and *Dirofilaria immitis.* Periodical retesting may be required based on risk of exposure.

Haemobartonella canis infection poses a unique concern as the organism is usually carried asymptomatically and only causes haemolysis in splenectomized dogs. In the carrier state it is rarely seen on the RBC, and no other test is available to detect infection. Nonetheless it can be transmitted by a blood transfusion from a carrier dog. For this reason it is sometimes recommended that canine blood donors be splenectomized to reveal infection, and to remove infected animals from a donor programme. Although there are cases reported of canine haemobartonellosis after transfusion, the prevalence of this occurrence is not known. Splenectomy reduces RBC mass and lowers the adoptability of a clinic-owned donor, and certainly client-owned donors will not be splenectomized. Furthermore, transfusion of *H. canis* infected blood is only likely to be a concern to dogs being treated by splenectomy, and the infection, if it occurs, is in most cases easily treated. As with all blood transfusion decisions, each clinic must make its own risk–benefit assessment. Clinic-owned dogs, including Greyhounds with extensive travel history, are not splenectomized at the OVC.

Splenectomy has also been recommended to reveal carriers of *Babesia* spp. However, serological tests and immunosuppressive therapy with prednisone can also be used to help identify carrier animals. Another approach is to treat donors empirically with imidocarb dipropionate (7.5 mg/kg i.m.). It should be noted than in areas with a high prevalence of babesiosis, there is a reasonable chance that the recipient is already infected, and one of the more common indications for RBC transfusion is acute anaemia due to this disease, where transmission of *Babesia* spp. from a carrier animal is not important.

Ideally blood donors should not be infested with endo- or ectoparasites, but this may not be achievable in some geographical areas. Severe flea infestations in donors will aggravate anaemia due to blood loss, but mild infestations do not seem to pose health risks to either donor or recipient. This applies as well to mild chronic *Ancylostoma caninum* infections.

Dogs with potential for bacteraemia should not be used as donors. These include dogs with wounds, abscesses, surgical implants, extensive skin lesions, advanced periodontal disease and diarrhoea. In addition, blood should not be collected from dogs with pyoderma affecting the collection sites.

Other disorders: Dogs with immune-mediated disorders, cancer, organ failure and other systemic disorders should not donate blood because of the potential for undesirable stress on the donor and negative effects on blood quality.

Drug therapy
Donors should not be receiving any drug therapy because of the potential for undesirable effects in the recipient and on blood quality, especially if blood is being stored. Donor dogs living in heartworm endemic areas must receive prophylaxis, but heartworm prophylaxis drugs should arguably not be given immediately preceding a donation. Donor dogs may also have routine flea control treatments, but such treatment immediately preceding donation is also discouraged.

Previous transfusions
Donors should not have received any transfusions because of the risks of developing antibodies that may cause minor incompatibility reactions (see Canine blood groups).

The feline donor
The ideal feline blood donor is a friendly clinically normal large cat (≥4.5 kg) with normal bodyweight. Males are preferred because of their larger size. At the OVC cats may donate blood up to 8 years of age. Because most feline transfusions are given to correct anaemia, a high donor PCV is preferred (≥35% at lower altitudes and ≥40% at higher altitudes). Pregnant queens should not be used for reasons given above. Previous pregnancy does not exclude a queen from donating blood.

Clinical evaluation
The same principles concerning exclusion of canine donors on the basis of systemic diseases apply to feline donors. Donor cats should be housed indoors to minimize fight wounds and infections. With respect to specific infectious diseases, feline donors should test negatively for feline leukaemia virus and feline immunodeficiency virus infections. Status of donor cats with respect to feline infectious peritonitis (FIP) virus titre is controversial. It is well recognized that many clinically normal cats with positive FIP titres

have had enteric coronavirus infections and never develop clinical FIP. Nonetheless, to minimize the chance of a donor transmitting FIP virus, cats with negative FIP titres are preferred.

The carrier state of *Haemobartonella felis* poses the same problems in the cat as does *H. canis* in the dog, although recipient cats more readily develop clinical disease without splenectomy. The recent availability of a polymerase chain reaction test for detection of *H. felis* should facilitate the removal of carriers from a donor population. Donor cats are not splenectomized at the OVC.

Cats should also be tested for *Bartonella henselae* and *Bartonella clarridgeiae* infection by serological and culture techniques. Although bartonellosis is sub-clinical or causes only mild clinical disease in cats, removing infected blood donors is recommended because of the organism's zoonotic potential.

Dirofilaria immitis and *Babesia* spp. infections should be ruled out in endemic areas.

Cats at the OVC are not routinely tested serologically for *Toxoplasma gondii* infection. Cats raised indoors and fed a commercial diet will have negative titres, whereas cats previously outdoors are likely to have been exposed. If a titre (IgG) is obtained and is positive, then either an IgM titre should be obtained or the IgG titre repeated in 2–4 weeks to rule out active infection. As with all cats, donor cats should not be fed uncooked meats.

BLOOD GROUPS

Blood groups are defined by inherited antigens on the surface of RBCs. They are important in transfusion medicine because of the risk of haemolytic reactions. Such reactions occur when there is antibody directed against a blood group antigen. The severity of a haemolytic reaction depends on several factors. Two key points are: firstly, for a given antibody type, generally the higher the titre the worse the reaction; secondly, IgM-mediated reactions tend to be more severe than IgG-mediated reactions because of superior complement fixation by IgM. A haemolytic transfusion reaction may occur as an acute intravascular crisis, dependent on complement activation by IgM or high-titre IgG, or as a delayed extravascular haemolytic event, dependent on IgG binding to RBCs (see Adverse Consequences of Transfusion).

Canine blood groups

Canine blood groups are classified by the DEA (Dog Erythrocyte Antigen) system. There are six DEAs (1.1, 1.2, 3, 4, 5 and 7) defined by currently available internationally standardized antisera, but 20 or more specificities have been described. DEAs have not been extensively characterized for composition and structure (Corato *et al.*, 1997).

Antigens

DEA 1.1 and 1.2 are alleles. A dog may be negative for both antigens or positive for only one of them. At the OVC, Golden Retrievers, Labrador Retrievers and Rottweilers tend to have DEA 1.1 or 1.2 blood type, whereas Greyhounds and German Shepherd Dogs tend to be DEA 1.1 and 1.2 negative.

There are no naturally occurring alloantibodies to DEA 1.1 or 1.2, so these antigens will not cause an acute reaction during a recipient's first transfusion. If, however, a DEA 1.1 negative dog receives a transfusion from a DEA 1.1 positive dog, anti-DEA 1.1 antibody formation (sensitization) will cause delayed haemolysis within 1–2 weeks. More importantly, on subsequent exposure to DEA 1.1 positive blood, an acute haemolytic transfusion reaction will occur, with destruction of all transfused RBCs within 12 hours. The reaction may be clinically moderate to severe, but is unlikely to be fatal (Giger *et al.*, 1995). The situation is similar for sensitization to DEA 1.2, except that the reaction is less severe, with destruction of transfused RBCs within 24 hours. A DEA 1.1/1.2 negative dog sensitized to 1.1 RBCs may also have a delayed haemolytic reaction when transfused with 1.2 positive RBCs.

Neonatal isoerythrolysis occurs when a sensitized DEA 1.1 negative female is bred to a DEA 1.1 positive male. Inheritance is autosomal dominant, therefore the likelihood is that some pups will be DEA 1.1 positive and have haemolytic disease.

A third allele in the DEA 1 group, DEA 1.3, has also been described (Symons and Bell, 1991). DEA 1.3 positive dogs are negative for DEA 1.1 and 1.2. Transfusing DEA 1.3 positive blood to a DEA 1.1, 1.2 and 1.3 negative dog will result in production of antibodies that will react with the 1.1, 1.2 and 1.3 antigens. However, dogs positive for DEA 1.3 may type as DEA 1.1 and 1.2 negative with conventional antisera. Thus it is possible for a transfusion of DEA 1.1 and 1.2 negative blood to sensitize a DEA 1.1 and 1.2 negative recipient. This is one reason why crossmatching is always recommended when a recipient has been previously transfused.

Dogs may also be sensitized to DEA 3, 5 and 7 by transfusion. In addition, naturally occurring alloantibodies, similar to the situation with the ABO blood groups in humans, are present in low prevalence to DEA 3 and 5. The prevalence of naturally occurring antibodies to DEA 7 is controversial but has been reported to be 15–50%. Antibodies to DEA 3, 5 and 7 usually result in delayed haemolysis. The prevalence of such transfusion reactions is not known, but it is probably fairly low.

Because most dogs are positive for DEA 4 and anti-DEA 4 antibodies do not cause haemolysis, this blood group has minimal transfusion significance.

An acute haemolytic reaction has also been described in a dog sensitized to an RBC antigen present in most dogs but distinct from the known DEAs (Callan *et al.*, 1995). If such a patient requires transfusion, a closely related dog should be sought, which may also be negative for that antigen.

Feline blood groups

The feline A, B and AB blood group system is discussed in more detail in Chapter 16. Other blood groups have not been described. There is no universal donor because, unlike dogs, cats have naturally occurring alloantibodies and no null type; therefore, RBC incompatibility reactions will occur in naïve recipients.

The reaction is typically peracute and sometimes fatal at the beginning of a transfusion of type A or AB RBCs to a type B recipient. An acute reaction more similar to the acute reaction seen in dogs followed completion of a transfusion of type A blood to a type B cat, with fever, icterus and destruction of transfused RBCs in 24 hours (Giger and Akol, 1990). This reaction may have been due to IgG rather than IgM. Delayed haemolysis occurs in type A recipients receiving type B or AB RBCs, and acute reactions may occur due to anti-A antibodies in type B donor plasma.

Type AB cats are universal RBC recipients but are also at risk of incompatibility reactions from donor plasma antibodies (so-called minor incompatibility reactions). Type AB cats are best transfused with type AB blood, but, given the low prevalence of this blood type, the likelihood of finding another AB donor is low. Type AB cats can be acceptably transfused with type A blood because the low titre of anti-B antibodies is unlikely to be harmful (RBC washing can be considered if large volume transfusions are needed). Type AB cats should not receive type B blood products because of the frequently high anti-A antibody titre.

BLOOD TYPING

Donor and recipient RBC compatibility should be considered when selecting a donor.

Blood typing in dogs

The best way to prevent DEA incompatibility reactions is by determining blood type using antisera. Blood typing is commercially available in some countries. Polyclonal antiserum is produced by alloimmunizing a dog negative for a given DEA by injecting it with small quantities of blood positive for that DEA. The RBCs to be typed are incubated with the antiserum in the presence of complement, with and without antiglobulin, in a similar fashion to that described for crossmatching below. Haemolysis or agglutination indicates presence of the antigen in

question. Antiserum produced by alloimmunizing a DEA 1.1/1.2 negative dog with 1.1 positive blood will react strongly with 1.1 positive RBCs and cross-react weakly with 1.2 positive RBCs.

To facilitate detection of DEA 1.2, DEA 1.2 RBCs are injected along with DEA 1.1 RBCs to produce non-specific anti-DEA 1.1/1.2 antiserum. Laboratories providing limited blood-typing services typically use such antiserum. A dog with a negative reaction is classified as DEA 1.1/1.2 negative. A dog with a positive reaction is classified as DEA 1.1/1.2 positive, but it is not known which antigen is present. (DEA 1.1/1.2 negative dogs have also been referred to as 'A-negative', and DEA 1.1/1.2 positive dogs as 'A-positive', based on the older terminology for dog blood group antigens. These terms are confusing and their continued use is not recommended.)

Further characterization of a positive DEA 1.1/1.2 reaction may be achieved by using antiserum specific for DEA 1.1. This antiserum is produced by alloimmunizing a DEA 1.2 positive dog with DEA 1.1 positive blood. A dog with positive DEA 1.1/1.2 and positive DEA 1.1 reactions has a DEA 1.1 blood type. A dog with positive DEA 1.1/1.2 and negative DEA 1.1 reactions has a DEA 1.2 blood type. Specific anti-DEA 1.2 antiserum may also be produced from anti-DEA 1.1/1.2 antiserum using DEA 1.1 red cell absorption techniques to remove anti-DEA 1.1 antibodies.

Some laboratories provide more complete characterization of blood type by using antisera for DEA 3, 4, 5 and 7. A typing card using a murine monoclonal antibody has recently become available for in-clinic use to determine DEA 1.1 status (RapidVet-H Canine 1.1, DMS Laboratories). The experience at the OVC and elsewhere is that false-positive reactions may occur with the typing cards resulting in a positive predictive value of about 75% (Moritz *et al.*, 1998). False-negative reactions may occur if the haematocrit is <10%.

RBC transfusions are commonly given to emergency or urgent cases, and historically blood typing has only been performed at reference laboratories. For these reasons blood typing has traditionally been used only to select clinic-owned and client-owned donors and not to type recipients in order to match donors and recipients.

Donor blood type

A universal donor is negative for DEA 1.1, 1.2, 3, 5 and 7. The minimal requirement to prevent an acute DEA-mediated haemolytic reaction is that a donor be negative for DEA 1.1 and 1.2. The minimal requirement to prevent a moderate to severe DEA haemolytic reaction is that a donor be negative for DEA 1.1. The clinical utility of more complete typing versus typing for DEA 1.1 alone is not known. At the OVC, clinic-owned donors are typed as universal donors by an outside specialist laboratory, and client-owned donors are typed as DEA 1.1/1.2 negative by using antisera produced in-house. The false-positive rate of the typing cards does not preclude their use for donor selection, but some potential DEA 1.1 negative donors will be excluded.

Recipient blood type

There is no universal recipient canine blood type. Determining the blood type of the recipient would be beneficial in that it would allow the use of DEA 1.1 positive and other non-universal donors. Although the availability of typing cards now permits rapid DEA 1.1 blood type determination, the cards should not be used to type recipients, because dogs falsely identified as DEA 1.1 positive will become sensitized after trans-fusion with DEA 1.1 positive blood.

Complete recipient blood type is occasionally de-termined for cases at the OVC where multiple trans-fusions are anticipated, in the event that non-universal donors can be used and thus prevent exhaustion of the regular blood supply. Merely typing recipients as DEA 1.1/1.2 positive and transfusing them with DEA 1.1/1.2 positive donor blood is not sufficient because it is possible that a DEA 1.2 positive recipient would become sensitized to DEA 1.1 and vice versa.

It is often stated that because a first transfusion can be given to any non-breeding dog without risk of acute haemolysis, it is unnecessary to type all donor blood and that it is acceptable to transfuse DEA 1.1/1.2 positive blood once. These practices are discouraged because it is possible that the recipient may require future transfusions. Certainly only universal donor, DEA 1.1/1.2 negative or DEA 1.1 negative blood should be transfused to:

- A dog transfused more than 4 days previously (anti-RBC antibodies develop within 4–14 days)
- A dog with a history of a transfusion reaction
- A dog whose transfusion history is not known
- A previously pregnant dog.

The availability of typing cards greatly facilitates proper donor selection. Even if donor selection is limited, the typing cards can be used to determine if the recipient was transfused with DEA 1.1 positive blood and thus if the dog is at increased risk of future haemolytic transfusion reactions.

Blood typing in cats

Feline blood typing is discussed in Chapter 16. A typing card is available for in-house determination of A, B, and AB blood types (RapidVet-H Feline, DMS Laboratories). Blood typing both donor and recipient in all cases is ideal. A crossmatch (see below) may identify blood type, especially if the blood type of either the donor or recipient is known. In the latter case the procedure is referred to as 'back typing'.

CROSSMATCHING

Crossmatching tests for anti-RBC antibodies by examining for agglutination and haemolysis. The technique is similar to blood typing, but in the latter a known antibody is used in the test to identify a specific RBC antigen. Crossmatching is an adjunct to, not a substitute for, blood typing, but it may be the only incompatibility test available. The major crossmatch detects recipient antibodies against donor RBCs. The minor crossmatch detects donor antibodies against recipient RBCs. A complete crossmatch is conducted at 37°C, room temperature (technically 25°C) and 4°C and includes an anti-globulin reagent (indirect Coombs' test).

Procedures

Numerous crossmatching procedures have been reported. Two methods are discussed, adapted to general practice from the methods used at the OVC. The rapid slide method (Figures 15.1 and 15.2) is roughly equivalent to phase I of the tube method. The tube method (Figures 15.3 and 15.4) is more cumber-some but superior as:

- Longer incubation is feasible with less rouleaux formation (pseudoagglutination), which facilitates detection of weak agglutinins
- It facilitates grading of agglutination
- It facilitates detection of haemolysis
- It can incorporate an antiglobulin test.

The author prefers the rapid slide test for cats and for dogs in an emergency. The tube test is recom-mended for dogs if time allows.

In both methods either serum or plasma can be used. The use of plasma is more convenient. The use of serum is preferred in dogs as the presence of fibrinogen and other proteins in plasma increases rouleaux formation. In cats, rouleaux formation is nearly as strong in serum as it is in plasma. In both species, rouleaux formation is increased in both serum and plasma in the presence of increased levels of immunoglobulins and fibrinogen and in the presence of synthetic colloids. In any case the use of donor and recipient controls is important to observe for rouleaux. The use of 4,4-diisothiocyanatostilbene-2,2-disulphonic acid has been investigated to block rouleaux formation in human compatibility testing.

Agglutination must be distinguished from rouleaux formation. This is easy to do with strong agglutination but may be difficult with weak agglutination when using the rapid slide method. The rouleaux formation may be strong, especially in cats and when using undiluted RBCs, and is macroscopically indistinguish-able from agglutination.

1. Collect 0.5-1 ml blood in an EDTA tube ± 1-2 ml in a clot tube from recipient and donor. Clearly label tubes.
2. Centrifuge tubes at standard speed for the centrifuge in use (usually about 1000-1500 *g* for 5-10 minutes) to separate RBCs from plasma and serum. If a centrifuge is not available, allow EDTA specimens to sit at room temperature for one to several hours until RBCs have sedimented. Using separate pipettes (or syringes and 18 G needles) for each sample, transfer serum and/or plasma to separate tubes. Clearly label tubes.
3. Prepare 4% donor and recipient RBC suspensions in tubes or syringes by mixing 0.2 ml packed RBCs and 4.8 ml saline. Use a separate pipette for each mixture and clearly label. This step is optional for the slide method. This dilution of RBCs in saline retards rouleaux formation and facilitates microscopic observation but results in less dramatic macroscopic agglutination. Further dilution may dilute alloantibodies to the point of non-reactivity and may still not completely eliminate rouleaux.
4. Label four glass slides as:

    *   donor control (donor RBCs and donor serum or plasma)
    *   major X-match (donor RBCs and recipient serum or plasma)
    *   minor X-match (recipient RBCs and donor serum or plasma)
    *   recipient control (recipient RBCs and recipient serum or plasma).

    On to each slide place either one drop of serum (or plasma) and one drop of RBC suspension or two drops of serum (or plasma) and one drop of undiluted RBCs. Rapidly mix together with an applicator stick.
5. Gently rock slides back and forth and observe for macroscopic agglutination within 2 minutes (see Figure 15.2). Place on a coverslip and observe the wet mounts with a 40 x objective lens ± a 100 x oil-immersion lens for microscopic agglutination within 5 minutes.

Figure 15.1: *Rapid slide method for crossmatching. The author prefers to use undiluted RBCs. If results are equivocal, the test is repeated with diluted RBCs. Repeating the test is preferred to adding several drops of saline to the slide. If saline is added to the slide, vigorous mixing is required to resuspend the RBCs, which may break up weak aggregates. If the test is still equivocal, it is repeated as described in phase I of the tube method.*

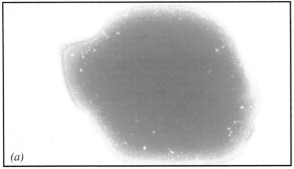

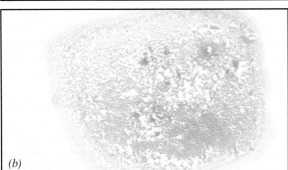

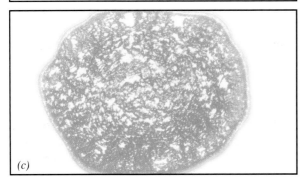

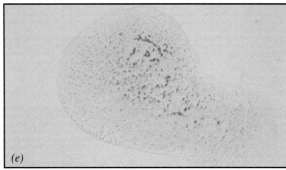

Figure 15.2: *Macroscopic agglutination and pseudoagglutination in a feline crossmatch. (a) Negative result at 2 minutes with undiluted type B red cells and type A plasma. (b) Positive result at 2 minutes with undiluted type A red cells and type B plasma. (c) Pseudoagglutination (strong rouleaux formation) at 10 minutes with undiluted type A red cells and type A plasma. (d) Positive result at 2 minutes with 4% suspension type A red cells and type B plasma. (e) Pseudoagglutination at 10 minutes with 4% suspension type A red cells and type A plasma.*

Phase I

1-3. As Figure 15.1 for rapid slide method. Typically 12 x 75 mm glass tubes are used, but any small glass tube will suffice. An optional recommended step with dogs is to wash the RBCs three times in saline before making the final 4% suspension. To perform this wash, add 0.5-1 ml of blood to the tube and fill the remainder of the tube with saline. Mix by inverting the tube and centrifuge at high speed for 1 minute (or longer if required to sediment the RBCs). Remove supernatant. Repeat twice more.

4. Label glass tubes as described for slides, and into each tube place two drops of RBC suspension and two drops of serum or plasma, and mix by flicking the bottom of the tube. In addition, two drops of guinea-pig complement may be added.* A complete set of major and minor crossmatch and control tubes is required for each temperature at which the test is conducted.**

5. Centrifuge at a low speed for 15-30 seconds, just enough to bring the cells together but not to pack tightly.

6. Gently shake tubes ('wiggle and tip') to resuspend the cells. Hold up to light (a radiograph viewing box works well) to observe for macroscopic agglutination and/or haemolysis (see Figure 15.4). Confirm agglutination microscopically.

7. If strong rouleaux formation is present, recentrifuge the serum/plasma–RBC mixture. Carefully remove supernatant with a pipette, replace with an equal volume of saline, and gently mix. Centrifuge the mixture once more, and then repeat step 6.

Phase II

8. If no agglutination is noted in step 6, incubate tubes for 30 minutes at test temperature(s).**
9. Repeat steps 5 and 6.

Phase III (dogs)

10. Antiglobulin test. Canine polyvalent antiglobulin (containing anti-IgG, anti-IgM and anti-C3) is added to each tube, incubated for 30 minutes and samples are centrifuged as above and observed for agglutination and/or haemolysis. This phase of the test is usually performed in reference laboratories.

Figure 15.3: *Tube method for crossmatching.*
Reference laboratories performing a complete crossmatch including an antiglobulin test will conduct the test at 37°C and room temperature and optionally at 4°C. Anti-DEA 1.1 and anti-DEA 1.2 antibodies have maximum reactivity at 37°C, but clinically relevant titres should react at room temperature. Many other anti-DEA antibodies have maximal reactivity at room temperature, which is in part why they are of less clinical significance. Blood for transfusion ideally should be compatible at 37°C and room temperature, but compatibility at 37°C is most important. Cold (4°C) incompatibilities do not cause transfusion reactions.
* Adding complement will promote detection of haemolysis. This is most likely to occur in the presence of anti-DEA 1.1 antibodies. A significant titre will, however, result in detectable agglutination in the absence of complement. Complement is unlikely to be used outside a reference laboratory, as the optimum storage temperature is –70°C.
** In a general practice the test is usually conducted at room temperature, but ideally it should also be conducted at 37°C.

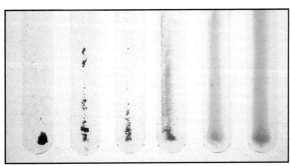

Figure 15.4: *Grading of agglutination reactions in a canine crossmatch. From left to right: 4+, one solid aggregate of red cells; 3+, several large aggregates; 2+, medium aggregates, clear background; 1+ small aggregates, turbid reddish background; +w, tiny or microscopic aggregates, turbid reddish background; negative.*

Microscopically, in aggregates of agglutinated RBCs, the cells are rafted together, randomly oriented and superimposed on each other (Figure 15.5). A three-dimensional structure is apparent, as RBCs of different layers of the aggregate come in and out of focus when the fine focus of the microscope is adjusted. The size and density of aggregates vary with the alloantibody titre, RBC density and location on the slide. Compared with higher density aggregates, individual RBCs can be discerned more easily in lower density aggregates, which may resemble 'bunches of grapes.' Aggregate clumps may be connected by linear aggregate formations. One-dimensional linear formations resemble 'strings of beads.'

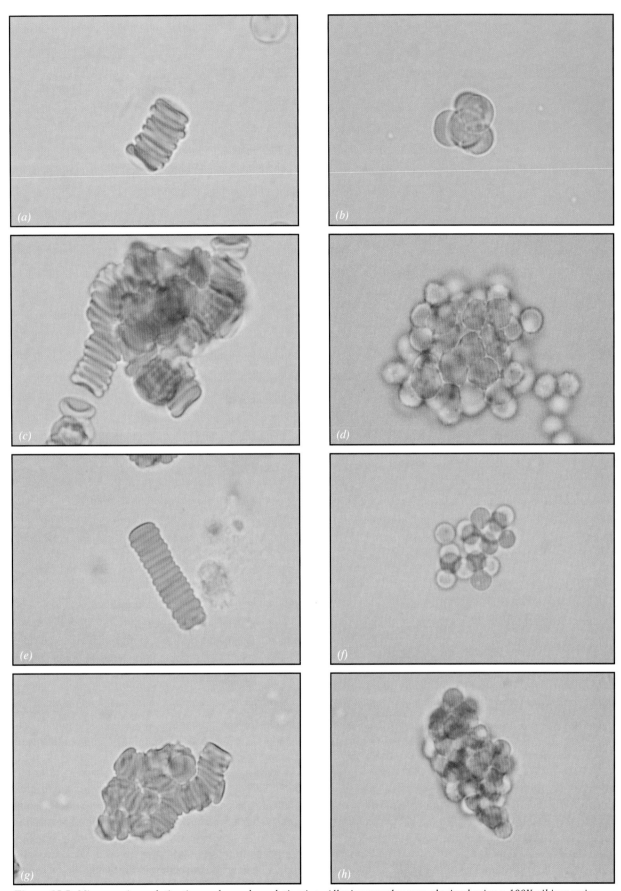

Figure 15.5: *Microscopic agglutination and pseudoagglutination. All micrographs were obtained using a 100X oil immersion objective lens unless otherwise indicated. (a) Canine single rouleaux formation. (b) Tiny canine aggregate. (c) Small canine rouleaux network. (d) Small canine aggregate. (e) Feline single rouleaux formation. (f) Feline medium density aggregate. (g) Small feline rouleaux network. (h) Small high-density feline aggregate.* **(continues overleaf)**

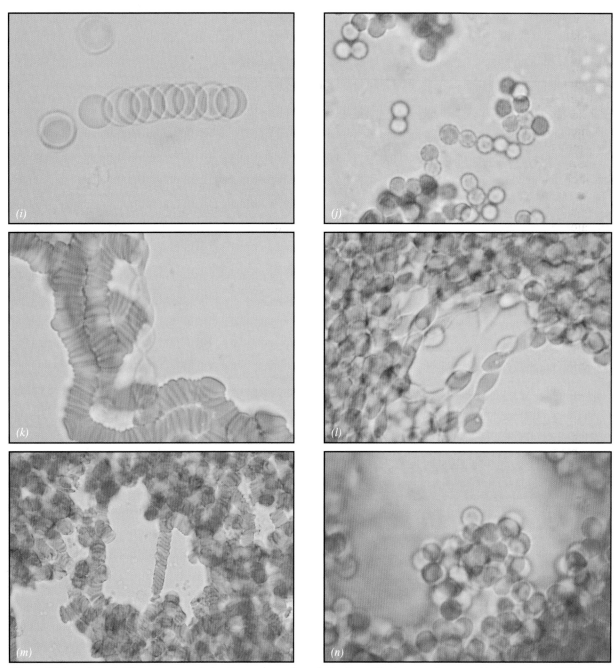

Figure 15.5 continued: *Microscopic agglutination and pseudoagglutination. All micrographs were obtained using a 100X oil immersion objective lens unless otherwise indicated. (i) Canine single rouleaux formation with the appearance of a fallen over stack of coins. Such formations form in thin layer wet mounts. (j) Low density feline aggregate resulting in a 'string of beads' effect. Red cell crenation is also present. (k) Medium size feline rouleaux network pulling apart forming a 'chain of lemons'. (l) Large feline aggregate pulling apart forming several 'chains of lemons'. (m) Large canine rouleaux networks bridged by a single rouleaux formation (40X high-power objective lens). (n) Large high-density feline aggregate. Close inspection of the edge of large, high-density formations aids in distinguishing between rouleaux formations and aggregates.*

Microscopically, in rouleaux the RBCs are aligned face to face and thus appear as 'stacks of coins' (see Figure 15.5). In some cases the stacks may seem to have 'fallen over,' appearing as chains of overlapping RBCs. Canine rouleaux may not be quite as 'tidy' as feline rouleaux. Strong rouleaux clump together and form rouleaux networks, which may be connected by single rouleaux formations. The size and density of rouleaux networks vary with the serum or plasma protein content, RBC density, location on the slide and time. Under 5 minutes using the rapid slide method most rouleaux will be single formations. Single rouleaux are predominantly one-dimensional in structure, and rouleaux networks are predominantly two-dimensional.

Small aggregates and single rouleaux and medium size and/or density aggregates and rouleaux networks, can usually be distinguished. However, the large high-density aggregates and rouleaux networks that may form when using undiluted RBCs in the rapid slide method may be difficult to distinguish. Examining other areas of the slide where smaller clumps may be present and close inspection of the edges of the clumps helps in making the distinction. Note, however, that rouleaux can form concurrently with aggregates and may stick to them. Also note that moving the slide on the microscope stage and using the oil immersion lens may mechanically break up both large rouleaux networks and aggregates, which can both be observed to be 'sticky' as they pull apart and form transient 'lemon chains.' If clumps of RBCs cannot be determined to be aggregates or rouleaux networks, the test should be repeated with diluted RBCs.

A rapid slide test using undiluted RBCs is superior for comparing strong macroscopic agglutination to rouleaux. Strong agglutination is usually evident within 1 minute and reaches a maximum reaction within 3 minutes. After 1-2 minutes in the cat and 2-3 minutes in the dog, desiccation of the sample on the slide results in rouleaux formation, beginning at the edges of the sample. However, rouleaux formation of equivalent intensity to strong agglutination requires 5-10 minutes to form. Microscopically large aggregates and rouleaux can be identified, but small aggregates cannot be identified because of the high density of RBCs.

A rapid slide test using diluted RBCs is superior for distinguishing agglutination and rouleaux microscopically and for detecting weak agglutination. In canine preparations, rouleaux will form in 3-4 minutes in plasma but will not form in serum with normal protein levels. However, as the slides are rocked the RBCs swirl and become unevenly distributed, mimicking macroscopic rouleaux. This effect may be more pronounced in serum than in plasma. In feline preparations, macroscopic rouleaux formation begins within 2-3 minutes.

Figures 15.6 and 15.7 show the interpretation of crossmatching in dogs and cats.

Any agglutination and/or haemolysis at 37°C and/or room temperature is a positive test.

Rapid slide or phase I–II of tube test:

- A *positive major crossmatch* indicates a significant antibody titre in the recipient against donor RBCs and precludes the use of that donor for RBC transfusion. Strong reactions are usually due to anti-DEA 1.1 antibodies. Weak reactions are usually due to anti-DEA 1.1 or 1.2, and perhaps anti-DEA 7, antibodies. The stronger the crossmatch reaction, the more severe will be the clinical reaction after transfusion.
- A *positive minor crossmatch* indicates the presence of antibodies in the donor against recipient RBCs, with the stronger reactions usually being due to anti-DEA 1.1 antibodies as in the major crossmatch. The significance of the antibodies depends on the titre in the donor and the volume of plasma transfused. If the minor crossmatch reaction is strong, even small volumes of donor plasma may cause a significant transfusion reaction and precludes the use of the donor unless the donor RBCs are washed. With weaker reactions, packed RBCs from the donor may be transfused. With very weak reactions, transfusion of large volumes of plasma should be avoided.
- A *positive recipient control* indicates that the patient is autoagglutinating. If the major crossmatch is positive with a similar strength of reaction, agglutination is probably due to non-specific anti-RBC antibodies and not a specific anti-DEA antibody.
- A *positive donor control* usually indicates a procedural error. It is also possible that the donor has subclinical immune-mediated haemolytic anaemia and should not be used.

Phase III of tube test:

- A *positive major crossmatch* indicates the presence of subagglutinating antibodies. These antibodies are most likely to be anti-DEA 1.2, 3, 5 or 7. These will not result in an acute transfusion reaction but may result in delayed haemolysis. The donor should not be used if a more compatible donor is available, especially if the reaction is strong. If a compatible donor is not available, the incompatible donor may be used to provide temporary RBC replacement, especially if there is life-threatening anaemia.
- A *positive minor crossmatch* is of minimal clinical importance, except, perhaps when large volumes of plasma are to be transfused.
- A *positive recipient or donor control* is a positive direct antiglobulin (Coombs') test, and should be interpreted as above.

The nature of the incompatibility may be further characterized by incubating recipient serum with RBCs of known antigenic composition. In humans this procedure is referred to as antibody screening. Antibody screening is performed before crossmatching and its use has reduced the value of the latter.

When transfusing multiple units of a blood product, incompatibility between donor units is of minimal concern, as long as all units are compatible with the recipient.

Figure 15.6: Interpretation of crossmatch results in the dog.

- Type B serum mixed with type A or AB RBCs results in typically strong macroscopic agglutination (see Figure 15.2).
- Type A serum mixed with type B or AB RBCs results in weak macroscopic, only microscopic or no agglutination. For practical purposes the rapid slide test is negative macroscopically whether using undiluted or diluted RBCs, because the possibility of rouleaux formation precludes positive identification of small aggregates. The test is also usually negative microscopically when using undiluted RBCs, because the high RBC density and rouleaux formation preclude identification of small aggregates.
- Type AB serum (uncommon blood type) mixed with type A or type B RBCs does not result in any agglutination.
- *Negative major and minor crossmatch:* donor and recipient are probably of the same blood type (A, B or AB). The donor can be used. It is also possible that a weak anti-A or anti-B titre is present in the donor or recipient. Some type B cats with weak anti-A titres have now been reported (Knottenbelt *et al.*, 1999). If the recipient has a weak anti-A or anti-B titre, use of an incompatible donor may cause a mild acute transfusion reaction, and delayed haemolysis will occur.
- *Positive major crossmatch:* strong macroscopic agglutination denotes type B recipient and type A or AB donor. Minor crossmatch will be negative or weakly positive with a type A donor and negative with a type AB donor. Use of this donor is likely to result in a severe transfusion reaction.
- *Positive minor crossmatch:* strong macroscopic agglutination denotes type A or type AB recipient and type B donor. Major crossmatch will be negative or weakly positive with a type A recipient and negative with a type AB recipient. In the likely event that the recipient is type A, use of this donor may cause a mild to moderate acute transfusion reaction, and delayed haemolysis will occur. If the recipient is type AB, use of this donor may cause a mild to moderate acute transfusion reaction.
- *Positive donor or recipient control:* This usually indicates a procedural error. It is also possible that the donor or recipient is autoagglutinating. In addition, some type B and AB cats have been reported to have weak anti-B antibodies (Knottenbelt *et al.*, 1999).

Figure 15.7: Interpretation of crossmatch results in the cat.

Crossmatching in dogs

Few studies have examined the utility of the complete crossmatch for dogs in the veterinary clinical setting. A complete crossmatch will detect all clinically important anti-RBC antibodies.

Specifically, a complete crossmatch is usually needed to detect anti-DEA 3, 5 and 7 antibodies and low titres of anti-DEA 1.1, 1.2 and 1.3 antibodies. A complete crossmatch is usually performed at reference laboratories as few clinics can justify purchasing the reagents. This is again a problem because many transfusions are given in emergency or urgent situations. Even for clinics affiliated to a reference laboratory, there is insufficient time in an emergency to perform a complete crossmatch. Furthermore, a complete crossmatch adds a substantial expense to the transfusion.

The abbreviated crossmatch is performed at room temperature and omits an antiglobulin test. It may be performed by either the rapid slide or tube method. It is quick and inexpensive and can be done in any clinic. As with the complete crossmatch it is subject to false-positive and false-negative findings when conducted by inexperienced staff. The abbreviated crossmatch will detect anti-RBC antibodies that are present in high enough titres to cause a clinically moderate to severe haemolytic reaction. Although

the antibodies may be stronger haemolysins than agglutinins, agglutination will be detected in the crossmatch. Complement can be added to improve detection of haemolysis. The abbreviated crossmatch is unlikely to detect antibodies that will cause delayed or mild acute reactions.

When should crossmatching be performed? A complete crossmatch can be justified scientifically in all cases, even where blood type of donor and recipient are known, since canine blood groups are not fully characterized. However, this is economically and practically not feasible for most clinics. Routine complete crossmatching is not performed at the OVC. An abbreviated crossmatch is recommended in all cases simply to maintain expertise in the procedure. A crossmatch (complete preferred) should always be performed when:

- The recipient has been previously transfused more than 4 days before the planned transfusion
- There is a history of a transfusion reaction
- The recipient's transfusion history is unknown
- The recipient has previously been pregnant.

In addition, complete crossmatching is recommended when a dog is likely to receive multiple transfusions or where any immunological stimulation is likely to be detrimental, even where donor blood is of universal type or known to be compatible with the recipient's blood type. The latter situation includes immune-mediated haemolytic anaemia (IMHA), but in many cases RBC autoantibody will result in an apparent incompatibility with all donors. The crossmatch may assist in selecting the 'most compatible' donor.

The minor crossmatch is less important than the major because of dilution of the donor antibodies in the recipient. Indeed, some authors have recommended elimination of the minor crossmatch. The only important minor incompatibility involves anti-DEA 1.1 antibodies reacting in phases I–II of the crossmatch, unless large volumes of plasma are to be transfused. However, even small amounts of donor plasma with a high titre of anti-DEA 1.1 antibodies can cause a significant transfusion reaction in a DEA 1.1 positive dog. Such a titre can only develop in a previously pregnant or transfused DEA 1.1 negative dog. As noted previously, such dogs should not be accepted as blood donors. Thus clinics with properly selected blood donors can eliminate a routine minor crossmatch. If a donor of uncertain background is being used, the minor crossmatch should be performed unless the recipient is known to be DEA 1.1 negative or the donor DEA 1.1 positive. The minor crossmatch is also recommended if large-volume plasma transfusions are anticipated or where any immunological reaction is considered deleterious.

DEA compatibility and plasma products
Because of the emphasis on having DEA 1.1/1.2 negative RBC donors, veterinarians commonly insist on plasma products from DEA 1.1/1.2 negative donors. There is no increased risk of an acute transfusion reaction with plasma from a DEA 1.1/1.2 positive dog. Indeed, such plasma is less likely to cause a minor incompatibility reaction as DEA 1.1/1.2 positive dogs are less likely to be sensitized. However, there is the potential for DEA alloimmunization owing to contaminating RBCs in plasma products, as only small volumes of incompatible RBCs are needed to stimulate antibody production. In humans, fresh frozen plasma contains only traces of RBC stroma and rarely causes sensitization. Plasma prepared from stored whole blood and platelet-rich plasma contains higher levels of contamination and occasionally causes sensitization. It is therefore recommended that DEA 1.1 or 1.1/1.2 negative blood be routinely used to prepare plasma by centrifugation of stored whole blood or by sedimentation of whole blood and to prepare platelet products. This is consistent with the recommendation that canine RBC donors should routinely be DEA 1.1 or 1.1/1.2 negative. However, since the occurrence of sensitization with fresh frozen plasma is probably rare, the use of fresh frozen plasma and plasma from expired fresh frozen plasma prepared from DEA 1.1 or 1.1/1.2 positive donors is acceptable. This practice substantially increases the donor pool, which is important because patients requiring plasma transfusions often require multiple units. After blood collection from a DEA 1.1 or 1.1/1.2 positive donor, the plasma is harvested and the RBCs are returned to the donor.

Crossmatching in cats
A crossmatch using the rapid slide method or phase I of the tube method at room temperature will detect RBC incompatibility in most cases. Crossmatching is recommended in all cases where donor and/or recipient blood type is not known, especially if a transfusion is to be given to a breed with a known high prevalence of B blood type. The utility of crossmatching in addition to blood typing donor and recipient is not known. Potential benefits include verification of blood-typing results and detection of non-AB anti-RBC antibodies.

Crossmatching in addition to blood typing is recommended if a cat has been previously transfused or is infected with feline leukaemia virus, because there are anecdotal reports of non-AB incompatibilities in these situations. Currently at the OVC donors are blood typed and are then crossmatched against naïve domestic shorthaired and domestic longhaired recipients by using a rapid slide method. This policy is followed to reduce costs because B and AB blood types are rare in the region's non-purebred cat population. Recipient blood type is, however, determined in purebred cat breeds with a reported prevalence of type B blood.

ANTICOAGULANT–PRESERVATIVE SOLUTIONS

The solutions into which blood is collected contain either heparin or citrate, which function as anticoagulants by binding Ca^{++}. The use of heparin should be restricted to blood collected for immediate transfusion. The citrate solutions may also contain agents that act as RBC preservatives. The purpose of these preservatives is to support the glycolytic energy metabolism (adenosine triphosphate production) of RBCs to maintain their viability during storage. Historically, dextrose was the first preservative added to citrate solution, followed by phosphate and then adenine. The additive nutrient solutions Adsol, Nutricel and Optisol were then developed. Composition and use of anticoagulant–preservative solutions in the dog and cat have been reviewed (Wardrop, 1995) and are summarized in Figure 15.8.

Phosphate is also a substrate for 2,3-diphosphoglycerate (2,3-DPG) production. 2,3-DPG decreases the affinity of haemoglobin for oxygen,

Solution	Components	Supplied* and use	Maximum whole blood storage time**	Maximum packed red cells storage time**	Comment
Heparin	Heparin 1000 IU/ml	Supplied: 10 ml bottles Use: 5-12.5 IU/ml of blood For a cat donation draw 300-750 IU (0.3-0.75 ml) into a 60 ml syringe	2 days (dog, cat)	Storage not recommended	Used most for cat donations No red cell preservative Readily available in most clinics Caution: do not confuse with 10 000 IU/ml solution May cause heparinization of smaller recipients (see Transfusion reactions)
Sodium citrate	Sodium citrate	Supplied: 3.8% solution, 500 ml bag*** or prepared by a pharmacy Use: 1 ml 3.8% solution:9 ml blood For a cat donation draw 6 ml into a 60 ml syringe For solutions of strength other than 3.8% use 0.5 g sodium citrate/100 ml blood	5 days (dog) Not known (cat)	Storage not recommended	No red cell preservative Obsolete in small animal medicine, but used extensively for plasma harvesting with large animals (red cells returned to donor)
Acid citrate dextrose Dextrose (ACD)	Solution A (ACD-A): Citric acid Sodium citrate Dextrose	Supplied: 500 ml or 1000 ml bag,*** human collecting bag containing 67.5 ml Use: 1 ml ACD-A: 7-9 ml blood For a cat donation draw 8 ml into a 60 ml syringe	Not known	Storage not recommended	Standard solutions for many years Citric acid was once thought to increase red cell preservation Used mostly for cat donations for fresh transfusion Preferable to heparin and sodium citrate for fresh transfusion Superseded by CPD-based solutions for blood banking ACD-A has higher concentrations of citric acid, sodium citrate, dextrose than ACD-B ACD-A preferred for fresh transfusions owing to larger volume of collected blood
	Solution B (ACD-B) Citric acid Sodium citrate Dextrose	Supplied: 500 ml bags*** Use: 1 ml ACD-B:4 ml blood For a cat donation draw 15 ml into a 60 ml syringe	3 weeks (dog) 4 weeks (cat)	Storage not recommended	
Citrate phosphate dextrose (CPD)	Citric acid Sodium citrate Phosphate Dextrose	Supplied: human collecting bag*** containing 63 ml or 70 ml Use: 0.14 ml/ml blood For a cat donation draw 7.5 ml into a 60 ml syringe	4 weeks (dog, cat)	Storage not recommended	63 ml bag is for collecting 450 ml of blood; 70 ml bag is for 500 ml
Citrate phosphate dextrose adenine₁ (CPDA₁)	Citric acid Sodium citrate Phosphate Dextrose Adenine	Supplied: human collecting bag*** containing 63 ml or 70 ml; 50 ml bottles Use: 0.14 ml/ml blood For a cat donation draw 7.5 ml into a 60 ml syringe	5 weeks (dog, cat)	3 weeks (dog, cat)	63 ml bag is for collecting 450 ml of blood; 70 ml bag is for 500 ml
AS-1 (Adsol)	Dextrose Adenine Mannitol Sodium chloride	Supplied: human collection pack,**** collecting bag contains 63 ml CPD, 100 ml Adsol added to 1 canine unit For cat blood, 10 ml of Adsol is added to 1 feline unit	Not applicable	5-6 weeks (dog) 6 weeks (cat)	Adsol should be added to red cells within 72 hours of collection
AS-3 (Nutricel)	Dextrose Adenine Phosphate Sodium chloride Sodium citrate Citric acid	Supplied: human collection pack,**** collecting bag contains 63 ml CPD2, 100 ml Nutricel added to 1 canine unit For cat blood, 10 ml of Nutricel is added to 1 feline unit	Not applicable	5-6 weeks (dog) 6 weeks (cat)	Nutricel should be added to red cells within 72 hours of collection
AS-5 (Optisol)	Dextrose Adenine Mannitol Sodium chloride	Supplied: human collection pack,**** collecting bag contains 63 ml CPD, 100 ml Optisol added to 1 canine unit For cat blood, 10 ml of Optisol is added to 1 feline unit	Not applicable	5-6 weeks (dog) 6 weeks (cat)	Optisol should be added to red cells within 72 hours of collection

Figure 15.8: *Anticoagulant–preservative solutions for blood collection and blood banking in the dog and cat.*
*Supply may vary with country. **This should be determined based on 75% in vivo red blood cell (RBC) viability at the end of the storage period, as determined by 24 hour post-transfusion survival in autologous recipients by using radiolabelling or biotinylation techniques. Recommendations here are based on in vivo viability studies, in vitro studies and clinical experience. The blood product may be used up to midnight on the expiry date. Refrigerated human RBCs may be rejuvenated by using a special solution up to 3 days after expiration. The rejuvenated red cells must be washed, refrigerated and transfused within 24 hours of rejuvenation. ***For collecting cat blood into a syringe by using solutions supplied in human collecting bags or bags used for haemapheresis and related procedures, a sampling site coupler (Figure 15.16) is used, and the desired volume of solution is aseptically withdrawn. ****The nutrient additive solutions (AS) are provided in special collection packs consisting of a bag containing the nutrient solution, satellite bags for plasma or platelet storage and a collecting bag containing CPD (citrate phosphate dextrose) solution (with Adsol and Optisol) or CPD2 solution (with Nutricel). CPD2 differs from CPD in having twice the amount of dextrose. The processing of these bags is described in Blood product preparation and storage. The collection packs routinely used with dogs contain 63 ml CPD/CPD2 and 100 ml of nutrient AS and are designed for collecting and processing 450 ml of blood. Collection packs are also available with 70 ml CPD/CPD2 and 110–111 ml of nutrient AS that are designed for collecting and processing of 500 ml of blood.

thereby promoting oxygen release to needy tissues. The concentration of 2,3-DPG gradually decreases during storage in ACD, so that blood at the end of the storage period is not as effective as fresh blood in delivering oxygen to needy tissues. Upon transfusion, up to 50% of normal 2,3-DPG levels are synthesized within 3–8 hours, and most within 24 hours, but this may not be sufficient in critical cases. CPD was developed in part to maintain better 2,3-DPG levels. However, 2,3-DPG levels still decline somewhat during storage in phosphate-containing solutions. In a dog with severe acute anaemia, blood with a sufficient level of 2,3-DPG for immediate tissue oxygenation is desirable. For such a case, packed RBCs stored less than 2 weeks and whole blood stored less than 4 weeks are preferred, assuming storage in CPD, CPDA$_1$, Adsol, Nutricel or Optisol. This is not as important in cats since this species normally has low levels of 2,3-DPG.

Dog and cat blood is most often collected into CPD, CPD2 or CPDA$_1$. For syringe collection in cats, the solutions supplied in bottles are less expensive to use than those supplied in collecting bags where the collecting system is wasted. Whenever a solution is being drawn into a syringe, the rubber diaphragm of the container should be wiped with alcohol and allowed to dry before needle puncture.

BLOOD DONATION

Dogs

Volume and frequency
Fifteen to 20% of estimated blood volume can be safely donated.

$$\text{Estimated blood volume (litres)} = 0.08\text{–}0.09 \times \text{Bodyweight (kg)}$$

Using the above formula, the maximum acceptable donation volume is about 16–18 ml/kg. By convention and for convenience, a standard blood donation in the dog is 450 ± 45 ml, which is referred to as 'one canine unit.'

Dogs can donate every 3 weeks as long as they receive good nutrition. The need for iron supplementation in the diet should be determined by measuring serum iron levels at least once a year. Microcytosis is a late change in iron deficiency and should not be used to monitor iron status. Serum total iron binding capacity is typically increased in dogs that frequently donate blood, reflecting increased erythropoiesis, and should not be interpreted as a sign of iron deficiency. At the OVC, clinic-owned donors may be given 100 mg of ferric pyrophosphate as part of a liquid vitamin–mineral supplement added to the ration every 1–2 months.

Repeat donor stress is preferable to patient death, and in emergencies a dog can donate again after 1 week. If a progressive decrease in a donor's PCV is noted, then the donor should be rested until the RBC count and indices have normalized. Client-owned dogs usually donate blood every 2–3 months, and nutritional supplementation is not required. Guidelines have not been established for how frequently dogs can donate blood for plasma and/or platelet harvesting if the RBCs are returned to the donor. It is suggested that whole blood donation guidelines be followed.

Collection system

Human blood collection packs: Modern human blood banking standards stipulate the use of closed blood collection systems. A closed system is one that has no potential for environmental contact of the blood as it flows from the vein to the collecting container. Any system involving the operator having to connect pieces together is an open system, which increases the risk of microbial contamination. Closed systems are ideal, especially when blood products are to be stored, since such products are excellent microbiological growth media. However, open systems have been used for many years and are acceptable as long as strict attention is given to avoiding contamination of connecting surfaces. Also, closed systems do not guarantee sterility as contamination from cutaneous organisms can occur, even with aseptic venepuncture technique.

Human blood collection packs are currently the most suitable closed collection systems for use in dogs (Figure 15.9). Such a pack is a self-contained unit consisting of a 16 G thin-walled needle, tubing and plastic collecting bag containing an anticoagulant–preservative solution. Packs are also available with 'satellite bags' for preparation of blood components. During the donation the blood flows into the collecting bag by gravity or vacuum assistance (Figure 15.10). High-rate infusion pumps have been used for blood collection in large animals but this method has not been reported in the dog.

Vacuum bottles: Vacuum bottles with anticoagulant, or to which anticoagulant may be added, are still available although obsolete. When a vacuum bottle is used it is an open collection system. A special tubing set is required that has an attached needle at one end (to pierce the diaphragm of the collecting bottle) and can accommodate a needle for venepuncture at the other end. As the blood enters the bottle it should be directed against the side, not the bottom, to minimize haemolysis. Alternatively the bottle may be held upside down so that the blood flows through the anticoagulant. Blood collected in this manner is not suitable for storage, and contact with glass deactivates platelets and factors VIII (FVIII) and XIII (FXIII).

Syringes: In an emergency situation, if a regular collection system is not available, multiple aliquots of blood can be collected by using 60 ml syringes and a winged-infusion set as described for cats below. Care must be taken to avoid contamination when attaching and

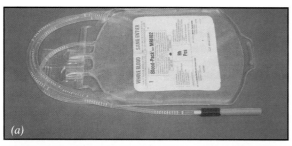

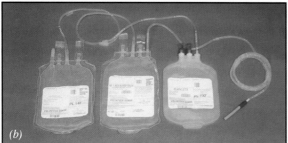

Figure 15.9: *Human blood collection packs. (a) Whole blood collection pack designed for collecting and processing 450 ml of blood. Packs designed for collecting and processing 500 ml of blood are also available but are not routinely used with dogs. (b) Collection pack with satellite bag suitable for preparing plasma and platelet products. This set also incorporates a bag containing Adsol (see Figure 15.8).*

Collection packs may be supplied in packages containing more than one pack. Manufacturer's instructions should be followed for length of time unused bags may be stored in opened packages. It is important that the package is tightly closed after removing a pack to prevent desiccation of the remaining packs, especially if the packs are not to be used within 1–2 months. Hands should be thoroughly washed before removing a pack from the package to minimize contamination of the pouch, which may result in fungal growth. The package should be inspected for fungal growth whenever a pack is removed, and contaminated packages should be discarded.

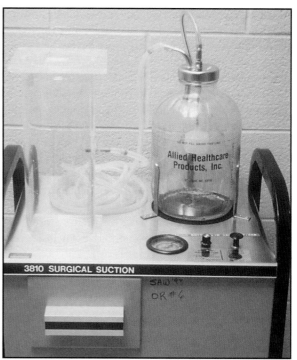

Figure 15.10: *Plexiglas vacuum chamber attached to surgical suction unit. The collecting bag is placed into the vacuum chamber to shorten the donation time. Such chambers were once commercially manufactured for human use and may be available from hospital surplus suppliers. Chambers for veterinary use are available from the Animal Blood Bank (Dixon, California, USA). A vacuum pressure of 125–175 mmHg (5–7 inchesHg, 170–238 cmH₂O)* *should be used. Vacuum pressures above this may result in collapse of the vein. If a collection set containing satellite bags is used, the bags are rolled up and placed beneath or behind the collecting bag, to ensure that they do not occlude the vacuum port.*

detaching the collecting syringes from the infusion set. Alternatively, a new intravenous saline bag can be emptied, anticoagulant added and a 16–18 G needle and fluid administration set used to fashion a collection system. In the author's opinion, it is preferable to use an irregular blood collection system than to withhold a potentially life-saving transfusion. Blood should not be stored, however, after having been collected by such methods.

Venepuncture and blood collection

Fasting: A 12-hour fast before donation is recommended in the event that sedation or anaesthesia is required or that hypotension causes nausea and vomiting. If the donor has not been fasted, for example, with an emergency donation, post-prandial lipaemia does not seem to affect the quality of fresh or stored blood products or to increase the risk of transfusion reactions. Lipaemia may increase rouleaux formation, which complicates crossmatching. Lipaemia may also cause some platelet activation, but the clinical importance of this is not known.

Blood vessels: Blood is usually collected by jugular venepuncture. The cephalic vein may be used in a large dog. The femoral artery may also be used, but this is technically more difficult, there is an increased chance of haematoma formation and repeat collection can lead to scarring of the vessel. Femoral artery puncture or cardiocentesis are the preferred methods of collection from terminal donors as these methods increase volume yield. Carotid–jugular fistulae may be created to facilitate haemoaccess, but are not recommended.

Procedure: Two people, a restrainer and a phlebotomist, are required for a blood donation. A third person is helpful to provide additional restraint and handle the collecting bag. Most dogs are restrained in lateral recumbency for jugular venepuncture; some dogs are more comfortable in sternal recumbency. Habituated donors can be manually restrained in a quiet location. If sedation is required, narcotics such as oxymorphone (0.05–0.2 mg/kg i.v. or i.m., maximum dose 4.5 mg) or butorphanol (0.05–0.4mg/kg i.v. or i.m., maximum dose 6 mg) are often sufficient, but diazepam (0.25–0.5 mg/kg i.v.) or a low dose of acepromazine (0.01–0.025 mg/kg i.v. or i.m.) may be given as well. Intractable dogs may have blood collected under anaesthesia with barbiturates, propofol and/or inhalation agents. Trace drug levels in the collected blood are of minimal concern, except acepromazine which impairs platelet function and should be avoided where blood is intended to be used in the treatment of thrombocytopenic dogs.

A 19 G winged infusion set or 20 G catheter placed aseptically into the cephalic or lateral saphenous vein is optional. The catheter facilitates prompt intravenous administration of sedative drugs and intravenous fluids should these be required.

A blood donation is illustrated in Figures 15.11– 15.15. During collection there must be strict adherence to asepsis, especially if blood is to be stored. Venepuncture should be minimally traumatic to minimize platelet clumping and coagulation. The injection of local anaesthesia at the venepuncture site is not recommended because it interferes with visualization and palpation of the vein. If local anaesthesia is desired, a topical preparation containing prilocaine and/or lignocaine is effective. A 'mini cut-down' can be performed but is not usually necessary.

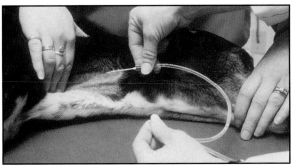

Figures 15.11: Canine blood donation. The skin over the venepuncture site is clipped and surgically prepared. Inexperienced phlebotomists should wear sterile gloves. The jugular vein is raised with gentle pressure placed over the jugular groove at the thoracic inlet by either the assistant (in this case the owner), the phlebotomist or by use of a tourniquet and a large wooden bead. It is important that the skin is taut over the vein.

Before removing the needle cover, the tubing is kinked or clamped to prevent the anticoagulant–preservative solution from emptying out of the tubing into the bag. To prevent damage to the collection tubing when clamping, clean bandage tape should be wrapped around the grooves of a haemostat, or a plastic intravenous tubing clamp should be used.

If the dog is in lateral recumbency, directing the needle towards the heart facilitates venepuncture. If the dog is in sternal recumbency, directing the needle towards the head facilitates venepuncture.

The needle should be held at 10–20 degrees to the skin. Alternatively, the skin may be penetrated at 45 degrees and the needle reoriented in line with the vein at 10–20 degrees. A sharper angle is likely to result in piercing of the opposite vessel wall.

In either case, a quick sharp thrust is less painful to the donor and less apt to push away the vessel wall than a gradual thrust. A popping sensation may be felt when the needle enters the vein.

Successful venepuncture is usually indicated by a flash of blood into the tubing. If the phlebotomist believes the needle is correctly placed, but no flash occurs, then the tubing clamp should be released. If blood does not flow into the tubing, the tubing should be clamped, the needle withdrawn and venepuncture attempted again.

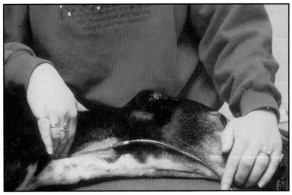

Figure 15.12: Canine blood donation. During collection the needle should be at least 1.5 cm within the vein to guard against dislodgement. The tubing is secured manually, either against the table or at the needle hub against the skin. In the author's experience, the former is preferable when the donor is in lateral recumbency, the latter resulting in more dislodgement during donation. If the donor is in sternal recumbency, the needle hub must be manually secured.

The bag is closely observed for continuous expansion during collection. If cessation of flow is suspected, the site of entry of the tube into the bag should be digitally compressed to wipe away residual blood and observed for flow. If blood flow stops, the venepuncture site should be examined for haematoma formation. If none is noted, the needle should be gently rotated. If blood flow does not resume, the needle should be slowly advanced in line with the vein. If this does not result in resumption of blood flow, the needle should be slowly withdrawn until blood flow resumes.

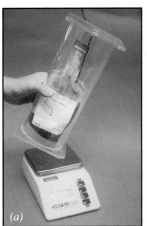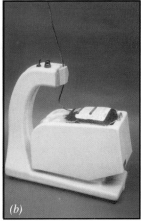

Figure 15.13: Canine blood donation. (a) The collecting bag is gently rocked as blood flows in, to ensure adequate mixing with the anticoagulant–preservative solution. An assistant most easily accomplishes this, but an experienced phlebotomist can stabilize the tubing with one hand and rock the collecting bag with the other. An alternative to rocking the chamber during vacuum collection is to hang the bag upside down in the chamber. This ensures that the blood flows through the anticoagulant-preservative solution. A laboratory blood tube rocker may be used with gravity collection.

A scale is tared to the combined weight of the collecting bag, anticoagulant-preservative solution and vacuum chamber if used, and the weight is checked periodically during the donation. The tube is clamped near the needle when the desired weight of 477 ± 48 g of blood is reached before removing the needle, to minimize air entry into the collecting bag.

(b) A blood shaker can be used, which rocks the blood during gravity collection and clamps the tubing when the bag reaches a desired weight.

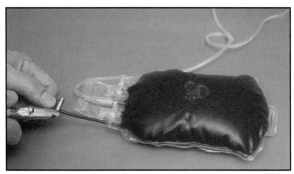

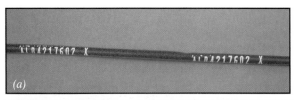

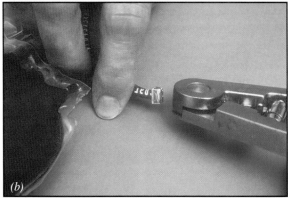

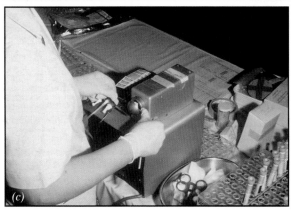

Figure 15.14: *Canine blood donation. Once the donation is completed, the blood remaining in the tubing is mechanically (preferably) or digitally stripped into the bag. The bag is gently rocked back and forth to ensure adequate mixing, and then the bag is gently manually compressed to refill the tubing.*

Figure 15.15: *Canine blood donation. (a) The tubing is sealed at the 'X' to provide aliquots of about 0.5 ml, which can be used to measure packed cell volume, total solids and other variables on the blood, and to perform compatibility testing, without invading the bag. The tubing is left attached to the bag, folded at the sealing points and secured to the bag with a rubber band. (b) Aluminium sealing clips are most cost-efficient for the quantity of blood bags processed by veterinary clinics. (c) Thermal sealers are more time efficient when large quantities of blood are being processed.*
If a sealing system is not available, firm knots may be tied, but these do not provide as secure a barrier against leakage and contamination.

Volume: The standard collection volume is 450 ± 45 ml. This volume is estimated by weight. Assuming 1.0 ml of blood weighs about 1.06 g, the standard collection weight is about 477 ± 48 g. The minimum acceptable 'underdraw' for blood collected into CPD (citrate phosphate dextrose) or $CPDA_1$ (citrate phosphate dextrose adenine$_1$) to be transfused as whole blood is 405 ml (429 g). The minimum acceptable underdraw for blood to be used to prepare packed RBCs is 300 ml (318 g), in which case the plasma is discarded. Underdrawing the bag below these values decreases RBC survival during storage and increases the risk of citrate intoxication (see Transfusion reactions). The maximum acceptable 'overdraw' is 495 ml (525 g). Overdrawing the bag beyond these values increases the risk of coagulation during collection and rupture of the bag during centrifugation and decreases RBC survival during storage.

Time: The entire donation process, if problem free, typically takes 20–30 minutes. Blood collection is completed within 5–15 minutes with gravity collection and 3–10 minutes with vacuum collection. A brief stoppage of flow during collection (e.g. <2 minutes) usually does not result in coagulation but may result in some platelet clumping. Collections of longer than 15 minutes do not result in coagulation if blood flow is continuous but may also result in platelet clumping.

Problems: If a haematoma develops or the needle becomes dislodged, blood collection must usually be discontinued and a new venepuncture site selected. If this occurs early in the procedure, it is best to begin again with a new collection set. If this occurs well into the procedure, it is unlikely that a new unit can be collected without excessive donor blood loss. Based on human standards, a blood bag should be discarded if donation is completely interrupted. However, if the veterinary clinic cannot afford to waste the donation, then as long as contamination of the needle did not occur, it is the author's opinion that completing the donation from a new venepuncture site is acceptable, especially if the blood is to be given as a fresh transfusion. If both jugular veins develop haematomata and completing the donation is essential, then anaesthesia of the donor and surgical exposure of the vein can be performed. The vein is always located in the middle of the haematoma.

Aftercare of the donor

Moderate pressure is placed over the venepuncture site for 2–5 minutes. A neck bandage is optional. The dog is observed for 15–30 minutes for weakness, pale mucous membranes, weak pulses and other signs of hypotension.

Volume replacement with saline or similar crystalloid solutions has been recommended after donation. This is no longer routinely practised at the OVC.

Volume replacement at two to three times the blood loss (i.e. about 1000–1500 ml) is given at 90 ml/kg/h i.v., if there are clinical signs of hypotension.

The dog may be fed after the post-donation observation period. The owner is advised to avoid exercising the dog excessively for several days.

Cats

The principles described above for the dog apply to the cat. Differences in feline blood donation are described below.

Volume and frequency

Fifteen to 20% of estimated blood volume can be safely donated.

$$\text{Estimated blood volume (litres)} = 0.055\text{–}0.065 \times \text{Bodyweight (kg)}$$

Using the above formula the maximum acceptable donation volume is approximately 11–13 ml/kg, referred to as 'one feline unit.' A standard donation in the cat at the OVC results in 60 ml of anticoagulated blood. Cats can donate once every 3–4 weeks and again in 2 weeks in times of emergencies. Cats that donate blood on a monthly basis, or more frequently, should be given regular iron supplementation in their diet (e.g. 10 mg/kg ferrous sulphate twice a week, 5 mg/cat ferrous fumarate daily). Iron supplementation in the form of daily vitamin-mineral tablets may be preferred since liquid iron supplements may be unpalatable. The level of supplementation should be adjusted based on laboratory assessment of iron deficiency.

Collection system

Infusion set: Blood is commonly collected from cats with a 19 G winged infusion set attached to a 60 ml syringe into which the anticoagulant–preservative solution has been drawn (Figures 15.16–15.18). For blood banking purposes, the blood is then transferred to a 100–150 ml storage bag. Alternatively, the anticoagulant–preservative solution may be added to the storage bag, the storage bag tubing attached to an 18 G needle for venepuncture and the blood collected by gravity or with vacuum assistance. These are open systems.

Closed systems: Closed systems with small bags and needles are currently not available. There are two options if a closed collection system is desired. Firstly, a closed system can be fabricated by using a sterile tube welding instrument designed for preparation of unique human paediatric blood collection sets (Springer *et al.*, 1998). Secondly, standard double bag human blood collection packs can be used to collect feline blood (Price, 1991).

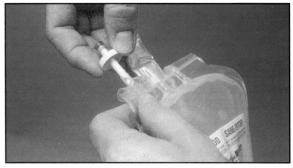

Figure 15.16: Feline blood donation. A sampling site coupler (e.g. Baxter 4C2405), that provides an injection port for blood product bags, is attached to a human collecting bag so that a small volume of anticoagulant–preservative solution may be withdrawn.

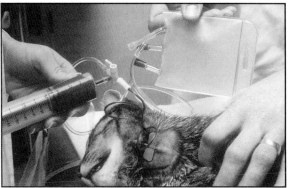

Figure 15.17: Feline blood donation. A 19 G winged infusion set ('butterfly') is attached to a 60 ml syringe into which the anticoagulant–preservative solution has been drawn. The same principles concerning venepuncture in the dog apply to the cat. The syringe is gently rocked during blood collection. The collection tubing may be gently manually secured against the donor's head when in lateral recumbency. Care is taken to avoid excessive negative pressure, which may cause haemolysis. Two 35 ml syringes may be used to increase donation volume from a large donor.

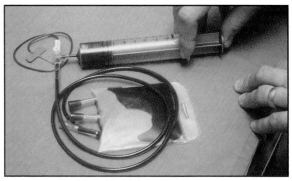

Figure 15.18: Feline blood donation. For blood banking purposes, a three-way stopcock is placed between the butterfly and the syringe, and a 100 ml capacity storage bag (Animal Blood Bank, Dixon, California, USA) is attached. After collecting the blood into the syringe, the stopcock is turned, and the blood is slowly injected into the storage bag. Any air that has entered the bag is withdrawn, along with sufficient blood to fill the tube to the desired amount; the tube is then sealed as described above.

An alternative storage bag is a 150 ml capacity paediatric transfer pack (e.g. Baxter 4R2001). In this case a sampling site coupler (see Figure 15.16) is attached to the bag, and the blood is slowly injected into the bag through an 18 G needle.

The feline jugular vein is as large as the human antecubital vein (the standard human venepuncture site) and can accommodate the 16 G needle. The length of the needle makes venepuncture more difficult than with shorter needles when the donor is in lateral recumbency, so sternal recumbency is recommended. If this system is used, the collecting bag is rolled up to express excess anticoagulant–preservative solution into the satellite bag, leaving 8 ml in the collecting bag (which may be verified by measuring bag weights). Blood is collected by gravity.

Sedation and anaesthesia

Almost all cats require sedation or anaesthesia. A 21–23 G winged infusion set or 20–22 G catheter aseptically placed into the cephalic or medial saphenous vein is recommended. Recommended sedation and anaesthesia protocols include:

- Ketamine 100 mg/ml mixed 1:1 or 1:2 with diazepam 5 mg/ml. Give 0.1 ml/kg i.v. Additional boluses of one-quarter to one-half the initial dose may be given to prolong anaesthesia
- Ketamine 10 mg/kg and midazolam 0.2 mg/kg, mixed together, i.m. Additional boluses of ketamine 1.0 mg/kg i.v., may be given to prolong anaesthesia
- Ketamine 2 mg/kg and midazolam 0.1 mg/kg, mixed together, i.v. Additional boluses of one-quarter to one-half the initial dose may be given to prolong anaesthesia.

The principal disadvantages of ketamine-based protocols are the prolonged post-anaesthesia effect and the possibility of arrhythmogenesis in cats with undiagnosed hypertrophic cardiomyopathy. For these reasons some prefer to use neuroleptanalgesia-based regimens:

- Oxymorphone 0.05–0.1 mg/kg and acepromazine 0.04–0.10 mg/kg, mixed together, i.m. or i.v.
- Butorphanol 0.2–0.4 mg/kg ± acepromazine 0.04–0.10 mg/kg, mixed together, i.m. or i.v.
- Butorphanol 0.1–0.2 mg/kg ± diazepam 0.5 mg/kg, mixed together, i.v.

The principal disadvantages of these neuroleptanalgesia regimens are potential exacerbation of hypotension by acepromazine during blood collection and insufficient sedation for blood collection. Some phlebotomists prefer to sedate donors with oxymorphone 0.1–0.2 mg/kg i.v., without acepromazine to minimize hypotension. If sedation is insufficient with acepromazine and/or a narcotic, then the following agents may be added:

- Propofol, calculated induction dose of 4 mg/kg i.v., with one-half the dose given as a rapid bolus and the remainder given to effect. Additional boluses of propofol 1.0 mg/kg i.v., are given to prolong anaesthesia
- Ketamine–diazepam, as previously described, 0.5–0.1 ml/kg i.v. Additional boluses of one-quarter to one-half the initial dose may be given to prolong anaesthesia. Sedation with intramuscular butorphanol–acepromazine followed by intravenous ketamine–diazepam is the protocol widely used at the OVC.

An oxygen mask may be placed over the cat's face during the donation, and an endotracheal tube should be available should ventilatory support be required. Endotracheal intubation is recommended if the cat has not been fasted before donation, although this does not eliminate the possibility of aspiration because of the need to extubate cats before developing a swallowing reflex. Inhalation anaesthesia with isoflurane can also be used for blood donation. The use of vascular access devices to facilitate feline blood donation without anaesthesia is being investigated.

Venepuncture and blood collection

Blood is collected by jugular venepuncture, with the cat restrained in either lateral or sternal recumbency (see Figure 15.17). Cardiocentesis may be used in terminal donors. Vasoconstriction is more pronounced in the cat than dog after venepuncture, making venepuncture more difficult if repeat attempts are necessary. Assuming the volume of anticoagulant-preservative solution was meant for a 60 ml donation, the minimum acceptable underdraw for blood collected into ACD-A (acid citrate dextrose-A), CPD, or CPDA$_1$ (see Figure 15.8) to be given as whole blood is a final volume of 55 ml. The minimum acceptable underdraw for blood to be used to prepare packed RBCs is a final volume of 42 ml, in which case the plasma is discarded. The maximum acceptable overdraw is a final volume of 65 ml. Blood collection is typically completed within 3–5 minutes. Routine post-anaesthesia monitoring is performed.

Aftercare of the donor

Hypotension, characterized variably by pale mucous membranes, tachycardia and weak pulses, is a common complication of feline donation, but its significance to donor health is not known. Rapid volume expansion during donation to correct hypotension is undesirable because of haemodilution. At the OVC, in the past, volume replacement after the donation with crystalloid solutions at three times the blood loss (i.e. 150–180 ml) was given intravenously over 15–20 minutes. Such rapid volume replacement occasionally resulted in bradycardia and rarely pulmonary oedema. The current fluid therapy protocol is to give 90 ml of saline subcutaneously immediately before the donation, and then to infuse 60 ml of saline over 15–20 minutes starting half-way through the donation.

BLOOD PRODUCT PREPARATION AND STORAGE

Editor's Note: In the UK, the storage of blood and the preparation of blood products for storage is not encouraged by the Royal College of Veterinary Surgeons. The 1996 RCVS Guide to Professional Conduct states that the taking of blood from healthy animals for the purposes of blood transfusion is only recognized in veterinary practice where there is an immediate or anticipated clinical indication for the transfusion. Blood storage and preparation of blood products is covered under the Animals (Scientific Procedures) Act 1986 and would require a specific Home Office Licence. Moreover, blood products would need to be licensed under the Medicines Act 1968.

Collected blood may be given as a fresh transfusion, stored and transfused at a later date or separated into various components for fresh transfusion or storage. Modern blood banking practice standards stipulate that only blood products prepared from blood collected in closed collection systems should be stored, to minimize risk of microbial growth. The open collection system illustrated in Figure 15.17 is used at the OVC for cat donations, and the blood products obtained have been stored successfully without microbial growth, but blood banking is practised at the OVC by experienced staff. For general practices that do not intend to develop a special interest in transfusion medicine, it is recommended that only fresh blood products be used for the cat or that a closed human collection system be used for storage.

The most important blood products in veterinary medicine are whole blood, packed RBCs, frozen plasma and fresh frozen plasma. Component therapy is more important in dogs than in cats, and feline components are more difficult to prepare because of the smaller volumes involved. Any component prepared from one unit of whole blood is referred to as one unit of that component. The various components may be washed, depleted of leucocytes and irradiated in an effort to reduce immunogenicity, but these techniques are rarely used in veterinary medicine.

A flow chart for the preparation of blood components is given in Figure 15.19. The collected blood should be held at room temperature while awaiting separation into fresh components. The blood product should be clearly labelled as to the type of product, collection date, expiry date, donor, blood type (if known), PCV (for whole blood and packed RBCs) and total solids protein (for whole blood, packed RBCs and plasma products).

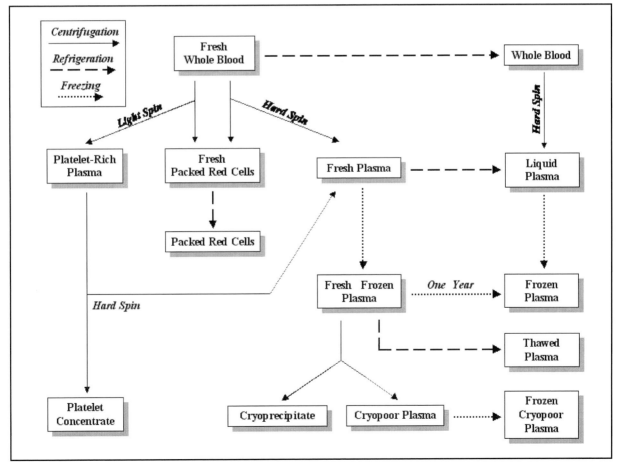

Figure 15.19: *Flowchart for the preparation of blood components by centrifugation.*

RBC products

Whole blood

Storage: Whole blood is stored under refrigeration at 1-6°C (see Figure 15.20). Ideally a dedicated refrigerator should be used. If a general-purpose refrigerator is used, a designated area should be set aside for blood products (not in the door), and the refrigerator door should be opened and closed as quickly as possible. A thermometer should be kept inside the refrigerator and examined a minimum of two times a day to ensure proper refrigeration. Continuous temperature recorders are available. If refrigeration is interrupted for more than 30 minutes, the blood product should be used within 24 hours. Maximum storage times reported with various anticoagulant–preservative solutions are presented in Figure 15.8. The bag should not be 'invaded,' i.e. no blood should be withdrawn or additive injected, during the storage period. The practice of storing feline whole blood in the collecting syringe is not recommended.

Haemostatic properties: Stored whole blood differs from fresh whole blood primarily with respect to haemostatic properties. Platelets refrigerated for up to 24 hours have normal to increased immediate function, but post-transfusion circulation time declines substantially after 6 to 8 hours of refrigeration, and is only 10% after 24 hours. After 72 hours of refrigeration, platelet haemostatic ability in vivo is lost, although platelets will retain some ability to aggregate in vitro.

Similarly, activity levels of the labile coagulation factors, i.e. FV (potentially useful in the treatment of disseminated intravascular coagulation) and FVIII (essential in the treatment of haemophilia A), and von Willebrand factor (vWf; important to the therapy of von Willebrand's disease) progressively decline in refrigerated whole blood due to proteolytic degradation. Human FVIII activity decreases by 50% after 24 hours, but effective haemostatic activity remains for 2 weeks. Canine FVIII is more stable than human FVIII, with about 85% of activity of the former present after 24 hours of refrigeration. Activity of vWf also decreases rapidly. In human blood, about 75% activity is present after 24 hours, 33% after 1 week, 22% after 2 weeks and 13% after 3 weeks of storage. This loss in activity is mostly owing to breakdown of large multimers into smaller multimers, and is not reflected in vWf antigen, which may actually increase during storage. Human FV retains most of its activity in refrigerated whole blood for about 1 week, and >50% activity has been found after 21 days. There is only mild loss of other coagulation factors and antithrombin III (ATIII).

Fresh blood use: The use of fresh whole blood has largely been abandoned in human medicine, leading some veterinarians to make similar recommendations. However, one of the main reasons for discouraging the use of fresh blood products in general in human medicine is that screening for infectious diseases and compatibility testing often take up to 24 hours to complete. In addition, the wide availability of component products permits the replacement of lost blood components to be tailored to individual patient needs. Blood components have more restricted availability in veterinary medicine. Proper donor selection and rapid compatibility testing (see Transfusion reactions) allow for safe transfusion of fresh whole blood (and other fresh blood products), which is likely to remain a necessity in animals.

Transfusion: The principal indication for transfusion of fresh or stored whole blood is substantial acute haemorrhage, since replacement of RBCs, plasma colloid and volume deficits is required. A guideline is to consider transfusion if volume replacement with crystalloids results in a PCV <20% or total protein <25 g/l (Wagner and Dunlop, 1993). Fresh whole blood may be preferred if haemorrhage is owing to disorders of haemostasis, unless other blood products and/or treatments can be given concurrently to address the haemostatic defects. It should also be noted that RBC transfusion in itself has some haemostatic benefit and may reduce bleeding time and activated partial thromboplastin time (Ho, 1998).

The volume of whole blood to transfuse is based on previous, ongoing and estimated future losses. Usually the volume will be between 10 and 22 ml/kg, and the volume transfused per day should not exceed this upper value unless there are severe ongoing losses. Reinfusion of shed blood may be useful under these circumstances (see Autotransfusion). Hypertonic (7.5%) saline, 4–5 ml/kg i.v. over 10 minutes, should also be considered if there is haemorrhagic shock. Its beneficial effects last about an hour. Once bleeding has been controlled, the remaining RBC deficit can be replaced as described below.

Whole blood is also frequently given to correct anaemia from causes other than acute haemorrhage, although packed RBCs are preferred. Guidelines for when to consider transfusion are discussed elsewhere in this manual. Simple rules of thumb to determine the volume to give are:

- 1.0 ml (transfused whole blood)/lb (recipient weight) raises the recipient PCV by 1%

- 2.0 ml (transfused whole blood)/kg (recipient weight) raises the recipient PCV by 1%

The volume to transfuse is more precisely calculated by the following formula:

$$\text{Volume of donor blood to be transfused (ml)} = \text{Recipient weight (kg)} \times \frac{85 \text{ (dog)}}{\text{or}} \times \frac{\text{Recipient desired PCV} - \text{Current PCV}}{\text{PCV of anticoagulated donor blood}}$$

This formula assumes that 60 and 85 represent ml/kg average blood volume for cat and dog, respectively.

Packed RBCs

Preparation and storage: Fresh whole blood is separated into packed RBCs and plasma by centrifugation (preferably) or sedimentation. Packed RBCs are stored under refrigeration at 1–6°C (Figure 15.20). Maximum storage times for packed RBCs reported with various anticoagulant–preservative solutions are given in Figure 15.8. Canine, but not feline, RBCs have also been stored by cryopreservation.

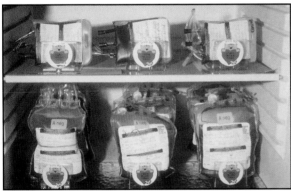

Figure 15.20: *Refrigerated storage of red blood cell (RBC) products. Whole blood and packed RBC bags should be stored vertically or sideways in plastic holders or boxes to reduce the risk of damage to the blood bags, and to facilitate organization and retrieval. Such storage also maximizes oxygen diffusion in to, and carbon dioxide diffusion out of, the bag, but the effect of this on RBC viability of dog and cat blood is not known. RBC products at the Ontario Veterinary College are gently mixed daily, but the importance of this practice is not known. The bag holders shown here are available from the Animal Blood Bank, Dixon, California, USA.*

Centrifugation: Centrifugation requires a centrifuge that is cost prohibitive to most veterinary clinics (Figure 15.21). Centrifugation at 5000 g for 5 minutes at 4°C is recommended. For slower centrifuges, 2000 g for 10 minutes has been found to be satisfactory at the OVC. Centrifugation times include time required for acceleration but not for deceleration. Rapid deceleration can result in resuspension of RBCs. Once RBCs are packed, the plasma is removed with a plasma extractor (Figure 15.22). Adsol, Nutricel or Optisol may then be added to the packed RBCs (Figure 15.23).

Sedimentation: For sedimentation of dog blood, the blood bag is suspended vertically in a refrigerator at 1–6°C for a minimum of 12 hours. Sedimentation from 3 days to 2 weeks, or addition of synthetic colloid, maximizes RBC and plasma separation and should be considered if a primary goal is to produce plasma with minimal RBC content. If a plasma extractor is not available, the blood bag can be suspended upside down for RBC sedimentation. The packed RBCs can then be transfused or transferred to a 300 ml transfer pack by gravity. For feline blood the 60 ml collecting syringe can be stored vertically or upside down and the plasma or packed RBCs transfused or transferred to a 150 ml transfer pack by injection. Feline RBCs sediment more rapidly and efficiently than do canine RBCs.

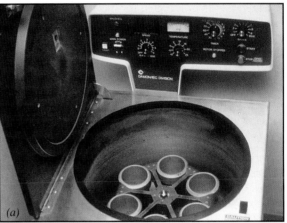

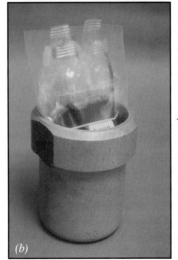

Figure 15.21: *Centrifugation of blood. (a) Large capacity swing-bucket floor-model refrigerated centrifuge suitable for the preparation of blood components. Tabletop fixed bucket centrifuges may also be used but are not ideal. Styrofoam and cork moulds can be made for the buckets to accommodate the smaller cat blood bags. Alternatively, the smaller bag can be placed into two thicknesses of standard bags with the tops cut off and secured with rubber bands to a bag of saline for support during centrifugation (Schneider, 1995). (b) Blood bags should be placed perpendicular to the rotation axis to reduce the chance of rupture. Satellite bags should be tucked in alongside the blood bags (they may be rolled up) and loose tubing occluded and secured to the bags with a rubber band. The centrifuge is best balanced with dry rubber material. If water is used, the blood bag should be placed in a plastic centrifuge bag and the centrifuge buckets thoroughly dried after each used to minimize growth of fungi and algae. If bags frequently rupture during centrifugation, then either the centrifugation rate should be decreased and centrifugation time increased, or water should be poured around the blood bags to support them during centrifugation.*

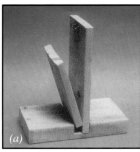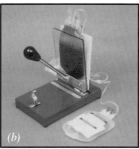

Figure 15.22: Expressing canine plasma. The primary (blood) bag is gently transferred to (a) a homemade extractor or, preferably, (b) a commercial spring-driven plasma extractor.

If a collection pack with a satellite bag was used, the plastic seal at the top of the primary bag is broken. Otherwise a 300 ml transfer pack is aseptically attached to the middle entry port of the primary bag. The plasma is then expressed into the secondary (plasma) bag. Pressure on the primary bag should be initially manually reduced to prevent rupture. Plasma expression is terminated by manually clamping the tubing.

Plasma extractors with electronic control of plasma expression are also available. If the packed red blood cells (RBCs) in the primary bag are to be stored in citrate phosphate dextrose adenine$_p$, the final packed cell volume should be <80%. This requires leaving at least 50 ml of plasma in the primary bag, which is accomplished by terminating plasma expression when the RBC–plasma interface is about 2 cm from the top. The resulting volume of packed RBCs is usually 250–300 ml. For packed RBCs to be stored in Adsol, Nutricel or Optisol, no residual plasma is required in the primary bag, and plasma expression is terminated before RBCs begin to enter the secondary bag. The tubing is sealed as described above and cut. One millilitre of plasma weighs 1.03 g, therefore the volume in the plasma bag is:

$$\frac{Plasma\ unit}{volume\ (ml)} = \frac{Weight\ of\ unit(g) - Weight\ of\ bag(g)}{1.03}$$

One unit of canine plasma usually contains 150–250 ml.

With feline blood, plasma expression is terminated when the RBC–plasma interface reaches the top of the bag. Alternatively, the plasma may be drawn off with a syringe and 18 G needle. One unit of feline plasma usually contains 25–35 ml.

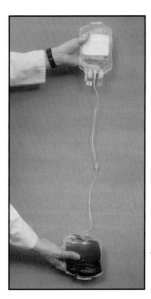

Figure 15.23: The seal on the Adsol, Nutricel or Optisol bag is broken and the solution is transferred by gravity into the primary bag containing the packed red blood cells (RBCs). The additive solution bag is then rolled up to maximize transfer of the solution. The RBCs and additive solution are gently mixed together by rocking. One half of the packed RBCs may then be transferred with the plasma extractor back into the additive solution bag to create two half units. For feline packed RBCs, the nutrient solution is injected into the storage bag via the injection port.

RBC transfusion: The principal indication for packed RBC transfusion is anaemia without hypovolaemia or deficits in other blood components. Packed RBCs are particularly useful with patients at an increased risk of volume overload (see Transfusion reactions). The transfusion volume is calculated with the formula given above. The rules of thumb for transfusion volume are:

- 1.0 ml (transfused packed RBCs)/lb (recipient weight) raises the recipient PCV by 2%

- 2.0 ml (transfused packed RBCs)/kg (recipient weight) raises the recipient PCV by 2%

Packed RBCs may also be used to treat acute haemorrhagic anaemia, with concurrent administration of plasma products, synthetic colloid solutions and crystalloid solutions.

RBC substitutes: Various RBC substitutes are under development, including perfluorochemicals, liposome-encapsulated haemoglobin and haemoglobin-based oxygen carriers (Wohl and Cotter, 1995).

Oxyglobin (Biopure, Cambridge, Massachusetts, USA), a polymerized bovine haemoglobin solution, is an example of the latter (Rentko, 2000). It is available for use in dogs in some countries and has also been given successfully to cats. The dose is 10–30 ml/kg, given at a maximum rate of 10 ml/kg/h. Haemoglobin concentration, not haematocrit, should be used to monitor anaemia after transfusion. The principal advantages of Oxyglobin are that it is convenient to use, avoids incompatibility reactions and is superior to RBCs in delivering oxygen to tissues. The principal disadvantage is its short duration of effect (11–82 hours, half-life of 18–26 hours) compared with RBCs (a typical transfusion lasts 4–6 weeks unless there is accelerated RBC destruction). Other disadvantages include interference with various serum chemistry analyses and development of haemoglobinaemia, haemoglobinuria and icterus. The last may interfere with monitoring of patients with haemolytic anaemia. Oxyglobin acts as a plasma volume expander and causes vasoconstriction – this increases systemic and pulmonary arterial blood pressure, which may be beneficial or detrimental depending upon the clinical situation.

Plasma products

After RBCs are separated from plasma as described above (or by automated plasmapheresis), the plasma may be processed into various products. All of these plasma products are poor in platelets, which remain in the packed RBC fraction.

Fresh plasma and fresh frozen plasma

- Fresh plasma is plasma that has been separated from RBCs within 8 hours of collection and immediately transfused
- Fresh frozen plasma is plasma that has been separated and placed at −18°C or colder within 8 hours of collection.

These time restrictions are based on the deterioration of human FVIII activity and reflect the importance of haemophilia A in human medicine. Fresh and fresh frozen plasma have maximal activity of all coagulation factors, also making them suitable for treating coagulopathies due to hepatic failure and DIC as well as other causes. Fresh and fresh frozen plasma likewise have maximum levels of vWf, as well as containing normal levels of albumin (see Liquid plasma and frozen plasma). Although not of proven benefit, fresh frozen plasma has been recommended for the treatment of acute pancreatitis to replace albumin and treat DIC, but more specifically to replenish α_2 macroglobulins. The α_2 macroglobulins are plasma protease inhibitors that bind to activated pancreatic proteases, which are then cleared from the circulation by macrophages. The original studies in rats and humans used fresh frozen plasma, but in fact α_2 macroglobulins seem to be stable in plasma under refrigeration.

Storage: Because of the time restriction, fresh and fresh frozen plasma are normally prepared by centrifugation. However, dog plasma separated after 12–48 hours of sedimentation still contains clinically useful levels of the labile proteins. Such plasma is best used as fresh plasma.

It is not known how long plasma prepared by sedimentation and then placed at −18°C can be stored while maintaining clinically useful levels of labile proteins, but a 3-month expiry date is suggested. Fresh frozen plasma is ideally stored at −30°C or colder (based on FVIII stability), but storage at −18°C is satisfactory (Figure 15.24). This is the intended temperature of a regular household refrigerator freezer, but it should be verified with a thermometer that the freezer is maintaining this temperature. Freezers with automatic defrost cycles should be avoided. If such a freezer is the only one available, the plasma bag should be stored between two artificial ice bags in an effort to minimize thawing during defrosting. A dedicated freezer is ideal, and the freezer door should be opened and closed as quickly as possible.

After a 1-year storage period, the product is relabelled as frozen plasma, which may be stored as such for an additional 4 years at −18°C or colder. The 1-year expiry date for fresh frozen plasma is also based on the deterioration of FVIII activity. If the freezer does not maintain −18°C, the expiry date should be at most 3 months.

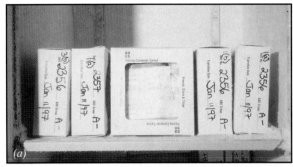

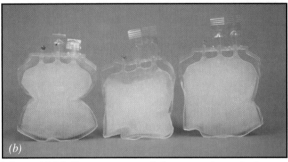

Figure 15.24: *Frozen storage of plasma products. At the Ontario Veterinary College fresh frozen plasma is stored at −70°C and frozen plasma is stored at −18°C. (a) Plasma products are properly frozen in bags (e.g. freezer bags) within a cardboard storage container to prevent breakage. (b) The bags are initially frozen lying flat in the freezer. After complete freezing the bags are stored vertically, resulting in the appearance of the bag on the right. Should inadvertent thawing and refreezing occur, the bag will change shape and any air bubbles will shift to the top (middle bag), indicating a storage problem. In addition a rubber band can be placed around the bag during freezing and then removed (left bag). An inadvertent thaw and refreeze results in loss of the rubber band mark (middle bag).*

Transfusion: The initial dose of fresh or fresh frozen plasma is 10–30 ml/kg, but larger volume transfusion may be required if haemorrhage or acquired coagulation defects persist. Transfusion of fresh and fresh frozen plasma should ideally be completed within 4 hours of separation or thawing, respectively.

Thawed plasma

If fresh frozen plasma is thawed but not immediately transfused, it should be refrigerated (1–6°C). If it is not transfused within 24 hours, the product is relabelled as thawed plasma and may be transfused for up to 5 days after thawing. It has somewhat decreased FVIII and vWf activities, but is otherwise equivalent, compared to fresh frozen plasma.

Liquid plasma and frozen plasma

Storage: Liquid plasma is plasma stored under refrigeration at 1–6°C for more than 8 hours after blood collection. The maximum storage time is 6 weeks, at which point the plasma should be placed at −18°C and labelled as frozen plasma. (It may, of course, be frozen sooner.)

The only reasons to keep refrigerated liquid plasma are if a freezer is not available or if there is an upcoming plasma transfusion, to eliminate thawing time.

Plasma is also prepared by centrifuging stored whole blood at any time during the storage period, and up to 5 days after the RBCs are outdated. The later in the storage period, the higher will be the plasma haemoglobin, potassium and ammonia levels. The RBCs are discarded. The plasma may be kept as liquid plasma for up to 5 days beyond the expiry date of the RBCs, at which time it should be frozen.

Fresh frozen plasma should also be relabelled as frozen plasma after 1 year of storage. The maximum storage time of frozen plasma at -18°C is 5 years.

Coagulation factors: Liquid and frozen plasma typically do not contain clinically adequate levels of FVIII or vWf, especially if prepared from outdated whole blood. Human FVIII activity declines at the same rate in refrigerated plasma as in whole blood, although the decline in vWf activity is slower. The vitamin K-dependent coagulation factors (II, VII, IX and X) are stable in liquid and frozen plasma, so these products may be used to treat bleeding due to anticoagulant rodenticide poisoning, vitamin K deficiency and haemophilia B. The initial dose for this purpose is 10–20 ml/kg. Fibrinogen, FV, ATIII and α_2 macroglobulin levels are also stable in liquid and frozen plasma.

Transfusion: Liquid and frozen plasma have historically been used most often to treat hypoalbuminaemia in dogs. Normally only 40% of total body albumin is in plasma. The remainder is in the interstitium, which acts as a reservoir. Plasma and interstitial albumin are in equilibrium, so hypoalbuminaemia owing to impaired production (from chronic liver failure or severe malnutrition) or external loss (via the intestinal tract, kidney or skin) is accompanied by a shift of albumin from the interstitium into the plasma. There is therefore a total body albumin deficit that is much greater than the plasma deficit. When plasma is transfused, about 60% of the transfused albumin shifts back into the interstitium. Thus large volumes of plasma are required to raise plasma albumin levels and to maintain them in the presence of ongoing losses. This is expensive, especially in big dogs, and increases the risk of transfusion reactions. Large plasma volumes are also required when hypoalbuminaemia is due to vasculitis, where the cause of hypoalbuminaemia is a shift in the equilibrium towards the interstitium.

Neither hypoalbuminaemia nor oedema is, in itself, an indication for transfusion. Transfusion is required when there are life-threatening complications of reduced plasma oncotic pressure such as severe pleural effusion or pulmonary oedema.

Transfusion is also recommended for the patient undergoing anaesthesia, where there are increased concerns with hypotension and altered protein drug binding. Transfusion has been recommended in critical care patients as hypoalbuminaemia has a negative correlation with survival in some studies of humans. However, this is controversial, and other studies have suggested that although transfusion corrects hypoalbuminaemia it may actually worsen clinical outcome. It is controversial how much low albumin levels relate to surgical healing. When poor surgical healing occurs in such patients it is a result of a general catabolic state but may also be due to tissue oedema.

In all the above indications there is usually no need to normalize plasma albumin levels. Plasma transfusion to maintain plasma albumin levels at 15–20 g/l will address physiological concerns while helping to contain costs. About 22.5 ml/kg plasma is required to raise the recipient's albumin level by 5 g/l. The volume to transfuse is more precisely calculated by using the following formula:

$$\text{Volume of donor plasma to be transfused (ml)} = \text{weight (kg)} \times 4.5 \times [\text{Desired} - \text{current recipient plasma albumin level (g/l)}]$$

This formula assumes that normal canine plasma volume is 4.5% kg bodyweight, albumin level in the donor plasma bags averages 25 g/l and the distribution of albumin is 40% in the plasma. The plasma transfusion volume (in millilitres) may be divided by 200 ml (average volume of one unit of canine plasma) to estimate the number of units required.

Albumin-rich products: The albumin-rich blood products of choice in humans are purified albumin (5% and 25% solutions) and plasma protein fraction, which are prepared by ethanol extraction. Equivalent canine products do not exist, but the human products have been used in dogs to correct hypoalbuminaemia and for volume resuscitation. At the OVC, 25% albumin is used at an initial maximum dose of about 2 ml/kg/day.

The rate of administration depends on the clinical situation:

- For the treatment of hypoproteinaemia, albumin is typically given as a constant rate infusion of 0.1 ml/kg/h for up to 3 days
- For urgent correction of hypotension, the dose is given over 4 hours or faster
- For volume resuscitation in severe hypotension, it has been given over 10–15 minutes.

A 25% albumin solution has an osmolality of 1500 mOsm/l and will cause an intravascular volume increase of five times the volume of transfused solution within 30–60 minutes. Rapid infusion must be avoided in conditions with increased risk of pulmonary oedema from volume overload (e.g. heart failure). Angioedema may occur during administration, and anaphylaxis is a potential concern on repeat administration.

Synthetic plasma expanders: The use of synthetic colloids instead of, or in addition to, plasma can also reduce the number of plasma transfusions and reduce costs. These include 6% dextran-70, 10% pentastarch and 6% hetastarch, given intravenously at a dose of 10–20 ml/kg/d in dogs and 5–10 ml/kg/d in cats for up to 3 days. The daily dose may be infused over 15 minutes to 24 hours depending on the need to maintain blood pressure and volume expansion. Pentastarch and hetastarch may have the additional benefit in vasculitis of helping to 'plug' the leaky vessels. Synthetic colloids and albumin solutions may aggravate haemostatic defects, requiring the transfusion of platelet-rich, fresh or fresh frozen plasma.

Colloidal volume expanders should be considered in the management of shock if crystalloid fluid infusion is inadequate or oedema develops. Liquid and frozen plasma may be used for this purpose at a dose of 10–20 ml/kg, but synthetic colloids or concentrated albumin solutions are preferred. It should also be remembered that RBCs act as colloidal volume expanders, and that one volume of RBCs has two to three times the volume expansion effect as an equivalent volume of plasma.

Cryoprecipitate

Preparation and storage: Cryoprecipitate is a precipitate of fresh frozen plasma. It is also known as cryoprecipitated antihaemophilic factor and CRYO. Canine cryoprecipitate is prepared by thawing a unit of fresh frozen plasma at 4°C until a slushy consistency is achieved (typically 3–4 hours). At that point the bag is centrifuged at 4°C, and the supernatant is expressed, decanted or siphoned into a satellite bag, leaving a small residual volume behind with the cryoprecipitate. Various centrifugation times and residual volumes have been reported, including 5000 g for 5 minutes with a residual volume of 10–15 ml (Schneider, 1995), 3500 g for 10 minutes with a residual volume of 30–40 ml (Stokol and Parry, 1998) and 4050 g for 15 minutes with the cryoprecipitate resuspended in 20 ml of 0.15M saline (Ching *et al.*, 1994).

Canine cryoprecipitate can also be prepared without centrifugation by expressing 90% of the supernatant when the fresh frozen plasma has thawed about 90% (Schneider, 1995). The bags are sealed as described previously and refrozen.

Cryoprecipitate may be stored at -18°C or colder for up to 1 year from the unit's collection date.

Transfusion: Cryoprecipitate is enriched in FVIII and vWf and is the veterinary product of choice for treating haemorrhage due to haemophilia A (uncommon) and vWD (more common). Treating the donor before blood collection with a desmopressin (DDAVP)

solution for intranasal use 0.6–1.0 µg/kg s.c. 30–120 minutes before donation is recommended. This increases the donor's vWf levels (see Chapter 14). A unit of cryoprecipitate contains on average 40–60% of the FVIII and vWf in the original fresh frozen plasma from which it was made, and the most active multimers of the latter may be selectively enriched. Cryoprecipitate also contains some of the fibrinogen, FXIII, fibronectin and α_2 macroglobulins of the original plasma.

The initial dose of cryoprecipitate is 1 unit/10 kg, which may be repeated every 4–12 hours as needed. The dose of cryoprecipitate (and other plasma products) required to treat a coagulopathy can be more specifically calculated if the concentration of the deficient factor in the recipient and plasma product can be rapidly determined (Wardrop, 1996).

$$\text{Plasma product (ml)} = \frac{\text{Recipient weight (kg)} \times \begin{array}{c}(85\,[\text{dog}]\\ \text{or}\\ 60\,[\text{cat}])\end{array} \times [\text{1-Haematocrit(l/l)}] \times [\text{Desired - current factor level (U/ml)}]}{\text{Factor level in plasma product (U/ml)}}$$

This formula assumes that 60 and 85 represent ml/kg average blood volume as a proportion of bodyweight for cat and dog, respectively.

A principal advantage of cryoprecipitate is that it allows repetitive transfusions of concentrated coagulation factors without large volume transfusions, thereby reducing the risk of transfusion reactions. The argument has been made that, because only about half of the FVIII and vWf in fresh frozen plasma is cryoprecipitated, maximum haemostatic utility of available blood units is achieved by transfusing either fresh whole blood or fresh or fresh frozen plasma. However, for equivalent amounts of FVIII or vWf activities in the blood products, transfusion of cryoprecipitate will result in higher activities in the recipient than will transfusion of fresh frozen plasma, at least when the products have been prepared from donors treated with DDAVP (Stokol and Parry, 1998). This improved efficacy in haemostatic activities compensates or overcompensates for the poor yield of these factors during cryoprecipitation.

Cryoprecipitate is, however, unavailable to many practitioners. The recommended initial dose of fresh or fresh frozen plasma to treat haemophilia A or vWD is typically 10 ml/kg, but doses up to 30 ml/kg may be required. The formula above can also be used to determine the required volume. If the factor level in the plasma product is not known, the following formula may be used as a rule of thumb:

- 1ml plasma contains about 1 unit of coagulation factor activity (Wardrop, 1996).

In a bleeding diathesis the likelihood is also high that the patient will require RBC replacement, therefore fresh whole blood is in many situations the most practical therapeutic option. An initial dose of 20 ml/kg is recommended. If this degree of RBC transfusion is too high, the dose may be lowered to a minimum of 10 ml/kg. As with cryoprecipitate transfusion, fresh whole blood transfusions may have to be repeated to control haemorrhage. Repeating fresh or fresh frozen plasma transfusions every 12 hours and fresh whole blood transfusions every 24 hours is recommended in an effort to obtain acceptable haemostasis while minimizing transfusion reactions. With transfusion therapy of vWD, regardless of the blood product to be used, treating the donor with DDAVP is recommended.

FVIII and vWf concentrates may be prepared by further purification of pooled units of cryoprecipitate or by recombinant DNA technology. These have been given to dogs in research facilities. Cryoprecipitate is also used to prepare a surgical sealant known as 'fibrin glue'.

Cryosupernatant

The supernatant expressed when making cryoprecipitate is known as cryosupernatant or cryopoor plasma. It contains the vitamin K-dependent clotting factors, albumin and ATIII from the original plasma and may be used to treat vitamin K antagonist poisoning or deficiency, haemophilia B and hypoalbuminaemia, as previously discussed. Cryosupernatant is particularly useful for the treatment of hypoalbuminaemia due to nephrotic syndrome, where dogs are at risk of thrombosis because of reduced ATIII levels and increased fibrinogen and FVIII levels. Cryosupernatant may also be preferred to fresh frozen plasma in some cases of DIC, where fibrinogen transfusion may increase thrombosis and production of fibrin degradation products. Cryosupernatant may be stored at -18°C or colder for up to 5 years from the unit's collection date.

Platelet products

Platelet-rich plasma

Canine platelet-rich plasma is prepared by the centrifugation of fresh whole blood (collected in CPD, CPD2 or CPDA₁) at a lighter gravitational force than normally used to separate packed RBCs and plasma. This concentrates the platelets in the plasma. The plasma is expressed into a satellite bag until the RBC–plasma interface is 1.0 cm from the top of the bag. Most of the platelets are thereby expressed with the plasma. Preparation of platelet-rich plasma can be difficult. Results depend on the donor, the technician, the centrifuge and the centrifugation protocol. Various centrifugation rates and times have been recommended. Most protocols use about 1000 g for 4–6 minutes or 2000–2500 g for 2.5–3 minutes. At the OVC the protocol is 1000 g for 4 minutes at room temperature, with an acceleration time of 30 seconds and braking time of 2.5 minutes.

Feline platelet-rich plasma has been prepared by using a 30 minute sedimentation period, followed by centrifugation at 150 g for 10 minutes (Cowles *et al.,* 1992). Anecdotally, platelet-rich plasma may also be prepared by sedimentation alone, although results have not been reported. A 1 hour sedimentation time is suggested for feline blood and 8 hours for canine blood.

Platelet concentrate

Preparation: Canine platelet concentrate is prepared by apheresis or by centrifugation of platelet-rich plasma. Centrifugation results in sedimentation of nearly all the platelets. If platelet-rich plasma is made by using 2000–2500 g for 2.5–3 minutes, it is typically centrifuged at 4000–5000 g to make platelet concentrate. If platelet-rich plasma is made by using 1000 g for 4–6 minutes, it is typically then centrifuged at 2000 g. At the OVC the centrifugation protocol is 2000 g for 10 minutes at room temperature, with an acceleration time of 1 minute and braking time of 2.5 minutes. The platelet-poor plasma is expressed, leaving 40–70 ml of plasma and the sedimented platelets behind. The resulting platelet concentrate is left undisturbed for 60 minutes to promote disaggregation, and the platelets are then resuspended by gentle manual agitation and kneading. Large leucocyte–platelet aggregates may be present, which require digital compression to aid in resuspension.

Feline platelet concentrate has been prepared by pooling three units of platelet-rich plasma, centrifuging them at 1100 g for 10 minutes, and resuspending the platelets in 5 ml of platelet-poor plasma (Cowles *et al.,* 1992). Canine and feline platelet-poor plasma may be used for fresh or fresh frozen plasma.

Storage: If platelet products are to be stored, collection sets with the appropriate plastic platelet satellite bag should be used. Platelet products should be stored at room temperature under constant agitation (Figure 15.25). Platelet storage bags of different composition are designed for 3- and 5-day storage. For canine platelet products, a maximum storage period of 3 days in a '5-day' bag is ideal. Cryopreserved and lyophilized canine platelet concentrates have been prepared but are not routinely available.

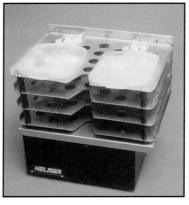

Figure 15.25:
Canine platelet products stored under continuous reciprocal agitation. End-over-end tumblers, elliptical rotators and blood sample rockers may also be used. If continuous agitation is not possible, then intermittent gentle manual agitation is recommended.

Transfusion: Platelet products are used in the treatment of haemorrhage due to thrombocytopenia and thrombocytopathy. Platelet transfusion is most beneficial for thrombocytopenia caused by decreased platelet production (e.g. leukaemia, aplastic anaemia). It is less beneficial with increased platelet consumption (DIC) and sequestration (splenomegaly). Platelet transfusion is least beneficial, but not useless, with increased platelet destruction (immune-mediated thrombocytopenia; IMT).

As IMT is the most common cause of thrombocytopenia in general practice, and dogs with other thrombocytopenic disorders are often euthanazed because of poor prognosis or cost of therapy, platelet transfusion is not frequently performed. However, with an increased willingness on the part of veterinarians and owners to treat complex haematological problems, platelet transfusion may become more frequent.

The initial dose for platelet transfusion is one unit of platelet-rich plasma or platelet concentrate/10 kg. Assuming an average unit contains 60×10^9 platelets, the recipient's platelet count 1 hour after transfusion should be increased by 35×10^9/l if there is no accelerated platelet destruction, consumption or sequestration. The expected platelet count 1 hour after transfusion in the dog is more precisely calculated with the formula:

$$\frac{\text{Expected 1-hour}}{\text{platelet count}} = \frac{\text{Platelet count before}}{\text{transfusion } (\times 10^9/l)} + \frac{\frac{\text{Unit platelet count } (\times 10^9/l)}{\times \text{ unit volume (l) } \times 0.51}}{\text{Recipient weight (kg) } \times 0.085 \text{ l/kg}}$$

In the above formula 0.085 x weight is the average blood volume for the dog, and 0.51 corrects for splenic sequestration of transfused platelets. If there is minimal platelet production but no accelerated platelet destruction, consumption or sequestration, the recipient's platelet count should drop by 33% each day after transfusion. When interpreting the success of a platelet transfusion, it should be remembered that platelet counts at low values are imprecise. Critical haemorrhage can usually be prevented by repeat transfusion to maintain the platelet count above $10-15 \times 10^9$/l.

The necessity for a centrifuge and the short shelf life make platelet products largely unavailable to most clinics. Cases requiring extensive platelet support are best referred to a facility that can provide the transfusions and other aspects of critical care that are needed. If platelet products are not available, fresh whole blood should be used. As a rule of thumb:

- 10 ml/kg of fresh whole blood will raise the recipient's platelet count by about 10×10^9/l.

If this is continued for more than a few days, polycythaemia will result. Hyperproteinaemia may also result from transfusion of large volumes of platelet-rich plasma (see Transfusion reactions).

If no platelet product is available, transfusion with 10 ml/kg fresh frozen plasma should be used because it contains functional platelet microparticles. Various platelet substitutes are under development.

Vinca-loaded platelets: A unique treatment for IMT is the use of 'vinca-loaded platelets,' which are prepared by adding supratherapeutic doses of vincristine or vinblastine to platelet concentrates, and, after incubation, discarding the supernatant plasma. The vinca alkaloids bind to platelet microtubules. On transfusion to patients with IMT, the vinca-loaded platelets are phagocytosed by splenic macrophages, which then suffer cytotoxic injury. The platelets thus act as 'Trojan horses,' permitting higher than usual doses of vinca alkaloids to be delivered to the macrophages while sparing the bone marrow.

Vincristine-loaded platelets have had limited use in veterinary medicine. Anecdotally, veterinarians have injected a therapeutic dose of vincristine into platelet-rich plasma or fresh whole blood, and, after an hour's incubation period, performed the transfusion. This method of vinca-loading platelets is incorrect. A reported protocol based on correct principles consists of incubating 100 ml of platelet-rich plasma (containing about 250×10^9 platelets/l) with 3 mg vincristine sulphate for 1 hour at 37°C with constant agitation (Helfand *et al.*, 1984). The platelet-rich plasma is then centrifuged to prepare a platelet pellet, and all the supernatant plasma is discarded. The platelets are resuspended into a total of 35 ml saline and transfused over 30–60 minutes.

Vincristine-loaded platelet therapy seems to have induced remission of disease in several dogs with IMT, but interpretation is obscured by concurrent therapy. The dogs so treated have ranged in weight from 9–30 kg, and thus received quite different vincristine-loaded platelet doses. There is no information on the pharmacokinetics of vincristine given to dogs in this manner or on the optimal platelet and vincristine doses.

Leucocyte products

Blood mononuclear cells may be collected by leucapheresis and modified for progenitor cell transplantation, adoptive immunotherapy and gene therapy. Neutrophils may be collected to prepare granulocyte concentrates (see Chapter 8).

Serum products

Pooled adult serum may be given to neonates as a colostrum substitute when there is failure of passive transfer. The dose reported in pups is 20 ml/kg orally or 20–40 ml/kg s.c. at birth (Bouchard *et al.*, 1992). Subcutaneous administration at the highest dose is most effective and does not interfere with feeding.

The injection should be given slowly to minimize pain. The dose reported in kittens is 150 ml/kg i.p. or s.c. divided into three treatments over 24 hours (Levy and Crawford, 2000). The treatment protocol in kittens was more effective and should be considered for pups. Serum treatment should also be considered in the treatment of a fading neonate because immunoglobulin therapy (see Intravenous immunoglobulin) is beneficial in the treatment of human neonatal sepsis. The preparation of pooled serum may not be practical in a general veterinary clinic, and the use of serum from a single donor is likely to be beneficial.

Other serum preparations used in dogs and cats include antitoxins and antivenins, immune serum for parvoviral infections and antithymocyte serum for immunosuppression.

Blood derivatives and blood substitutes

Intravenous immunoglobulin

Concentrated preparations of human immunoglobulins were initially developed for the treatment of human immunodeficiency states. Intramuscular preparations have been superseded by intravenous immunoglobulin (IVIG), which is purified monomeric IgG. Human IVIG may also be used to treat IMT in humans and has been used to treat dogs with immune-mediated haemolytic anaemia (IMHA) at a dose of 0.5–1.5 g/kg as a 12-hour infusion (Scott-Moncrieff and Reagan, 1997). The mechanisms of action include immunosuppression and inhibition of macrophage erythrophagocytosis by saturation of immunoglobulin receptors. Human IVIG therapy has corrected anaemia in some dogs with chronic non-regenerative IMHA. It has not had a major impact on survival in severe acute IMHA and is often cost prohibitive. Human IVIG has also been used to treat canine IMT in a limited number of cases, with variable results. Anaphylaxis is a potential concern, especially with repeated administration, but has not been reported.

Lyophilized canine IgG has been prepared and used in the management of parvovirus infection (Macintire et al., 1999). Digoxin immune Fab fragments may be used to treat digoxin toxicosis.

Other products

Other blood derivatives and blood substitutes have been discussed previously in the appropriate sections.

ADMINISTRATION OF WHOLE BLOOD AND BLOOD COMPONENTS

Warming and mixing

Refrigerated whole blood and blood components do not need to be routinely warmed before administration. The products gradually warm to room temperature during administration, and excessive warming may decrease RBC viability and increase the risk of microbial growth. Refrigerated products should, however, be warmed to room or body temperature for recipients at risk of hypothermia and when large-volume and/or rapid transfusions are planned, because the rapid infusion of cold fluids is arrhythmogenic.

To warm to room temperature, the blood product may be allowed to sit at room temperature for 30–60 minutes before beginning the transfusion. To warm to body temperature, the intravenous line may be passed through a bowl of water or sandwiched between oat bags warmed to 37–38°C. Electrical infusion warmers are also available. The blood bag may also be warmed by immersion in a 37–38°C water bath, although this increases the risks of contamination and decreased RBC viability compared with warming the infusion line. Microwave warming is not recommended because of the risks of haemolysis.

Stored whole blood should be mixed by gentle inversion (at least 60 times) before transfusion. With canine packed RBCs stored in CPDA$_1$, the PCV is often 70–80% and the product may be too viscous to transfuse easily, and RBC clumps may be present. This problem may be corrected by adding 100 ml of 37°C saline to the unit and resuspending the RBCs by gentle manual agitation and kneading. Adding more than 100 ml unnecessarily increases transfusion volume. Although feline packed RBCs have a lower PCV, dilution with 20–30 ml of saline facilitates passage through the smaller filters recommended for use in cats. Canine and feline packed RBCs stored in Adsol, Nutricel or Optisol do not usually require further dilution before transfusion. Calcium-containing fluids such as lactated Ringer's should not be used for dilution because the calcium may initiate coagulation.

Frozen plasma products should be thawed in a 37–38°C water bath or incubator. Thawing time is 30 minutes or more for a unit of canine plasma. Agitation and manually kneading the bag to break up ice crystals speed ups thawing. Higher temperatures may result in denaturing of proteins. The plasma unit should be left in the freezer bag and box during thawing to prevent contamination of the entry ports, although this slows down thawing time.

Frozen plasma products may be more rapidly thawed in a microwave oven. A reported protocol for microwave thawing of canine plasma resulted in thawing times of less than 10 minutes (Hurst et al., 1987). The bag was placed in 37°C water for 1 minute and then microwaved at the highest setting in a 700W oven for 14–17 cycles of 10-second cooking intervals and 5-second intervals of manual agitation. When ice particles less than 1.0 cm long remained, the bag was inverted several times for 30 seconds to complete the thaw. Thawing at the defrost setting has also been recommended (Kristensen and Feldman, 1995a). Caution is advised when microwaving plasma because of variations between microwave ovens. Short cooking times and intermittent agitation are recommended to minimize non-uniform heating and protein denaturation. Bags with aluminum clips should not be microwaved.

Frozen plasma products should not be thawed in a refrigerator as this results in formation of cryoprecipitate. Units of cryoprecipitate may be thawed as described above or by adding 10 ml of 37°C saline per unit and gently kneading the bag for 3 minutes. Multiple units should be pooled in one bag for transfusion (Kristensen and Feldman, 1995a).

Venous access

A transfusion may be given via any vein. Viscosity of transfused whole blood may slow or stop transfusions with smaller catheters. In the dog, a 16–19 G jugular catheter or 18–20 G peripheral vein catheter is satisfactory, with the larger gauge catheters preferred for packed RBC transfusions. In cats, a 22 G peripheral vein catheter also works because of the lower PCV and smaller RBC size.

If venous access is not possible, the intraosseous (intramedullary) route is best, with an 18–20 G needle or bone marrow aspiration needle placed into the trochanteric fossa (Otto and Crowe, 1992). The transfusion will be rapidly absorbed into the systemic circulation. Intraosseous transfusion is particularly useful in neonatal transfusion, where a 22 G needle can also be placed into the tibial crest.

Neonates can also be transfused by intraperitoneal injection. About 50% of transfused RBCs will be absorbed into the circulation from the peritoneal space in 24 hours, and 70% within 48–72 hours, but they will have a shorter life span.

Transfusion rate

As a general rule, whole blood and its components may be transfused at a rate of 5–10 ml/kg/h. The initial rate should be 0.25 ml/kg/h for the first 15–30 minutes to allow for early detection of potentially severe transfusion reactions. This step may have to be omitted if emergency transfusion is required.

The maximum rate of transfusion is 22 ml/kg/h, which is usually only used in an emergency situation. Electrocardiographic monitoring is recommended during higher transfusion rates (especially with large volumes) since arrhythmias may occur from various mechanisms.

Transfusion rates must be slowed down in the presence of increased risks of volume overload. To minimize the risk of bacterial proliferation in RBC and plasma products, human standards stipulate that a transfusion should be completed within 4 hours.

In some cases this may not be possible, and in the author's opinion it is acceptable for a transfusion to extend over a longer period so long as strict attention is given to preventing contamination when the transfusion is set up. Alternatively, some blood products may be divided into subunits and the subunits refrigerated until transfused. This practice, however, involves additional manipulation of the blood product, increasing the risks of contamination and in vitro haemolysis.

Filter

Special administration sets for blood transfusion are commercially available, which contain in-line filters to remove clots, platelet aggregates and some fat (Figures 15.26 and 15.27). However, if an animal is in need of an emergency transfusion and a filter set is not available, then an unfiltered transfusion of fresh whole blood or plasma can be given so long as the collection is smooth and rapid and there are no grossly visible clots. Filters should always be used with stored whole blood and blood components. Filters are recommended for plasma products as they may contain particulate matter.

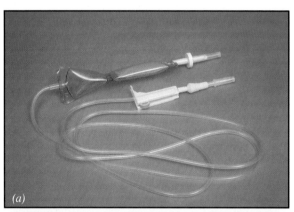

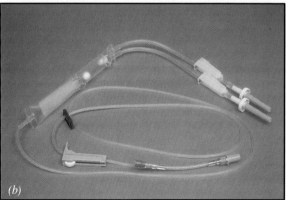

Figure 15.26: *Standard transfusion sets containing a 170 μm filter for use in blood transfusions to middle and large breed dogs. Sets come as (a) 'straight' (single line) and (b) 'Y', which allows for concurrent fluid therapy with saline. When blood products are being given to deliver platelets or clotting factors, transfusion sets without latex bulbs should be used, as latex may bind these components.*

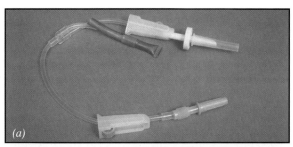

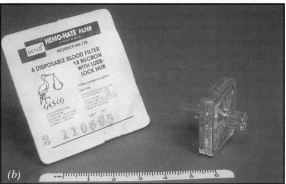

Figure 15.27: The standard transfusion sets are too large to use with cats, toy breeds and paediatric patients, as much of the transfusion remains in the set and must be flushed through with saline, thus increasing the risk of volume overload. Human paediatric filters and small infusion sets are suitable for small volume transfusions. (a) Blood component infusion set (Baxter 4C2223) containing an 80 μm filter. (b) Hemo-Nate (Gesco) containing a 20 μm filter. The smaller pore filters are designed to remove microaggregates of degenerating platelets, leucocytes and fibrin, which will pass through standard 170 μm filters. Microaggregate filtration is of most benefit in cardiopulmonary bypass and blood scavenging (see Autotransfusion). Microaggregate filtration may also ameliorate the thrombocytopenia that may occur after transfusion owing to splenic sequestration of microaggregates. The microaggregate filters are used here for the advantage of the small volume infusion sets.

Delivery

In most veterinary clinics canine transfusions are delivered by gravity. Newer infusion pumps can be used. Some older models cause haemolysis, and the manufacturer should be consulted. For feline and paediatric transfusions, a 60 ml syringe can be used to slowly deliver the transfusion by intermittent injection. Syringe infusion pumps are also available. If the small volume blood product is in a bag, a smaller volume transfusion set should be used (Figure 15.27a). Alternatively the blood product may be gently drawn out of the bag with an 18 G needle and 60 ml syringe and then injected. If a standard canine unit is being used to transfuse a small patient, a biuret can be placed between the bag and the filter set to regulate the delivered volume.

Record keeping

A transfusion log should be kept noting the information from the blood product label, recipient, transfusion date, and transfusion reactions. A highly visible notation should be added to the medical record to show the patient has received a transfusion.

ADVERSE CONSEQUENCES OF TRANSFUSION (TRANSFUSION REACTIONS)

Transfusion reactions are categorized as immunological and non-immunological and as acute and delayed. The major transfusion reactions are listed in Figure 15.28. Immunological reactions are due to RBC, plasma protein, white cell and platelet antigens. The non-specific signs that may occur with an acute immunological reaction to any blood product are shown in Figures 15.29 and 15.30. More specific clinical signs are discussed with each type of reaction. Some of the information concerning causes and manifestations of transfusion reactions is based on experimental evidence and extrapolated from human medicine. The reported rates of acute transfusion reactions in dogs and cats range from 3 to 8%. These rates are expected to decline with improved compatibility testing and increasing experience in veterinary transfusion medicine.

Immunological transfusion reactions
RBC incompatibility reactions
Reactions to plasma proteins
Reactions to white blood cells and platelets
Other immunological reactions
Non-immunological transfusion reactions
Anaphylactoid reactions
Volume (circulatory) overload
Hypothermia
Citrate intoxication (hypocalcaemia)
Heparinization
Coagulopathy and thrombosis
Microbial contamination
Hyperammonaemia
Hypophosphataemia
Hyperkalaemia
Acidosis
Pretransfusion (in vitro) haemolysis
Haemosiderosis

Figure 15.28: Transfusion reactions in the dog and cat.

Weakness, depression, recumbency
Tremors, agitation, vocalization
Polypnoea, dyspnoea
Tachycardia, bradycardia (cats), arrhythmias, pale mucous membranes, weak pulses (hypotension)
Cardiopulmonary arrest (may be the only sign present during anaesthesia)
Salivation (and other signs of nausea), vomiting, diarrhoea
Urination
Seizures, coma
Angioedema and urticaria (see Figure 15.30)

Figure 15.29: Non-specific clinical signs that may occur with an acute immunological reaction to a transfused blood product.

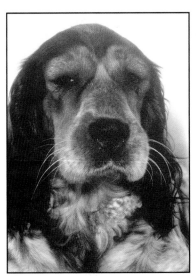

Figure 15.30: Angioedema in a dog occurring within minutes of giving a test dose of whole blood at 0.25 ml/kg/h.

Immunological transfusion reactions

RBC incompatibility reactions (haemolysis)

The pathogenesis of haemolytic reactions has been discussed above (see Canine blood groups and Feline blood groups). The clinical signs of an acute haemolytic crisis in dogs include one or more of the signs listed in Figure 15.29 plus haemoglobinuria and haemoglobinaemia. Fever is common but urticaria and angioedema are not. Acute renal failure and DIC are uncommon sequelae. The severity of the reaction is directly correlated with the number of RBCs destroyed. The reaction is predominantly IgG mediated.

The severe acute haemolytic reaction of cats is IgM mediated and resembles anaphylaxis more than the reaction in dogs. It is divided into two phases (Auer and Bell, 1986; Griot-Wenk and Giger, 1995). Recumbency, stretching of limbs, hypotension, bradycardia and apnoea are the most common signs in phase I, occurring within 2 minutes of starting the transfusion and lasting up to 5 minutes. Other acute signs may also occur. Less severe reactions are associated with milder hypotension, tachycardia and polypnoea. Haemoglobinuria and haemoglobinaemia may be undetectable since small volumes of blood, as little as 1 ml, can initiate a severe reaction. Phase II (the recovery phase) is characterized by tachycardia and polypnoea, which may last for several hours. Hypertension and ventricular arrhythmias follow a severe reaction for about 30 minutes. Pulmonary oedema may develop within several hours.

In a delayed haemolytic reaction there are no acute clinical signs, but the post-transfusion PCV declines rapidly over 3–5 days. In dogs and cats a transfusion is expected to 'last' 4–6 weeks, because the half-life of transfused compatible RBCs is about 21 days in the dog and 35 days in the cat.

Pretransfusion treatment with antihistamines and corticosteroids will not prevent an acute or delayed RBC incompatibility reaction in either dogs or cats.

Reactions to plasma proteins

Immunological reactions to plasma proteins (usually gamma globulins) are allergic in nature (i.e. IgE mediated), resulting in urticaria and angioedema or, rarely, anaphylaxis. Pruritus, salivation, vomiting and diarrhoea, and dyspnoea from bronchoconstriction may occur, but fever is not typical. The hallmark of anaphylaxis is hypotension, characterized by weakness, weak pulses and pale mucous membranes. In allergic reactions there is loss of fluid and albumin from the circulation, which partly abrogates any benefit from the transfusion in this regard. With severe reactions, ascites, pleural effusion and pulmonary oedema may occur. Allergic reactions to plasma proteins typically occur within 1–15 minutes but may occur at any time during a transfusion, even if there has been no reaction to a test dose. The risk of such reactions increases with the rate of transfusion, possibly because some are anaphylactoid.

In humans, anaphylaxis occurs when a sensitized IgA deficient individual with anti-IgA antibodies receives a transfusion containing IgA (i.e. most donor blood). The author has seen one anaphylactic reaction in a dog that was IgA deficient, but circulating anti-IgA antibodies could not be demonstrated. Allergic reactions do not seem to occur frequently in dogs and cats, but they can occur in a naïve recipient. There is some evidence that the risk of allergic reactions increases with multiple transfusions in dogs and cats, and that an animal that has had a previous allergic reaction is at increased risk of a subsequent one. An urticarial reaction in humans is not typically repeated on subsequent transfusion, whereas anaphylaxis becomes more severe. Dogs and cats, unlike humans, may be transfused more than once from a certain donor, and this may increase the risk of allergic reactions.

For animals receiving multiple transfusions, use of a new donor for each transfusion (donor rotation) and pretreatment with antihistamines with or without corticosteroids can be considered, especially if there is a history of allergic reactions. Pretreatment with antihistamines and corticosteroids should be used if a rapid transfusion rate is necessary. However, such pretreatment does not guarantee that an allergic reaction will not occur. For an antihistamine, either diphenhydramine or tripelennamine 1.0 mg/kg i.m. 30 minutes before transfusion can be used. These drugs can be given intravenously if necessary, but in some cases administration by this route results in transient hypotension and agitation. For a corticosteroid, dexamethasone sodium phosphate 0.5–1.0 mg/kg i.v. 5–15 minutes before transfusion is recommended.

If a recipient requiring a RBC transfusion has a history of severe allergic reactions or is known to have a plasma protein incompatibility with the only available donor, RBCs should be washed with saline before transfusion. Washing may be performed either with apheresis equipment or by centrifugation. With the latter technique, packed RBCs are prepared as previously described, except that as much plasma as possible is expressed. A volume of saline equivalent to the volume of plasma expressed is added to the RBCs, which are resuspended by gentle manual agitation. The saline–RBC suspension is then centrifuged as before to produce packed RBCs, and the saline–plasma supernatant is expressed. The procedure is repeated two more times.

Reactions to white blood cells

In humans, reactions to leucocytes occur owing to incompatibilities of major histocompatibility complex (MHC) antigens. Platelets also express these antigens. Reactions between recipient antibodies and donor leucocytes are characterized primarily by fever, chills and vomiting. Such reactions are not usually clinically dangerous but interfere with patient wellbeing and with monitoring for sepsis in critically ill patients. In addition, when fever occurs haemolysis must be ruled out. Non-haemolytic febrile reactions may also occur in response to cytokines and other bioactive substances that accumulate in the stored blood. With either cause, the rate of transfusion does not seem to be important.

Non-haemolytic febrile reactions in dogs and cats after whole blood and platelet transfusions are presumed to be due to recipient immune responses to donor leucocyte antigens and bioactive substances. In the author's experience, such fevers (accompanied variably by tremors and vomiting) may occur during or within several hours of transfusion, range from mild to greater than 41.0°C and may take up to 12 hours to fully resolve. Animals typically do not seem to be as clinically ill as do animals with an equivalent fever due to a bacterial infection. In humans, the risk of subsequent reactions is 12.5–50%. The risk in dogs and cats is not known, but it is presumably high if the same donor is used.

Pretreatment with antihistamines will not prevent febrile reactions. Pretreatment with dexamethasone sodium phosphate 0.5–1.0 mg/kg i.v. 5–15 minutes before transfusion, or non-steroidal anti-inflammatory drugs at standard doses or paracetamol (dogs only) 10–15 mg/kg orally 1 hour before transfusion may help to prevent a febrile reaction. Pretreatment is only recommended if the recipient has a history of deleterious febrile reactions. Donor rotation may also reduce the risk of febrile reactions. Leucocyte-absorption filters for various blood products are available but expensive (Brownlee *et al.*, 2000). Leucocyte content of packed RBCs may be reduced less expensively although less efficiently by using 20–40 μm filters and/or by inverted centrifugation, where the whole blood bag is centrifuged upside down when preparing packed RBCs and 70–80% of the RBCs (determined by weight) are removed by gravity. Platelet concentrates may be depleted of leucocytes by using a special centrifugation system (Leukotrap Platelet Pooling System, Cutter). All methods of white blood cell removal result in some loss of RBCs or platelets.

A severe acute respiratory distress syndrome may also occur in humans after transfusion. This is characterized by non-cardiogenic pulmonary oedema and is believed to be due to donor antibodies reacting with recipient leucocytes. This specific reaction in dogs and cats has not been reported, although pulmonary oedema may occur in phase II of the reaction of a type B cat receiving type A blood.

Reactions to platelets

Platelet alloimmunization may occur with repetitive transfusions and results in platelet transfusions becoming ineffective (Slichter, 2000). The onset of platelet alloimmunization may be delayed by using a new unrelated donor for each transfusion and may be prevented by treating the recipient with cyclosporin, but not with prednisone or cyclophosphamide. Leucocyte reduction combined with ultraviolet irradiation may also prevent alloimmunization, but it is unavailable to most veterinary clinics.

Post-transfusion thrombocytopenia may rarely occur in humans and dogs within 1–2 weeks after transfusion and last up to 2 months (Wardrop *et al.*, 1997). Antibody response to transfused platelets is generalized to an attack on the recipient's own platelets. Immunosuppressive therapy with prednisone may hasten recovery.

Other immunological reactions

Immunosuppression resulting from blood transfusion is most important in organ transplantation, enhancing allograft survival except with marrow allografts. It is controversial whether or not transfusion-associated immunosuppression increases the risk of infection and neoplasia. The effect of transfusion on the course of canine and feline immune-mediated diseases is not known.

Transfusion-related graft-versus-host disease refers to pancytopenia caused by an immunological attack on the recipient's bone marrow by lymphocytes in the transfused blood. In dogs and cats it is a problem mostly in bone marrow transplantation but may be a concern in severely immunosuppressed cancer patients. If available, irradiation of blood products with 25–50 Gy should be considered for such patients.

A transfusion may have an antineoplastic effect. This has been reported with lymphoid leukaemia in a dog (MacEwen *et al.*, 1981).

Non-immunological transfusion reactions

These reactions occur from excessive volumes or rates of transfusion or from changes during storage.

Anaphylactoid reactions

Anaphylactoid reactions usually occur from too rapid a transfusion rate and resemble allergic reactions to plasma proteins. Non-IgE-mediated mast cell degranulation occurs, probably triggered by plasma proteins.

Volume (circulatory) overload
Transfusion often involves the administration of relatively high fluid rates and/or volumes. Volume overload is most often a problem in cats, animals with concurrent cardiac or renal failure and animals with chronic anaemia. The resulting polypnoea and dyspnoea – and occasionally ascites – may be confused with a RBC incompatibility reaction or anaphylactic/anaphylactoid reaction to plasma proteins. The radiographic changes associated with volume overload and anaphylaxis/anaphylactoid reactions may also be similar, in that the latter may result in pulmonary oedema or pleural effusion secondary to increased vascular permeability.

In addition to history, cardiovascular findings are helpful in distinguishing volume overload from anaphylactic/anaphylactoid reactions. With volume overload, the heart rate tends to be normal to low (unless tachycardia is present due to heart disease or another disorder), arterial pressure tends to be normal to high and central venous pressure is high (e.g. jugular distension may be evident). If pulmonary oedema is due to volume overload, pulmonary venous distension will be present on radiographs, and cardiomegaly may be evident. In contrast, anaphylactic/anaphylactoid reactions cause distributive shock and are characterized by tachycardia, arterial hypotension (weak pulses) and poor central venous pressure. Pulmonary veins are normal to small on radiographs, and microcardia may be present (unless there is cardiomegaly due to heart disease).

Polycythaemia and hyperproteinaemia
Polycythaemia may occur when repetitive transfusions of fresh whole blood are used to treat a haemostatic disorder. The increased blood viscosity and altered rheology may be detrimental in animals that are septic (ideal PCV=30%) or prone to thrombosis and ischaemia. Phlebotomy (20 ml/kg) may be necessary, and the plasma and platelets may be returned to the donor to minimize loss of haemostatic function. Hyperproteinaemia may also occur with repetitive transfusions of plasma products. In the event that hyperproteinaemia causes an unacceptable increase in blood viscosity, phlebotomy and reinfusion of RBCs should be used before transfusion to remove a volume of recipient plasma equal to the volume to be transfused.

Hypothermia
Administration of cold blood products may result in hypothermia. This occurs most often with rapid large-volume transfusions, transfusions to paediatric and small patients and transfusions during anaesthesia. Transfusion-induced hypothermia may aggravate hypothermia due to shock, cause tremors and result in arrhythmias, which may in turn cause acute cardiopulmonary arrest.

Citrate intoxication (hypocalcaemia)
When large volumes of citrated blood products are given rapidly, the citrate anticoagulant (which is present in excess) can chelate calcium in the patient resulting in signs of hypocalcaemia, including muscle tremors, twitching of ears, tetanic seizures, vomiting and arrhythmias. The problem is only likely to occur if more than one recipient blood volume is transfused. Lesser volumes can cause citrate intoxication if blood collection bags have been underfilled or if there is liver failure, severe hypotension or hypothermia, impairing the metabolism of citrate to bicarbonate. Tremors due to hypocalcaemia can be confused with those due to hypothermia, which may also result from rapid large volume transfusion.

Confirmation of citrate-induced hypocalcaemia requires measurement of ionized calcium, because the citrate-bound calcium will be measured if total serum calcium is measured. Unfortunately, ionized calcium levels are not available as a 'stat' value in most veterinary clinics. Electrocardiographic changes may be supportive. The most common change is prolongation of the Q-T interval; other changes include depression of P and T waves and ventricular arrhythmias. Treatment is 10% calcium gluconate 0.5–1.5 ml/kg i.v. over 5–10 minutes, to effect. The injection of calcium gluconate should be interrupted if vomiting or arrhythmias occur.

Citrate intoxication may also cause hypomagnesaemia. With the recent interests in the role of magnesium in critical care, this effect may receive more attention in the future.

Heparinization
An animal is considered to be heparinized when it has received a heparin dose greater than 100 IU/kg, but marked haemorrhagic tendencies are not likely to occur until doses greater than 300 IU/kg have been given. Heparin is rapidly metabolized (plasma half-life is 1.5 hours) so bleeding is rarely a problem. In the event of an inadvertent massive overdose of heparin, protamine sulphate may be given at a maximum dose of 1.0 mg/100 IU of heparin intravenously, although few veterinary clinics routinely carry this product. It is important to err on the side of underdosing protamine, since protamine itself is an anticoagulant with no antidote.

Coagulopathy and thrombosis
Dilutional coagulopathy may occur from rapid transfusion of large volumes (usually greater than one blood volume) of stored whole blood or liquid/frozen plasma, which are deficient in platelets and have reduced levels of coagulation proteins. This is most likely to occur in catastrophic trauma patients, and the situation is aggravated by aggressive fluid therapy. Transfusion with platelet-rich blood products and fresh frozen plasma may be required.

Blood transfusion may increase the risk of pulmonary thromboembolism in dogs with IMHA (Klein *et al.*, 1989). Transfusions of fresh or fresh frozen plasma may increase the risk of thrombosis in some situations (see Cryoprecipitate and Cryosupernatant).

Microbial contamination (transfusion-associated sepsis)

Transfusion of blood products contaminated with bacteria or fungi can result in acute vomiting, diarrhoea, dyspnoea, collapse, cardiopulmonary arrest and haemolysis, thus mimicking immunological reactions. Fever may occur, but its absence does not rule out blood product contamination. The peracute signs result from transfused endotoxins rather than bacterial proliferation in the recipient. However, the transfused bacteria may also cause later signs of systemic or localized infections. Contaminated blood may appear darker than usual or brown and/or contain air bubbles or clots, and such blood should not be used.

Sources of microorganisms include donors (bacteraemia and skin flora) and contaminated blood collection, banking and transfusion supplies. Infections resulting from a fresh transfusion are unlikely to occur unless there is gross contamination during collection. The problems occur most often when microorganisms proliferate in stored blood products. The risk of transfusion-associated sepsis with modern human blood banking is low. The risk is higher with leucocyte-depleted products, since leucocytes phagocytose microorganisms during storage, and with platelet products stored at room temperature.

The organisms implicated most often in humans are psychrophilic environmental contaminants and faecal flora, which can typically use citrate as a carbohydrate source. The most common RBC contaminants are *Yersinia enterocolitica* and *Pseudomonas* spp., whereas platelet products are most commonly contaminated with *Staphylococcus* spp., *Streptococcus* spp. and various Gram-negative organisms.

The prevalence of microbial contamination and organisms involved in veterinary transfusion medicine are poorly documented. Sepsis after transfusion of *Klebsiella* spp. contaminated blood occurred in one dog at the OVC. Contamination of cat blood with *Serratia marcescens* has been reported (Hohenhaus *et al.*, 1997). In this report sepsis resulted from use of a contaminated intravenous solution and not from use of an open collection system. When a practice is first developing blood banking, blood products should be routinely cultured using blood-culture media before and after storage. Routine culturing was discontinued at the OVC in 1991 since there had not been a positive isolate in 5 years, and no infections owing to transfusions have been documented since that time.

Hyperammonaemia

Ammonia builds up during RBC storage, and only RBC products stored for less than 2 weeks should be given to animals with liver failure.

Hypophosphataemia

Phosphate levels decrease progressively during RBC storage, and RBC fragility increases. This is not normally a problem. However, transfusion of whole blood or packed RBCs nearing the end of their storage periods may aggravate hypophosphataemia. Transfusion of RBC products stored for less than 2 weeks is recommended in hypophosphataemic animals, especially if the transfusion is being given because of haemolysis secondary to hypophosphataemia.

Hyperkalaemia

RBCs leak potassium during storage, and transfusions greater than one recipient blood volume may cause hyperkalaemia in humans with renal failure or pretransfusion hyperkalaemia. This is not as likely to be a problem in dogs and cats, which have lower RBC potassium levels. Purebred and crossbred Akitas are an exception and should therefore not be used as donors. Shiba Inus also have increased RBC potassium levels but are not usually used for blood donation because of their small size.

Acidosis

There is a progressive decrease in the pH of stored RBC and platelet products. Large-volume transfusion could, therefore, potentially aggravate metabolic acidosis. This rarely occurs, especially since transfused lactate and citrate are usually rapidly metabolized to bicarbonate.

Pretransfusion (in vitro) haemolysis

In vitro haemolysis may occur from microbial contamination, poor RBC viability during storage, rough handling, freezing, overheating of blood or mixing with hypotonic solutions. RBC-rich blood products should not be diluted in a 5% dextrose solution. A 5% dextrose solution is isotonic, but when mixed with whole blood or packed RBCs, the red cells will metabolize the dextrose, and the resulting hypotonic solution will cause haemolysis. Signs of pretransfusion haemolysis are identical to IgG-mediated haemolysis. At the OVC two transfusion reactions to canine packed RBCs stored in CPDA$_1$ were attributed to poor in vitro viability and rough handling; no such problems have occurred with transfusions of packed RBCs stored in Adsol, Nutricel or Optisol.

Even under ideal storage conditions, some haemolysis occurs. In IMHA transfused RBCs are likely to undergo immediate immunological attack. RBCs with increased fragility are likely to be more susceptible to immunological injury, so transfusions of RBCs less than 2 weeks old are preferred.

Haemosiderosis

Liver damage may rarely occur as a complication of iron overload from numerous transfusions. It has been reported as a complication of transfusion therapy with some congenital haemolytic anaemias.

MANAGEMENT OF ACUTE TRANSFUSION REACTIONS

The management of acute transfusions reactions has been reviewed by Auer and Bell (1986), Harrell and Kristensen (1995) and Mathews (1996).

General measures

1. Monitor the patient closely during transfusion to facilitate early detection. The patient should be observed 'at the bedside' for the first 15 minutes and then 'at a distance' throughout the transfusion for any signs of a possible reaction. Temperature, heart rate and respiratory rate should be obtained every 5–10 minutes for the first 15–30 minutes and every 15–30 minutes thereafter.
2. Stop the transfusion at the first sign of a possible reaction. This may be the only specific measure required with mild reactions. With a severe peracute reaction (e.g. anaphylaxis, type B cat receiving type A blood), aspirate any blood product remaining in the catheter before infusing fluids or drugs. Verify that the correct blood product was given to the intended recipient. Identify the volume that has been transfused and the rate at which that volume has been transfused. Do not discard the blood product – it may be needed for full investigation or it may be possible to resume the transfusion. During interruption of a transfusion, platelet-poor blood products should be refrigerated. Interruption of a transfusion may violate the 'complete transfusion within 4 hours rule'. In the author's opinion, this is acceptable as long as care was taken not to contaminate the transfusion during set up, and it is preferable to wasting a blood product.
3. If a reaction is suspected, assess the recipient's temperature, pulse rate and quality, respiration rate and character, mucous membrane colour and capillary refill time and alertness. Monitor these variables closely. If hypotension is suspected, measure blood pressure if possible. If arrhythmias are present or there is a high risk of occurrence, establish continuous electrocardiographic monitoring if possible.
4. Begin artificial respiration if respiratory arrest has occurred and cardiopulmonary resuscitation if cardiopulmonary arrest has occurred. Resuscitation should be attempted as the situation is not hopeless. Resuscitation may result in recovery without drug therapy.

Address angioedema and anaphylactic/anaphylactoid shock

5. If urticaria, angioedema or pruritus is present, rule out haemolysis and examine for signs of shock (e.g. recumbency, tachycardia, weak pulses, pale mucous membranes). Give an antihistamine (e.g. diphenhydramine 0.5–2.0 mg/kg i.m., tripelennamine 1.0 mg/kg i.m.) and dexamethasone sodium phosphate 0.5–1.0 mg/kg i.v. over 20 minutes. The antihistamine and corticosteroid should not be given as rapid intravenous boluses as both such treatments can promote hypotension. If a reaction to plasma proteins is stable or subsiding, the transfusion can be started again at 25–50% of the previous rate.
6. If anaphylactic or anaphylactoid shock has occurred:
   - Ensure an open airway and administer oxygen
   - If peracute give 1:10 000 adrenaline 0.1 ml/kg i.v.
     1:10 000 adrenaline is prepared by taking 1 ml adrenaline 1:1000 (1 mg/ml) and diluting in 9 ml saline
   - If severe give 1:100 000 adrenaline 0.1 ml/kg i.v.
     1:100 000 adrenaline is prepared by taking 0.1 ml adrenaline 1:1000 (1 mg/ml) and diluting in 9 ml saline
   - If mild to moderate give 1:100 000 adrenaline 0.05 ml/kg i.m. and 0.05 ml/kg s.c. Adrenaline may be repeated every 2–30 minutes as required
   - Begin saline or similar fluid at 90 ml/kg/h (1.5 ml/kg/min) in dogs and 60 ml/kg/h (1.0 ml/kg/min) in cats. This high fluid rate should be discontinued as soon as possible to avoid exacerbation of pulmonary oedema
   - Give an antihistamine as in (5)
   - Give an H_2 blocker, for example, cimetidine 5 mg/kg i.v. or ranitidine 0.5–2.0 mg/kg i.v. (dog), 2.5 mg/kg i.v. (cat)
   - Once hypotension has been reversed, give prednisolone sodium succinate 5–30 mg/kg i.v. or dexamethasone sodium phosphate 0.5–4.0 mg/kg i.v. over 20 minutes. More rapid administration may exacerbate hypotension
   - If there are signs of increased vascular permeability (e.g. increasing PCV with decreasing total solids, ascites, pulmonary oedema, pleural effusion) or hypotension is persisting, give pentastarch or hetastarch at a dose of 10–20 ml/kg (dogs) and 5–10 ml/kg (cats) over 15–30 minutes
   - If hypotension is persisting, give adrenaline or dopamine by constant rate infusion (CRI). For adrenaline CRI, add 5 mg adrenaline to 1.0 litre saline (final concentration = 5 µg/ml); start at 0.1 µg/kg/min (0.02 ml/kg/min, 1.2 ml/kg/h) and titrate up or down to effect. For dopamine CRI, add 200 mg dopamine to

500 ml 5% dextrose solution (final concentration = 400 µg/ml) and give at 2–10 µg/kg/min (0.005–0.025 ml/kg/min, 0.3–1.5 ml/kg/h) and titrate up or down to effect

- If dyspnoea is present (from pulmonary oedema or bronchoconstriction), give aminophylline 5 mg/kg i.v. over 20 minutes. The dose may be repeated in 6 hours if necessary. Do not use aminophylline with cimetidine
- Once an anaphylactoid reaction has subsided, the transfusion may be resumed at 10–25% of the previous rate. If a transfusion has resulted in anaphylaxis, the recipient should never be transfused from that donor again and must be transfused from a new donor with extreme caution in the future.

Rule out haemolysis

7. If RBCs are being transfused, collect a microhaematocrit tube of blood from the recipient and from the blood bag. Examine plasma from each for evidence of haemolysis. Check the recipient's urine for haemoglobinaemia. Remember that cats in particular can have a haemolytic reaction without evidence of haemoglobinaemia and haemoglobinuria. If a haemolytic reaction has occurred, blood typing of donor and recipient and crossmatching should be performed to elucidate the incompatibility or repeated to rule out pretransfusion laboratory error.

8. Canine haemolytic reaction: If haemolysis is present in a dog, regardless of cause, obtain baseline serum urea and/or creatinine level and activated clotting time. Begin intravenous fluid therapy with a replacement fluid to maintain adequate hydration and treat hypotension. In moderate to severe cases give frusemide 2–4 mg/kg i.v. to help maintain urine production. If the dog has severe haemolysis and is acidaemic, it may also be beneficial to treat with intravenous sodium bicarbonate; this may facilitate excretion of RBC stroma, although it is not of proven benefit. Monitor urine production. In the unlikely event that acute renal failure develops, give dopamine at 5 µg/kg/min i.v. as in (6), and institute standard therapy. If massive haemolysis or overwhelming sepsis has occurred, consider giving heparin 70–200 IU/kg s.c. tid as prophylaxis for DIC.

9. Feline haemolytic reaction (type B cat receiving type A blood): Treatment of short-term (phase I) hypotension is the cornerstone for managing this reaction. Giving crystalloids as described in (6) and 'waiting out' the reaction may be all that is necessary. Antihistamines and corticosteroids are not routinely given. If cardiopulmonary arrest occurs, the most important treatment is cardiopulmonary resuscitation. If cardiac function has not returned within 90 seconds, give 1:10 000

(0.1 mg/ml) adrenaline 0.1–0.3 ml/kg i.v., and repeat in 2–3 minutes if necessary. Persistent phase I hypotension should be treated with synthetic colloids (preferably) or crystalloids and drugs if necessary, as described in (6). Persistent phase I bradycardia may be treated with atropine 0.04 mg/kg i.v., or 0.08 mg/kg intratracheally. The latter route reduces the risk of ventricular fibrillation. Treatment for hypotension must be discontinued when phase II hypertension develops.

10. Management of pretransfusion haemolysis in both dogs and cats is similar to the management of haemolysis in dogs described in (8). The dose of frusemide in the cat is 1–2 mg/kg. Potential causes should be investigated.

Rule out microbial contamination of blood product

11. If signs are compatible with transfusion-associated sepsis, microbial contamination should be ruled out by testing the blood remaining in the bag. Gram-stained or Wright's-stained blood smears should be examined for microorganisms, and the blood should be cultured at 1–6°C, 25–30°C and 37°C. Two simultaneous samples for blood culture from different veins should also be obtained from the recipient, who should then be treated with enrofloxacin 5 mg/kg i.v. and either cefazolin 30 mg/kg i.v. or clindamycin 10 mg/kg i.v., all given over 20 minutes. This approach is not necessary with simple urticarial reactions.

Address dyspnoea

12. Rule out haemolysis, sepsis and allergic reactions and treat these as described above. If dyspnoea is due to volume overload, give frusemide 2–4 mg/kg (dog) or 1–2 mg/kg (cat) i.v. Oxygen therapy is usually beneficial regardless of the cause of dyspnoea. Aminophylline (see 6) may also be beneficial. Mechanical ventilation may be required in severe cases of non-cardiogenic pulmonary oedema, such as may occur in phase II of an acute feline haemolytic reaction.

Address fever

13. If fever is the only sign, rule out haemolysis and bacterial contamination as previously discussed. If the transfusion is not completed and the fever is believed to be due to leucocyte antigens, the transfusion may be resumed. If the temperature is higher than 41.0°C, consider giving an antipyretic drug if not contraindicated by concurrent disorders. Drugs include dipyrone 25 mg/kg (dogs) or 10 mg/kg (cats) by slow intravenous bolus, intramuscularly or subcutaneously; aspirin 10 mg/kg orally (dog only) and other non-steroidal anti-inflammatory drugs at standard doses; paracetamol 10–15

mg/kg orally (dog only); and dexamethasone sodium phosphate 0.5–1.0 mg/kg i.v.

Address other problems

14. Arrhythmias should be treated by standard therapy. Note that the most common arrhythmia in phase II of an acute feline haemolytic reaction is ventricular bigeminy, which does not normally require treatment.
15. Seizures are usually self-limiting. Frequent seizures or status epilepticus should be treated by standard therapy with diazepam with or without phenobarbital.
16. Gastrointestinal signs are usually self-limiting and do not require specific treatment. An exception is with allergic reactions, where treatment with an H_2 blocker as listed in (6) should be considered if moderate to severe vomiting and diarrhoea are present.

AUTOTRANSFUSION

In autotransfusion the patient's own blood is collected and reinfused. This approach, which is underutilized in veterinary medicine, avoids disease transfer, the need for a donor and incompatibility. There are three types of autotransfusion: preoperative donation, haemodilution and scavenging.

Preoperative donation and haemodilution

These procedures refer to elective donation of blood from a patient before a procedure where there is a high likelihood of transfusion requirement. These procedures are particularly useful with dogs that have a history of transfusion reactions and with type B cats where donor availability may be limited. A case series of preoperative donation has been recently reported in cats (Fusco *et al.*, 2000).

Preoperative donation may be performed at any time within the maximum RBC storage period, but is ideally performed about 2–3 weeks in advance of surgery. This allows time for the marrow to regenerate the lost RBCs while minimizing the decrease in stored RBC viability. Iron supplementation is recommended in humans. If sufficient regeneration has occurred, predonation may be combined with haemodilution.

With haemodilution the donation is performed immediately before surgery. The withdrawn blood volume is replaced by three times that volume with crystalloid solutions. Colloid solutions may also be used, with the replacement volume equal to the withdrawal volume. In acute blood loss, the haemodynamic problem is one of volume depletion and not RBC loss. With this procedure volume depletion is corrected and intraoperative RBC loss is minimized. If the donation precedes volume replacement, the maximum donation volume is 25% of estimated blood volume. If volume replacement occurs concurrently with blood withdrawal, the target haematocrit is 20–28% in an otherwise healthy animal. The volume to remove is calculated as:

$$\text{Phlebotomy volume} = \text{Estimated blood volume} \times \frac{\text{Initial PCV - Final PCV}}{\text{Average of initial and final PCV}}$$

The blood is stored at room temperature and reinfused within 8 hours to preserve haemostatic properties.

Haemodilution is more complicated than preoperative donation. The main advantage of haemodilution over preoperative donation is that the blood contains normal levels of platelets and coagulation factors. Haemodilution is also useful where blood banking is not possible.

Although immunological transfusion reactions are avoided, anaphylactoid reactions, non-haemolytic febrile reactions to bioactive compounds and non-immunological reactions may still occur.

Salvage (scavenging)

This refers to collecting intrathoracic or intra-abdominal blood and reinfusing it. It is usually performed with trauma and surgery patients, and is a particularly useful procedure in veterinary emergency clinics where blood supply can easily be exhausted and there is insufficient time for a fresh donation (Purvis, 1995).

Commercial scavenging systems, and in-line collecting bags for use with commercial suction chest drainage systems, are available. Scavenging systems using readily available equipment have been described (Crowe, 1980). Large volumes of shed blood may be suctioned through a Poole suction tip, peritoneal dialysis catheter or large-bore tube into a sterile collecting bottle. Another method is to attach an injection cap ('INTS', 'PRN adapter') to a collection catheter. The needle of a blood collection set is pierced through the injection cap, and blood is collected by vacuum as described previously for jugular collection. The salvaged blood may be reinfused as rapidly as possible. For small dogs and cats, aspiration of blood with a 60 ml syringe and sterile intravenous tubing will suffice. Three-way stopcocks and intravenous tubing may be attached to allow direct reinfusion and anticoagulation. Because it takes 1 hour or more of serosal contact for blood to become fully defibrinated, anticoagulation is recommended at a rate of 0.05 ml CPD (or $CPDA_1$)/ml salvaged blood.

Salvaged blood is more prone to haemolysis and must be handled gently. Vacuum pressures should be 40–60 mmHg (1.6–2.4 inchesHg, 54–82 cmH_2O) for intraoperative collection and 10–15 mmHg (0.4–0.6 inchesHg, 14–20 cmH_2O) for collection from closed body cavities. Aspiration of air should be minimized as this can worsen haemolysis. Autotransfusion should not be performed if haemorrhage occurred more than 6 hours previously, because contact of blood with traumatized serosa increases haemolysis. Excessive pressure must be avoided when reinfusing by injection. Infusion pumps should not be used.

Coagulation and fibrinolysis are activated on contact of blood with serosal surfaces, and platelets are reduced in number and function. This has several implications. Firstly, salvaged blood cannot be expected to correct hypocoagulable states. Indeed, large-volume autotransfusion may result in a hypocoagulable state. This is most likely to occur with volumes greater than 50% of patient blood volume, and haemostasis usually normalizes within 3 days. Secondly, salvaged blood contains microthrombi (as well as other microemboli) and should be given through a filter. Ideally a 40 μm filter should be used.

The risk of sepsis resulting from an autotransfusion of salvaged blood is potentially greater than that from a regular transfusion. Microbial contamination of salvaged blood may occur as open collection systems are used and sterility may be broken in the rush of emergency patient care. Intestinal rupture may result in contamination of intra-abdominal blood. Autotransfused patients are frequently immunocompromised because of shock or underlying disorders. For these reasons empirical therapy with broad-spectrum antibiotics (see Chapter 8) should be considered.

Dissemination of neoplasia is a theoretical concern with salvage after rupture of a haemangiosarcoma. Dissemination of neoplasia does not seem to be a major concern with scavenging in human medicine, but haemangiosarcoma is an uncommon tumour. Not all cells shed from a tumour have metastatic potential, and the likelihood is that a ruptured haemangiosarcoma has already metastasized, so autotransfusion should be considered if no other transfusion is available. Perhaps a more important concern with salvage of blood shed from a haemangiosarcoma is that the blood may have been pooling in body cavities for more than 6 hours. However, the serosal surfaces would not be traumatized, and autotransfusion should be performed if the dog requires transfusion and no other blood is available.

REFERENCES AND FURTHER READING

Auer LK and Bell K (1986) Feline blood transfusion reactions. In: *Current Veterinary Therapy IX Small Animal Practice,* ed. RW Kirk, pp. 515-521. WB Saunders, Philadelphia

Bouchard G, Plata-Madrid H, Youngquist RS, Buening GM, Ganjam VK, Krause GF, Allen GK and Paine AL (1992) Absorption of an alternate source of immunoglobulin in pups. *American Journal of Veterinary Research* **53,** 230-233

Brownlee L, Wardrop KJ, Sellon RK & Meyers KM (2000) Use of prestorage leukoreduction filter effectively removes leukocytes from canine whole blood while preserving red blood cell viability. *Journal of Veterinary Internal Medicine* **14,** 412-417

Callan MB, Jones LT and Giger U (1995) Hemolytic transfusion reaction in a dog with an alloantibody to a common antigen. *Journal of Veterinary Internal Medicine* **9,** 277-280

Ching YNLH, Meyers KM, Brassard JA and Wardrop KJ (1994) Effect of cryoprecipitate and plasma on plasma von Willebrand factor multimers and bleeding time in Doberman Pinschers with type-I von Willebrand's disease. *American Journal of Veterinary Research* **55,** 102-110

Corato A, Mazza G, Hale AS, Barker RN and Day MJ (1997) Biochemical characterization of canine blood group antigens: immunoprecipitation of DEA 1.2, 4 and 7 and identification of a dog erythrocyte membrane antigen homologous to human Rhesus. *Veterinary Immunology and Immunopathology* **59,** 213-223

Cotter SM (1991) *Comparative Transfusion Medicine,* ed. SM Cotter. Academic Press, New York

Cowles BE, Meyers KM, Wardrop KJ, Menard M and Sylvester D (1992) Prolonged bleeding of Chédiak-Higashi cats corrected by platelet transfusion. *Thrombosis and Haemostasis* **67,** 708-712

Crowe DT (1980) Autotransfusion in the trauma patient. *Veterinary Clinics of North America: Small Animal Practice* **10,** 581-597

Feldman BF, Zinkl JG and Jain NC (2000) *Schalm's Veterinary Hematology, 5th edn,* ed. BF Feldman, JG Zinkl and NC Jain. Lippincott Williams and Wilkins, Hagerstown

Fusco JV, Hohenhaus AE, Aiken SW, Joseph RJ and Berg JM (2000) Autologous blood collection and transfusion in cats undergoing partial craniectomy. *Journal of the American Veterinary Medical Association* **216,** 1584-1588

Giger U and Akol KG (1990) Acute hemolytic transfusion reaction in an Abyssinian cat with blood type B. *Journal of Veterinary Internal Medicine* **4,** 315-316

Giger U, Gelens CJ, Callan MB and Oakley DA (1995) An acute hemolytic transfusion reaction caused by dog erythrocyte antigen 1.1 incompatibility in a previously sensitized dog. *Journal of the American Veterinary Medical Association* **201,** 1358-1362

Griot-Wenk ME and Giger U (1995) Feline transfusion medicine: blood types and their clinical importance. *Veterinary Clinics of North America: Small Animal Practice* **25,** 1305-1322

Harrell KA and Kristensen AT (1995) Canine transfusion reactions and their management. *Veterinary Clinics of North America: Small Animal Practice* **25,** 1323-1361

Helfand SC, Jain NC and Paul M (1984) Vincristine-loaded platelet therapy for idiopathic thrombocytopenia in a dog. *Journal of the American Veterinary Medical Association* **185,** 224-226

Ho C-H (1998) The hemostatic effect of packed red cell transfusion in patients with anemia. *Transfusion* **38,** 1011-1014

Hohenhaus AE (1992) Transfusion medicine. *Problems in Veterinary Medicine* **4,** 555-670

Hohenhaus AE, Drusin LM and Garvey MS (1997) *Serratia marcescens* contamination of feline whole blood in a hospital blood bank. *Journal of the American Veterinary Medical Association* **210,** 794-798

Hurst TS, Turrentine MA and Johnson GS (1987) Evaluation of microwave-thawed canine plasma for transfusion. *Journal of the American Veterinary Medical Association* **190,** 863-865

Klein MK, Dow SW and Rosychuk RAW (1989) Pulmonary thromboembolism associated with immune-mediated hemolytic anemia in dogs: 10 cases (1982-1987). *Journal of the American Veterinary Medical Association* **195,** 246-250

Knottenbelt CM, Day MJ, Cripps PJ and Mackin AJ (1999) Measurement of titres of naturally occurring alloantibodies against feline blood group antigens in the UK. *Journal of Small Animal Practice* **40,** 365-370

Kristensen AT and Feldman BF (1995a) Blood banking and transfusion medicine. In: *Textbook of Veterinary Internal Medicine, 4th edn,* ed. SJ Ettinger and EC Feldman, pp. 347-360. WB Saunders, Philadelphia

Kristensen AT and Feldman BF (1995b) Canine and feline transfusion medicine. *Veterinary Clinics of North America: Small Animal Practice* **25,** 1231-1490

Levy JK and Crawford PC (2000) Failure of passive transfer in neonatal kittens: correction by administration of adult cat serum. *Journal of Veterinary Internal Medicine* **14,** 362

MacEwen EG, Patnaik AK, Hayes AA, Wilkins RJ, Hardy WD, Kassel RL and Old LJ (1981) Temporary plasma-induced remission of lymphoblastic leukemia in a dog. *American Journal of Veterinary Research* **42,** 1450-1452

Macintire DK, Smith-Carr S, Jones R and Swango L (1999) Treatment of dogs naturally infected with canine parvovirus with lyophilized canine IgG. *Journal of Veterinary Internal Medicine* **13,** 255

Mathews KA (1996) *Emergency and Critical Care Protocols,* ed. KA Mathews. Lifelearn V, Guelph, Canada

Mollison PL, Contreras M and Engelfield CP (1997) *Blood Transfusion in Clinical Medicine, 10th edn*. Blackwell Science, Oxford

Moritz A, Widman T and Hale AS (1998) Comparison of current typing techniques for evaluation of dog erythrocyte antigen 1.1. *Journal of Veterinary Internal Medicine* **12**, 226

Novinger MS, Sullivan PS and McDonald TP (1996) Determination of the lifespan of erythrocytes from greyhounds using an in vitro biotinylation technique. *American Journal of Veterinary Research* **57**, 739-742

Otto CM and Crowe DT (1992) Intraosseous resuscitation techniques and applications. In: *Current Veterinary Therapy XI Small Animal Practice,* ed. RW Kirk and JD Bonagura, pp. 107-112. WB Saunders, Philadelphia

Petz LD, Swisher SN, Kleinman S, Spence RK and Strauss RG (1996) *Clinical Practice of Transfusion Medicine, 3rd edn*, ed. LD Petz, SN Swisher, S Kleinman, RK Spence and RG Strauss. Churchill Livingstone, New York

Price LR (1991) A method for collecting and storing feline whole blood. *Veterinary Technician* **7**, 561-563

Purvis D (1995) Autotransfusion in the emergency patient. *Veterinary Clinics of North America: Small Animal Practice* **25**, 1291-1304

Rentko V (2000) Practical use of a blood substitute. In: *Current Veterinary Therapy XIII Small Animal Practice,* ed. JD Bonagura, pp. 424-427. WB Saunders, Philadelphia

Schneider A (1995) Blood components: collection, processing, and storage. *Veterinary Clinics of North America: Small Animal Practice* **25**, 1245-1261

Scott-Moncrieff JCR and Reagan WJ (1997) Human intravenous immunoglobulin therapy. *Seminars in Veterinary Medicine and Surgery (Small Animal)* **12**, 178-185

Slichter SJ (2000) Platelet transfusions and platelet alloimmunization. *Proceedings of the 18th Annual Veterinary Medical Forum,* pp. 477-478. American College of Veterinary Internal Medicine, Seattle

Springer T, Hatchett WL, Oakley DA, Niggemeir A and Giger U (1998) Feline blood storage and component therapy using a closed collection system. *Journal of Veterinary Internal Medicine* **12**, 248

Stokol T and Parry BW (1998) Efficacy of fresh-frozen plasma and cryoprecipitate in dogs with von Willebrand's disease or hemophilia A. *Journal of Veterinary Internal Medicine* **12**, 84-92

Symons M and Bell K (1991) Expansion of the canine A blood group system. *Animal Genetics* **22**, 227-235

Vengelen-Tyler V (1999) *Technical Manual, 13th edn*, ed. V Vengelen-Tyler. American Association of Blood Banks, Bethesda

Wagner AE and Dunlop CI (1993) Anesthetic and medical management of acute hemorrhage during surgery. *Journal of the American Veterinary Medical Association* **203**, 40-45

Wardrop J (1996) Medical indications for plasma therapy. *Proceedings of the 14th Annual Veterinary Medical Forum,* pp. 31-33. American College of Veterinary Internal Medicine, Lakewood

Wardrop KJ (1995) Selection of anticoagulant-preservatives for canine and feline blood storage. *Veterinary Clinics of North America: Small Animal Practice* **25**, 1263-1276

Wardrop KJ, Lewis D, Marks S and Buss M (1997) Posttransfusion purpura in a dog with hemophilia A. *Journal of Veterinary Internal Medicine* **11**, 261-263

Wohl JS and Cotter SM (1995) Blood substitutes: oxygen-carrying acellular fluids. *Veterinary Clinics of North America: Small Animal Practice* **25**, 1417-1440

Blood Groups in Cats

Andrew Sparkes and Tim Gruffydd-Jones

INTRODUCTION

Blood groups are established by identifying major antigenic differences between erythrocytes from different individuals. In cats, a well established A–B blood group system based on naturally occurring alloantibodies has been described that has important clinical implications. Recent work suggests that the antigenic differences between erythrocytes in cats forming this grouping system relates to the form of neuraminic acid present on the glycolipids of the erythrocyte cell membrane (Andrews *et al.*, 1992).

THE A–B BLOOD GROUP SYSTEM IN CATS

The A–B blood group system in the cat seems to be inherited in a simple dominant form via two alleles at the same gene locus. The allele for group A is dominant over that for group B, and thus cats expressing the group A phenotype have a homozygous (A/A) or heterozygous (A/B) genotype, whereas cats expressing the group B phenotype are invariably homozygous for the B allele (B/B). In addition to the A and B phenotype, a small proportion of cats (generally less than 1%) have been identified that express both A and B antigens on the erythrocyte membrane (i.e. are of AB phenotype), although a recent study from the United Kingdom identified a higher proportion of AB cats (5%) in the population studied (Knottenbelt *et al.*, 1999). These AB cats are assumed to have an A/B genotype but with a third allele that prevents the normal A dominance being expressed, the genes therefore acting as a co-dominant pair.

CLINICAL SIGNIFICANCE OF BLOOD GROUPS IN CATS

The clinical significance of blood groups in cats relates mainly to the high levels of naturally occurring alloantibodies found in many cats against the heterologous blood group (a situation that does not occur in dogs). Most cats of blood group B (more than 95%) contain moderate to high titres of both haemagglutinating (mainly IgM) and haemolytic (IgM and IgG) alloantibodies against group A antigens, whereas a

much smaller proportion (about 25%) of group A cats have corresponding alloantibodies against the B group antigen, and when they are found these are of very low titre. The rare AB group cats contain neither alloantibody. These alloantibodies are of particular significance in two situations, firstly, blood transfusions where there are implications for immediate transfusion reactions and also for the survival of transfused erythrocytes and, secondly, the phenomenon of neonatal isoerythrolysis.

Major transfusion reactions

The high levels of anti-A alloantibodies in most group B cats means that these individuals carry a high risk of a major transfusion reaction if they receive blood from a group A donor. Fortunately this is not common, as there is a low prevalence of group B cats in the general population. Nevertheless, certain breeds have a much higher prevalence of group B cats (Figure 16.1) and consequently the risk of major reactions in these breeds is much higher.

Pedigree breed	Group A (%)	Group B (%)
British Shorthair	41	59
Devon Rex	57	43
Persian	76	24
Somali	78	22
Abyssinian	80	20
Himalayan (Colourpoint)	80	20
Birman	82	18
Scottish Fold	85	15
Siamese	100	0
Tonkinese	100	0
Oriental Shorthair	100	0
American Shorthair	100	0
Burmese	100	0
Norwegian Forest	100	0

Figure 16.1: Frequency of types A and B blood groups in pedigree cats from the United States. (Giger et al., 1991a; Bücheler and Cotter, 1993)

If a group B cat receives type A blood, the donated erythrocytes are destroyed within minutes to hours depending on the antibody titre, and clinical signs of transfusion reaction may develop. The initial clinical signs of a severe reaction (seen within seconds of receiving even 1–2 ml of type A blood) are typical of acute anaphylaxis, with restlessness, vocalization, urination, vomiting, salivation, collapse, mydriasis, apnoea/hypopnoea, bradycardia (sometimes with atrioventricular block), dysrrhythmia, and profound hypotension. These signs typically last for 1–5 minutes and are followed by tachycardia, dysrrhythmia, hypertension and tachypnoea, with gradual return to normality in about an hour. In addition, haemoglobinaemia and haemoglobinuria occur owing to acute intravascular haemolysis. Although such transfusion reactions are potentially fatal, the severity of the reaction will be related to the titre of anti-A alloantibodies, and some cats will therefore experience less severe subacute reactions.

Major transfusion reactions have not been reported in group A cats receiving type B blood, but the short half-life of the transfused erythrocytes in this situation is an important concern.

Survival of transfused erythrocytes

The half-life of transfused erythrocytes in cats given autogenous blood is typically 30–38 days. A similar half-life is also seen in group A and B cats given matched allogeneic transfusions, indicating the effectiveness of these transfusions in clinical practice. Erythrocytes from mismatched transfusions have a much shorter half-life. Depending on the anti-A titre, as already noted type A erythrocytes transfused to a group B cat might have an extremely short half-life (minutes to hours), whereas type B erythrocytes transfused to a group A cat typically have a half-life of 2 days (Giger, 1992). The survival of the transfused cells is an important reason why matched transfusions should be given, in addition to the need to avoid major transfusion reactions.

Neonatal isoerythrolysis

Neonatal isoerythrolysis is an immune-mediated haemolytic disease of neonates that can occur when a kitten of blood group A (or AB) is born to a queen of blood group B. The potential for this to occur is present in any mating of a group A tom to a group B queen, and the chances of such a mating occurring are much higher in the breeds with a higher prevalence of group B cats (Figure 16.1).

The group B queen secretes anti-A alloantibodies in her colostrum and milk and, after sucking, the IgG antibodies can be absorbed from the intestine of the neonate during the first 24 hours of life. Depending therefore on the antibody titre in the blood and colostrum of the queen and the amount absorbed by the kitten, haemolytic anaemia and death can occur in group A phenotype kittens within the first 2 to 3 days after birth. Although relatively few cases of neonatal isoerythrolysis have been reported, the true incidence is difficult to define as many affected kittens may die without a specific diagnosis being made (death being attributed to the 'fading kitten syndrome'). Affected cats typically show haemoglobinuria, bilirubinuria and jaundice and should be separated from the queen and artificially reared or fostered until they are 48–72 hours old.

PREVALENCE OF BLOOD GROUPS IN CATS

Relatively little information is available on the prevalence of the different blood groups in cat populations, but what there is suggests there may be noticeable geographical variations and certainly profound differences between pedigree breeds.

As the allele for group A is dominant, there should be a low prevalence of type B cats among large relatively free-breeding cat populations. Indeed, in most countries where studies have been made of domestic (both shorthair and longhair) cats, the prevalence of group A cats is between 94% and 100% (Figure 16.2).

Country	Group A domestic cats (%)
Australia	73
Austria	96
England	87–97
Finland	100
France	85
Germany	94
Holland	96
Italy	87
Japan	90
Scotland	97
Switzerland	>99
United States	>99

Figure 16.2: *Frequency of type A blood group in domestic cats in various countries. (Giger et al., 1989; Lubas and Continanza, 1995; Knottenbelt et al., 1999).*

At present the only substantial published information on the prevalence of blood groups in different pedigree breeds comes from the United States (Giger *et al.*, 1991a), with some additional data from Italy (Lubas and Continanza, 1995) and the United Kingdom (Knottenbelt *et al.*, 1999). As the production of pedigree breeds involves selective breeding (sometimes from a limited starting gene pool) it is not surprising to find that many breeds have a much higher proportion of group B cats than the domestic (non-pedigree) cat population. It is, however, unwise to assume that the distribution of blood groups in cats from the United States will be similar in all countries. For example, in Italy (Lubas and Continanza, 1995) the prevalence of group A cats among Siamese was found to be 96% and among Persians was 97%, compared with 100% and 76% respectively in the United States. Even within countries, regional variations are likely to exist in the prevalence of blood groups in both pedigree and non-pedigree cats (Giger *et al.*, 1991b).

The general picture for the distribution of blood groups in pedigree breeds in the United Kingdom seems to be similar to that described in the United States. Most breeds identified as having a high prevalence of type B cats in the United States also have a high prevalence in the United Kingdom (e.g. Devon Rex, British Shorthairs). The major difference is that group B cats are rare in UK Abyssinians (TJ Gruffydd-Jones, unpublished observations). In the study of UK cats by Knottenbelt *et al.* (1999), information was available from 121 British Shorthairs (59% were type B), 24 Birmans (29% were type B) and 17 Persians (12% were type B). Other breeds were tested but the numbers were small (≤10).

BLOOD TYPING

Although naturally occurring blood transfusion reactions are uncommon in cats, it is clear certain breeds run a much higher risk of a major reaction. Knowledge of the overall prevalence of group B cats within a breed helps to quantify the risks involved but may be inaccurate owing to geographical and local regional variations. Blood typing before transfusion is therefore routinely recommended as the safest approach. In addition, blood typing of pedigree cats with a known

high prevalence of B group in the breed may facilitate planned breeding programmes to avoid the possibility of neonatal isoerythrolysis (i.e. avoid mating a type B queen to a type A tom).

The recent introduction of a simple rapid card-agglutination test for typing cat blood makes these procedures much simpler, and is available to all practitioners (Rapid Vet-H Feline, DMS Laboratories). It should be noted, however, that major and minor crossmatching of blood may still have to be performed in cats receiving more than one transfusion, as the first transfusion (even with matched blood) may induce production of antibodies against red cell antigens other than those involved in the A-B blood group system (Giger, 1992; Lubas and Continanza, 1995).

REFERENCES

Andrews GA, Chavey PS, Smith JE and Rich L (1992) N-glycolylneuraminic acid and acetylneuraminic acid define feline blood group A and B antigens. *Blood* **79**, 2485-2491

Bücheler J and Cotter S (1993) Setting up a feline blood donor program. *Veterinary Medicine* **88**, 838-845

Giger U (1992) The feline AB blood group-system and incompatibility reactions. In: *Current Veterinary Therapy XI*, eds. RW Kirk and JD Bonagura, pp. 470-474. WB Saunders, Philadelphia

Giger U, Bucheler J and Patterson DF (1991a) Frequency and inheritance of A and B blood types in feline breeds of the United States. *Journal of Hereditary* **82**, 15-20

Giger U, Griot-Wenk M, Bucheler J, Smith S and Diserens D (1991b) Geographical variation of the feline blood type frequencies in the United States. *Feline Practice* **19**, 21-27

Giger U, Kilrain CG, Filippich LJ and Bell K (1989) Frequencies of feline blood groups in the United States. *Journal of the American Veterinary Medical Association* **195**, 1230-1232

Knottenbelt CM, Addie DD, Day MJ and Mackin AJ (1999) Determination of the prevalence of feline blood types in the UK. *Journal of Small Animal Practice* **40**, 115-118

Lubas G and Continanza R (1995) Recent advances in our understanding of the immunohaematological characteristics of cats and their clinical application. *European Journal of Companion Animal Practice* **5**, 47-54

Reference Values for Haematology and Haemostasis

The reference values in the following table have been taken from the BSAVA *Small Animal Formulary, 2nd edition* (1997; edited by Bryn Tennant). These values reflect those commonly used by small animal veterinary surgeons. The ranges given in individual chapters may vary because of the geographical spread of the authors.

It should always be remembered that any table of reference values of this kind is for guidance only. Whenever a sample is sent to a laboratory for analysis, the laboratory should be asked to provide a reference value for the specific laboratory, the specific test and the specific patient type so that interpretation of the results can be done fairly.

HAEMATOLOGY		
Value	**Dog**	**Cat**
PCV (l/l)	0.35–0.55	0.26–0.46
Hb (g/l)	120–180	80–150
RBC (x 10^{12}/l)	5.4–8	5–11
MCV (fl)	65–75	37–49
MCH (pg)	22–25	12–17
MCHC (g/l)	340–370	320–350
Reticulocytes (%)	0–1	0–1
Reticulocytes (x 10^9/l)	20–80	20–60
RBC life (days)	100–120	66–78
ESR (mm/h)	0–2	0–10
M:E ratio	0.75–2.5:1	0.6–3.9:1
Platelets (x 10^9/l)	150–400	150–400
WBC (x 10^9/l)	6–18	5.5–19.5
Neutrophils: bands	0–0.3	0–0.3
Neutrophils: mature	3–12	2.5–12.5
Lymphocytes	0.8–3.8	1.5–7
In young dogs up to 6 months old lymphocyte number may be increased by as much as 50%.		
Monocytes	0.1–1.8	0–0.85
Eosinophils	0.1–1.9	0.1–1.5
Basophils	0–0.2	0–0.2
MCV (fl) = (PCV x 1000) ÷ RBC.		
MCHC (g/l) = (Hb concentration) ÷ PCV		
HAEMOSTASIS		
Value	**Dog**	**Cat**
One stage prothrombin time (OSPT) (seconds)	7–12	7–12
Activated partial thromboplastin time (APTT) (seconds)	12–15	12–22
Bleeding time (ear) (min)	1–2	1–5
Whole blood coagulation time		
Glass (min)	6–7.5	8
Silicone (min)	2–15	
Capillary tube (min)	3–4	5–5.4
Activated coagulation time (seconds)	60–129	
Fibrinogen (g/l)	2–4.5	1–4
Fibrin degradation products (µg/ml)	<10	<10

List of Abbreviations

ACD	acid citrate dextrose		DIC	disseminated intravascular coagulation
ACT	activated clotting time		2,3-DPG	2,3-diphosphoglycerate
ADP	adenosine diphosphate		DSH	domestic shorthaired (cat)
AIHA	autoimmune haemolytic anaemia			
AITP	autoimmune thrombocytopenia		ECF-A	eosinophil chemotactic factor of anaphylaxis
ALL	acute lymphoblastic leukaemia			
AML	acute myeloid leukaemia		EDTA	ethylenediamine tetra-acetic acid
AMoL	acute monocytic leukaemia		ELISA	enzyme-linked immunosorbent assay
ANA	antinuclear antibody		EPO	erythropoietin
APTT	activated partial thromboplastin time			
ARC	AIDS-related complex		FAD	flea allergy dermatitis
ARDS	acute respiratory distress syndrome		Fc	immunoglobulin heavy chain (fragment crystallizable)
ARF	acute renal failure			
ATIII	antithrombin III		FDPs	fibrinogen degradation products
ATP	adenosine triphosphate		FeLV	feline immunodeficiency virus
AZT	zidovudine		FeSFV	feline syncytium-forming virus
			FeSV	feline sarcoma virus
BFU-E	burst-forming unit – erythroid		FIA	feline infectious anaemia
BMBT	buccal mucosal bleeding time		FIP	feline infectious peritonitis
BUN	blood urea nitrogen		FIV	feline immunodeficiency virus
			FVIII:Ag	factor VIII antigen
C3	third component of complement			
cAMP	cyclic adenosine monophosphate		G-CSF	granulocyte colony stimulating factor
CBC	complete blood count		GM-CSF	granulocyte–macrophage colony stimulating factor
CFU-Bas	colony-forming unit – basophil			
CFU-E	colony-forming unit – erythroid		GP	glycoprotein
CFU-Eos	colony-forming unit – eosinophil			
CFU-G	colony-forming unit – granulocyte		HES	hypereosinophilic syndrome
CFU-GM	colony-forming unit – granulocyte–macrophage		HIV	human immunodeficiency virus
			HUS	haemolytic uraemic syndrome
CFU-M	colony-forming unit – macrophage			
CLAD	canine leucocyte adhesion deficiency		IFN-γ	interferon gamma
CLL	chronic lymphocytic leukaemia		Ig	immunoglobulin (IgG, IgM, IgA)
CML	chronic myeloid leukaemia		IL	interleukin (e.g. IL-1 to IL-18)
CNS	central nervous system		IL-2R	interleukin 2 receptor
CPD	citrate phosphate dextrose		IMHA	immune-mediated haemolytic anaemia
CPDA	citrate phosphate dextrose adenine$_1$			
CRI	constant rate infusion		IMT	immune-mediated thrombocytopenia
CRD	chronic renal disease		ITP	idiopathic thrombocytopenic purpura
CRF	chronic renal failure		IVIG	intravenous immunoglobulin (therapy)
CSF	colony stimulating factor			
DAT	direct antiglobulin test			
DDAVP	1-deamino-8-D-arginine vasopressin		LGL	large granular lymphocyte
DEA	Dog Erythrocyte Antigen		LPD	lymphoproliferative disease

MCHC	mean corpuscular haemoglobin concentration	rHuEPO	recombinant human erythropoietin
M-CSF	macrophage colony stimulating factor	rHuG-CSF	recombinant human granulocyte colony stimulating factor
MCV	mean corpuscular volume	rHuGM-CSF	recombinant human granulocyte–macrophage colony stimulating factor
M/E	myeloid:erythroid		
MGDF	megakarocyte growth and development factor	RVVT	Russell's viper venom test
MODS	multiple organ dysfunction syndrome		
MPD	myeloproliferative disease	SCID	severe combined immunodeficiency
MPS	mononuclear phagocytic system	SID	strong ion difference
MPV	mean platelet volume	SIRS	systemic inflammatory response syndrome
NBT	nitroblue tetrazolium (test)	SLE	systemic lupus erythematosus
NK	natural killer (cell)		
		T4	thyroxine
OSPT	one-stage prothrombin time	TCT	thrombin clot time
OVC	Ontario Veterinary College	TF	tissue factor
		TFPI	tissue factor pathway inhibitor
PAI-1	plasminogen-activator inhibitor 1	TIBC	total iron binding capacity
PCR	polymerase chain reaction	TNF	tumour necrosis factor
PCV	packed cell volume	tPA	tissue-type plasminogen activator
PF3	platelet factor 3 (test)	TPI	tissue plasmin inhibitor
PFK	phosphofructokinase		
PGL	persistent generalized lymphadenopathy	uPA	urokinase-type plasminogen activator
PIE	pulmonary infiltrates with eosinophils		
PIVKA	proteins induced by vitamin K absence	VPIS	Veterinary Poisons Information Service
PRCA	pure red cell aplasia	vWD	von Willebrand's disease
PT	prothrombin time	vWf	von Willebrand factor
PTH	parathyroid hormone	vWf:Ag	von Willebrand factor antigen
RBC	red blood cell	WBC	white blood cell (count)
RDW	red cell distribution width	WBCT	whole blood clotting time

Index